The Menopause at the MILLENNIUM

The Menopause at the MILLENNIUM

The Proceedings of
the 9th International Menopause Society
World Congress on the Menopause

Yokohama, Japan
October 17-21, 1999

Edited by
Takeshi Aso, Takumi Yanaihara &
Seiichiro Fujimoto

The Parthenon Publishing Group
International Publishers in Medicine, Science & Technology
NEW YORK LONDON

Library of Congress Cataloging-in-Publication Data

World Congress on the Menopause (9th : 1999 : Yokohama-shi, Japan)
The menopause at the Millennium : proceedings of the 9th World Congress on the Menopause/ edited by T. Asō, Takumi Yanaihara and Seiichiro Fujimoto
p. : cm.
Includes bibliographical references and index.
ISBN 1-85070-709-X (alk. paper)
1. Menopause - Congresses. I. Asō, Takeshi. II. Yanaihara, Takumi. III. Fujimoto, Seiichiro. IV. Title.
[DNLM: 1. Menopause–Congresses. WP 580 W927m 2000]
RG186. W675 1999
618.1′75–dc21 00-033647

British Library Cataloguing in Publication Data

The menopause at the millennium : proceedings of the 9th World Congress on the Menopause
1. Menopause - Congresses I. Aso, Takeshi II. Yanaihara, Takumi III. Fujimoto, Seiichiro IV. International Menopause Society World Congress on the Menopause (9th : 1999 : Yokohama, Japan)
612.61′65

ISBN 1-85070-709-X

Published in the USA by
The Parthenon Publishing Group Inc.
One Blue Hill Plaza
PO Box 1564, Pearl River
New York 10965, USA

Published in the UK and Europe by
The Parthenon Publishing Group Limited
Casterton Hall, Carnforth
Lancs. LA6 2LA, UK

Typeset by AMA DataSet Ltd., Preston, UK
Printed and bound by Bookcraft (Bath) Ltd., Midsomer Norton, UK

Contents

Section 3 Quality of life in the menopause

Section 4 Aging process of endocrine organs

Section 5 Emerging biological actions of steroidal hormones

Section 6 Breast cancer and the menopause

Section 7 Primary care in the menopause: an international perspective

List of principal contributors

A. Amsterdam
Department of Molecular Cell Biology
The Weizmann Institute of Science
Rehovot 76100
Israel

T. Aono
Department of Obstetrics & Gynecology
School of Medicine
The University of Tokushima
3-18-15, Kuramoto-cho
Tokushima 770-8503
Japan

T. Aso
Department of Obstetrics & Gynecology
Tokyo Medical & Dental University
School of Medicine
1-5-45, Yushima
Bunkyo-ku
Tokyo 113-8519
Japan

M. Birkhäuser
Division of Gynecology
Universitäts-Frauenklinik Bern
Schanzeneckstrasse 1
CH-3012 Bern
Switzerland

M. Brincat
Faculty of Medicine & Surgery Medical School
Medical School
Msida
Malta

H. G. Burger
Prince Henry's Institute of Medical Research
Monash Medical Centre
PO Box 5152
Clayton
Victoria 3168
Australia

A. Cano
Department of Pediatrics, Obstetrics and Gynecology
Facultad de Medicina
Av. Blasco Ibanex 17
E-46010 Valencia
Spain

S. H. Cho
Department of Obstetrics & Gynecology
College of Medicine
Hanyang University
#17 Haengdangdong
Sungdongku
Seoul 133-792
Korea

C. Christiansen
Centre for Clinical & Basic Research
Ballerup Byvej 222
DK-2750
Ballerup
Denmark

A. Collins
Department of Clinical Neuroscience
Karolinska Hospital
Stockholm 171 76
Sweden

S. R. Davis
The Jean Hailes Foundation for Women
173 Carinish Road
Clayton
Victoria 3168
Australia

B. de Lignieres
Department of Endocrinology and Reproductive Medicine
Hôpital Necker - Pavillon Apert
149 rue de Sevres
Paris 75015
France

L. Dennerstein
Office for Gender & Health
Department of Psychiatry
University of Melbourne
6th Floor, Charles Connibere Building
Royal Melbourne Hospital
Victoria 3050
Australia

J. Donát
Department of Obstetrics and Gynecology
University Hospital
500 05 Hradec Králové
Czech Republic

B. L. Drinkwater
Pacific Medical Center, Q10
1200 12th Avenue
Seattle
WA 98144
USA

J. A. Eden
School of Obstetrics & Gynecology
University of New South Wales
Royal Hospital for Women
Randwick, NSW 2031
Australia

E. F. Eriksen
University Department of Endocrinology
Aarhus Amtssygenhus
DK-8000 Aarhus C
Denmark

T. Fujibayashi
Department of Oral & Maxillofacial Surgery
Dokkyo University School of Medicine
880 Kitakobayashi
Mibu-machi
Shimotsuga-gun
Tochigi 321-0293
Japan

S. Fujimoto
Department of Obstetrics and Gynecology
Hokkaido University
School of Medicine
Sapporo
Japan

A. R. Genazzani
Department of Reproductive Medicine and Child Development
Division of Obstetrics & Gynecology
Via Roma 35
Pisa 56100
Italy

D. B. Georgiev
Sheinovo Hospital
II Obstetrics & Gynecology Hospital
19 Sheinovo str.
1504 Sofia
Bulgaria

A. Graziottin
Via San Secondo 19
10128 Torino
Italy

J. G. Greene
The Medical Centre
1 High Street
Neilston
Glasgow
UK

C. A. Gurucharri
University of Buenos Aires
Ave Santa Fe 1531
Buenos Aires 1060
Argentina

J. R. Guthrie
Office for Gender & Health
Department of Psychiatry
University of Melbourne
6th Floor, Charles Connibere Building
Royal Melbourne Hospital
Victoria 3050
Australia

C. J. Haines
Department of Obstetrics & Gynecology
The Chinese University of Hong Kong
Prince of Wales Hospital
Shatin, NT
Hong Kong
SAR China

V. W. Henderson
Department of Neurology
University of Southern California (PMB-B105)
1420 San Pablo Street
Los Angeles
California 90089
USA

H. Honjo
Department of Obstetrics & Gynecology
Kyoto Prefectural University of Medicine
Kawaramachi-Hirokoji
Kamigyo-ku
Kyoto 602-8566
Japan

F. Horiguchi
35 Shinanomachi
Shinjuku-ku
Tokyo 160-0016
Japan

K.-E. Huang
Department of Obstetrics and Gynecology
Chang Gung Memorial Hospital
123 Ta-Pei Road
Niao-Sung Hsiang
Kaohsiung, Taiwan 833

D. Hudita
University of Medicine & Pharmacy
Str. Ion Movila, Nr. 5-7
Sector 2
Bucharest 70.266
Romania

J. A. Kanis
University of Sheffield
WHO Collaborating Centre
Beech Hill Road
Sheffield S10 2RX
UK

J. M. Kaufman
University Hospital Ghent
Endocrinology 9K 121E
De Pintelaan 185
B-9000 Ghent
Belgium

K. Kawakubo
Department of Health Promotion Sciences
Tokyo University Graduate School of Medicine
7-3-1, Hongo
Bunkyo-ku
Tokyo 113-0033
Japan

P. W. Kincade
Oklahoma Medical Research Foundation
825 NE 13th Street
Oklahoma City
OK 73104
USA

L. Kovács
Department of Obstetrics & Gynecology
Albert Szent-Györgyi Medical University
Semmelweis str. 1
Szeged H-6725
Hungary

F. Labrie
Oncology and Molecular Endocrinology
Research Center
Laval University Medical Center (CHUL)
2705 Laurier Boulevard
Quebec City
Quebec G1V 4G2
Canada

B.-M. Landgren
Department of Obstetrics & Gynecology
Huddinge University Hospital
Karolinska Institute
14186 Huddinge
Sweden

J. Y. Lee
Department of Obstetrics & Gynecology
Seoul National University Hospital
28 Yungun-Dong
Chongno-ku
Seoul 110-744
Korea

Khunying K. Limpaphayom
Department of Obstetrics & Gynecology
Faculty of Medicine
Chulalongkorn University
Prathumswan
Bangkok 10330
Thailand

M. Lock
Department of Social Studies of Medicine
McGill University
3655 Drummond Street
Room 416
Montreal, Quebec H3G 1Y6
Canada

B. Lunenfeld
7 Harav Ashi Street
69395 Tel Aviv
Israel

K. A. Matthews
Department of Psychiatry
University of Pittsburgh
3811 O'Hara Street
Pittsburgh, PA 15213
USA

M. McClung
Oregon Osteoporosis Center
5050 NE Hoyt
Suite 651
Portland, Oregon 97213
USA

N. L. McCoy
San Francisco State University
4252 Newberry Court
Palo Alto
CA 94306-4138
USA

J. B. McKinlay
New England Research Institutes, Inc.
9 Galen Street
Watertown
MA 02472
USA

N. R. Melo
Latin American Federation of Climacterium and Menopause Societies (FLASCYM)
Av. Indianopolis, 2700 Indianopolis
Sao Paulo 04062-003
Brazil

M. J. Messina
Nutrition Matters, Inc.
1543 Lincoln Street
Port Townsend, WA 98368
USA

G. V. Miranda
Rua Do Ouro 686 Serra
Belo Horizonte MG 30 220 000
Brazil

T. Moskovic
University Hospital for Obstetrics & Gynecology
'Narodni Front'
Narodnog Fronta 62
Belgrade 11000
Yugoslavia

P. M. Motta
Instituto di Anatomia Umana Normale
University of Rome 'La Sapienza'
Via A. Borelli, 50
00161 Rome
Italy

E. A. Musgrove
Cancer Research Program
Garvan Institute of Medical Research
St. Vincent's Hospital
384 Victoria Street
Darlinghurst, NSW 2010
Australia

E. Namihira
Department of Letters & Education
Ochanomizu University
2-1-1 Ohtsuka
Bunkyo-ku
Tokyo 112-0012
Japan

M. Neves-e-Castro
Clinic of Reproductive Medicine
Portuguese Diabetic Association
Av. Antonio Augusto Aguiar, 24, 2° Dto
Lisbon 1050-016
Portugal

E. Nieschlag
Institute of Reproductive Medicine of the University
Domagkstr. 11
D-48129 Münster
Germany

A. Noji
Department of Nursing, School of Health Sciences
Sapporo Medical University
South 1, West 17
Chuo-ku
Sapporo 060-8556
Japan

H. E. O'Connell
Private Medical Centre
Royal Melbourne Hospital
Suite 12
Parkville
Victoria 3050
Australia

T. Ohkura
Department of Obstetrics & Gynecology
Koshigaya Hospital
Dokkyo University School of Medicine
2-1-50, Minamikoshigaya
Koshigaya
Saitama 343-8555
Japan

H. M. Park
Chung-Ang University
65-207, 3-ka, Hangang-ro
Yongsan-ku
Seoul 140-757
Korea

I. R. Persson
Department of Medical Epidemiology
Karolinska Institute
SE-171 77
Stockholm
Sweden

A. Pines
Department of Medicine 'T'
Ichilov Hospital
6 Weizman Str.
Tel Aviv 64239
Israel

D. W. Purdie
Centre for Metabolic Bone Disease
H S Brocklehurst Building
Hull Royal Infirmary
220–236 Anlaby Road
Hull
HU3 2RW
UK

M. F. Ramashala
University of Durban-Westville
Private Bag X54001
Durban 4000
South Africa

S. T. Reece
C. G. Jung Institute of Los Angeles
1741 Silver Lake Blvd
Room 2A
Los Angeles
CA 90026
USA

J.-Y. Reginster
University of Liege
45 Quai G. Kurth
Liege 4020
Belgium

S. Rozenberg
Interdisciplinary Group on Osteoporosis
Free Universities of Brussels VUB-ULB
St. Peter Hospital
Rue Haute 322
B-1000 Brussels
Belgium

J. Rymer
HRT Research Unit
Department of Gynaecology
Guy's, King's & St. Thomas' School of Medicine
6th Floor North Wing
St. Thomas' Hospital
London
UK

C. M. Sampselle
University of Michigan School of Nursing
400 North Ingalls
Ann Arbor
MI 48109-0482
USA

M. O. Sator
Division of Endocrinology & Reproductive Medicine
Department of Obstetrics & Gynecology
University Hospital of Vienna
Währinger Gürtel 18-20
A-1090 Vienna
Austria

S. S. Sherman
National Institute of Aging
National Institute of Health
Gateway Building, Suite 3E327
7201 Wisconsin Avenue
Bethesda, MD 20892-9205
USA

N. O. Siseles
Av. Santa Fe 3802 P.11
Buenos Aires 1425
Argentina

A. J. C. Slooter
Department of Neurology
University Medical Centre
Room G 03-228
PO Box 85500
3508 GA Utrecht
The Netherlands

V. Smetnik
Scientific Center of Obstetrics, Gynecology and Perinatology
Oparin Street 4
Moscow
Russia 117815

T. Sone
Department of Nuclear Medicine
Kawasaki Medical School
577 Matsushima
Kurashiki
Okayama 701-0192
Japan

T. C. Spelsberg
Department of Biochemistry & Molecular Biology
Mayo Clinic and Mayo Medical School
200 First Street SW
Rochester
MN 55905
USA

J. Studd
Lister Hospital
Chelsea Bridge Road
London SW1N 8RH
UK

C. A. Stuenkel
University of California, San Diego
9500 Gilman Drive, 0659
La Jolla
CA 92037-0659
USA

T. Ushiroyama
Department of Obstetrics & Gynecology
Osaka Medical College
2-7, Daigaku-machi
Takatsuki
Osaka 569-8686
Japan

W. H. Utian
NAMS
5900 Landerbrook Drive
Suite 195
OH 44124
USA

B. von Schoultz
Department of Obstetrics & Gynecology
Karolinska Hospital
Stockholm 171 76
Sweden

M. L. Wahlqvist
International Health & Development Unit
Monash University
8th Floor, Menzies Building
Wellington Road
Clayton
Victoria 3168
Australia

N. K. Wenger
Emory University School of Medicine
69 Butler Street, SE
Atlanta
GA 30303
USA

N. F. Woods
University of Washington School of Nursing
Box 357260
Seattle
WA 98195-7260
USA

B. G. Wren
Sydney Menopause Centre
Royal Hospital for Women
Barker Street
Locked Bag 2000
Randwick NSW 2031
Australia

B. Xiao
National Research Institute for Family Planning
No. 12 Da Hui Si
Haidian District
Beijing 100 081
China

T. Yanaihara
Department of Obstetrics and Gynecology
Showa University
School of Medicine
1-5-8 Hatanodia
Shinagawa-ku
Tokyo 142
Japan

L. Zichella
I Institute of Obstetrics & Gynecology
University of Rome 'La Sapienza'
Viale del Policlinico, 155
Rome 00161
Italy

R. Ziegler
Department of Internal Medicine I
University of Heidelberg
Bergheimer STr. 58
Heidelberg D-69115
Germany

Preface

The need to address issues surrounding the menopause is gaining more and more importance as the population of most societies around the world ages. We believe, therefore, that now is the time to re-evaluate the significance of the menopause from various angles. Although the biologically programmed aging processes have a great impact on women during the menopause, many of the effects at this early stage may not be subjectively recognized. The overt clinical manifestations, some of which may develop into life-threatening conditions, usually appear much later, in the elderly. In addition to these alterations in physical functions, menopausal women encounter various situations of mental stress that arise from the conflicting relationships between younger and older generations living together in the current complicated society. Facing this global situation, the International Menopause Society is rightly expected to play a key role, particularly in the promotion of better health care and improved quality of life for the elderly, including menopausal and aging women and also men.

In October 1999, as we were leaving behind the 20th century and entering the new millennium, the 9th International Menopause Society World Congress on the Menopause was organized under the concept of 'Global and Multidisciplinary Approaches to Menopausal Care'. More than 2200 delegates from 68 countries gathered in Yokohama, Japan and many excellent presentations from various fields and different cultural background were given. As a consequence of the active discussions among specialists, the holistic direction for healthy aging based on human dignity and quality of life in the next century was demonstrated. Most of the lectures delivered at the plenary sessions and symposia are summarized in this Proceedings and appear in the order in which they were presented in the scientific program of the Congress. It is our hope that this volume will be of considerable value for readers who engage in menopausal health care. We are extremely grateful to the authors for contributing their outstanding papers and also to The Parthenon Publishing Group for agreeing to publish this book.

Takeshi Aso
Takumi Yanaihara
Seiichiro Fujimoto

The hypothalamo–pituitary–ovarian axis during the perimenopause

1

H. G. Burger, E. Dudley, P. Mamers, D. M. Robertson, N. Groome and L. Dennerstein

INTRODUCTION

The perimenopause includes the period immediately prior to the menopause (when the endocrinological, biological and clinical features of approaching menopause commence) and the first year after the menopause[1]. The hypothalamo-pituitary-ovarian axis is a classic example of a closed-loop negative-feedback endocrine system. Hypothalamic gonadotropin-releasing hormone (GnRH) is secreted in a pulsatile fashion and stimulates the release of the gonadotropins follicle stimulating hormone (FSH) and luteinizing hormone (LH) from the anterior pituitary. Both hormones stimulate ovarian function, including the secretion of both steroids and peptide hormones. The major steroids estradiol and progesterone exert predominantly negative feedback effects on the hypothalamus and pituitary to restrain GnRH and gonadotropin secretion. The major gonadal peptides involved in the feedback loop are the inhibins A and B. The inhibins are secretory products of the follicular granulosa cells and act as negative feedback signals suppressing the synthesis and secretion of FSH, and acting directly on the pituitary without significant effects at the hypothalamic level[2]. Both inhibins are dimeric glycoproteins, consisting of an α-subunit linked to a hormone-specific β-subunit, either βA or βB[3]. Studies of the localization of each of the inhibin subunits within the ovary[4], together with analysis of their secretory patterns during the menstrual cycle[5], support the postulate that inhibin A is primarily a product of the granulosa cells from the dominant follicle and the granulosa lutein cells of the subsequently developed corpus luteum. Inhibin B, on the other hand, is a product of small antral follicles in the cohort from which the dominant follicle is selected. Inhibin A concentrations are therefore expected to reflect dominant follicle and corpus luteal function, while inhibin B reflects the size and/or function of the ovarian follicular pool, particularly the cohort of small antral follicles found during the follicular phase of the cycle.

Ovarian follicle numbers decline steadily and exponentially from birth until the late 30s, when the rate of decline increases substantially[6], although this interpretation of the data has been challenged recently[7]. During the perimenopause there are typically a few hundred follicles in the ovary, and at the time of the final menstrual period or menopause, few if any follicles remain. Ultrasonographic studies of follicle numbers also show a decline with increasing age[8].

OVERALL CONCEPTS OF FEMALE REPRODUCTIVE AGING

While a major focus of studies of the endocrine changes which occur in association with the perimenopause and menopause has been on changes in ovarian function associated with the declining follicle numbers, there has also been considerable emphasis on the fact that both animal studies and human observations provide evidence for the occurrence of significant changes in the central nervous system, and particularly the hypothalamic pulse generator, as aging occurs[9]. Whether these are primary events, or whether they are secondary to the gradual decline in the ovarian feedback signals, has not been clearly resolved. A major and recently recognized change in ovarian function with age is the declining secretion of the inhibins, particularly inhibin B[10]. It is also clear that a decrease in fertility is observable long before the total loss of ovarian follicles occurs and long before there are any changes in menstrual cyclicity.

It must be emphasized strongly that, while much of the data that have been collected have been analyzed on the basis of results in groups of women or groups of animals, there is a great deal of individual variation in hormonal patterns, making it difficult to make overall generalizations.

FOLLICLE STIMULATING HORMONE CHANGES WITH AGE

A clear-cut feature of reproductive aging is the observation of increased concentrations of FSH during the early follicular and early luteal phases of the menstrual cycle[11]. The precise age at which FSH increases commence is not fully established, although one large study, involving women presenting at an infertility clinic, shows that the FSH increase commences in the late 20s[12]. An important study which documents the endocrine changes associated with reproductive aging in regularly cycling women showed that if a young group, less than 35 years of age, is used as controls, women aged 36–40 already manifest some increase in FSH levels which becomes much more obvious in the fifth decade[11]. Careful inspection of that data indicates a high degree of variability between subjects. Of significance is the fact that the increasing FSH levels are accompanied by no change or, if anything, a small increase in the levels of estradiol, minor changes in LH and no change in luteal progesterone concentrations. Studies of the endocrinology of reproductive aging have therefore concentrated on exploring the explanation for the monotropic rise in FSH.

CENTRAL NERVOUS SYSTEM CHANGES WITH REPRODUCTIVE AGING

The possibility that alterations in hypothalamic function play a role in reproductive aging was raised by the observation that ovarian transplants from old animals, under the kidney capsule of regularly cycling but previously ovariectomized female hosts, was followed by follicular development and ovulation when the ovaries of the old animals were exposed to the neuroendocrine stimuli of the young recipients[13]. This suggested that ovarian function could continue normally, even in animals in which disturbances of cyclicity had occurred. Normal ovarian function could also be induced in old female rats through the administration of drugs which reinstated hypothalamic monoaminergic activity[14] or by stimulation of the preoptic area of the hypothalamus[15]. These experiments provided evidence for changes in the GnRH pulse generator which might contribute to the reproductive aging phenomenon. An increase in FSH, particularly during the secondary FSH surge, in cycling female rats is a feature of reproductive aging in that species which also shows changes in LH pulsatility. Some human studies suggest that changes may occur in LH pulsatility in older, regularly cycling women with increased FSH levels. Increases in LH pulse duration and decreased LH pulse frequency have been reported in regularly cycling middle-aged women during the mid- to late follicular phase of the menstrual cycle, at a time when estradiol levels are similar to those of young controls[16]. These findings are not, however, universal. In summary, both animal studies and human observations support the possibility that central nervous system changes may contribute to the phenomenon of reproductive aging. Furthermore, it has been postulated that the increase in FSH may, in older women, lead to accelerated follicular development and may have a causative role in the increased rate of loss of ovarian follicles in the late 30s[17].

OVARIAN CHANGES WITH REPRODUCTIVE AGING

Because circulating estradiol concentrations tend to increase rather than decrease with aging[11], it is clear that a decrease in steroid feedback cannot explain rising FSH levels. Much evidence has now been obtained to indicate that it is a selective decrease in the ovarian secretion of the inhibins, particularly inhibin B, which may explain the increase in FSH. Klein and colleagues[10] reported important observations in a group of women aged 40–45 years, selected because their serum FSH levels on day 3 of the cycle were > 2 SD above the mean day-3 FSH concentration found in a group of 12 normal women aged 20–25 years. Using the follicular phase FSH peak as a reference point, these investigators showed that estradiol concentrations in the older women were higher than those in the younger women, and there was no difference in inhibin A but inhibin B levels were significantly lower in the older women. These observations have been confirmed in several studies, in some of which it has also been shown that luteal phase inhibin A concentrations are lower in older than in younger subjects[18,19]. It has additionally been suggested that the levels of activin A, an FSH stimulating gonadal peptide, are higher in older women and may contribute to the rising FSH levels[20]. The present authors have conducted a study in which the circulating concentrations of FSH, estradiol and the inhibins were measured between days 3 and 5 of the menstrual cycle in a group of 60 normal subjects ranging in age from 20 to 50 and all continuing to cycle regularly. The data showed that there was a significant age-related increase in the circulating levels of FSH, estradiol and inhibin A and a non-statistically significant decline in the levels of inhibin B. When the subject groups were divided into those younger and older than 40 years, it was shown that in the over 40 age group there was a statistically significant inverse relationship between the levels of inhibin B and FSH. The data were consistent with the primary regulatory role of inhibin B in determining the rising FSH concentrations in older women.

ENDOCRINE CHANGES IN THE PERIMENOPAUSE

Perhaps the most striking feature of the perimenopause from an endocrine viewpoint is the high degree of variability and unpredictability of hormone levels in individual subjects. In the longer cycles often characteristic of this period of reproductive life, levels of the gonadotropins and the gonadal steroids are highly variable both within and between subjects[21]. The Melbourne Women's Midlife Health Project is a longitudinal study of a cohort of women randomly selected from the Australian community as they pass through the perimenopause and menopause[22]. The study has completed its eighth year of observations. A cross-sectional analysis of data was undertaken in the third year of the study, where subjects were divided into those continuing to cycle regularly (the premenopausal group), those who had reported the onset of cycle irregularity but had had menses within the preceding 3 months (the early-perimenopausal group), a group who had had no menses for 3 months but had menstruated within the preceding 12 months (late-perimenopausal group) and those in whom no menses had occurred for at least 12 months (the postmenopausal group)[23]. The most striking result of this analysis was that the concentrations of inhibin B in the early to mid-follicular phase of the cycle fell dramatically when the early-perimenopausal group was compared with the premenopausal group. This fall occurred without any significant change in the levels of estradiol and inhibin A and with a small although not statistically significant rise in FSH levels. It was concluded that the most important event characterizing the endocrinology of entry into the menopausal transition was a selective decrease in circulating inhibin B levels, presumably reflecting the attainment of a critically low number of ovarian follicles or a critical decline in their function, or both.

While the analysis of hormonal changes in the perimenopause seems most logical in relation to the pattern of menstrual cyclicity, data can also be examined in relation to final menses. Data from the Melbourne Women's Midlife Health Project[24] indicate that, in a group of 150 women in whom the date of final menses was established prospectively, circulating FSH levels at the time of final menses had reached approximately 50% of their final postmenopausal concentrations, while estradiol levels had fallen by approximately 60% to a mean level of 113 pmol/l. At that time, levels of inhibin A and B were either undetectable or low.

SUMMARY, CONCLUSIONS AND INTERPRETATION

Reproductive aging is marked by increasing circulating concentrations of FSH when group data are examined. There is clearly a high degree of individual variability, with some late-reproductive-aged women showing no change whatever in circulating FSH[22]. The changes in gonadotropin secretion are explicable in terms of changes in the secretion particularly of inhibin B from ovarian follicular granulosa cells, but it is also likely, based on results of animal and human studies, that primary changes in the GnRH pulse generator may contribute to the ovarian changes. It is postulated that the increasing FSH concentrations stimulate increased follicular secretion of estradiol, which is maintained until the late perimenopause[23], and accelerated follicular development[17].

There is currently much interest in the use of endocrine markers in the prediction of potential fertility, particularly in women who have delayed initiation of pregnancy into their late 30s or early 40s and who present for assisted reproductive technologies[25]. Continued uncertainty surrounds the precise place of measurements of serum FSH and/or inhibin B in the early follicular phase of the cycle. The marked variability of hormone concentrations during the perimenopause gives such measurements little if any diagnostic value in assessing the 'menopausal status' of individual subjects, whose history of menstrual cyclicity provides the strongest evidence about their current situation[26].

ACKNOWLEDGEMENTS

The authors acknowledge with gratitude the contributions of Mr Nick Balazs and his staff in the Department of Chemical Pathology, Monash Medical Centre for their assays of total inhibin, FSH and estradiol. We are grateful to Mr Nick Cahir and Mrs Enid Pruysers for measuring inhibins A and B. The support of the Australian National Health and Medical Research Council and the Victorian Health Promotion Foundation was essential for this work, and the costs of some hormone assays were covered by a grant from Organon Australia Pty. Ltd.

References

1. World Health Organization. *Research on the Menopause.* Report of a WHO Scientific Group. Technical Report Series. Geneva: WHO, 1981:670
2. Burger HG, Igarashi M. Inhibin: definition and nomenclature, including related substances. *J Clin Endocrinol Metab* 1988;66:885
3. Burger HG. Inhibin. *Reprod Med Rev* 1992;1:1–20
4. Roberts VH, Barth S, El-Roeiy A, Yen SSC. Expression of inhibin/activin subunits and follistation messenger ribonucleic acids and proteins in ovarian follicles and the corpus luteum during the human menstrual cycle. *J Clin Endocrinol Metab* 1993;77:1402–10
5. Groome NP, Illingworth PJ, O'Brien M, *et al.* Measurement of dimeric inhibin B throughout the human menstrual cycle. *J Clin Endocrinol Metab* 1996;81:1401–5
6. Richardson SJ, Senikas V, Nelson JF. Follicular depletion during the menopausal transition: evidence for accelerated loss and ultimate exhaustion. *J Clin Endocrinol Metab* 1987;65:1231–7
7. Leidy LE, Godfrey LR, Sutherland MR. Is follicular atresia biphasic? *Fertil Steril* 1998;70:851–9
8. Ruess ML, Kline J, Santos R, *et al.* Age and the ovarian follicle pool assessed with transvaginal ultrasonography. *Am J Obstet Gynecol* 1996;174: 624–7
9. Wise PM, Smith MJ, Dubal DB, *et al.* Neuroendocrine influences and repercussions of the menopause. *Endocr Rev* 1999;20:243–8
10. Klein NA, Illingworth NP, Groome NP, *et al.* Decreased inhibin B secretion is associated with the monotropic FSH rise in older, ovulatory women: a study of serum and follicular fluid levels of dimeric inhibin A and B in spontaneous menstrual cycles. *J Clin Endocrinol Metab* 1996;81:2742–5
11. Lee SJ, Lenton EA, Sexton L, *et al.* The effect of age on the cyclical patterns of plasma LH, FSH, oestradiol and progesterone in women with regular menstrual cycles. *Hum Reprod* 1988;3:851–5
12. Ahmed Ebbiary NA, Lenton EA, Cook ID. Hypothalamic-pituitary aging: progressive increase in FSH and LH concentrations throughout the reproductive life in regularly menstruating women. *Clin Endocrinol* 1994;41:199–206
13. Peng M-T, Huang H-H. Aging of hypothalamic-pituitary-ovarian function in the rat. *Fertil Steril* 1972;232:535–42
14. Clemens JA, Amenomori Y, Jenkins T, *et al.* Effects of hypothalamic stimulation, hormones, and drugs

on ovarian function in old female rats. *Proc Soc Exp Biol Med* 1969;132:561-3

15. Clemens JA, Bennett DR. Do aging changes in the preoptic area contribute to loss of cyclic endocrine function? *J Gerontol* 1977;32:19-24
16. Matt DW, Kauma SW, Pincus SM, *et al.* Characteristics of luteinizing hormone secretion in younger vs. older premenopausal women. *Am J Obstet Gynecol* 1998;178:504-10
17. Klein NA, Battaglia DE, Fujimoto VY, *et al.* Reproductive aging: accelerated ovarian follicular development associated with a monotropic FSH rise in normal older women. *J Clin Endocrinol Metab* 1996;81:1038-45
18. Danforth DR, Arbogast LK, Mroueh J, *et al.* Dimeric inhibin: a direct marker of ovarian aging. *Fertil Steril* 1998;70:119-23
19. Welt CK, McNicholl DJ, Taylor AE, *et al.* Female reproductive aging is marked by decreased secretion of dimeric inhibin. *J Clin Endocrinol Metab* 1999;84:105-11
20. Reame NE, Wyman TL, Phillips DJ, *et al.* Net increase in stimulatory input resulting from a decrease in inhibin B and an increase in activin A may contribute in part to the rise in follicular phase follicle-stimulating hormone of aging cycling women. *J Clin Endocrinol Metab* 1998;83: 3302-7
21. Hee J, MacNaughton J, Bangah M, *et al.* Perimenopausal patterns of gonadotrophins, immunoreactive inhibin, oestradiol and progesterone. *Maturitas* 1993;18:9-20
22. Burger HG, Dudley EC, Hopper JL, *et al.* The endocrinology of the menopausal transition: a cross-sectional study of a population-based sample. *J Clin Endocrinol Metab* 1995;80:3537-45
23. Burger HG, Cahir N, Robertson DM, *et al.* Serum inhibins A and B fall differentially as FSH rises in perimenopausal women. *Clin Endocrinol* 1998;48: 809-13
24. Burger HG, Dudley EC, Hopper JL, *et al.* Prospectively measured levels of serum FSH, estradiol and the dimeric inhibins during the menopausal transition in a population-based cohort of women. *J Clin Endocrinol Metab* 1999;in press
25. Sharara FI, Scott RT Jr, Seifer DB. The detection of diminished ovarian reserve in infertile women. *Am J Obstet Gynecol* 1998;179:804-12
26. Burger HG. Diagnostic role of follicle-stimulating hormone (FSH) measurements during the menopausal transition - an analysis of FSH, oestradiol and inhibin. *Eur J Endocrinol* 1994;130:38-42

Menopause: implications for women's health care in aging societies

2

N. F. Woods

INTRODUCTION

The population of women who are of postmenopausal age is growing dramatically throughout the world. Data about the population of the USA and other countries with similar economies suggest that contemporary midlife women are living to nearly 80 years of age and outliving men by nearly 7 years. In the USA, the population of women over the age of 65 years will double over the next 30 years. Nearly half of the women who survive to age 65 live to be age 85[1]. These data indicate that most women will live approximately one-third of their lifespan after the menopause.

LEADING CAUSES OF MORTALITY AND MORBIDITY FOR WOMEN IN THE USA

Leading causes of death include heart disease, cancer, cerebrovascular disease, pneumonia, influenza, chronic obstructive pulmonary disease, diabetes mellitus, accidents, Alzheimer's disease, nephritis, nephrosis and septicemia. Causes of significant morbidity and institutionalization include these, as well as fractures, hypertension, diabetes mellitus, osteoarthritis, cataracts and dementias.

Despite their longevity, women live a greater number of years with disability than do men. On average, US women live for 2.7 years with a serious limitation in comparison to men, who live for 1.4 years with such a limitation. Living with severe disability requires assistance with activities of daily living (eating, dressing, bathing, toileting, transferring), which increases with age. Three per cent of those 65–74 years of age, but 22% aged 85 years and older, need such assistance. Women also experience an increased need for assistance with instrumental activities of daily living (meal preparation, shopping, money management, telephoning and light housework) as they age: 6.3% of those aged 65–74 years, but 40.8% of those 85 years of age and older, need such assistance.

Reviews of contemporary literature on primary prevention of major causes of mortality and morbidity for women as they age indicate that women should be counselled during midlife, around the time of the menopause, with respect to several prevention strategies.

The review of La Croix and colleagues[2] concerning strategies for health aging recommended:

(1) Assessing risk factors for fractures and falls and modifying those that can be changed;

(2) Ensuring an adequate intake of calcium and vitamin D;

(3) Engaging in shared decision-making processes about hormone therapy for the prevention of fractures, considering the risks and benefits;

(4) Evaluating weight changes of more than 5% over a 6–12 month period and discouraging weight loss for women who are not at risk for other conditions;

(5) Encouraging the consumption of five or more fruits and vegetables each day, a diet low in total and saturated fat, and the use of a daily multivitamin supplement;

(6) Engaging in enjoyable physical activity for 30 min most days of the week;

(7) Getting regular screening for breast, cervical and colorectal cancer.

Taken together, this program would address cardiovascular disease risk, risk for osteoporotic fractures and falls, and the early detection of cancer[2].

Policy makers, researchers and clinicians alike are concerned about the increasing cost of treating diseases of advanced age in the growing population of midlife women and the possible role of the menopause in their future morbidity and mortality. The menopause provides an important occasion for health promotion and disease prevention efforts, which can influence a woman's health throughout her remaining lifespan.

The purposes of this paper are, first, to explore the significance of the menopause for women in an aging society with respect to morbidity and mortality, and, second, to examine the menopause as an occasion for health promotion and disease prevention efforts.

SIGNIFICANCE OF MIDLIFE AND THE MENOPAUSE TO WOMEN IN AN AGING SOCIETY

Midlife

Contemporary women view midlife and the menopause both similarly and differently from their mothers' generation. Data from in-person interviews with a random sample of women enrolled in the Seattle Midlife Women's Health Study[3] ($n = 131$) during 1990–93 indicated that their imagery of midlife focused on change. Although their most common image of midlife was getting older, they associated changes of every kind with midlife. Many alluded to transitions with respect to their physical bodies, emotions, feelings about getting older, outlook on life, relationships and 'change of life'. A few referred to their changing health and vulnerability. These women described midlife similarly to women from earlier birth cohorts, with one important exception: the centrality of work and personal achievement in their lives. As women's roles have changed, so have the experiences that women count as important. Personal achievement and work-related events have assumed a central place, along with family events, in how women describe their lives. With a life course that is made more complex than their mothers' by lifelong employment, contemporary midlife women are not wondering what to do with the rest of their lives as much as they are wondering how to juggle the demands of family and work-related responsibilities. Being able to function in their daily roles is a central concern[3].

Menopause

As part of the longitudinal Seattle Midlife Women's Health Study[4], women ($n = 508$) participated in in-person interviews between 1990 and 1993 about their definitions of the menopause and their expectations and concerns about their own menopausal experiences. At that time, of women ranging in age from 35 to 55 years (median = 41), most were premenopausal or in an early stage of the menopausal transition. Most (80%) were Euro-American and were well educated (median = 15 years).

Women's definitions of the menopause clustered in ten categories and most women offered multiple definitions. The most frequently cited definitions included cessation of menstrual periods, the end of reproductive capacity, and hormonal changes. In addition, many women described the menopause as a change of life or a new life stage. Some referred explicitly to changing bodies or changing emotions. Others spoke about the menopause as an element of the aging process. Only a small proportion of women linked their definitions of the menopause to symptoms, disease risk (e.g. osteoporosis) or the need for medical care. Although some women had negative or positive expectations of the menopause, most women expressed uncertainty about their own menopause or had no expectations. This cohort of midlife women did not seem to have adopted a medical model of the menopause and were most likely to view the menopause as a normal developmental process. Their uncertainty about what to expect provides an opportunity for health teaching and anticipatory guidance[4].

In a study commissioned by the North American Menopause Society, the Gallup organization conducted a poll of 752 postmenopausal US women aged 50–65 years of age[5]. Standardized interviews were conducted, with women identified by using random-digit telephone dialling. Women reported that they were happier and more fulfilled now, at ages 50–65 years, than in their 20s, 30s or

40s. These data indicated that postmenopausal women considered midlife and menopause to be the beginning of many positive changes in their lives. In addition, when they were asked about the personal experiences of the menopause they would like to discuss, their responses included long-term risks (such as those for cardiovascular disease and osteoporosis), medical treatment options and symptoms such as hot flushes[5].

Taken together, these studies provide evidence that premenopausal women do not view the menopause as linked to disease or medical care, but postmenopausal women identify a need for discussion of health risks around the time of the menopause. Uncertainty about the menopausal transition provides opportunities for health education efforts for this population of women for whom being able to function is a significant concern.

HEALTH RISKS

Given that women express a desire to discuss long-term health risks, it is important to understand how women view their own risks. Participants in a large sample survey of postmenopausal women aged 50 years and older, with access to health care and living in Washington State, rated their personal risk of developing diseases of advanced age consistently with their concern about risk. They expressed the highest perceived likelihood of developing heart disease, osteoporosis and bladder problems (scale of 1–7, 7 = high likelihood), but they expressed greatest concern (scale of 1–7, 7 = high concern) about breast cancer, heart disease, osteoporosis and bladder problems[6]. These data suggest that what worries women most about their own health does not correspond directly with mortality data for women in general as they age. This is not surprising, given that women's heightened awareness about breast cancer is consistent with their personal experiences with age-peer women who are being diagnosed and treated for breast cancer, and their lack of direct experience with age peers who have osteoporosis and cardiovascular disease. These data suggest a need for public health education efforts to raise women's awareness of diseases of advanced age as well as their roles in lifestyle modification and screening efforts for the early detection of disease.

MENOPAUSE AS AN OCCASION FOR HEALTH PROMOTION AND DISEASE PREVENTION

In the USA, several consensus statements about menopause care have called for health-care providers to provide high-quality education about the menopausal transition for midlife women and have encouraged professionals to discuss strategies for preventing diseases of advanced age as well as the advantages and disadvantages of hormone therapy. Recently, the National Committee for Quality Assurance has recommended that managed care organizations report on the percentage of insured women who receive counselling about menopause issues[7]. The Health Employer Data and Information Set (HEDIS) criteria for evaluating the quality of health care will include elements related to menopause counselling beginning in the year 2000. Informed health-care choice is one area of health-plan performance that will be assessed using the menopause counselling indicators. Selection of menopause counselling as part of the measurement of performance reflects the essential nature of supporting informed decision-making about the menopause under conditions of uncertainty about the best course of action for managing menopausal symptoms and preventing diseases such as osteoporosis and other diseases of advanced age. Moreover, inclusion of the menopause counselling indicators reflects the importance of women's participation in their health-care decisions and expectations that health-care providers will discuss the menopause, symptom management and prevention strategies with midlife women.

There is growing evidence that women make lifestyle changes around the time of the menopause and that women who have the opportunity to discuss hormone therapy as one part of menopause counselling are also likely to be those making lifestyle changes. Under the direction of the North American Menopause Society (NAMS), the Gallup organization conducted a poll of 752 postmenopausal US women aged 50–65 years of age identified by using random-digit telephone dialling[5]. Women responded to the question: 'What type of health-related lifestyle changes, if any, have you, yourself, made at middle age or menopause?' Results of the NAMS survey indicated that the majority of women made lifestyle changes around the time of the menopause. Approximately 75% of the women surveyed reported making one or more such change at middle age or the menopause. Only 23% said that they had not made any health-related lifestyle changes. Changes in diet and nutrition were the most frequent responses, mentioned by 51% of those surveyed. Next most frequent were starting or increasing the amount of exercise (34%) and reducing stress levels by taking vacations, getting massages or making more time for themselves (25%). Nearly 9% of women said they reduced their alcohol intake, and a similar proportion said they stopped smoking. About one in ten women said they tried alternative or holistic remedies and treatments.

Moreover, women who had discussed using hormone therapy with a health-care provider were more likely to have modified their diets, increased their exercise, reduced stress and were slightly more likely to have reduced alcohol intake and tried therapeutic alternatives. They were less likely to have reduced smoking, perhaps because fewer smoked in the first place[5].

One of the benefits of counselling about hormone therapy, despite the uncertainty about its efficacy for heart disease prevention, is that such counselling may cue women to consider preventive activities they may wish to institute in conjunction with hormone therapy or as an alternative strategy. Moreover, given the cross-sectional nature of these data, it seems important to acknowledge that women who have access to health care in the USA and who receive menopause counselling belong to a subset of the population that also may have incorporated preventive practices into their lives prior to the menopause.

In addition to having the opportunity to discuss hormone therapy, women who had seen a health-care provider also had the opportunity to participate in screening for the early detection of diseases likely to limit their lifespans. Those who had the opportunity to discuss hormone therapy with their health-care provider were also more likely to have had a mammogram within the past 2 years, a pelvic examination and cholesterol measurement. They were somewhat more likely to have had a bone density measurement than women who did not have the opportunity to discuss hormone therapy with their health-care providers.

FACTORS LIMITING WOMEN'S ACCESS TO GOOD HEALTH IN OLD AGE

Despite the positive indications that women find the menopause to be an occasion for health promotion and prevention efforts, and receive prevention counselling and screening, these benefits do not accrue uniformly to all women. Data from a study of clinicians practicing in a large health-maintenance organization revealed that barriers to their providing menopause counselling included lack of information about risks and benefits, unique challenges of counselling, and lack of resources to conduct counselling[8]. Suggested strategies included development of patient education materials, including written materials, use of discussion groups, and organizational support for counselling.

In addition to organizational barriers, data from the NAMS survey revealed that both education and income level were related to whether a woman received counselling about hormone therapy. Moreover, women who have insurance that covers hormone therapy are more likely to use it[9]. Thus, socioeconomic status may influence women's chances of:

(1) Having access to insurance to cover the cost of visits and hormone therapy prescription;

(2) Being sufficiently informed to ask about menopause counselling or hormone therapy;

(3) Having access to a primary care provider.

This study and others support a persistent pattern that suggests women of lower socioeconomic status (education and income), without insurance and without a primary care provider, are less likely to benefit from counselling about options for disease prevention in advanced age[10]. In the USA, the organization and financing of health care has had important effects on women's access to services, including counselling and prevention during midlife.

In addition to socioeconomic effects on menopause counselling and hormone therapy use, being white also increased women's chances of receiving hormone therapy counselling. Race may affect women's likelihood of using hormone therapy, because osteoporosis risk may be higher for white women than for other groups. Thus, the prescription of hormone therapy by providers may be influenced by disease risk, which they believe is linked to race. Another explanation is that race is linked to socioeconomic status and, through income and education, race affects exposure to menopause counselling and hormone use[11]. Still others have found that the meaning of menopause varies across racial and ethnic groups[12-15]. Future studies that sample specific racial/ethnic groups of women within various socioeconomic groups are needed to disentangle the significance of the relationship between race and access to counselling and hormone therapy use.

CONCLUSION

In conclusion, the significance of midlife and the menopause to women is consistent with their being in the prime of life and staying healthy. The menopause is not viewed as a medical event, but does create an opportunity for women to evaluate their health. Evidence suggests that women make lifestyle changes and engage in new health-promoting and disease-preventing behaviors. Women who have access to health care also get counselling from professionals regarding their health at the menopause and beyond, and obtain screening for diseases. Those who adopt hormone therapy are more likely to get these counselling and screening opportunities. These data also reveal the inequity in women's access to health care and warrant a re-examination of the effects of rationing health care in the USA on the health of midlife and older women. Clinical services to enhance health promotion and disease prevention should be available to all if the entire society is to benefit from the contributions of older women. Moreover, intensive public-health education efforts for midlife women can support their efforts at lifestyle modification and provide access to screening in countries lacking a national health plan.

References

1. *US Vital Statistics*, 1992
2. La Croix A, Newton K, Leveille S, Wallace J. Healthy aging: a women's issue. *Western J Med* 1997;167:220–32
3. Woods N, Mitchell E. Women's images of midlife: observations from the Seattle Midlife Women's Health Study. *Health Care Women Int* 1997;18: 439–53
4. Woods N, Mitchell E. Anticipating menopause: observations from the Seattle Midlife Women's Health Study. *Menopause* 1999;6:167–73
5. Utian W, Boggs P. The North American Menopause Society 1998 Menopause Survey. Part I. Postmenopausal women's perception about menopause and midlife. *Menopause* 1999;6:122–8
6. Woods N, Saver B, Taylor T. Attitudes toward menopause and hormone therapy among women with access to health care. *Menopause* 1998;5:178–88
7. National Committee for Quality Assurance. *HEDIS 2000 Technical Specifications*, vol 3. Washington, DC: National Committee for Quality Assurance, 1999
8. Anderson L, Caplan L, Buist D, *et al.* Perceived barriers and recommendations concerning hormone replacement therapy counseling among primary care providers. *Menopause* 1999;6:161–6
9. Ettinger B, Woods N, Barrett-Connor E, Pressman A. The North American Menopause Society 1998 Menopause Survey. Part II. Counseling about hormone replacement therapy: association with socioeconomic status and access to medical care. *Menopause* 2000; in press

10. Cauley J, Cummings S, Black D, *et al.* Prevalence and determinants of estrogen replacement therapy in elderly women. *Am J Obstet Gynecol* 1990;163: 1438–44
11. Brett K, Madans J. Differences in use of postmenopausal hormone replacement therapy by black and white women. *Menopause* 1997;4:66–70
12. Mebans-Sims I. Menopause - different meanings for different women. *Menopause* 1997;4:63–5
13. Standing T, Glazer G. Attitudes of low income clinic patients toward menopause. *Health Care Women Int* 1992;13:271–80
14. Pham K, Freeman E, Grisso J. Menopause and hormone replacement therapy: focus groups of African American and Caucasian women. *Menopause* 1997; 4:71–9
15. Holmes-Rovner M, Padonu G, Kroll J, *et al.* African American women's attitudes and expectations of menopause. *Am J Prev Med* 1996;12:420-3

Mechanisms of action of estrogens and antiestrogens

3

F. Labrie, C. Labrie, A. Bélanger, J. Simard, V. Luu-The and B. Candas

INTRODUCTION

The progress being achieved in the field of antiestrogens is simply remarkable. Some new compounds possess characteristics which could never have been predicted by even the most optimistic scientist. With the recent progress achieved, these new compounds could well become the best example of the success achievable by biomedical and pharmaceutical research and of the efficient complementarity between university and industry.

The new chemically produced antiestrogens induce three-dimensional structural changes of the estrogen receptor (ER), which lead to a multitude of activities of the ER–antiestrogen complex that are specific for each target cell type and gene. Such ligand-induced modifications of the three-dimensional structure of ER, which are unique to each antiestrogen, lead, at one extreme, to a complete blockade of the normal action of estrogens in some tissues while, in other tissues, the same ER–ligand complex completely mimics or even surpasses the natural action of estrogens.

While being of major importance for preventive and therapeutic medicine, the unexpected cell-specific and even gene-specific properties of the new antiestrogens offer unique tools to investigate and further understand the mechanisms of action of estrogens and antiestrogens, including the structural domains of ER responsible for their delicate interactions with the numerous other intracellular regulatory proteins (co-activators and co-repressors) that culminate in the cell-specific stimulation or inhibition of the expression of each estrogen-sensitive gene under both normal and pathological conditions.

Estrogens, especially 17β-estradiol, have long been recognized as playing a key role in the development, growth and function of the female sex organs and mammary gland, as well as in the development of female sex characteristics[1,2]. An important role of estrogens has also been identified in the bones, the cardiovascular system and the central nervous system[3–5].

Although estrogen replacement therapy at the menopause can prevent bone loss and cardiovascular disease, there is evidence that estrogens are associated with an increased risk of breast cancer and endometrial cancer[6], thus seriously limiting the use of estrogen replacement therapy. The ideal compound for women's health should be able to decrease the risk of the most important causes of morbidity and mortality in women, namely breast cancer, uterine cancer, osteoporosis, bone fractures and cardiovascular disease. Heart disease is, in fact, the leading cause of death in postmenopausal women[7]. The ideal compound should also have an excellent safety profile in order to ensure compliance over the 20–40 years of a woman's postmenopausal life.

MENOPAUSE, OSTEOPOROSIS AND CARDIOVASCULAR DISEASES

Despite the well-known beneficial effects of estrogen therapy on menopausal symptoms[8–10] and their role in reducing bone loss and coronary heart disease[11–16], compliance is low. Women decide not to take estrogens or stop treatment early because of the fear of breast cancer and uterine cancer[10] and because of symptoms associated with their therapy, namely uterine bleeding, breast tenderness and fluid retention.

The menopause is thus the condition in most urgent need of tissue- or cell-targeted endocrine therapy. In fact, estrogen-like compounds are required for the prevention of both bone loss and cardiovascular disease. On the other hand, for the breast and endometrium, the ideal approach is a pure antiestrogen which would inhibit the development and growth of breast and endometrial carcinomas. The effects required in the bones and cardiovascular system (estrogenic) are thus the opposite of those required in the breast and endometrium, where antiestrogenic activity is recommended.

The availability of such a compound would be a major step forward compared to standard estrogen-based replacement therapy. Such a compound could be called a pure response-specific ER regulator, with responses ranging from pure antiestrogenic to full estrogenic activities, depending upon the responses and tissues involved, instead of mixed agonist–antagonist activities. The acronym SERM (selective estrogen receptor modulator) does not appropriately describe compounds such as EM-652, since it describes compounds having a wide range of ratios of antiestrogenic and estrogenic properties, with no indication of any completely specific activity in individual tissues. As an example, both tamoxifen and raloxifene are SERMs, but they are very different compounds, thus indicating the need for a more explicit terminology. In fact, the acronym SERM does not identify the compounds which are pure antiestrogens in the mammary gland and endometrium and are thus the compounds most likely to have the highest efficacy in preventing both breast and endometrial cancer.

THE ESTROGEN RECEPTORS AND THEIR MULTIPLE GENE ACTIVATION MECHANISMS

ER-α and ER-β

The ER is the only known member of the family of steroid receptors that has multiple subtypes. This diversity of ERs offers unique possibilities for the modulation of estrogen-responsive genes.

The human ER was first cloned and its structure determined from human breast cancer MCF-7 cells[17,18]; ER-α was found to consist of 595 amino acids divided into six functional domains[19]. Over the past decade, all the studies on the elucidation of the molecular events underlying the mode of ER action, as well as antiestrogen-designed therapies, have focused on the ER-α identified and cloned several years ago[17,18,20]. Recently, a second estrogen receptor, designated ER-β, has been described and shown to share common structural and functional characteristics with ER-α[21–23]. Based on a comparison of amino acid sequences, ER-β shares with ER-α the same modular structure composed of six domains (A–F)[24]. Domain C, which contains the two zinc fingers responsible for DNA binding, is the most conserved, followed by domain E, which is responsible for ligand binding, homodimerization and nuclear localization. Domain E also contains a ligand-dependent activation function (AF-2) involved in *trans*-activation by the ERs. As mentioned above, a second activation function, AF-1, resides in the A/B domain and acts in a ligand-independent manner[19,25,26]. Both ERs recognize a specific estrogen response element (ERE) composed of two AGGTCA motif half-sites configured as a palindrome spaced by three nucleotides[23]. ER-α has also been shown to interact with a number of co-regulators via the AF-2 domain, and these protein–protein interactions promote the transcriptional regulation of target genes[27–30].

A most important question is the distribution of ER-α and ER-β in different tissues in order to explain the tissue-specific effects of estrogens and, especially, the new antiestrogens. ER-β has a high level of expression in the bone, prostate, hypothalamus and specific areas in the central nervous system[21,31,32]. As illustrated in Figure 1, the ER-α–17β-estradiol and ER-β–17β-estradiol complexes can form homodimers (ER-α–ER-α and ER-β–ER-β) or heterodimers (ER-α–ER-β). Such a diversity of ER-α and ER-β interactions provides additional means of exerting gene-specific actions.

AF-1 and AF-2 functions of ER

ERs are members of a family of ligand-inducible transcriptional regulators that include steroids, thyroid hormones, retinoids and vitamin D.

Estrogen-induced AF-2 activation

Classically, 17β-estradiol binds to the ER, thus leading to conformational changes which result in the dimerization of 17β-estradiol–ER complexes, with subsequent binding to a specific ERE located within the promoter area of genes responsive to estrogen (Figure 2). The classical ERE element is an inverted hexanucleotide repeat separated by three nucleotides[33]. Such binding of the dimerized ER–17β-estradiol complex to the ERE results in the activation of transcription.

Kinase-induced AF-1 activation

The ER, in analogy with many other nuclear receptors, plays a double life, since it can be activated by kinase cascades independently of estrogens or of the activation of the estrogen binding site by an estrogenic ligand (Figure 2).

Polypeptide growth factors have been proposed as autocrine or paracrine mediators of classically estrogen-regulated mitogenesis[34,35]. For example, the exogenous administration of epidermal growth factor (EGF) mimics the effect of estrogens on the differentiation and proliferation of the reproductive tract in mice[36]. Much evidence has accumulated to indicate that such action of EGF is mediated by the ER[35–37]. We will describe in more detail later the activation of AF-1 by Ras and EGF and, most interestingly, the complete inhibition of such action by the pure antiestrogen EM-652 (Figure 3).

In fact, AF-1 is thought to be responsible for the partial estrogenic activity of tamoxifen in cells which express ER-α[38]. Moreover, it should be mentioned that tamoxifen, in contrast to EM-652, is unable to interfere with the activation of genes by factors acting through AF-1[25]; such activation can be blocked by pure antiestrogens such as EM-652. As an example, the stimulatory effects of EGF and diethylstilbestrol on DNA synthesis and phosphatidylinositol turnover in the ovariectomized mouse uterus were blocked to the same extent by the simultaneous administration of the pure antiestrogen ICI 164,384, thus indicating that both EGF and diethylstilbestrol act through the ER, the effects of these two very different compounds being completely blocked by a pure antiestrogen[35].

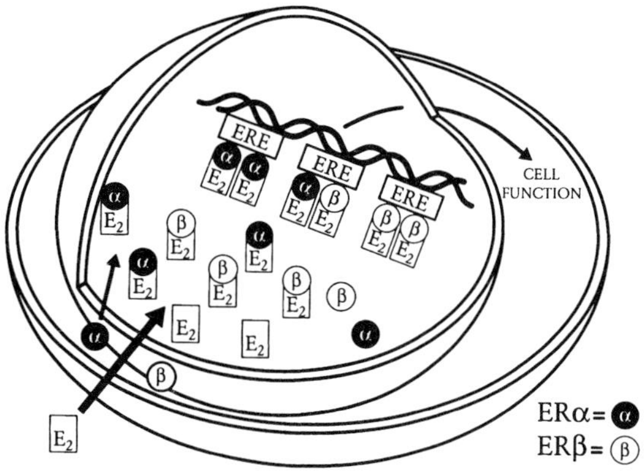

Figure 1 Formation of the homodimers estrogen receptor (ER)-α-17β-estradiol (E_2)-ER-α-E_2 and ER-β-E_2-ER-β-E_2 as well as the heterodimer ER-α-E_2-ER-β-E_2, in cells which express both ER-α and ER-β. ERE, estrogen response element

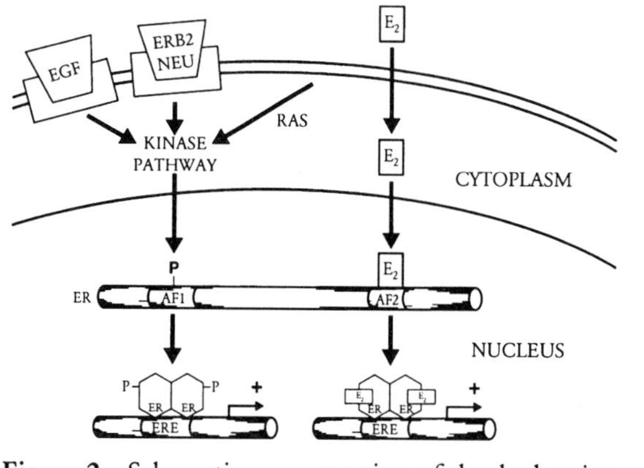

Figure 2 Schematic representation of the dual activation mechanisms of the estrogen receptor (ER) by the activation function (AF)-1 and AF-2 sites. EGF, epidermal growth factor; P, progesterone; E_2, 17β-estradiol

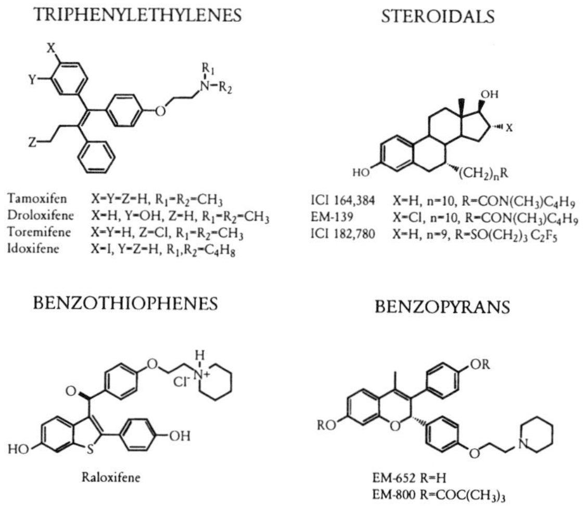

Figure 3 Molecular structures of antiestrogens

It can be mentioned that EGF, in the absence of estrogen, caused a translocation of ER to the nucleus in a way analogous to the effect of estrogen itself. Such data show that EGF can induce proliferative effects that are undistinguishable from the action of estrogens.

AP-1 response element

Not all genes responsive to estradiol possess an ERE element in their promoter but, instead, possess other specific DNA sequences. The AP-1 response element is such a specific DNA sequence, requiring the protein transcription factors c-jun and c-fos for activity (Figure 4).

The tissue specificity of an estrogenic, antiestrogenic or a mixed estrogenic–antiestrogenic response can thus be explained by two different sites of DNA action of ER-α and ER-β. The classical ERE (Figure 4a) binds both ER-α–17β-estradiol and ER-β–17β-estradiol, with a positive response in both cases[39]. With ER-α or ER-β and a reporter gene under the transcriptional control of an ERE, tamoxifen and raloxifene, as well as ICI 164,384, inhibit the stimulatory effect of 17β-estradiol.

When the reporter gene was controlled by an AP-1 instead of an ERE element, 17β-estradiol, diethylstilbestrol, tamoxifen, raloxifene and ICI 164,384 all stimulated transcription with ER-α. When ER-β was transfected instead of ER-α, 17β-estradiol and diethylstilbestrol had an inhibitory effect, while the three antiestrogens exerted a stimulatory effect. Most interestingly, 17β-estradiol could reverse the stimulatory effect of raloxifene mediated by ER-β and the AP-1 element in a dose-dependent manner. While these experiments were performed in Hela cells, it is most relevant to mention that, in human breast cancer MCF-7 and uterine cancer Ishikawa cells[39], ER-β acting at an AP-1 element led to the same observations: stimulation by antiestrogens and inhibition by estrogens, these effects being opposite to the classical action of estrogens and antiestrogens on the transcription of genes controlled by an ERE element. In agreement with these data, tamoxifen has been reported to inhibit ERE-mediated estrogen action, while stimulating transcription by ER-regulated genes through the AP-1 element[40].

The above-mentioned data indicate that the ratio of ER-α and ER-β (Figure 1), as well as the ratio of ERE and AP-1 sites in the cell, can lead to markedly different and even opposite responses to the same agents, thus adding to cell- and even gene-specific types of response to any ER ligand.

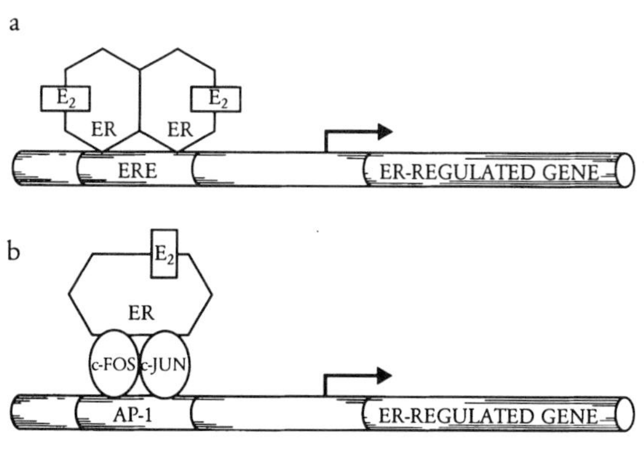

Figure 4 Schematic representation of the activation of estrogen receptor (ER)-regulated genes by classical interaction of dimerized ER–17β-estradiol (E_2) with an estrogen response element (ERE) in the promoter (a) and by interaction of ER–E_2 in association with c-fos and c-jun with the AP-1 element of the promoter (b) of ER-regulated genes

Co-activators and co-repressors

While the simple mechanisms of estrogen action illustrated schematically in Figure 5a can offer a highly simplified explanation of the multiple effects mediated by estrogens, it has become clear that the stimulation or inhibition of transcription by ER-regulated genes is a highly complex phenomenon that involves the interaction of dozens of proteins that enhance or inhibit the activity of the ER–17β-estradiol complex.

Rapid progress is being made in the identification and understanding of function of the large series of co-activators and co-repressors that are expressed at various levels (from zero to high values) in a cell-specific fashion[41]. Only when all these determinants of ER-α and ER-β function are known for each ligand in each cell type will it be possible to predict with some confidence the agonist, antagonist and mixed agonist-antagonist effects of each ligand on each gene in each cell type.

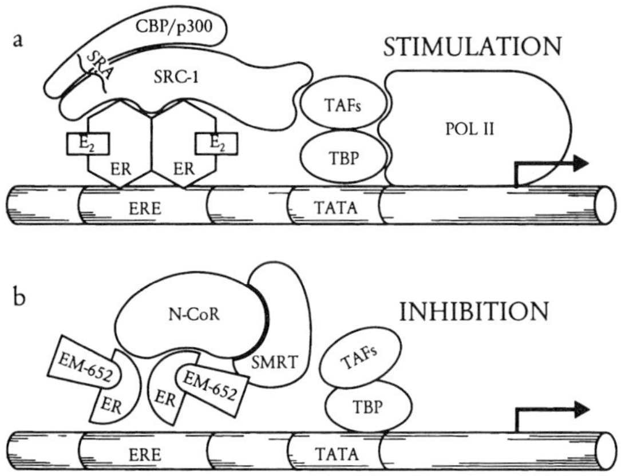

Figure 5 Model for activation by co-activators (a) and inhibition by co-repressors (b) of transcription. CBP/p300, cAMP response element binding protein; SRA, steroid receptor RNA activator; SRC-1, steroid receptor co-activator 1; TBP, TATA-binding protein; TAF, TBP-associated factor; pol II, RNA polymerase II; N-CoR, nuclear receptor co-repressor; SMRT, silencing mediator of retinoic and thyroid hormone receptors; E_2, 17β-estradiol; ER, estrogen receptor; ERE, estrogen response element

Co-activators

The most widely studied co-activators of the ER are steroid receptor co-activator (SRC)-1 and p300 or CBP (cAMP response element [CREB] binding protein) (Figure 5). Since co-activators bind to the ligand-binding domain of nuclear receptors, the ligand-binding domain has been used as a bait to isolate co-activator proteins represented by the families SRC-1/nuclear receptor co-activator (NCoA)-1, transcription intermediary factor (TIF)-2, glucocorticoid receptor interacting protein (GRIP)-1/NCoA-2 and CREB binding protein-interacting protein (pCIP)/nuclear receptor co-activator (ACTR)/amplified in breast cancer 1 (AIB1)[42,43]. These co-activators have been shown to have in common multiple LXXLL motifs which interact with the ligand-binding domain of nuclear receptors. As an example, in Hep 62 (human hepatocellular carcinoma) cells, in which 4-hydroxytamoxifen is an agonist, the addition of SRC-1[44], but not GRIP-1, could enhance the 4-hydroxytamoxifen-induced transcription. As another example, AIB1, a member of the SRC-1 family, has been found to be elevated in 70% of breast cancers[45]. On the other hand, the disruption of the SRC-1 gene in mice has been shown to lead to partial hormone resistance[46].

CBP/p300 has been found to interact directly with nuclear receptors and with SRC-1, thus acting synergistically to stimulate transcription[47,48]. CBP/p300 and other co-activators possess histone acetyltransferase activity, which could induce remodelling of the DNA structure, thus facilitating specific gene transcription. CBP also interacts with RNA polymerase II[49], as well as with transcription factor IIb (TFIIB)[50]. CBP could thus help to recruit polymerase II to the promoter of specific genes. CBP overexpression can increase estrogen-stimulated ER-mediated transcriptional activity approximately ten-fold[49].

Recently, a complex called vitamin D receptor interacting protein (DRIP) or thyroid hormone receptor-associated protein (TRAP) has been identified as binding to many members of the nuclear receptor family. The single subunit DRIP-205/TRAP-220 binds to the ligand-binding domain AF-2 core following binding of the receptor to its cognate ligand[43,51], before attracting the other 15–20 proteins which form the DRIP/TRAP complex. The formation of this complex is an absolute requirement for the ligand-induced transcriptional activity of the receptor–ligand complex.

In addition to the highly complex battery of protein co-activators, an RNA co-activator has recently been identified and its interaction with some other co-activators has been studied[52]. The RNA co-activator, termed SRA, interacts with the AF-1 domain of the progesterone receptor and it has been suggested that SRA could serve as a ligand to recruit SRC-1 in the activation complex of steroid receptors.

Co-repressors

On the other hand, transcription induced by nuclear receptors can be inhibited by protein molecules called co-repressors. The silencing mediator of retinoic and thyroid hormone receptors (SMRT)[53] and the nuclear receptor co-repressor (N-CoR)[54] are among the best known of this class of proteins that inhibit transcription (Figure 5). In fact, in their inactive state, ERs are thought to be bound by inactivating co-repressors. Upon binding of the cognate ligand, or activation by kinases

(Figure 2), the co-repressors are released while co-activators are recruited, thus potentiating the transcriptional capacity of ER.

At least for some nuclear receptors, in the absence of agonists, the co-repressors N-CoR and SMRT interact with Sin3 and RPD3 (a protein showing histone deacetylase activity), thus tightening the chromatin structure and inhibiting access to the genes[44,55,56].

The exact mechanisms by which ER AF-2 functions remain to be elucidated, but it is clear that the activation by estrogen of ER AF-2 involves multiple interactions of ER with a long series of co-activators and co-repressors. It has also become clear that the interaction of a co-repressor or a co-activator with the ER–ligand complex depends not only upon the ligand, but also upon the cell type or intracellular environment, as well as the element responsive to ER in the promoter of each gene. Different compounds will thus all have different agonist/antagonist activities, depending upon the promoter and cell content of various co-activators and/or co-repressors[57].

Binding of the ligand to the ligand-binding domain of the ER induces changes in the three-dimensional conformation of the ER, which is well illustrated in studies with 17β-estradiol and raloxifene[58]. In addition, the interaction of ER with co-activators and co-repressors specific for each cell type permits the induction of a complete estrogenic effect in some tissues, while, in other tissues, a pure antiestrogenic activity is obtained (Figure 6). In the endometrium, full estrogenic activity is produced by 17β-estradiol (Figure 6a), while tamoxifen presents relatively strong agonistic effects (Figure 6b) and raloxifene possesses low estrogenic activity (Figure 6c), an opposite effect being observed in terms of antiestrogenic activity. EM-652 (SCH 57068) or ICI 18280, on the other hand, show pure antiestrogenic activity in the mammary gland and endometrium (Figure 6d).

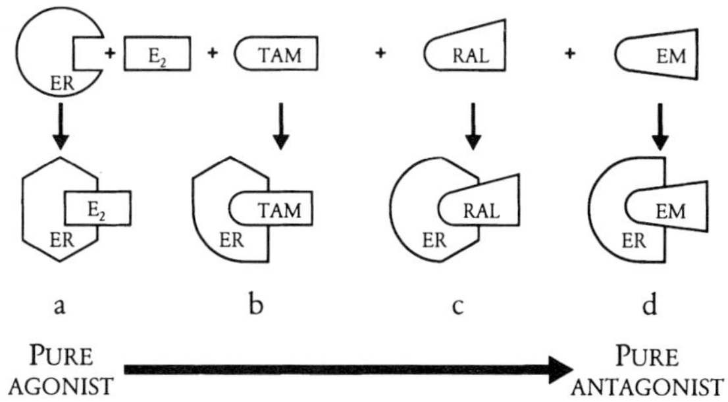

Figure 6 Schematic representation of the ligand-induced changes in the conformation of the estrogen receptor (ER) which lead to activities ranging from pure estrogenic (a) to pure antiestrogenic (d) effects. In addition to the ligand-induced changes in the three-dimensional structure of ER, the multiple interactions with cell-specific co-activators and co-repressors determine the final activity of each ER–ligand complex in each cell. E_2, 17β-estradiol; TAM, tamoxifen; RAL, raloxifene; EM, EM-652

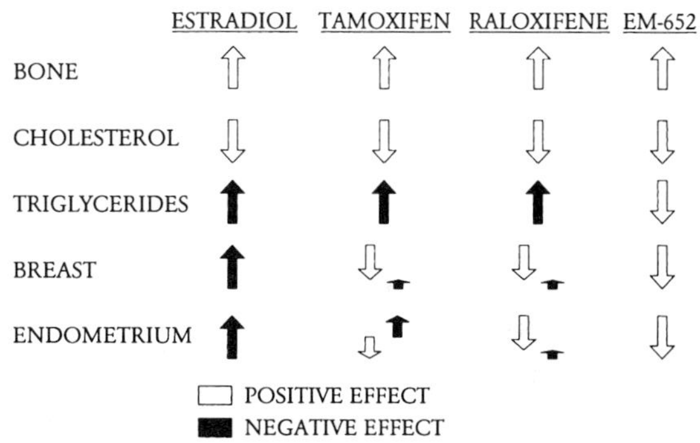

Figure 7 Schematic representation of the estrogenic and/or antiestrogenic action of estradiol, tamoxifen, raloxifene and EM-652 on the main parameters important for women's health, namely the breast, endometrium, bone and serum lipids

ANTIESTROGENS

Figure 7 summarizes the activities characteristic of 17β-estradiol and of the three classes of antiestrogens so far available, namely tamoxifen (first-generation SERM), raloxifene (second-generation SERM) and EM-652 (pure SERM), on the best-known parameters of women's health. As can be seen in this schematic figure, tamoxifen, while exerting beneficial effects on serum cholesterol, bone loss and breast cancer, possesses a relatively strong estrogenic activity in the endometrium as well as some stimulatory effect on breast cancer proliferation. Raloxifene, on the other hand, represents an important improvement in terms of a decrease of the stimulatory activity in the endometrium, although some small estrogenic activity persists in the endometrium as well as in breast cancer cell proliferation. EM-652, on the other hand, is the only compound having pure antiestrogenic activity in the breast and endometrium while decreasing serum cholesterol and triglycerides and protecting against bone loss.

An ideal therapy at the menopause should prevent bone loss and simultaneously reduce cardiovascular risks, without producing significant estrogenic effects in the endometrium and mammary gland, which seriously limit the acceptance of the current estrogen replacement therapy. EM-800 lacks a stimulatory effect on the endometrium, as demonstrated by histopathological examination[59-61]. Similarly, EM-800 shows pure antiestrogenic activity in human endometrial Ishikawa carcinoma cells[62]. It should also be mentioned that raloxifene, droloxifene and tamoxifen stimulate, to various degrees, the estrogen-sensitive parameter alkaline phosphatase in human endometrial Ishikawa carcinoma cells, the stimulatory effect of these compounds being fully reversible by EM-800[62,63], thus confirming the intrinsic estrogenic activity of these compounds.

ACKNOWLEDGEMENTS

The expert and devoted collaboration of all the personnel of the Oncology and Molecular Endocrinology Research Center who have been associated with this project is deeply appreciated.

References

1. Henderson BE, Ross R, Bernstein L. Estrogens as a cause of human cancer: The Richard and Hinda Rosenthal Foundation Award Lecture. *Cancer Res* 1988;48:246–53
2. Grese TA, Dodge JA. Selective estrogen receptor modulators (SERMs). *Curr Pharm Des* 1998;4: 71–92
3. Smith EP, Boyd J, Frank GR, *et al.* Estrogen resistance caused by a mutation in the estrogen-receptor gene in a man [see Comments] [published erratum appears in *N Engl J Med* 1995;332:131]. *N Engl J Med* 1994;331:1056–61
4. Ciocca RG, Choi J, Graham AM. Antiphospholipid antibodies lead to increased risk in cardiovascular surgery. *Am J Surg* 1995;170: 198–200
5. Ciocca R, Roig L. Estrogen receptors in human nontarget tissues: biological and clinical implications. *Endocr Rev* 1995;16:35–62
6. Gambrell RD Jr. The menopause: benefits and risks of hormone replacement therapy. *Compr Ther* 1994;20:580–5
7. Lerner DJ, Kannel WB. Patterns of coronary heart disease morbidity and mortality in the sexes: a 26-year follow-up of the Framingham population. *Am Heart J* 1986;111:383–90
8. Lomax P, Schonbaum E. Postmenopausal hot flushes and their management. *Pharmacol Ther* 1993;57:347–58
9. Greendale GA, Judd HL. The menopause: health implications and clinical management. *J Am Geriatr Soc* 1993;41:426–36
10. Grady D, Rubin SM, Petitti DB, *et al.* Hormone therapy to prevent disease and prolong life in postmenopausal women. *Ann Intern Med* 1992;117: 1016–37
11. Lobo RA. Clinical review 27: Effects of hormonal replacement on lipids and lipoproteins in postmenopausal women. *J Clin Endocrinol Metab* 1991; 73:925–30
12. Harris ST, Genant HK, Baylink DJ, *et al.* The effects of estrone (Ogen) on spinal bone density of postmenopausal women. *Arch Intern Med* 1991;151: 1980–4
13. Stampfer MJ, Colditz GA, Willett WC, *et al.* Postmenopausal estrogen therapy and cardiovascular disease. Ten year follow up from the Nurses' Health Study [see Comments]. *N Engl J Med* 1991;325: 756–62
14. Barrett-Connor E, Bush TL. Estrogen and coronary heart disease in women [see Comments]. *J Am Med Assoc* 1991;265:1861–7
15. Lindsay R. Hormone replacement therapy for prevention and treatment of osteoporosis. *Am J Med* 1993;95:37s–9s
16. Field CS, Ory SJ, Wahner HW, *et al.* Preventive effects of transdermal 17 beta estradiol on osteoporotic changes after surgical menopause: a two year placebo controlled trial. *Am J Obstet Gynecol* 1993;168:114–21
17. Green S, Walter P, Kumar V, *et al.* Human oestrogen receptor cDNA: sequence, expression and homology to *v-erb*-A. *Nature (London)* 1986;320: 134–9

18. Greene GL, Gilna P, Waterfield M, *et al.* Sequence and expression of human estrogen receptor complementary DNA. *Science* 1986;231:1150–4
19. Kumar V, Green S, Stack G, *et al.* Functional domains of the human estrogen receptor. *Cell* 1987; 51:941–51
20. White R, Lees JA, Needham M, *et al.* Structural organization and expression of the mouse estrogen receptor. *Mol Endocrinol* 1987;1:735–44
21. Kuiper GGJM, Enmark E, Pelto-Huikko M, *et al.* Cloning of a novel estrogen receptor expressed in rat prostate and ovary. *Proc Natl Acad Sci USA* 1996;93:5925–30
22. Mosselman S, Polman J, Dijkema R. ERβ: identification and characterization of a novel human estrogen receptor. *FEBS Lett* 1996;392:49–53
23. Tremblay GB, Tremblay A, Copeland NG, *et al.* Cloning, chromosomal localization and functional analysis of the murine estrogen receptor β. *Mol Endocrinol* 1997;11:353–65
24. Krust A, Green S, Argos P, *et al.* The chicken oestrogen receptor sequence: homology with *v-erb*A and the human oestrogen and glucocorticoid receptors. *EMBO J* 1986;5:891–7
25. Berry M, Metzger D, Chambon P. Role of the two activating domains of the oestrogen receptor in cell-type and promoter-context dependent agonistic activity of the anti-oestrogen 4-hydroxytamoxifen. *EMBO J* 1990;9:2811–18
26. Metzger D, Ali S, Bornert JM, *et al.* Characterization of the amino-terminal transcriptional activation function of the human estrogen receptor in animal and yeast cells. *J Biol Chem* 1995;270: 9535–42
27. Cavaillès V, Dauvois S, L'Horset F, *et al.* Nuclear factor RIP140 modulates transcriptional activation by the estrogen receptor. *EMBO J* 1995;14: 3741–51
28. Halachmi S, Marden E, Martin G, *et al.* Estrogen receptor-associated proteins: possible mediators of hormone-induced transcription. *Science* 1994;264: 1455–8
29. Horwitz KB, Jackson TA, Rain DL, *et al.* Nuclear receptor coactivators and corepressors. *Mol Endocrinol* 1996;10:1167–77
30. Onate SA, Tsai SY, Tsai M-J, *et al.* Sequence and characterization of a coactivator for the steroid hormone receptor superfamily. *Science* 1995;270: 1354–7
31. Laflamme N, Nappi RE, Drolet G, *et al.* Expression and neuropeptidergic characterization of estrogen receptors (ERα and ERβ) throughout the rat brain: anatomical evidence of distinct roles of each subtype. *J Neurobiol* 1998;36:357–78
32. Kuiper GG, Carlsson B, Grandien K, *et al.* Comparison of the ligand binding specificity and transcript tissue distribution of estrogen receptors α and β. *Endocrinology* 1997;138:863–70
33. Beato M, Truss M, Chavez S. Control of transcription by steroid hormones. *Ann NY Acad Sci* 1996; 784:93–123
34. Dickson RB, Lippman ME. Estrogenic regulation of growth and polypeptide growth factor secretion in human breast carcinoma. *Endocr Rev* 1987;8: 29–43
35. Ignar-Trowbridge DM, Nelson KG, Bidwell MC, *et al.* Coupling of dual signaling pathways: epidermal growth factor action involves the estrogen receptor. *Proc Natl Acad Sci USA* 1992;89:4658–62
36. Nelson KG, Takahashi T, Bossert NL, *et al.* Epidermal growth factor replaces estrogen in the stimulation of female genital-tract growth and differentiation. *Proc Natl Acad Sci USA* 1991;88:21–5
37. Power RF, Mani SK, Codina J, *et al.* Dopaminergic and ligand-independent activation of steroid hormone receptors. *Science* 1991;254:1636–9
38. McInerney EM, Katzenellenbogen BS. Different regions in activation function-1 of the human estrogen receptor required for antiestrogen- and estradiol-dependent transcription activation. *J Biol Chem* 1996;271:24172–8
39. Paech K, Webb P, Kuiper GGJM, *et al.* Differential ligand activation of estrogen receptors ERα and ERβ at AP1 sites. *Science* 1997;277:1508–10
40. Webb P, Lopez GN, Uht RM, *et al.* Tamoxifen activation of the estrogen receptor/AP-1 pathway: potential origin for the cell-specific estrogen-like effects of antiestrogens. *Mol Endocrinol* 1995;9: 443–56
41. O'Malley BW Jr, Li D, Buckner A, *et al.* Limitations of adenovirus-mediated interleukin-2 gene therapy for oral cancer. *Laryngoscope* 1999;109:389–95
42. Xu L, Glass CK, Rosenfeld MG. Coactivator and corepressor complexes in nuclear receptor function. *Curr Opin Genet Dev* 1999;9:140–7
43. Freedman LP. Increasing the complexity of coactivation in nuclear receptor signaling. *Cell* 1999; 97:5–8
44. Smith CL, Nawaz Z, O'Malley BW. Coactivator and corepressor regulation of the agonist/antagonist activity of the mixed antiestrogen, 4-hydroxytamoxifen. *Mol Endocrinol* 1997;11: 657–66
45. Anzick SL, Kononen J, Walker RL, *et al.* AIB1, a steroid receptor coactivator amplified in breast and ovarian cancer. *Science* 1997;277:965–8
46. Xu J, Qiu Y, DeMayo FJ, *et al.* Partial hormone resistance in mice with disruption of the steroid receptor coactivator-1 (SRC-1) gene. *Science* 1998; 279:1922–5
47. Kamei Y, Xu L, Heinzel T, *et al.* A CBP integrator complex mediates transcriptional activation and AP-1 inhibition by nuclear receptors. *Cell* 1996;85: 403–11
48. Yao TP, Ku G, Zhou N, *et al.* The nuclear hormone receptor coactivator SRC-1 is a specific target of p300. *Proc Natl Acad Sci USA* 1996;93:10626–31

49. Smith CL, Onate SA, Tsai MJ, *et al.* CREB binding protein acts synergistically with steroid receptor coactivator-1 to enhance steroid receptor-dependent transcription. *Proc Natl Acad Sci USA* 1996;93:8884–8
50. Kwok RP, Lundblad JR, Chrivia JC, *et al.* Nuclear protein CBP is a coactivator for the transcription factor CREB [see Comments]. *Nature (London)* 1994;370:223–6
51. Rachez C, Suldan Z, Ward J, *et al.* A novel protein complex that interacts with the vitamin D3 receptor in a ligand-dependent manner and enhances VDR transactivation in a cell-free system. *Genes Dev* 1998;12:1787–800
52. Lanz RB, McKenna NJ, Onate SA, *et al.* A steroid receptor coactivator, SRA, functions as an RNA and is present in an SRC-1 complex. *Cell* 1999;97: 17–27
53. Chen JD, Evans RM. A transcriptional co-repressor that interacts with nuclear hormone receptors [see Comments]. *Nature (London)* 1995;377:454–7
54. Horlein AJ, Naar AM, Heinzel T, *et al.* Ligand-independent repression by the thyroid hormone receptor mediated by a nuclear receptor co-repressor [see Comments]. *Nature (London)* 1995; 377:397–404
55. Jackson TA, Richer JK, Bain DL, *et al.* The partial agonist activity of antagonist-occupied steroid receptors is controlled by a novel hinge domain-binding coactivator L7/SPA and the co-repressors N-CoR or SMRT. *Mol Endocrinol* 1997; 11:693–705
56. Wagner BL, Norris JD, Knotts TA, *et al.* The nuclear corepressors NCoR and SMRT are key regulators of both ligand- and 8-bromo-cyclic AMP-dependent transcriptional activity of the human progesterone receptor. *Mol Cell Biol* 1998;18:1369–78
57. Lefstin JA, Yamamoto KR. Allosteric effects of DNA on transcriptional regulators. *Nature (London)* 1998;392:885–8
58. Brzozowski AM, Pike AC, Dauter Z, *et al.* Molecular basis of agonism and antagonism in the oestrogen receptor. *Nature (London)* 1997;389: 753–8
59. Luo S, Sourla A, Gauthier S, *et al.* Effect of 24-week treatment with the antiestrogen EM-800 on estrogen-sensitive parameters in intact and ovariectomized mice. *Endocrinology* 1998;139:2645–56
60. Couillard S, Labrie C, Bélanger A, *et al.* Effect of dehydroepiandrosterone and the antiestrogen EM-800 on the growth of human ZR-75-1 breast cancer xenografts. *J Natl Cancer Inst* 1998;90:772–8
61. Sourla A, Luo S, Labrie C, *et al.* Morphological changes induced by six-month treatment of intact and ovariectomized mice with tamoxifen and the pure antiestrogen EM-800. *Endocrinology* 1997;138: 5605–17
62. Simard J, Sanchez R, Poirier D, *et al.* Blockade of the stimulatory effect of estrogens, OH-tamoxifen, OH-toremifene, droloxifene and raloxifene on alkaline phosphatase activity by the antiestrogen EM-800 in human endometrial adenocarcinoma Ishikawa cells. *Cancer Res* 1997;57:3494–7
63. Gauthier S, Caron B, Cloutier J, *et al.* (*S*)-(+)-4-[7-(2,2-dimethyl-1-oxopropoxy)-4-methyl-2-[4-[2-(1-piperidinyl)ethoxy]phenyl]-2*H*-1-benzopyran-3-yl]-phenyl-2,2-dimethylpropanoate (EM-800): a highly potent, specific, and orally active non steroidal antiestrogen. *J Med Chem* 1997;40:2117–22

Bone loss and bone gain: how to handle them 4

R. Ziegler

INTRODUCTION

Optimal growth and maintenance of the human skeleton depend on three principal factors. The construction elements and substrates stem from nutrition; physical exercise is a determinant of stability and strength; and the sex hormones add to the skeleton an additional layer of bone mass that is needed for reproduction and which is maintained as long as reproduction is possible (Figure 1). Like our other organs, the skeleton is subject to aging; the life program of the skeleton is not endless. Genetic influences may regulate the speed of aging, they may be responsible for a better or poorer quality of bone mass itself, and they may strengthen or weaken the three previously mentioned supports: nutrition, physical activity and sex hormones[1].

Diseases may weaken the supports. Syndromes of malnutrition, maldigestion or malabsorption can be followed by lower bone mass and quality; diseases that are followed by immobility lead to bone loss; and conditions of sex hormone deficiency are accompanied by the lack of bone gain at the time of puberty or by an accelerated bone loss due to acquired hypogonadism later.

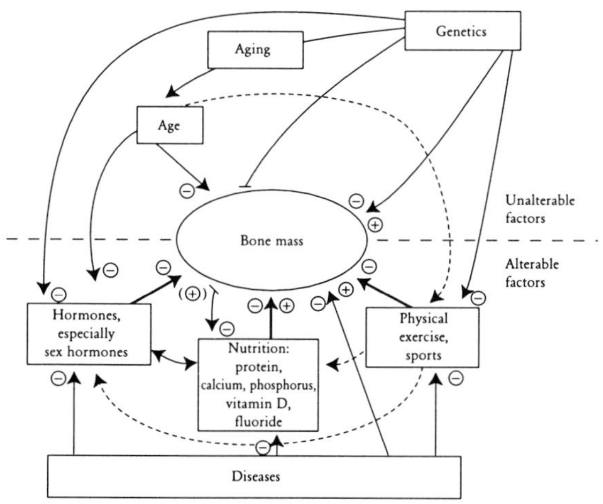

Figure 1 The main supports of optimal development and maintenance of bone mass: nutrition, physical stress and sex hormones. Genetic influences may produce variants of the supports. Diseases may impair the three supports, or they may attack the bone directly

All these factors interfere with the continuous turnover of bone tissue. The basic multicellular units (BMUs)[2] move through the bone tissue, resorbing older parts and leaving newly formed tissue behind. On their way, they may diminish or augment bone mass, depending on the general and local conditions. Their program is determined by the previously mentioned three factors. Some of their potentials need to be kept in mind by physicians. BMUs of trabecular bone replace and renew it in about 4 years; the turnover of compact bone requires double this time for renewal. This explains why all noxae leading to bone loss impair trabecular bone twice as fast as compact bone – and why therapeutic efforts may show positive effects faster at the trabecular sites than in compact bone.

The tools for measuring bone mass and bone turnover are densitometric techniques that include ultrasound; laboratory parameters indicative of bone formation such as bone-specific alkaline phosphatase, osteocalcin, collagen-1-propeptides; or resorption markers such as collagen cross-links or telopeptides, released when bone tissue is resorbed. Of course, parameters describing the function of the supports (Figure 1) may be useful.

The following paragraphs describe the relationship between the supports, typical risks and special points of attention during a woman's lifetime as a program for the medical practitioners who are responsible for the individual's health.

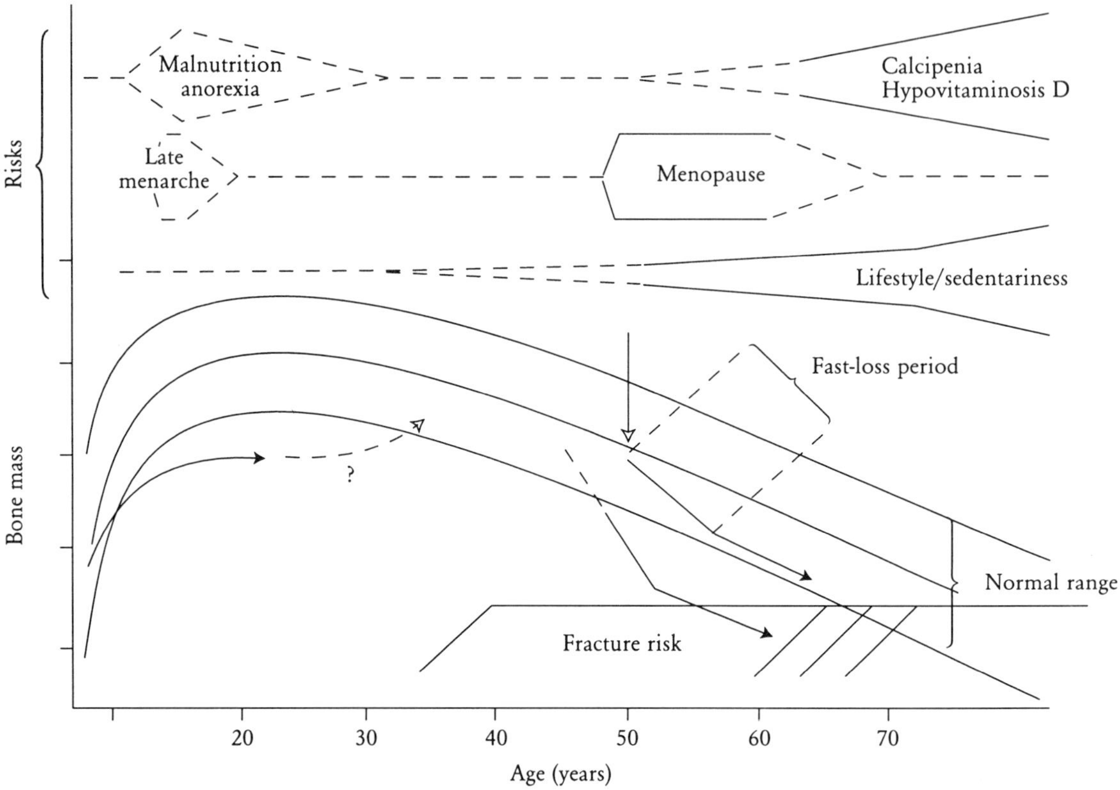

Figure 2 The course of bone mass during a woman's life. The risks are different during the life periods

CHILDHOOD

The skeletons of prepubertal boys and girls grow in a similar way. Sexual dimorphism is not yet visible; determinants are optimal nutrition and the avoidance of immobility (and of bone-related diseases). The main risk stems from malnutrition. Optimalization of calcium in-take leads to an increase in bone mineral density (BMD), as has been shown in twin studies in the USA[3] and Australia[4]. It is remarkable that prepubertal children showed up to 5% increase in BMD when the calcium intake was increased from 900 mg/day to 1600 mg/day. It remained open how long the bone gain was maintained, because the difference faded as puberty started.

ADOLESCENCE AND PUBERTY

As already mentioned, the exposure of the skeleton to sex hormones is accompanied by an increase in BMD aiming at an additional calcium store for reproduction. It is still an open question whether early menarche yields higher peak bone mass[5] or not[6]. Perhaps spontaneous variation of the time of menarche in the context of otherwise normal conditions for the development of bone masks the influence of the age of menarche. In parallel, the finding of lower peak bone mass in men with late puberty[7] has not always been confirmed[8].

However, there is no doubt that the manipulation of menarche due to lifestyle seems to be relevant. Ballet-dancing girls who had a late menarche presumably due to excess physical activity in combination with maintaining a slim body shape had stress fractures much more often than other girls passing through menarche in earlier years[9]. Therefore, there seems to be a difference between spontaneous late menarche and late menarche due to an unfavorable lifestyle.

The correlation between lean body mass as an index of muscle strength and whole-body bone mineral content is parallel in boys and girls up to the age of about 10 years. Thereafter, the curves show dimorphism. The same increase in lean body mass generates a larger increase in bone mineral content in girls up to the age of 18[10]. In boys, the slope bends at about 15 years of age, showing larger increase in bone mineral content later. The observation that after puberty more bone is formed in relation to the increase in muscle mass can be interpreted as sensitization of the mechanostat. Sex hormones ensure that more bone is built up per unit of physical stress.

ADULTHOOD

Peak bone mass is achieved in the decade between 20 and 30 years. BMD at 30 years is taken as the 100% level when calculating the *T* score of (BMD)[11]. There are typical risk factors that may influence peak bone mass in women, especially those of lifestyle. In principle, sport is favorable for the development of the skeleton. Active individuals have higher BMD than the inactive population. However, if sport is performed in excess, this stress may lead to a decrease in estrogen production. Women with amenorrhea due to excessive exercise present lower BMD values than female athletes who are less active but maintain their menstruation[12]. There seems to be a hierarchy among the bone-protecting factors: the decline in estrogens cannot be compensated for by more activity.

Anorexia mentalis is another condition that may diminish BMD. Several studies have shown that this psychological abnormality leading to diminished caloric intake, impaired ovarian function and sometimes physical inactivity is accompanied by a relevant deficit in BMD[13]. The fate of the skeleton is connected with the prognosis of anorexia: poor outcome implies distinctly lowered BMD values.

Smoking is another risk factor. It has been shown that women who smoke one pack of cigarettes per day throughout adulthood will have a deficit of 5–10% in BMD at the time of the menopause, combined with an increased fracture risk[14]. Presumably tobacco and its products accelerate estrogen metabolism, leading to the enhanced formation of inactive catechol estrogens[15]. Smoking women seem to reach the menopause earlier than non-smoking women.

There are many other risks due to diseases such as hyperthyroidism, hyperparathyroidism and intestinal and skeletal diseases, which also require observation of the bone status, in order to avoid early bone loss before aging begins to be relevant.

MENOPAUSE

Early menopause is a well-known risk factor for later osteopenia or osteoporosis. If manifest osteoporosis with fractures occurs, a longer 'estrogen exposition time' is advantageous, so that the first fracture happens later in life. (There is a positive correlation between the estrogen exposition time and the time when fractures occur.) The main event in bone metabolism after the drop in plasma estradiol is fast turnover. The loss of estrogens leads to accelerated bone resorption due to an increased activity of osteolytic cytokines such as interleukin (IL)-1 and IL-6. In the second half of life, fast turnover means bone loss, in contrast to the same situation at puberty, when fast turnover is accompanied by bone gain. The time of postmenopausal high turnover lasts for about one decade, then bone metabolism slows down (provided there is no secondary hyperparathyroidism; see below). It has been shown that estrogen replacement therapy has a higher efficiency at a time of high bone loss compared with slow bone loss[16].

All risk factors for bone loss are of greater importance if they are present after the menopause. For example, hyperthyroidism, which may be tolerated by the skeleton of premenopausal women as well as of men, may be detrimental after the menopause[17].

SENESCENCE

Senescence is often characterized by declining mobility and decreasing supply of calcium and vitamin D. A negative selection seems to take place in society. Compared to people who were 80 years of age around 1950, such people in the same population showed many more hip fractures 30 years later (as was shown in Sweden[18] and elsewhere). It is clear that such curves do not follow a lowering in BMD. Correspondingly, at older age, BMD is no longer the determinant of fracture risk[19]. Aged people eat less and thereby less calcium. They get less sunshine and many of them present with lowered levels of 25-OH-vitamin D in the blood. Based on these observations, preventive studies supplementing moderate doses of calcium and vitamin D have proved very efficient[20].

Whether the senescent skeleton profits from sex hormones when they are re-initiated remains to be determined.

CONCLUSIONS AND RECOMMENDATIONS

It is evident that there are no general rules for the prevention and treatment of bone loss and osteoporosis, except to give the following message to people throughout their lifetime. Choose your food according to the need of your bones, be physically active at a reasonable level even when growing older, discuss with your doctor the status of your sex hormones as well as any episodic or chronic disease that could be relevant for the maintenance of bone mass and quality.

There are special periods in life when a theoretical risk should be addressed by the doctor. Healthy nutrition should be stressed before and during puberty. When observing BMD at the time of the menopause: is the starting level of BMD higher or lower when the fast-loss period starts? Is bone loss fast or slow at the time of examination? The recommendation of hormone replacement therapy can also be based on the status of the skeleton. Taking an exact history and physical examination aiming at the skeletal condition is mandatory. Recommendations should be risk-factor related: the inactive person should get an exercise program; the undernourished person needs calcium and perhaps vitamin D supplements. Special programs, e.g. glucocorticoid treatment, are available for unfavorable conditions.

The same data analysis is needed for patients with existing osteoporosis. For the choice of the most promising medication, the doctor needs to know: is bone turnover high or low? Are recommendations regarding activity or prescriptions of calcium and vitamin D promising or not? The best diagnosis of bone turnover is made by bone histology, especially if the history does not yield the necessary information. Bone turnover markers may be indicative. However, present fractures may throw up questions: in the case of a fresh vertebral fracture, is a moderately elevated level of bone turnover markers due to the developing callus, with the remainder of the skeleton in a low-turnover status, or do the markers reflect the general skeletal condition? The efficiency of antiresorptive drugs depends on the activity of bone turnover[21]. The definition of the patient's bone status is decisive for the choice of treatment (Table 1).

Fascinating findings have emerged with respect to genetics. For many determinants of bone mass,

Table 1 Life period-related risk factors for the development of bone loss or osteoporosis and measures for specific prevention

	Predominant risk			
Period	*Calcipenia (hypovitaminosis D)*	*Sedentary occupation*	*Hypogonadism*	*Recommendation*
Childhood	+	(+)	–	optimize calcium supply
Adolescence/puberty	+	(+)	+	optimize calcium supply avoid delay of puberty
Adulthood (peak bone mass)	+	+	+	optimize calcium, exercise, sex hormone exposure
After the menopause	++	+	+++	consider HRT optimize calcium, physical exercise
Senescence	+++	++	(+)	optimize calcium *and* vitamin D, physical exercise (HRT? anabolics?)

HRT, hormone replacement therapy

Table 2 Osteoporosis: potential influence of genetics

Compartment	*Genetic variation*
Ground substance, collagens	collagen type I gene alleles (COL 1A1/A1) TGFβ polymorphism (mutations/deletions in osteogenesis imperfecta)
Constitution	athletic vs. asthenic habitus
Nutrition	
calcium	lactase deficiency (nutrition habits?)
vitamin D	vitamin D receptor gene alleles (B/b)
(vitamin K?)	APO E*4 polymorphism
Sex hormones	late puberty (females and males) early menopause (females) relative estrogen deficiency in males? relative androgen deficiency in females? estrogen receptor gene alleles (VNTR polymorphisms)
after menopause	interleukin-6 gene alleles
Physical forces	program of mobility? sedentary occupation? threshold of the mechanostat?

TGFβ, transforming growth factor-β; APO, apolipoproteins; VNTR, variable number of tandem repeats

quality and metabolism, variants of favorable and unfavorable conditions have been found (Table 2). Collagen genes seem to have alleles for better or poorer quality. The bone promoting factor transforming growth factor-β shows polymorphism, leading to different potency. The constitutional types of the athletic or the asthenic human being could be relevant for the later risk of osteoporosis.

Calcium metabolism may be genetically influenced by handicaps such as lactase deficiency. The exploding field of the vitamin D receptor gene alleles does not provide a clear picture at the moment[22].

The field of sex hormones shows broad variance related to heredity, including early or late puberty and early menopause. It remains to be determined whether a relative estrogen deficiency is relevant for the male skeleton, and whether a relative androgen deficiency is a risk factor in females. The effectiveness of estrogens themselves may depend on the 'quality' of estrogen receptor gene alleles[23]. When the level of IL-6 rises after the menopause, alleles for its gene may determine more aggressive or milder resorption.

Recently, the alleles for apolipoprotein E4 were related to the hip fracture risk in older women: women with an APO E*4 allele had a higher rate of hip fractures in the presence of more than three additional risk factors than women in whom this allele was absent[24].

Finally, the effectiveness of physical forces could be genetically influenced. From animal experiments it is known that sedentary mice present with lighter bones than more active mice[25]. The question is justified whether the mechanostat presents with genetic variances.

The analysis of genetic risk factors[26] will be an additional reason for switching from generalized and therefore not very efficient recommendations to an individualized program. Asthenic people might require a program for gymnastics and sports, starting in childhood; people with impaired calcium absorption may need larger recommended daily allowances for calcium and vitamin D; women with the 'aggressive' IL-6 gene allele may be best treated with a potent bisphosphonate. The medical society responsible for the prevention and treatment of osteoporosis should wisely enforce the individual approach instead of following the false dream of simple and uniform handling of osteoporosis.

References

1. Ziegler R, Scheidt-Nave C, Scharla S. Pathophysiology of osteoporosis: unresolved problems and new insights. *J Nutr* 1995;125:2033S-7S
2. Frost HM. Bone 'mass' and the 'mechanostat': a proposal. *Anat Rec* 1987;219:1-9
3. Johnston CC, Miller JZ, Slemenda CW, *et al.* Calcium supplementation and increases in bone mineral density in children. *N Engl J Med* 1992;327;82-7
4. Nowson CA, Green RM, Larkins RG, *et al.* The effect of calcium supplementation on bone mass in adolescent female twins. In Burckhardt P, Heaney RP, eds. *Nutritional Aspects of Osteoporosis '94. Challenges of Modern Medicine.* Rome: Ares-Serono Symposia Publications, 1995;7:169-75
5. Johnell O, Nilsson BE. Life-style and bone mineral mass in perimenopausal women. *Calcif Tissue Int* 1984;36:354-6
6. Melton LJ III, Bryant SC, Wahner HW, *et al.* Parity, lactation and hip fracture. *Osteoporosis Int* 1993;3: 76-83
7. Finkelstein JS, Neer RM, Biller BMK, *et al.* Osteopenia in men with a history of delayed puberty. *N Engl J Med* 1992;326:600-4
8. Bertelloni S, Baroncelli GI, Ferdeghini M, *et al.* Normal volumetric bone mineral density and bone turnover in young men with histories of constitutional delay of puberty. *J Clin Endocrinol Metab* 1998;83:4280-3
9. Warren MP, Brooks-Gunn J, Hamilton LH, *et al.* Scoliosis and fractures in young ballet dancers. Relation to delayed menarche and secondary amenorrhea. *N Engl J Med* 1986;314:1348-53
10. Schiessl H, Frost HM, Jee WSS. Perspectives: estrogen and bone-muscle strength and 'mass' relationships. *Bone* 1998;22:1-6
11. World Health Organization. Assessment of fracture risk and its application to screening for postmenopausal osteoporosis. Report of a WHO Study Group. Geneva: WHO, 1994
12. Lloyd T, Myers C, Buchanan JR, Demers LM. Collegiate women athletes with irregular menses during adolescence have decreased bone density. *Obstet Gynecol* 1988;72:639-42
13. Herzog W, Minne H, Deter C, *et al.* Outcome of bone mineral density in anorexia nervosa patients 11.7 years after first admission. *J Bone Miner Res* 1993;8:597-605
14. Hopper JL, Seeman E. The bone density of female twins discordant for tobacco use. *N Engl J Med* 1994;330:387-92
15. Baron JA, LaVeccia C, Levi F. The antiestrogenic effect of cigarette smoking in women. *Am J Obstet Gynecol* 1990;162:502-14
16. Quigley MET, Martin PL, Burnier AM, Brooks P. Estrogen therapy arrests bone loss in elderly women. *Am J Obstet Gynecol* 1987;156:1516-23
17. Ziegler R, Wüster C. Thyroid hormones and bone in perimenopausal women. In Orgiazzi J, Leclère J, eds. *The Thyroid and Tissues.* Schattauer, Stuttgart, New York: Merck European Thyroid Symposium, 1994:107-13
18. Obrant KJ, Bengner U, Johnell O, *et al.* Increasing age-adjusted risk of fragility fractures: a sign of increasing osteoporosis in successive generations? *Calcif Tissues Int* 1989;44:157-67
19. Cummings SR, Kelsey JL, Nevitt MC, O'Dowd KJ. Epidemiology of osteoporosis and osteoporotic fractures. *Epidemiol Rev* 1985;7:178-208
20. Dawson-Hughes B, Harris SS, Krall EA, Dallall GE. Effect of calcium and vitamin D supplementation on bone density in men and women 65 years of age and older. *N Engl J Med* 1997;337:670-6
21. Dambacher MA, Neff M, Kissling R, Qin L. Highly precise peripheral quantitative computed tomography for the evaluation of bone density, loss of bone density and structures. Consequences for prophylaxis and treatment. *Drugs Aging* 1998; Suppl 1:15-24
22. Gong G, Stern HS, Cheng S-C, *et al.* The association of bone mineral density with vitamin D receptor gene polymorphisms. *Osteoporosis Int* 1999;9:55-64
23. Rosenkranz K, Hinney A, Ziegler A, *et al.* Systematic mutation screening of the estrogen receptor beta gene in probands of different weight extremes: identification of several genetic variants. *J Clin Endocrinol Metab* 1998;83:4524-7
24. Cauley JA, Zmuda JM, Yaffee K, *et al.* Apolipoprotein E polymorphism: a new genetic marker of hip fracture risk - the study of osteoporotic fractures. *J Bone Miner Res* 1999;14:1175-81
25. Kaye M. Strain, bone mass and physical activity in mice. *J Bone Min Res* 1994; Suppl 1:386
26. Ralston SH. The genetics of osteoporosis. *Q J Med* 1997;90:247-51

Culture and the menopause 5

M. Lock

It is probably fair to say that the majority of researchers and clinicians who have an interest in the menopause tend to assume that the biological changes associated with the end of menstruation are essentially universal, and that differences in the subjective reporting of symptoms by individual women can be fully accounted for by variation among psychological, social and cultural factors that, in effect, obfuscate the facts of biology.

Although, of course, reproductive senescence among human females is universal, considerable evidence now exists indicating that the menopausal transition and its postulated long-term sequelae exhibit much more variation than has been previously recognized. These findings suggest that it is appropriate to think of biology and culture as in a continuous feedback relationship of ongoing interaction, in which *both* exhibit variation. The environment in which individuals subsist, lifestyles, language and culture are crucial in accounting for this variation, but the effects of evolutionary and historical changes on human populations must also be taken into account.

Cross-cultural research in connection with menopausal symptomatology has shown consistently that the incidence of symptoms taken as characteristic of the menopause in North America and Europe, in particular hot flushes and night sweats, is not distributed equally among populations of peri- and postmenopausal women. Beyene, in her work among rural Mayans living in the Yucatan, Mexico, where women have numerous pregnancies and extended cycles of amenorrhea associated with prolonged lactation and malnutrition, found no reporting of hot flushes or cold sweats[1].

Research carried out in India[2], Indonesia[3,4], among Africans living in Israel[5], in Taiwan[4,6], Hong Kong[4,7], Japan[8], Singapore[4,9], China[10], Korea[4], the Philippines[4], Thailand[11] and Malaysia[4,12] all revealed low reporting of hot flushes and night sweats, although there was considerable variation in incidence among these studies. The response of some researchers has been to suggest that women's reporting biases the research findings. It is argued that, because individual responses to the menopause are culturally dependent, inattention to hot flushes is essentially learned behavior. The headaches, shoulder stiffness, dizziness and other non-specific symptoms commonly associated with the menopausal transition in Japan, and the 'atypical' symptoms of anxiety, irritability and headaches that Boulet and colleagues uncovered in their research in seven south-east Asian countries are, they argue, 'a form of communication' on the part of women[4]. These researchers speculate that vasomotor distress may be 'translated' by women into symptoms of psychological distress.

I am exceedingly uncomfortable with this kind of interpretation, as would be other anthropologists. The assumption made is that measurable facts reside in the body and that when subjective reporting does not coincide with these facts then subjectivity distorts the truth. I do not seek to privilege subjectivity - there are times when scientific tests detect pathology about which individuals are unaware, high blood pressure being the classic example. But I will argue that *both* forms of knowledge, objective and subjective, must count as valid and as truthful (aside from error in measurement, and lies). If a woman reports that she has not had a hot flush then, if the research has been reasonably well done, she has not had a hot flush. She is not a victim of her culture, nor does she convert hot flushes into something else.

The Mayans have been found to have endocrine changes at menopause similar to those reported for women in the USA, but we know that plasma, urinary and vaginal levels of estrogens are not correlated directly with hot flushes[13]. Changes in sweat rates, peripheral vasodilatation and deregulation of core body temperature provide valuable information in the laboratory about physiological changes associated with hot flushes, but if these changes do not coincide with the subjective reporting of a hot flush, as they often do not, what exactly *do* they reveal? A hot flush that is not a hot flush? A stupid woman? The power of culture? Or some leaps in inference?

Symptoms such as anxiety, headaches and, in Japan, shoulder stiffness, are very commonly reported at the menopause, but they are by no means limited to women alone, or to women of middle age. I would predict that Japanese men suffer as much from shoulder stiffness as do women. If a woman is asked to report on symptoms over the previous few weeks, she is likely to note common symptoms that may have nothing to do specifically with the end of menstruation. Until it is shown that significant elevations in reporting of these so-called 'atypical' symptoms of the menopause are confined to the perimenopause, it cannot be inferred that they are associated with the end of menstruation, or for that matter with the climacteric. Hypothesizing that symptoms such as headaches are a form of non-verbal communication is reasonable, although most headaches would not fall into this category. But to imagine that non-specific and atypical symptoms are actually hot flushes in disguise is not. It is a grave mistake in my estimation to try to explain away the low reporting of hot flushes. On the other hand, it is reasonable to speculate that, with urban migration and increased education, women might experience hot flushes more frequently, perhaps because of dietary changes, because of a more sedentary life style, or even because of changed expectations about this mid-life transition.

The physiological mechanism of the hot flush, although much better understood than formerly, has been by no means fully explained. Systematic compilation of subjective reporting, gathered in the language of the women being studied and analyzed simultaneously with objective measurement of biological changes during the perimenopause, is urgently needed, but one dataset should not be subsumed into or treated as secondary to another. Multidisciplinary teams will undoubtedly produce the best results.

JAPAN, CANADA AND THE USA: A COMPARATIVE STUDY

Analysis of datasets comprising 7802 Massachusetts women (Sonja McKinlay), 1307 Manitoban women (Patricia Kaufert) and 1225 Japanese women, all aged between 45 and 55 inclusively, reveal some remarkable differences in symptom reporting at the menopause (Table 1). The Japanese data were collected from three parts of Japan - southern Nagano, a rural area, where most women either manage or work on farms; the southern part of the city of Kyoto, from women employed in factories and in other blue-collar jobs; and in a suburb of Kobe, where women are for the most part housewives, although many of them hold down part-time jobs. There was a 76% response rate to the questionnaire used in Japan designed to be directly comparable with the Massachusetts and Manitoba studies. In all three sites, samples were selected from a general and not a clinical population of women. Those women who had undergone gynecological surgery were treated as a separate category in the analyses. I was responsible for the Japanese part of the study, the survey data of which was supplemented by numerous open-ended interviews with women who had filled out questionnaires, physicians and Japanese feminists, as well as by wide reading in the Japanese professional and popular literature on the subject[8].

Given that language and culture significantly shape the experience and subjective reporting of symptoms of all kinds, translation of concepts and terms across cultures is a demanding task, and presents a limitation on data collection that can never be entirely overcome. For example, the

Table 1 Percentage distribution of menopause status in each study

Menopause status	*Japan*	*Canada*	*USA*
Surgical menopause	9.9	20.5	28.6
Total (100%)*	1225	1307	7802
Natural menopause	35.7	35.5	43.9
Perimenopause	31.5	26.2	38.2
Premenopause	32.8	38.3	17.9
Total (100%)†	1104	1039	5568

*Totals exclude subjects with missing data; †totals exclude subjects with surgical menopause

Japanese word *kônenki*, usually translated into English as menopause, does not convey the same meaning as does menopause. At the time I did the research, Japanese women did not consider the end of menstruation to be a significant marker of female middle age - in part, I came to realize after completing the research, because very few women associated that event with distressing symptoms.

Kônenki is similar to the concept of the climacteric; that is, it is understood as a long, gradual process to which the end of menstruation is just one contributing factor. The term was deliberately created at the beginning of the century when Japanese physicians were in close contact with German colleagues. Most Japanese respondents in the present study placed its timing at age 45 or even earlier, lasting until nearly 60. One-quarter of the questionnaire respondents who were postmenopausal and had ceased menstruation for over 1 year reported that they had no sign of *kônenki*. It was important, therefore, before creating the questionnaire, to establish just what is in people's minds when the term *kônenki* is used, otherwise considerable miscommunication would have been a likely outcome.

A second difficulty arose because there is no word in Japanese that refers uniquely to the hot flush, even though Japanese is a language in which very fine discriminations can be made in connection with bodily states. One can simply say, 'to suddenly become hot'. Some women and physicians use the word *nobose* when speaking of hot flushes, but this term is also used to convey sensations of vertigo or dizziness, or when talking about someone who is 'hot-headed', or who has an infatuation. A second term, *hoteri*, translates simply as feeling hot or flushed, and is usually used when an individual, lacking the enzyme aldehyde dehydrogenase, becomes red faced after drinking alcohol. This term, too, is used by some women and medical professionals when talking about hot flushes. It was decided to use both *hoteri* and *nobose* in the questionnaire, together with a third term, *kyû na nekkan*, meaning to have a sudden feverish feeling, a term that had already been made use of in a small survey. Research in China, Indonesia and the Yucatan, among other places, also found no local terms for the hot flush. It is of note that there has been a highly specific popular term for hot flushes in English, 'hot blooms', for at least the past 150 years and quite possibly for a lot longer - long before the medicalization of the menopause in Europe.

Care also had to be taken when selecting the term for depression to be used in the Japanese questionnaire, because description of this state cannot be translated easily into an equivalent Japanese term. Furthermore, I found that numerous symptoms that do not appear on a standardized North American list of menopausal symptoms such as the Blatt Menopausal Index had to be included: in particular shoulder stiffness, ringing in the ears, a heavy feeling in the head and others. These are symptoms that Japanese women and their doctors commonly associate with *kônenki*.

In order not to bias the study and elicit only stereotyped responses about this stage of the life cycle, common illness symptoms associated with neither menopause (in the case of the United States and Canada) or *kônenki* (in the case of Japan) were included on the symptom reporting list. Women were asked to recall symptoms they had experienced over the previous 2 weeks. Research shows that longer periods of recall are very inaccurate. A list of core symptoms was created that revealed significant differences in the rates of reporting across the three subject groups. The results show that the Japanese responses were consistently different from those in the USA and Canada[14]. For 13 of the 16 core symptoms, Canadian and US women reported (sometimes markedly) higher rates than did the Japanese women (Table 2). For only one symptom (combined for purposes of the analysis as diarrhea/constipation) was Japanese reporting somewhat higher, and this probably has something to do with the high consumption of white rice.

In addition, the rates of multiple symptom reporting by Japanese women were consistently low (Table 3). No association was evident between menopausal status and symptom reporting in general among Japanese respondents, although among both Canadian and American women there was an increase of symptom reporting during the peri- and early postmenopause. Japanese reporting of hot flushes in the previous 2 weeks was low, 13.5% and 15.2% for peri- and postmenopausal women, respectively; although low in incidence,

Table 2 A comparison of the rates of core symptom reporting by study

Symptom	*Japan*	*Canada*	*USA*	χ^2 *(2 df)*
Diarrhea/constipation	24.5	12.8	21.4	62.8*
Persistent cough	4.2	5.2	10.1	68.4*
Upset stomach	6.3	12.9	16.1	85.1*
Shortness of breath	3.1	8.2	15.6	177.6*
Sore throat	10.5	9.1	10.7	2.9
Backaches	24.2	26.8	29.6	17.7*
Headaches	27.5	33.8	37.2	45.2*
Aches/stiffness in joints	14.5	31.4	38.6	279.1*
Dizzy spells	7.1	12.3	11.1	21.4*
Lack of energy	6.0	39.8	38.1	503.3*
Irritability	11.5	17.1	29.9	246.6*
Feeling blue/depressed	10.3	23.4	35.9	365.1*
Trouble sleeping	11.7	30.4	30.6	189.8*
Lack of appetite	4.6	4.0	5.4	5.8
Hot flushes	12.3	31.0	34.8	246.6*
Cold or night sweats	3.8	19.8	11.4	158.2*
Hot flushes/sweats (combined)	14.7	36.1	38.0	252.5*
Total (100%)	1225	1307	7802	

*$p < 0.01$

hot flushes were associated with menopausal status. Reporting of night sweats was extremely low and not associated with menopausal status (Table 4). Only 19% of Japanese women in this study had experienced a hot flush at some time in the past, and reporting of both frequency and intensity was much lower than among American and Canadian respondents. Reporting of sleep disturbance by Japanese women, at 11.5%, was low, corroborating their reports about lack of severity of hot flushes. I have gone to great lengths to establish that these results are not simply due to under-reporting. Follow-up interviews with women suggested to me that, if anything, the women in the Japanese study over-reported symptoms, including tiny subjective changes, in their eagerness to co-operate fully with the research.

The majority of Japanese women, when asked in interviews to describe their experience of *kônenki*, responded along the following lines:

> I've had no problems at all, no headaches or anything like that . . . I've heard from other women that their heads felt so heavy that they couldn't get up.

> The most common problems I've heard about are stiff shoulders, headaches, and aching joints.

Table 3 A comparison of the number of core symptoms reported by study

Number of symptoms reported	*Japan*	*Canada*	*USA*
0	26.7	13.8	15.4
1–4	63.4	60.0	50.3
5+	9.7	26.2	34.1
Total (100%)	1225	1307	7305

> I get tired easily, that's *kônenki* for sure, and I get stiff shoulders.

A small number of women, 12 out of 105 interviewed, made statements that sound much more familiar to North Americans and Europeans:

> The most noticeable thing was that I would suddenly feel hot; it happened every day, three times or so. I didn't go to the doctor or take any medication, I wasn't embarrassed and I didn't feel strange. I just thought it was my age.

The questionnaire findings indicated that shoulder stiffness was the most common symptom reported, followed by headaches. This research carried out in the mid-1980s and Japanese gynecologists, when interviewed, noted that women

Table 4 Vasomotor symptoms, reported by menopausal status

Menopausal status	*Japan**	*Canada†*	*USA†*
Hot flushes			
Premenopause	6.4	13.8	17.9
Perimenopause	13.5	39.7	38.1
Postmenopause	15.2	41.5	43.9
Total (100%)	1104	1039	5505
	$\chi^2 = 15.77$	$\chi^2 = 84.17$	$\chi^2 = 269.510$
Night sweats			
Premenopause	4.1	10.6	5.5
Perimenopause	4.0	27.6	11.7
Postmenopause	3.0	22.2	11.3
Total (100%)	1104	1039	5484
	$\chi^2 = 0.772$	$\chi^2 = 33.71$	$\chi^2 = 31.335$

The number in the American study differs because of missing data. Cases of surgical menopause have been removed.
* $p = 0.00$ and 0.68; †$p = 0.00$

complained most often of these symptoms. Some physicians did not list hot flushes at all when asked to describe the symptoms of *kônenki*. Over the past decade, of course, changes have taken place, and the subject of the menopause has been medicalized and now appears frequently in Japanese women's magazines, where hot flushes are often described as the 'typical' symptom of the menopause. It is interesting to note that the word sometimes used to describe this symptom is 'hotto furashu' taken directly from the English. The time is now right to undertake another round of research in Japan to ascertain to what extent, if any, symptom reporting by women has changed as a result of these publications and the simultaneous medicalization of *kônenki*. Such a study would have to be done, as was the previous one, making use of a non-clinical sample.

Similar to vasomotor symptoms, Japanese reporting in connection with feeling 'blue' or depressed was low, and not associated with menopausal status, since it was highest among premenopausal women (Table 5). Canadian reporting, although higher than the Japanese, also showed little change across menopausal status. These different patterns of reporting argue strongly against any *simple* causal link between declining endogenous estrogen levels and the reporting of depression, or even hot flushes - findings that have been corroborated by Sonja McKinlay in her longitudinal Massachusetts study[15].

Table 5 The percentage of women feeling blue/depressed, reported by menopausal status

Menopausal status	*Japan*	*Canada*	*USA*
Premenopause	12.7	24.1	29.1
Perimenopause	9.5	23.2	38.1
Postmenopause	8.9	23.0	33.8

It is well known that Japanese women currently enjoy the longest life expectancy in the world - a mean of nearly 82 years. The incidence of breast cancer, and of heart disease in men and women, is about one-third of that in North America. The ongoing work of Ross and co-workers[16] shows that the incidence of osteoporosis for both Chinese and Japanese women is less than half that of Caucasian women in North America, even though Asian women usually have a lower bone density. The present research also showed that only 28% of Japanese respondents suffer from a chronic health problem (diabetes, allergies, asthma, arthritis, high blood pressure), as opposed to 45% of Manitoban women and 53% of Massachusetts women. Taken together these figures suggest that middle-aged Japanese women enjoy good health in comparison to those in North America.

Women who were around 50 years of age when this study was done were born at the beginning of the war, and many experienced nutritional deprivation as very small children. However, virtually none of them have smoked, alcohol and coffee consumption is low, and the diet is low in fat and rich in soy beans and vegetables. Soy beans, as is now well known, are a source of phytoestrogens and may well contribute to the lower symptom reporting of hot flushes on the part of Japanese women[17]. So, too, may the herbal teas that many women drink, some of them also rich in phytoestrogens. This cohort of women have, as part of their daily lives, always done considerable exercise and weight bearing. Obviously this picture will change as succeeding generations of Japanese women become middle aged in their turn.

The longitudinal studies of McKinlay and Kaufert[15,18] indicate that, for the majority of North American women, the menopause is not a difficult time. Together with the Japanese findings and other cross-cultural work, their research suggests that we would do well to ask what it is that *protects* the majority of women from experiencing discomfort at menopause - a question that has rarely been asked. Moreover, the longevity and overall good health of Japanese women invites further systematic investigation. I conclude that healthy longevity can probably be attributed in large part to the relatively even distribution of wealth in Japanese society, little poverty and equal access to good health care and social benefits, added to which is universal public education of a high quality, and a long tradition of both public and familial investment in preventive medicine. In addition, it seems highly likely that the Japanese diet - low in fat, high in protein and natural estrogens - plays an important role in the relatively low symptom reporting at the end of menstruation and in longevity. Genetics may, of course, also make a contribution.

Some additional findings of interest come from the recent work of Jean Shea with 400 Chinese women. Vasomotor symptom reporting was low and resembled that of the Japanese sample cited above. However, the overall symptom reporting of the Chinese women was considerably higher than that of the Massachusetts, Manitoba and Japanese samples, leading Shea to conclude that sweeping generalizations about East Asia should be avoided[10]. Clearly, if the long-term health of aging women is of prime interest, then factors such as relative deprivation, chronic occupational stress and political turmoil, such as the majority of Chinese women have experienced, must be entered into the equation.

RETHINKING POSTMENOPAUSAL RISK

It is often assumed that, because mean life expectancy until the turn of the century in North America and Northern Europe was just under 50 years of age, virtually no women lived much past the menopause until the very recent past; postmenopausal life is understood, in effect, as a cultural artifact, often attributed to improved health care. However, data from hunter gatherer societies show that 20% of all individuals survive to age 60, and about 10% survive to age 70 or longer[19]. Figures to consider, however, are not life expectancy at birth, because in all societies until very recently infant mortality accounted for most deaths, and maternal mortality was also very high. Kertzer and Laslett have shown that mean life expectancy of mature adults has changed relatively little throughout human history[20]. However, periodic fluctuations in mean life expectancy take place, which can shift rather dramatically as a result of political and environmental changes. Research indicates that the ancient Greeks lived longer than did the Romans of classical times[21], and recently a decline in life expectancy of more than 3 years in Russia over a very short time provides strong evidence that longevity is primarily dependent upon social and political conditions.

Poverty undoubtedly plays a greater role in determining health in later life than do estrogen levels, and the data presented in this paper suggest that culturally mediated lifestyles make a major contribution to aging. We would do well to investigate these variables further, keeping in mind that culture and biology are interdependent and that not every aspect of this exquisitely intricate relationship is susceptible to measurement. As the surgeon/author Richard Selzer once put it: 'The facts are not always where the truth lies.'

References

1. Beyene Y. Cultural significance and physiological manifestations of menopause: a biocultural analysis. *Cult Med Psychiatry* 1986;10:47–71
2. Flint M. *Menarche and menopause of Rajput women.* PhD dissertation, City University of New York, 1974
3. Flint M, Suprapti Samil R. Cultural and subcultural meanings of the menopause. In Flint M, Kronenberg F, Utian W, eds. *Multidisciplinary Perspectives on Menopause. Ann NY Acad Sci* 1990;592: 134–48
4. Boulet MJ, Oddens BJ, Lehert P, *et al.* Climacteric and menopause in seven south-east Asian countries. *Maturitas* 1994;19:157–76
5. Walfish S, Antonovsky A, Maoz B. Relationship between biological changes and symptoms and health behavior during the climacteric. *Maturitas* 1984;6:9–17
6. Yeh A. The experience of menopause among Taiwanese women. Honors thesis, Department of East Asian Languages and Civilizations, Harvard University, Boston, 1989
7. Haines CJ, Chung TKH, Leung DHY. A prospective study of the frequency of acute menopausal symptoms in Hong Kong Chinese women. *Maturitas* 1994;18:175–81
8. Lock M. *Encounters with Aging: Mythologies of Menopause in Japan and North America.* Berkeley: University of California Press, 1993
9. McCarthy T. The prevalence of symptoms in menopausal women in the Far East: Singapore segment. *Maturitas* 1994;19:199–204
10. Shea J. Revolutionary women at middle age: an ethnographic survey of menopause and midlife aging in Beijing, China. Cambridge, MA: Harvard University, 1998
11. Chompootweep M, Tankeyoon K, Yamarat P, *et al.* The menopausal age and climacteric complaints in Thai women in Bangkok. *Maturitas* 1993;17:63–71
12. Ismael NN. A study of the menopause in Malaysia. *Maturitas* 1994;19:205–9
13. Martin M, Block J, Sanchez S, *et al.* Menopause without symptoms: the endocrinology of menopause among rural Mayan Indians. *Am J Obstet Gynecol* 1993;168:1839–45
14. Avis NE, Kaufert PA, Lock M, *et al.* The evolution of menopausal symptoms. In Burger H, ed. *Baillière's Clinical Endocrinology and Metabolism.* London: Harcourt, Brace Jovanovich, 1993;7:17–32
15. Avis NE, McKinlay SM. A longitudinal analysis of women's attitudes towards the menopause: results from the Massachusetts Women's Health Study. *Maturitas* 1991;13:65–79
16. Ross PD, Norimatsu H, Davis JW, *et al.* A comparison of hip fracture incidence among native Japanese, Japanese Americans, and American Caucasians. *Am J Epidemiol* 1991;133:801–9
17. Adlercreutz H, Hämäläinen E, Gorbach S, *et al.* Dietary phytoestrogens and the menopause in Japan. *Lancet* 1992;339:1233
18. Kaufert P, Gilbert P, Tate R. The Manitoba Project: a re-examination of the link between menopause and depression. *Maturitas* 1992;14:143–55
19. Weiss KM. Evolutionary perspectives on human aging. In Amoss P, Harrell S, eds. *Other Ways of Growing Old.* Palo Alto: Stanford University Press, 1989:25–58
20. Kertzer D, Laslett P. *Aging in the Past: Demography, Society and Old Age.* Berkeley: University of California Press, 1995
21. Montagu JD. Length of life in the ancient world: a controlled study. *J R Soc Med* 1994;87:25–6

Brain function, menopause and aging 6

A. R. Genazzani, M. Stomati and P. Monteleone

INTRODUCTION

Experimental and clinical trials have demonstrated that sex steroids are involved in the modulation of female neurobiology, and the identification of estrogen, progestin and androgen receptors in numerous regions of the central nervous system (CNS) confirms the pivotal role of sex steroid hormones in controlling different brain functions[1-4]. The mechanisms of action in the different brain areas are similar to those observed in the peripheral target organs: several actions are mediated via estrogen receptors by genomic activation, while other effects are rapid and direct, through non-genomic-mediated mechanisms[5]. The slow, long-term classical genomic effects are produced by the activation of specific intracellular receptors that modulate gene transcription and protein synthesis. Thus, gonadal steroids modulate the synthesis, release and metabolism of many neuropeptides and neurotransmitters, as well as the expression of their receptors[4-6]. In particular, among the neurotransmitters, noradrenaline, dopamine, γ-aminobutyric acid (GABA), acetylcholine, serotonin and melatonin are regulated by sex steroid hormones. Neuropeptides directly modulated by gonadal hormones include opioid peptides, gonadotropin releasing hormone, corticotropin releasing factor, neuropeptide Y and galanin. Steroid hormones also exert very rapid effects, both on the neuronal membrane and within the nucleus, that cannot be attributed to genomic mechanisms. In fact, estrogens, androgens and progestogens modulate non-specific steroid membrane receptors (GABA, *N*-methyl-D-aspartate, σ-receptors), producing effects on the neuronal membrane (electric excitability, synapse functioning and morphological features)[5-8]. The interaction of genomic and non-genomic mechanisms allows for the wide range of sex steroid actions in the regulation of cerebral functions.

In the postmenopause, neuroactive transmitters undergo important modifications as a consequence of the insufficient production of gonadal hormones, leading to CNS derangement and the onset of specific symptoms. Hot flushes, sweating, mood changes, anxiety and insomnia are consequences of neuroendocrine changes occurring in the early postmenopause, while the alterations of cognitive functions, such as short- and long-term memory impairment and attention decline, are related to changes occurring in the late postmenopause (Figure 1). Estrogen, progestin and androgen administration positively influences the postmenopausal modifications at the central level.

In the past 10 years, epidemiological and clinical studies have shown an important interaction between the withdrawal of sex steroids and the physiological and pathological aging processes, producing cognitive disturbances and degenerative chronic diseases such as Alzheimer's-type dementia and Parkinson's disease. Aging women are more frequently affected by chronic and degenerative diseases, such as senile dementia and Alzheimer's disease, than age-matched men[9]. The cholinergic neurons, which are critically involved in learning and memory cognitive processes, are particularly involved in the physiopathological mechanism of Alzheimer's disease[10,11]. Alzheimer's disease is characterized by neuronal loss and the accumulation of β-amyloid, with increased numbers of intracellular neurofibrillary tangles and extracellular senile plaques in the hippocampus and association neocortex. Epidemiological and clinical studies suggest that hormone replacement therapy (HRT) probably protects against neurodegenerative diseases. Prospective randomized trials are currently needed to confirm the preventive or ameliorative effect of HRT on Alzheimer's disease.

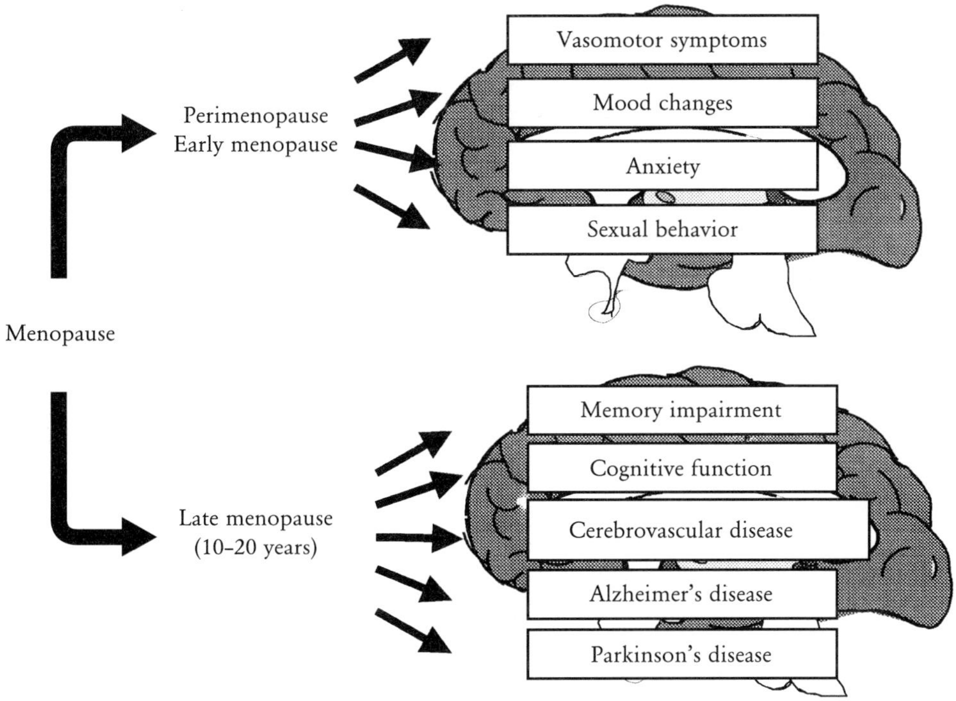

Figure 1 Symptoms occurring in the early postmenopause and the late postmenopause

The physiological model of the climacteric and postmenopause represents an interesting opportunity to investigate the fascinating functions of the CNS and the interactions with gonadal hormones.

BRAIN FUNCTION AND MENOPAUSE

In the early postmenopause, a large number of women complain about mood changes and generalized anxiety. Numerous studies investigating climacteric depression have shown that mood significantly improves in depressed postmenopausal women treated with estrogen[12–14].

The positive effects of estrogens on mood in postmenopausal women may relate to their effects on the adrenergic, serotoninergic and opiatergic tone (Figure 2). Sex steroid hormones modulate the noradrenergic and dopaminergic systems of the hypothalamus, as well as of the extrahypothalamic regions of the brain controlling movement and behavior, in both animals and humans. Studies in castrated female rats have shown an impairment of catecholaminergic neurons, with an increase in noradrenaline release and a decrease in dopamine[15]. Estrogen administration decreased noradrenaline release from the hypothalamus, while it increased dopaminergic neuronal activity and its release in the mediobasal hypothalamus[15]. When progesterone administration was combined with estrogen treatment in ovariectomized female rats, a suppression of the estrogen effects on the noradrenergic neurons in the pineal gland was observed. In another animal model, estradiol and progesterone enhanced noradrenaline release, leading to increased excitability of ventromedial hypothalamic neuronal activity and to the expression of lordosis behavior[15]. Regarding the modulation of the different subtypes of adrenergic receptor, *in vitro* studies suggest that estrogens upregulate α_1-adrenergic and downregulate β-adrenergic receptor activity. The serotoninergic system is also modulated by endogenous gonadal hormones or modified by their exogenous administration. Several findings indicate a sex difference in the central serotoninergic system: female

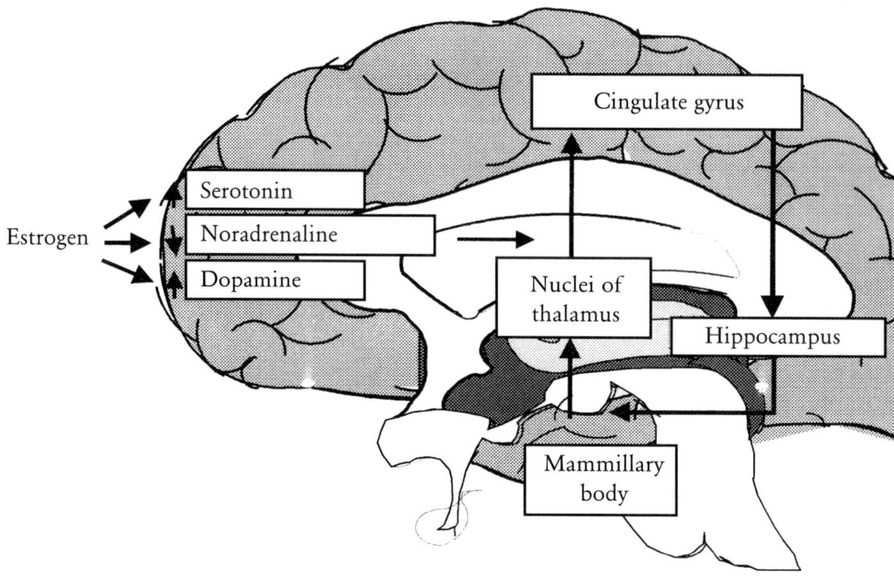

Figure 2 Modulation by estrogen of neurotransmitter systems in the brain, resulting in a positive effect on mood in postmenopausal women

rats have elevated synthesis, turnover rate and concentration of serotonin in the hypothalamus, cortex, hippocampus, forebrain and raphe, compared to male rats[16]. Brain serotonin concentration and activity are modified during the estrous cycle or other periods of ovarian hormone fluctuation[17]. Estrogen, progesterone or combined treatments in ovariectomized rats positively affect the serotoninergic system[18]. Estrogens can also modify the concentration and the availability of serotonin by increasing the rate of degradation of monoamine oxidase, the enzyme that catabolizes serotonin[19].

In humans, several studies performed in postmenopausal women have confirmed the modulation of gonadal steroids on mood, behavior and anxiety. A large number of studies regarding the effects of estrogen replacement therapy on climacteric depression showed a significant amelioration of mood in depressed postmenopausal women treated with estrogen[12-14,20], although other studies have not found a similar response to estrogen[21-23]. These different results may be due to a lower estrogen dosage or to the progestogen component of the combined preparations that were employed[24,25]. Generally, the different doses and regimens of estrogens conventionally used do not improve mood in women with major depression, but have a strong influence on mood and feeling of well-being in healthy, non-depressed, postmenopausal women[12,20-22,26-29]. The positive effects of estrogens on mood in postmenopausal women may relate to their effects on the adrenergic and serotoninergic tone. In fact, estrogen acts as a serotoninergic agonist by increasing serotonin synthesis and levels of its main metabolite, 5-hydroxyindoleacetic acid[19,27].

Moreover, estrogens directly modulate endogenous opioid activity and stimulate the expression of opioid receptors. The most important and biologically active endogenous opioid peptide, β-endorphin, may be considered one of the markers of neuroendocrine function. In rats, ovariectomy leads to a significant reduction in pituitary β-endorphin levels in comparison with fertile rats; estradiol administration produces a restoration of pituitary β-endorphin content[30,31]. The administration of progestins modifies estrogen effects in different ways: norethisterone acetate and norgestimate increase hypothalamic and circulating β-endorphin, while medroxyprogesterone acetate and desogestrel do not induce significant changes[30,31]. It is reasonable to hypothesize that these different effects are the consequence of the availability of synthetic progestin compounds that bind to several receptors. In fact, each progestin molecule is able to bind to the progesterone receptor and exert its specific progestative effect, but the different kinds of molecules may interfere with the receptors of other sex steroid hormones or other substances, thus exerting multiple effects in each target tissue.

Clinical studies demonstrate that, in humans, the modifications in circulating β-endorphin levels may be considered as one of the markers of neuroendocrine function[31,32]. A decrease in plasma β-endorphin levels has been shown in postmenopausal women after surgical or spontaneous menopause[32]. The postmenopausal reduction in circulating β-endorphin has been suggested to have a role in the mechanisms of hot flushes and sweat episodes[33,34]. The decrease in plasma β-endorphin levels has also been related to the pathogenesis of mood, behavior and nociceptive disturbances of the postmenopausal period[35,36]. Indeed, a positive role of HRT in vasomotor and subjective psychobehavioral symptoms may be mediated by its action on the opiatergic pathway[31,32]. In fact, oral estrogen replacement therapy subsequent to spontaneous or surgically induced menopause is followed by a significant increase in circulating β-endorphin levels[37].

Recent studies performed by our group show for the first time that, in postmenopausal women, HRT with transdermal estradiol, independently of the type of progestin used, induces a significant increase in plasma β-endorphin levels to premenopausal values[37]. Previous experimental and clinical evidence suggests that β-endorphin synthesis and release are modulated by noradrenaline, dopamine, serotonin, acetylcholine, GABA and corticotropin releasing factor[38,39]. In fertile women, we have found a β-endorphin response (i.e. an increase in the circulating levels) to specific noradrenergic and opiatergic stimuli: clonidine, an α_2-noradrenergic presynaptic receptor agonist, and naloxone, an opiate receptor antagonist. On the contrary, in postmenopausal women, a lack of response of β-endorphin to both these stimuli was shown, suggesting a postmenopausal impairment of the adrenergic and opiatergic systems in modulating β-endorphin release[37]. The restoration of the β-endorphin response to naloxone and clonidine tests in women undergoing transdermal estradiol treatment with different progestin molecules represents a valid tool that expresses a restored neuroendocrine regulation of the opioid peptide in postmenopausal women undergoing HRT[5,37,40–42].

The increased use of therapies employing sex steroid hormones has led to the study of the biochemical and metabolic properties of different progestin molecules available in hormonal therapies. In particular, attention has been focused on the interactions between estrogens and progestins in the neuroendocrine control of brain functions and their clinical implications. Some studies have investigated the effects of exogenous progestogen treatment, used in postmenopausal women undergoing hormone replacement therapy, on mood and cognitive functions. The estrogen–progestogen sequential replacement therapy restores the pattern of hormonal variation during an ovulatory menstrual cycle, while estrogen treatment alone has effects that are similar to an anovulatory cycle. Women on sequential treatments develop a cyclicity in their mood and physical signs. Many of these studies have reported negative effects of progesterone on the brain, producing, in some patients, a state of dysphoric mood[43,44]. Women undergoing only estrogen replacement therapy do not show any variation of mood during the treatment. A negative influence on mood by progestogens has been demonstrated in clinical trials using different combinations of estrogen and progestin compounds: conjugated equine estrogens and medroxyprogesterone acetate[45]; estrogen implants and norethisterone[44]; percutaneous estradiol and lynestrenol[24]; and ethinylestradiol and levonorgestrel[46]. These depressant actions are most likely due to the active metabolites of progesterone, such as allopregnenolone, 17-hydroxypregnenolone and 17α-hydroxyprogesterone. These metabolites are produced systematically or locally from progesterone. It is possible to speculate that progestogens and their metabolites may negatively influence mood by enhancing monoamine oxidase activity and GABA inhibitory action, and thus brain excitability. Regarding the effects of progestins on neurovegetative symptoms and cognitive functions, the few available data suggest that progestins do not modify the positive effects of estrogen[37,45,47].

MENOPAUSE AND AGING

In women, the effects of aging appear mostly in the late postmenopause, and sex steroid hormone withdrawal can play a role in the development of brain aging processes, producing cognitive disturbances and degenerative chronic diseases such as Alzheimer's-type dementia.

Clinical studies carried out in women in the late postmenopause have reported a frequent decrease in cognitive efficiency[48]. Estrogen administration improves cognitive functions by exerting a positive effect, especially on memory and reaction-time tests[11,49–55]. The employment of objective psychometric instruments to assess cognitive function has suggested that physiological levels of estrogen help in maintaining short- and long-term verbal memory, but have no effect on visual spatial memory. Although a majority of studies on estrogen and cognition have found a positive effect of estrogen on memory processes, other studies have failed to demonstrate this effect[56,57]. The explanations for these discrepant findings are both the differences in the selection of subjects and methodology, and the differences in the type and route of administration of hormonal preparations. Different oral preparations are differentially absorbed and metabolized by the stomach and liver, whereas parenteral or transdermal administration of estrogen bypasses initial hepatic metabolism. It is therefore reasonable to postulate that the mode of administration and the doses are responsible for some of the variance in the results. Another important factor may explain the different effects: in the postmenopausal period, estrogen administration enhances mood and subjective well-being. A depressed mood can produce a negative impact on psychometric performance. Although several studies have demonstrated a secondary influence of estrogen on cognition through its effects on mood, others have not found a direct correlation[54,55,58]. Recent studies have demonstrated specific memory impairment in surgically postmenopausal women[53,55], independently from the presence of affective disorders or other symptoms related to the menopause. In conclusion, it seems that estrogen may affect mood and cognition in both an indirect and a direct manner.

Findings from epidemiological studies on the correlation between estrogen use and the incidence of Alzheimer's disease indicate that HRT may reduce the relative risk of developing Alzheimer's disease[59–64] (Figure 3). In these studies, there appears to be a dose–response relationship between estrogen and the incidence of Alzheimer's disease, so that the relative risk decreases significantly with increasing doses and duration of therapy[9,10]. The neuroprotective effects of estrogen on memory functions probably become more important in elderly women, in whom the natural aging process induces neuronal death. Although the etiology of

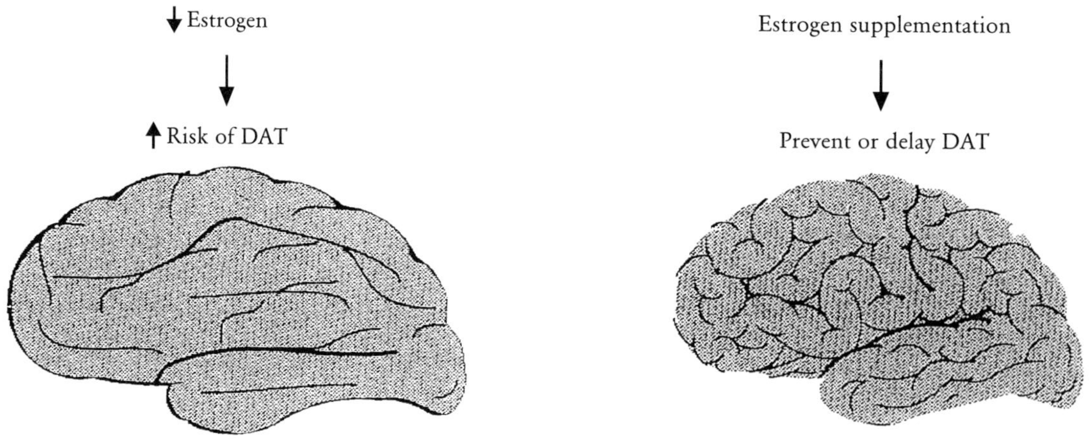

Figure 3 Effect of estrogen on Alzheimer's disease risk

the memory deficits associated with Alzheimer's disease is multifactorial, it is possible that estrogen may prolong the latency time to the onset of the memory loss. The biological mechanisms by which estrogens may influence cognitive functions and Alzheimer's disease are as yet unknown. Estrogen administration increases total cerebral and cerebellar blood flow by 30% and augments cerebral glucose utilization[64]. Sex steroids influence growth proteins that are associated with axonal elongation and promote synapse formation, particularly in the CA1 region of the hippocampus, an important area for memory processes[10,65]. Furthermore, estrogens are involved in the control of the cholinergic system by increasing choline *O*-acetyltransferase, the enzyme responsible for acetylcholine synthesis[65–67]. Acetylcholine is a key neurotransmitter in learning and memory, and a disturbance of the cholinergic system is the most significant neurochemical defect of Alzheimer's disease. Estrogens affect basal forebrain cholinergic neurons that project to the cerebral cortex and hippocampus in the rat brain. Studies of steroid effects on the expression of cholinergic enzymes have demonstrated that estrogens act as cholinergic agonists by inducing the synthesis and activation of choline *O*-acetyltransferase, the rate-limiting enzyme for acetylcholine formation. Estrogens may also blunt the neurotoxic effects of β-amyloid by promoting the breakdown of the amyloid precursor protein.

ADRENOPAUSE AND AGING

Aging is also accompanied by adrenopause, which is characterized by the progressive age-related decline of adrenal Δ5-steroid production. Dehydroepiandrosterone (DHEA) and its sulfate-conjugated ester, dehydroepiandrosterone sulfate (DHEAS), are the major circulating adrenal cortex products[68,69]. DHEAS is synthesized from the conversion of free DHEA, which is secreted in large amounts (70–80%) by the adrenals. Twenty per cent of DHEA is produced by the ovaries. Both Δ5-androgens (DHEA and DHEAS) are peripherally converted into androstenedione, testosterone, dihydrotestosterone and estrogens[68,69].

Less attention is commonly focused on the activity of androgens in normal female physiology or on the consequences of their deficiency. Women with an androgen deficiency may experience a variety of physical symptoms or psychological changes as consequence of their endocrine state. After the menopause, the principal source of circulating testosterone is from the peripheral conversion of androstenedione and DHEA(S). Circulating Δ5-androgens decrease linearly with age, starting from the third decade of life, and the decline is independent of the menopausal transition[70,71]. After 70 years of age, DHEA(S) levels are maintained at 20% or less of the maximum plasma concentrations, while cortisol levels remain unchanged[70,71].

Several epidemiological, experimental and clinical trials have focused on the actions of Δ5-androgens. Epidemiological studies have shown a relationship between the progressive decrease in circulating DHEA(S) levels and the increases in cardiovascular morbidity in men[72] and breast cancer in women[73,74], and the decline of immunocompetence in both sexes[75]. Experimental studies in rodents have demonstrated a protective role of DHEA on the development of spontaneous carcinomas, and an upregulation of the immune system has also been reported[76,77].

Only a few studies have investigated the effect of DHEA(S) on the CNS in humans (Figure 4). Clinical studies performed in postmenopausal women have shown that DHEA supplementation at 50 mg/day induces an improvement in psychological and physical well-being[78]. Moreover, DHEA(S) seems to have an antidepressant function (30–90 mg/day for 4 weeks) in middle-aged and elderly patients with major depression and low basal DHEA(S) levels[79,80]. On the other hand, DHEAS may directly affect the CNS. In fact, DHEA and DHEAS are considered to be neurosteroids, because they are also produced in the CNS. The concentration of DHEA(S) in the CNS is 5–10 times greater than DHEA(S) plasma levels. Experimental studies indicate that the mammalian brain contains steroid precursors, such as cholesterol and lipid derivatives, but it is also able to metabolize other steroids coming from the peripheral circulation[81,82]. The enzyme involved in the cleavage of cholesterol to pregnenolone and progesterone, localized in the mitochondria of glial cells, is cytochrome P450. This enzyme is encoded by the same P450 gene that is expressed in the

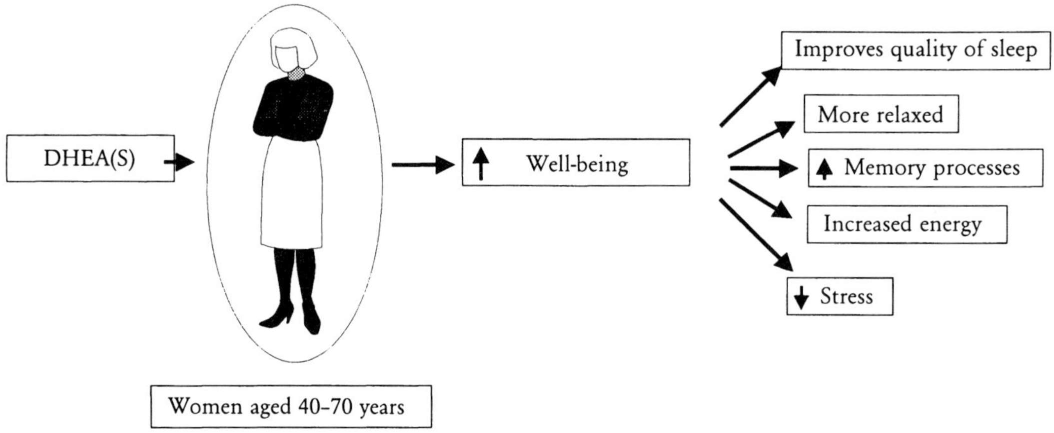

Figure 4 Effect of dehydroepiandrosterone (DHEA) and its sulfate-conjugated ester (DHEAS) in women aged 40–70 years

adrenals and gonads, and has been identified in rodents, cows and the human brain. The origin of DHEA in the brain is unknown, since the adult rat brain does not have 17α-hydroxylase activity and cannot convert pregnenolone or progesterone to hydroxylated compounds, nor can it convert C21 or C19 steroids[83]. However, the concentrations of DHEA(S) in the rat brain remain unchanged for a long time after the removal of the gonads and adrenals. The synthesis of classical neurosteroids, including DHEA, probably proceeds through different pathways with respect to those present in the adrenals or gonads. In fact, glial cells contain additional steroid-metabolizing enzymes that transform the classical steroid hormones into a variety of compounds[81–83]. Experimental evidence suggests that the effects of DHEA and DHEAS on the CNS occur directly through specific binding to the $GABA_A$ receptor, thus blocking the GABA-induced chloride transport or current in synaptosomes and neurons in a dose-dependent manner, resulting in an increase in neuronal excitability[84]. Moreover, a potentiating effect of DHEA on *N*-methyl-D-aspartate and σ-receptors has been reported in the rat brain[83].

Recently, the neuroendocrine effects of 3 months of DHEAS supplementation on the opiatergic tonus in postmenopausal women has been investigated by our group. In particular, our attention was focused on β-endorphin. Baseline plasma β-endorphin levels increased after the first month of therapy with DHEAS (50 mg), and even more so after the second and third months. Moreover, while there was no response before treatment, women treated with DHEA(S) showed a significant increase in plasma β-endorphin levels following naloxone injection ($p < 0.01$ at 15 and 30 min), clonidine injection ($p < 0.01$ at 15 and 30 min) or fluoxetine oral administration ($p < 0.01$ at 60 and 90 min) after 3 months of treatment[85]. These findings suggest that the neuroendocrine control of opioidergic, α_2-adrenergic and serotoninergic receptors in β-endorphin secretion from the anterior pituitary is restored following DHEAS supplementation. The modulation of neuroendocrine pathways after DHEAS supplementation may be mediated by a specific estrogenic action of DHEAS metabolites or, alternatively, by a similar specificity of DHEAS and HRT on opiatergic and adrenergic neurons[85].

CONCLUSION

Gonadal hormones exert several effects on brain functions and they are of primary importance for physiological brain function, acting both on the development and on the maintenance of female mood tone, cognition and reproductive function. Several diseases related to physiological and pathological aging processes are becoming more and more frequent and increase social costs. On the other hand, every year, different kinds of molecules, as well as numerous routes and regimens of administration, become available for HRT. As a result of these findings, epidemiological and large-scale longitudinal studies are required to explain the specific role of endogenous and exogenous sex steroids on CNS functioning and aging processes.

References

1. Genazzani AR, Petraglia F, Purdy RH, eds. *The Brain: Source and Target for Sex Steroid Hormones.* Carnforth, UK: Parthenon Publishing, 1996
2. Speroff L, Glass RH, Kase NH. *Clinical Gynecological Endocrinology and Infertility*, 5th edn. Baltimore, MD: Williams and Wilkins, 1995
3. Alonso-Soleis R, Abreu P, Leopez-Coviella I, Hernandez G, Fajardo N. Gonadal steroid modulation of neuroendocrine transduction: a transynaptic view. *Cell Mol Neurobiol* 1996;3:357–82
4. Panay N, Sands RH, Studd JWW. Estrogens and behavior. In Genazzani AR, Petraglia F, Purdy RH, eds. *The Brain: Source and Target for Sex Steroid Hormones.* Carnforth, UK: Parthenon Publishing, 1996: 257–76
5. Fuxe K, Gustafsson JA, Wetterberg L. *Steroid Hormone Regulation of the Brain.* Oxford: Pergamon, 1981:27–56
6. Kalra SP. Gonadal steroids promote interactive communication. In Genazzani AR, Petraglia F, Purdy RH, eds. *The Brain: Source and Target for Sex Steroid Hormones.* Carnforth, UK: Parthenon Publishing, 1996:153–64
7. Matsumoto A. Synaptogenic action of sex steroids in developing and adult neuroendocrine brain. *Psychoneuroendocrinology* 1991;16:25–40
8. McEwen BS, Wooley CS. Estradiol and progesterone regulate neuronal structure and synaptic connectivity in adult as well as developing brain. *Exp Gerontol* 1994;29:431–6
9. Tang M-X, Jacobs D, Stern Y, *et al.* Effect of oestrogen during menopause on risk and age at onset of Alzheimer's disease. *Lancet* 1996;348:429–32
10. Paganini-Hill A, Henderson VW. Estrogen deficiency and risk of Alzheimer's disease in women. *Am J Epidemiol* 1994;140:256–61
11. Sherwin BB. Estrogen effects on cognition in menopausal women. *Neurology* 1997;48(Suppl 7): S21–6
12. Studd JWW, Smith RNJ. Estrogen and depression in women. *Menopause* 1994;1:33–7
13. Ditkoff EC, Crary WG, Cristo M, Lobo RA. Estrogen improves psychological function in asymptomatic postmenopausal women. *Obstet Gynecol* 1991; 78:991–5
14. Daly E, Gray A, Barlow J, *et al.* Measuring the impact of menopausal symptoms on quality of life. *Br Med J* 1993;307:836–40
15. Etgen AM, Karkanias GB. Estrogen regulation of noradrenergic signaling in the hypothalamus. *Psychoneuroendocrinology* 1994;19:603–10
16. Dickinson SL, Curzon G. 5-Hydroxytryptamine-mediated behavior in male and female rats. *Neuropharmacology* 1986;25:771–6
17. Biegon A, Bercovitz H, Samuel D. Serotonin receptor concentration during the estrous cycle of the rat. *Brain Res* 1980;187:221–5
18. Mendelson SD, McKittrick CR, McEwen BS. Autoradiographic analyses of the effects of estradiol benzoate on (3H)-paroxetine binding in the cerebral cortex and dorsal hippocampus of gonadectomized male and female rats. *Brain Res* 1993; 601:299–301
19. Luine VN, McEwen BS. Effect of estradiol on turnover of type A monoamine oxidase in the brain. *J Neurochem* 1977;28:1221–7
20. Limouzin-Lamothe M, Mairon N, LeGal J, *et al.* Quality of life after the menopause: influence of hormone replacement therapy. *Am J Obstet Gynecol* 1994;170:618–24
21. Best N, Rees M, Barlow D, *et al.* Effect of estradiol implants on noradrenergic function and mood in menopausal patients. *Psychoneuroendocrinology* 1992;17:87–93
22. Klaiber EL, Broverman DM, Vogel W, *et al.* Estrogen replacement therapy for severe persistent depression in women. *Arch Gen Psychiatry* 1979;36: 550–4
23. Coope J. Is oestrogen therapy effective in the treatment of menopausal depression? *J R Coll Gen Pract* 1981;31:134–40
24. Holst J, Backstrom T, Hammarback S, von Schoulz B. Progestogen addition during estrogen replacement therapy - effects on vasomotor symptoms and mood. *Maturitas* 1989;11:13–20
25. Furuhjelm M, Feder-Freybergh P. The influence of estrogens on the psyche in climacteric and postmenopausal women. In van Keep PA, Albeaux M,

Greenblatt R, eds. *Consensus on Menopause Research.* London: MTP Press, 1976:84–93
26. Palinkas LA, Barrett-Connor E. Estrogen use and depressive symptoms in postmenopausal women. *Obstet Gynecol* 1992;80:30–6
27. Michael C, Kantor H, Shore H. Further psychometric evaluation of older women – the effect of estrogen administration. *J Gerontol* 1970;25:335–41
28. Ayward M. Estrogen and plasma tryptophan levels in perimenopausal patients. In Campbell S, ed. *The Management of the Menopause and Postmenopausal Years.* Baltimore, MD: University Park Press, 1976: 135–47
29. Furuhjelm M, Carlstrom K. Treatment of climacteric and postmenopausal women with 17-beta-oestradiol and norethisterone acetate. *Acta Obstet Gynecol Scand* 1977;56:351–61
30. Genazzani AR, Petraglia F, Cleva M, *et al.* Norgestimate increases pituitary and hypothalamic concentrations of immunoreactive beta-endorphin. *Contraception* 1989;5:605–13
31. Genazzani AR, Petraglia F, Mercuri N, *et al.* Effect of steroid hormones and antihormones on hypothalamic beta-endorphin concentrations in intact and castrated female rats. *J Endocrinol Invest* 1990; 13:91–6
32. Aleem FA, McIntosh T. Menopausal syndrome: plasma levels of β-endorphin in postmenopausal women using a specific radioimmunoassay. *Maturitas* 1985;13:76–84
33. Genazzani AR, Petraglia F, Facchinetti F, *et al.* Increase of proopiomelanocortin-related peptides during subjective menopausal flushes. *Am J Obstet Gynecol* 1984;149:775–9
34. Linghtman SL, Jacobs HS, Maguire AK, *et al.* Climacteric flushing: clinical and endocrine response to infusion of naloxone. *Br J Obstet Gynaecol* 1981;88:919–24
35. Adler MW. Minireview: opioid peptides. *Life Sci* 1980;26:496–510
36. O'Donouhe TL, Dorse DM. The opiomelanotropinergic neuronal and endocrine system. *Peptides* 1982;3:383–95
37. Stomati M, Bersi C, Rubino S, *et al.* Neuroendocrine effects of different oestradiol–progestin regimens in postmenopausal women. *Maturitas* 1997;28:127–35
38. McLoughin L, Grossman A, Tomlin S, *et al.* CRF-41 stimulates the release of beta-lipotropin and beta-endorphin in normal human subjects. *Neuroendocrinology* 1984;38:282–4
39. Petraglia F, Comitini G, Genazzani AR, *et al.* β-Endorphin in human reproduction. In Herz A, ed. *Opiods II.* Berlin: Springer-Verlag, 1993:763–80
40. Advis J, McConn S, Negro-Vilar A. Evidence that catecholaminergic and peptidergic (luteinizing hormone-releasing hormone) neurons in suprachiasmatic-medial preoptic, medial basal hypothalamus and median eminence are involved in estrogen negative feed back. *Endocrinology* 1980; 107:892–901
41. McEwen B. Steroid hormones are multifunctional messengers in the brain. *Trends Endocrinol Metab* 1991;12:62–7
42. Piva F, Limonta P, Dondi D, *et al.* Effects of steroids on the brain opioid system. *J Steroid Biochem Mol Biol* 1995;53:343–8
43. Hammarback S, Backstrom T, Holst J, von Schoultz B, Lyrenas S. Cyclical changes as in premenstrual tension syndrome during sequential estro-progestin postmenopausal replacement therapy. *Acta Obstet Gynecol Scand* 1985;64:393–7
44. Magos AL, Brewster E, Singh R, O'Dowd TM, Brincat M, Studd JWW. The effect of norethisterone in postmenopausal women on estrogen therapy: a model for premenstrual syndrome. *Br J Obstet Gynaecol* 1986;93:1290–6
45. Sherwin BB. The impact of different doses of estrogen and progestin on mood and sexual behavior in postmenopausal women. *J Clin Endocrinol Metab* 1991;72:336–43
46. Dennerstein L, Burrows GD, Hyman G, Sharpe K. Hormone therapy and affect. *Maturitas* 1979;1: 247–54
47. Sherwin B, Gelfand MM. A prospective one-year study of estrogen and progestin in postmenopausal women: effects on clinical symptoms and lipoprotein lipids. *Obstet Gynecol* 1989;73: 759–66
48. Halbreich U. Role of estrogen in postmenopausal depression. *Neurology* 1997;48(Suppl 7):S16–20
49. Caldwell BM, Watson RI. Evaluation of psychological effects of sex hormone administration in aged women: results of therapy after 6 months. *J Gerontol* 1952;7:228–44
50. Hackman BW, Galbraith D. Six month study of oestrogen therapy with piperazine oestrone sulphate and its effect on memory. *Curr Med Res Opin* 1977;4(Suppl):21–7
51. Campbell S, Whitehead M. Oestrogen therapy and the menopausal syndrome. *Clin Obstet Gynecol* 1977; 4:31–47
52. Fedor-Freybergh P. The influence of oestrogen on well being and mental performance in climacteric and postmenopausal women. *Acta Obstet Gynecol Scand* 1977;64(Suppl):5–69
53. Sherwin BB. Estrogen and/or androgen replacement therapy and cognitive functioning in surgically menopausal women. *Psychoneuroendocrinology* 1988;13:345–57
54. Sherwin BB, Phillips S. Estrogen and cognitive functioning in surgically menopausal women. *Ann NY Acad Sci* 1990;592:474–5
55. Phillips S, Sherwin BB. Effects of estrogen on memory function in surgically menopausal women. *Psychoneuroendocrinology* 1992;17:177–87

56. Rauramo L, Lagerspetz K, Engblom P, Punnonen R. The effect of castration and peroral estrogen therapy on some psychological functions. *Front Horm Res* 1975;13:94–104
57. Vanhulle R, Demol R. A double-blind study into the influence of estriol on a number of psychological tests in post-menopausal women. In van Keep PA, Greenblatt RB, Albeaux-Fernet M, eds. *Consensus on Menopausal Research*. London: MTP Press, 1976:94–9
58. Kampen D, Sherwin BB. Estrogen use and verbal memory in healthy postmenopausal women. *Obstet Gynecol* 1994;83:979–83
59. Birge SJ. The role of estrogen deficiency in the aging central nervous system. In Lobo RA, ed. *Treatment of the Postmenopausal Woman: Basic and Clinical Aspects*. New York: Raven Press, 1994:153–7
60. Henderson VW, Paganini-Hill A, Emanuel CK, Dunn ME, Buckwalter JG. Estrogen replacement therapy in older women: comparisons between Alzheimer's disease cases and nondemented control subjects. *Arch Neurol* 1994;51:896–900
61. Mortel KF, Meyer JS. Lack of postmenopausal estrogen replacement therapy and the risk of dementia. *J Neuropsychiatry Clin Neurosci* 1995;7:334–7
62. Lerner A, Cole R, Debanna S, *et al.* Immunological and endocrine condition in an Alzheimer's disease case-control study [Abstract]. *Neuropidemiology* 1995;14:307
63. Honjo H, Ogino Y, Naitoh K, *et al. In vivo* effects of estrone sulfate on the central nervous system – senile dementia (Alzheimer's type). *J Steroid Biochem* 1989; 34:521–5
64. Ohkura T, Teshima Y, Isse K. Estrogen increases cerebral and cerebellar blood flows in postmenopausal women. *Menopause* 1995;2:13–18
65. Gould E, Wolley CS, Frankfurt M, McEwen BS. Gonadal steroids regulate dendritic spine density in hippocampal pyramidal cells in adulthood. *J Neurosci* 1990;10:1286–91
66. Coyle JT, Price DL, DeLong MR. Alzheimer's disease: a disorder of cortical cholinergic innervation. *Science* 1983;219:1184–90
67. Lawrence AD, Sahakian BJ. Alzheimer disease, attention, and the cholinergic system. *Alzheimer Dis Assoc Disord* 1995;9:43–9
68. Parker LN, Odell WD. Control of adrenal androgen secretion. *Endocr Rev* 1980;4:392–410
69. Yamaji T, Ibayashi H. Serum dehydroepiandrosterone sulphate in normal and pathological conditions. *J Clin Endocrinol Metab* 1969;29:273–8
70. Hopper BR, Yen SSC. Circulating concentrations of dehydroepiandrosterone and dehydroepiandrosterone sulphate during puberty. *J Clin Endocrinol Metab* 1975;40:458–61
71. Davis SR, Burger HG. Androgens and the postmenopausal woman. Clinical review 82. *J Clin Endocrinol Metab* 1996;81:2759–63
72. Barrett-Connor E, Khaw K, Yen SSC. A prospective study of DS mortality and cardiovascular disease. *N Engl J Med* 1986;315:1519–24
73. Helzlsouer KJ, Gordon GB, Alberg A, Bush TL, Comstock GW. Relationship of prediagnostic serum levels of DHEA and DS to the risk of developing premenopausal breast cancer. *Cancer Res* 1992;52:1–4
74. Bulbrook RD, Hayward JL, Spicer CC. Relation between urinary androgen and corticoid excretion and subsequent breast cancer. *Lancet* 1971;2:395–8
75. Thoman ML, Weigle WO. The cellular and subcellular bases of immunosenescence. *Adv Immunol* 1989;46:221–61
76. Blauer KL, Rogers WM, Bernton EW. Dehydroepiandrosterone antagonizes the suppressive effects of glucocorticoids on lymphocyte proliferation. In *Proceedings of the 71st Annual Meeting of the Endocrine Society*, 1989
77. Rogers WM, Blauer KL, Bernton W. Dehydroepiandrosterone protection against dexamethasone induced thymic involution: flow cytometric and mechanism studies. In *Proceedings of the 71st Annual Meeting of the Endocrine Society*, 1989
78. Morales AJ, Nolan JJ, Nelson JC, Yen SSC. Effects of replacement dose of dehydroepiandrosterone in men and women of advancing age. *J Clin Endocrinol Metab* 1994;78:1360–7
79. Wolf OT, Neumenn O, Helhammer DH, *et al.* Effects of a two-week physiological dehydroepiandrosterone substitution on cognitive performance and well-being in healthy elderly women and men. *J Clin Endocrinol Metab* 1997;82:2363–7
80. Wolkowitz OM, Reus VI, Roberts E, *et al.* Dehydroepiandrosterone (DHEA) treatment of depression. *Biol Psychiatry* 1997;41:311–18
81. Majewska MD. Neurosteroids: endogenous bimodal modulators of the GABA-A receptor. Mechanism of action and physiological significance. *Prog Neurobiol* 1992;38:379–95
82. Corpechot C, Young J, Calvel M, *et al.* Neurosteroids: 3α-hydroxy-5α-pregan-20-one and its precursors in the brain, plasma, and steroidogenic glands of male and female rats. *Endocrinology* 1993; 133:1003–9
83. Mellon SH. Neurosteroids: biochemistry, modes of action, and clinical relevance. *J Clin Endocrinol Metab* 1994;78:1003–8
84. Majewska MD, Demirgoren S, Spivak CE, London ED. The neurosteroid DHEA is an allosteric antagonist of the GABA-A receptor. *Brain Res* 1990;526:143–6
85. Stomati M, Rubino S, Spinetti A, *et al.* Endocrine, neuroendocrine and behavioural effects of oral dehydroepiandrosterone sulphate supplementation in postmenopausal women. *Gynecol Endocrinol* 1999;13:15–25

Menopause and sexual functioning 7

L. Dennerstein, P. Lehert, H. G. Burger, C. Garamszegi and E. Dudley

INTRODUCTION

Women attending menopause clinics often complain of sexual problems[1]. Clinicians have been concerned to sort out whether any aspect of female sexual functioning is linked to hormonal change as this may indicate that hormone therapy would have a role in the treatment of such disorders. While double-blind randomized trials of hormone therapy provide results of the pharmacological properties of various compounds, often used in supraphysiological doses, they indicate little about the physiological etiology of any changes in sexual behavior experienced by women in midlife. Clinicians are also concerned about the relative role of hormonal factors to those of aging, health and psychosocial factors on human sexuality. Population-based surveys can help address the question of a link between aging, menopause and sexuality. Yet relatively few of the population-based studies of the menopausal transition in mid-aged women have assessed sexual functioning. Even fewer have used a validated questionnaire to assess the different aspects of sexuality. Differing measures of sexual functioning have been used with studies often failing to offer any data on the validity or reliability of these measures in their local population. Some of the assessments have been very vague constructs indeed. For example, Osborn and colleagues[2] asked a general practice population if they suffered from 'sexual dysfunction' while Koster and Garde[3] asked women whether sexual desire was decreased or infrequent compared with 11 years previously. Even fewer studies have undertaken any hormonal determinations and these have either been of small sample size[4] or are still in progress. Studies of the role of menopausal status often use a comparison of the health outcome measure before and after women have reached menopause (12 months of amenorrhea). Yet endocrine change occurs for some years prior to cessation of menopause so it would seem important to examine for changes in health outcomes also some years before menses cease. Exogenous hormones may mask the effects of changing ovarian function so that women taking the oral contraceptive pill or any sort of hormone therapy must be documented when the objective is to examine the role of the natural menopausal transition. Population-based studies often suffer from being cross-sectional in design. Cross-sectional studies can only indicate whether associations exist and are unable to determine the direction of causality. Cross-sectional studies are also unable to establish a difference between cohort membership (effects of social change on different age groups) and aging. Aging and length of the relationship are known to affect sexual functioning of both men and women. For example, James[5] used cross-sectional and longitudinal data to show that coital rate halved over the first year of marriage and then took another 20 years to halve again. The role of aging *per se* has to be disentangled from that of menopause, with which it is confounded. Longitudinal studies of samples derived from the general population are in the best position to sort out whether there is a change in sexual functioning, and if so whether this reflects aging, health status, or hormonal or psychosocial factors.

Other methodological issues include the need for an appropriate age band which covers the menopausal transition (45–55 years); use of standardized objective definitions of menopausal status; distinctions between women in the natural menopausal transition and those with an induced menopause; limitations imposed on women by questionnaire design; and need for appropriate data analysis techniques[6]. Most studies have only utilized univariate analysis and thus have been unable to take into account the role of confounding or interacting factors.

With these limitations in mind, this chapter utilizes the results of a population-based study of mid-aged Australian-born women to explore the impact of the menopause on women's sexual functioning.

THE MELBOURNE WOMEN'S MIDLIFE HEALTH PROJECT

The Melbourne Women's Midlife Health Project is one of the few longitudinal population-based studies to have measured the relationship between sexuality, mood, menopausal status and a range of other variables, including hormone levels and psychosocial factors.

Study design and sampling

The Melbourne Women's Midlife Health Project involves a community-based cohort of mid-aged women. The study began in 1991 with population sampling by random telephone digital dialling to find 2001 Australian-born women aged between 45 and 55 years and resident in Melbourne. There was a 71% response rate to participation in a telephone interview used to acquire baseline data[7,8]. The study was approved by the Human Research Ethics Committee of the University of Melbourne. All subjects provided written informed consent for their participation in the study. All those women who had experienced menses in the prior 3 months and who were not taking the oral contraceptive pill or hormone therapy were invited to participate in a longitudinal study. Of those eligible to enter the longitudinal study, only 56% chose to do so (n = 438) (see Figure 1).

Volunteers for the longitudinal study were more likely than non-participants to report: better self-rated health, paid employment, more than 12 years of education, having ever had a Papanicolaou smear, exercising at least once a week, and having undergone dilatation and curettage[9].

The retention rate of the 438 women who volunteered for the longitudinal study was 97% for year 2, 94% for year 3, 91% for years 4 and 5 and 90% for year 6.

Measures and procedures

The Melbourne research team was allowed access to questionnaires carefully constructed by the groups of Kaufert and McKinlay and used in cross-sectional and longitudinal studies in North America[10,11]. The core questionnaire was modified for use in Australia after advice from co-investigators and a community advisory committee. Additional references are given below for specific variables and for those questions or instruments which supplemented the core questionnaire.

The cross-sectional questionnaire utilized in the initial telephone interview included sociodemographic data, health status, history of premenstrual complaints, lifestyle behaviors, and attitudes to aging and to menopause. Questions pertaining to bothersome symptoms were included in a list of other health-related symptoms[7]. Menstrual status and use of any hormone therapy was determined. Premenopausal status was assigned to women who reported no change in menstrual frequency. Perimenopausal status was used when women reported change in menstrual frequency. Women were deemed to be postmenopausal when there had been amenorrhea for at least 12 months. Separate categories were assigned to women who were taking hormone therapy or had an induced menopause. Well-being was assessed by a validated scale[12,13]. Three questions related to sexual functioning[8]. Women were asked whether, with regard to the last 12 months: sexual intercourse had occurred at all; whether sexual intercourse had been associated with unusual pain or discomfort; or whether there had been any

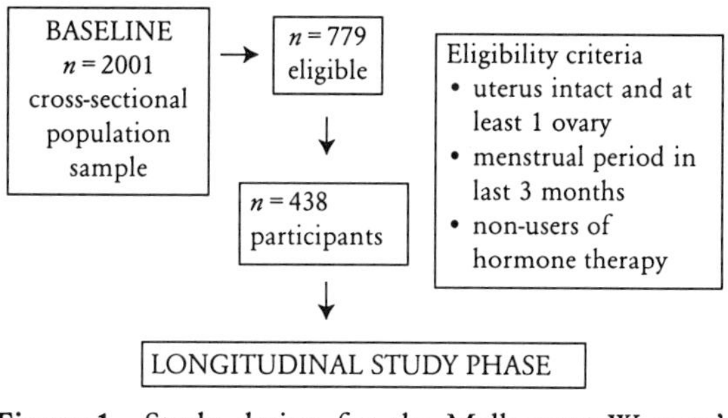

Figure 1 Study design for the Melbourne Women's Midlife Health Project

change in sexual interest (increased, no change, or decreased).

The longitudinal study involves annual face-to-face assessments in the women's own homes, with interviews and physical measures. Interview information is collected annually on the following variables: menstrual status; sociodemographic factors (age, marital status, paid work status); health status; symptoms (total score used)[7]; daily hassles[14,15]; stress[13]; well-being[12,13]; and use of hormone replacement therapy (HRT). The longitudinal study provided the opportunity to include a detailed assessment of sexual functioning. The Personal Experiences Questionnaire (PEQ)[16], derived from the McCoy Female Sexual Questionnaire[17], was handed to women to self-complete and return to field workers in a closed envelope. The PEQ focuses on current sexual experience and uses a 5-point Likert scale. Women were also asked to indicate their sexual preference and whether or not they had a sexual partner. Using cross-sectional data from the third year of study, the psychometric properties of the PEQ were assessed[16]. Six factors were extracted by principal components factor analysis and these explained 70% of the variance. Two of these factors related to possible determinants of sexual functioning: Feelings for partner; and Partner problems. The other four factors were considered to be indicators of different aspects of sexual functioning. These were named: Sexual responsivity, Sexual frequency, Libido and Vaginal dryness/dyspareunia. Internal consistency was considered adequate with a Cronbach's alpha of 0.71. Items included in each factor are shown in Table 1.

Blood samples for hormone assays and measurement of cholesterol were taken between days 4 and 8 for those still cycling or after 3 months of amenorrhea. Estradiol, follicle stimulating hormone (FSH) and immunoreactive inhibin were determined by radioimmunoassay[9].

RESULTS

Cross-sectional baseline study

The majority of women for whom data were available ($n = 1879$) reported no change in sexual interest over the 12 months in question (62.3%), although 31.1% reported a decline in sexual interest and a smaller group reported an increase (6.6%). Most women engaged in sexual intercourse in the previous year (84.2%) and, of these, only 11.9% reported experiencing unusual pain on intercourse. The natural menopausal transition was significantly associated with a decline in sexual interest, decreased likelihood of sexual intercourse and increased dyspareunia. Of the reasons offered for a decline in sexual interest, most were vague (e.g. no desire, bored, no interest) whereas increase

Table 1 The Personal Experiences Questionnaire (PEQ)

PEQ factor	*Item*
Factor 1 Feelings for partner	Companionable love for partner
	Satisfied with partner as friend
	Passionate love for partner
	Satisfied with partner as lover
	Resentment towards partner
	Hostility towards partner
Factor 2 Sexual responsivity	Arousal during sexual activities
	Orgasm during sexual activities
	Enjoyment of sexual activities
Factor 3 Frequency of sexual activities	Sexual intercourse in last month (frequency)
	Sexual activities in the last two weeks (frequency)
	Satisfied with frequency of sexual activity
Factor 4 Libido	Sexual thoughts/fantasies in last month (frequency)
	Masturbation (frequency)
Factor 5 Partner problems	Partner difficulties in sexual performance
Factor 6 Vaginal dryness/dyspareunia	Lack vaginal wetness during sexual activity
	Pain during intercourse

in sexual interest was most commonly associated with a new partner[8]. Logistic regression was used to identify explanatory variables for change in sexual interest. Decline in sexual interest was significantly associated with natural menopause, decreased well-being, decreasing employment and presence of bothersome symptoms. Eleven to 12 years of education was associated with a lower risk of decreased sexual functioning.

Longitudinal study

Longitudinal data from the first 6 years of annual assessments were included in the following analysis. Women were excluded from the analysis for the following reasons: drop-outs ($n = 49$), surgical menopause during the study ($n = 29$), oral contraceptive use during any year ($n = 6$). This left a sample size of 354 women.

Measures were selected for inclusion in this analysis based on significant relationships with sexual interest in the baseline cross-sectional study[8] and review of the literature. Structural equation modelling (SEM)[19,20] was chosen as a particularly suitable technique for assessing the whole model by means of a unique global goodness-of-fit test. This enables the relative role of hormonal, physical and psychosocial factors to be assessed. The results are summarized below from Dennerstein and colleagues[18].

Changes in sexuality factors with aging

The following factors significantly diminished ($p < 0.001$) with time (years in study): Feelings for Partner; Sexual Responsivity; Frequency of Sexual Activities; Libido. The following factors significantly increased ($p < 0.001$) with time (years in study): Vaginal Dryness/Dyspareunia; Partner Problems.

Structural modelling

Using the set of 354 women, we tested a global model using *a priori* hypotheses which included the sexual outcome factors measured by the PEQ, and possible determinants: aging, menopausal status, HRT use, symptoms, hormone levels, social factors (education, paid work, stress, daily hassles), well-being, Feelings about Partner and Partner Problems.

The best-fit model is shown in Figure 2, reprinted with permission from Dennerstein and co-workers[18]. The Normal-Fit Index was 0.92, which means that the fit was not too far from the perfect fit, taking the independence model as the zero fit. Rectangles represent the measured variables. The circle denotes the latent variable (ovarian functioning) and arrows designate a causal path and its direction. Two directional arrows indicate covariance between two variables. Age was confounded with menopausal status and has thus not been included in Figure 2. Menopausal status does directly affect two aspects of sexual functioning (Vaginal dryness/dyspareunia and Sexual responsivity). The effect on Sexual responsivity appears to be indirect, with significant effects of menopausal status on bothersome symptoms, which then affect well-being, which in turn influences Sexual responsivity. No direct effects of hormonal variables or HRT on sexual outcome measures were evident.

Social factors, such as stress, daily hassles, educational level and paid work, have only indirect effects on sexual functioning, through effects on well-being and experience of problematic symptoms, both of which affect parameters of sexual functioning. Women's increasing positive Feelings for partner have significant and powerful positive effects on their Libido, Sexual responsivity and well-being, and protect against experience of symptoms. The covariance between Feelings for partner and menopausal status may indicate a vulnerability during the menopausal transition. This close relationship during the menopausal transition is also evident for experience of stress. Similarly, covariance is evident between stress and daily hassles, stress and paid work, and paid work and educational status. Decreasing Sexual responsivity and increasing Vaginal dryness/dyspareunia increase partner problems. The presence of Partner problems leads to lower Frequency of Sexual activities but increased Libido (a measure of autoeroticism). Increasing Vaginal dryness/dyspareunia has a significant negative effect on Sexual responsivity and Libido. The reader is referred to Dennerstein and colleagues[18] for details

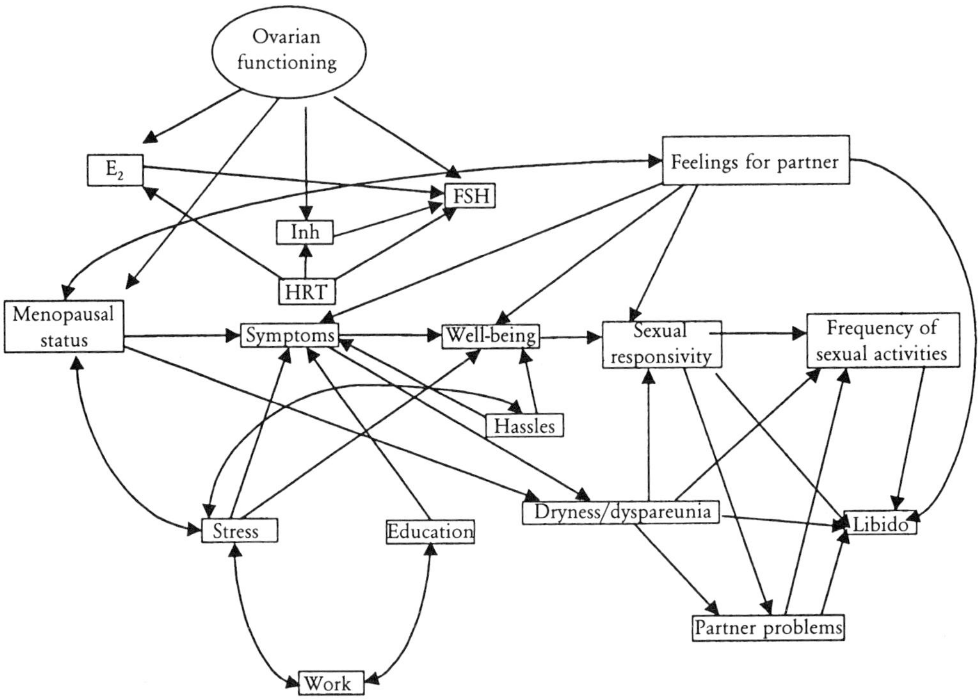

Figure 2 Global model of factors affecting sexual functioning. Reprinted with permission from reference 18. FSH, follicle stimulating hormone; E_2, estradiol; Inh, inhibin; HRT, hormone replacement therapy

of the regression weights which indicate the strength of each set of equations.

DISCUSSION

This study set out to determine whether women's sexual functioning declined in midlife, and if so the relative roles of biological and psychosocial factors. The initial cross-sectional analysis suggested that a substantial minority of women were aware of a decline in their sexual interest and that sexual interest, intercourse occurrence and dyspareunia were affected by the natural menopausal transition. Psychosocial and health status variables, including well-being and experience of bothersome symptoms, were also found to be significantly associated with a decline in sexual interest. The baseline study used only three questions about sexual functioning and a long recall period. The prospective study was able to include a detailed questionnaire (PEQ), a shorter recall period and annual hormone measures. The statistical analysis (SEM) chosen allowed an overall appraisal of the relative roles of various factors as well as pathways of interrelationships to be demonstrated. The SEM model provides an adequate way of controlling confounding, concomitant factors which may affect separate linear regressions. When this is done and most of the important determinants included in the model, the effects of hormone levels are relatively weak. Some effects of hormone levels are still present (indicated through a significant effect of menopausal status on Vaginal dryness/dyspareunia and direct effects of menopausal status on the number of bothersome symptoms. The number of symptoms then affects well-being, which influences Sexual responsivity, which in turn influences Frequency of sexual activities and Libido. This highlights the need for analytic models to include most of the variables rather than just a few. A powerful effect of Feelings for partner on Libido was found, confirming our preliminary analysis which found that the effect of Feelings about partner on Libido was much more significant ($p = 0.003$) than that of hormones ($p = 0.02$)[21]. Other social factors, such as educational level, experience of interpersonal stress and daily hassles, affect sexual functioning indirectly, by influencing symptoms and/or well-being.

Previous longitudinal analysis using repeated measures for multivariate analysis of covariance also found no direct effect of menopausal status, FSH, estradiol, or inhibin on the negative mood subscale of the well-being score[15]. However, negative mood was significantly adversely affected by bothersome symptoms, negative feelings for the partner, daily hassles and high interpersonal stress. The menopausal transition had an indirect effect in amplifying the effect of stressors and poor health[15].

The findings of the preliminary analysis[21] taken together with the current findings indicate that any effects of the hormones estradiol, FSH and inhibin on female sexual functioning are relatively weak compared to the effects of other variables, such as feelings for partner, symptoms, well-being and partner problems. Only a single blood sample for each woman was collected on an annual basis. Given the variability of menstrual cycles at this time and the associated variability of hormonal levels during the perimenopause[9], a great deal of variance in hormone levels would be expected. This, and the level of sensitivity of the estradiol assay, may limit the ability of annual single plasma hormone assays to detect relationships with parameters of sexual functioning. Furthermore, the current statistical modelling involves pooling data and this involves a loss of power. Future longitudinal modelling using change measures in structural equation modelling will provide a more sensitive confirmatory analysis. Techniques such as cluster analysis may identify particular groups of women who may be vulnerable to change in sexual functioning during the transition.

No relationship was evident between HRT use and any of the parameters of sexual functioning, even Vaginal dryness/dyspareunia. This may suggest that the type of HRT used may not be well adapted towards providing optimal sexual outcomes. The same seems to be true for effects of HRT on well-being and symptoms. However, we did not have measures of these health status variables just prior to use of HRT. Measures taken immediately prior to use of HRT and then some months into the use of HRT would be needed to adequately determine the effects of HRT. Clearly, double-blind controlled trials remain the best way to assess the effects of HRT.

Qualitative data

How do these findings relate to what women themselves say? The PEQ does have a place for further comments. All the comments provided by the women relating to changes in their sexual behavior during the longitudinal phase of the study were downloaded and subjected to a preliminary content analysis. There were a variety of responses listed but these fell predominantly into four groups. Some comments which are typical of women in each of these groups are described below.

No partner

'No current partner.'

'I have been widowed for 2 years.'

'Have been divorced for some time – no partner for the last 5 years.'

Husband's problems

'My partner is impotent so I don't have sex with him.'

'Some things have changed since my husband's operation for bowel cancer 1 year ago.'

'Husband currently working overseas with infrequent visits home.'

Her decreased interest

'The last 5 years have been quieter in the sex department than were the previous years.'

'We seldom have sex. Our relationship is good but not sexual these days.'

'Sexual intercourse is less exciting now than earlier years and I seem to find other things take time that my partner and I spend together e.g. children, friends, work. Put less effort into making it fun.'

'At 47 I don't feel like instigating sex.'

Increased interest

'I was separated 3 years ago. I have a new partner (9 months' duration). My new partner has transformed my life and love life.'

'I don't think I have changed. The difference between now and 5 years ago is that I have a different partner.'

'My sex life with the same partner has improved greatly from being satisfactory before in the past 5 years because we have deliberately made time for each other, such as going away for weekends once or twice a year.'

IMPLICATIONS FOR CLINICIANS

Population-based studies such as the Melbourne Women's Midlife Health Project suggest a deterioration in several aspects of female sexual functioning associated with the midlife years. This study provides further evidence about the direct and indirect roles of the hormonal changes of the menopausal transition. The analysis also demonstrates that hormonal change is only one aspect of the many factors that impact on sexual functioning. These include the woman's own premorbid level of sexual functioning, presence of bothersome symptoms, well-being, stress and the presence and quality of the sexual relationship with a partner.

When mid-aged women report sexual problems, the clinician must engage in detailed history taking involving the woman and her partner, alone and together. Given the range of factors affecting sexual functioning and the significantly more powerful effect of partner factors over that of hormonal factors, a broadly based biopsychosocial approach is needed. Bothersome symptoms which are known to be responsive to hormone therapy should be treated, as these impact on aspects of sexual functioning as well as causing distress in their own right. But hormonal prescription alone is rarely enough! Attention is needed to the relationship with the partner, and other stressors in the woman's life. Inspection of women's own comments reveals that the midlife transition allows the opportunity for positive change in relationships, if couples increase their intimacy at this time.

ACKNOWLEDGEMENTS

This study was supported by grants from the Public Health & Research Development Committee of the National Health & Medical Research Council and the Victorian Health Promotion Foundation. Prince Henry's Institute of Medical Research, Monash Medical Centre, received grants from Organon Pty Ltd, for hormone assays, and Pharmacia & Upjohn, grant-in-aid.

References

1. Sarrel P, Whitehead M. Sex and menopause: defining the issues. *Maturitas* 1985;7:217–24
2. Osborn M, Hawton K, Gath D. Sexual dysfunction among middle aged women in the community. *Br Med J* 1988;296:959–62
3. Koster A, Garde K. Sexual desire and menopausal development. A prospective study of Danish women born in 1936. *Maturitas* 1993;16: 49–60
4. McCoy N, Davidson J. A longitudinal study of the effects of menopause on sexuality. *Maturitas* 1985;7:203–10
5. James W. Decline in coital rates with spouses' ages in duration of marriage. *J Biosoc Sci* 1983;15:83–7
6. Dennerstein L. Well-being, symptoms and the menopausal transition. *Maturitas* 1966;23:147–57
7. Dennerstein L, Smith A, Morse C, *et al.* Menopausal symptoms in Australian women. *Med J Aust* 1993;159:232–6
8. Dennerstein L, Smith A, Morse C, *et al.* Sexuality and the menopause. *J Psychosom Obstet Gynaecol* 1994;15:59–66
9. Burger H, Dudley M, Hopper J, *et al.* The endocrinology of the menopausal transition: a cross-sectional study of a population-base sample. *J Clin Endocrinol Metab* 1995;80:3537–45
10. Kaufert P, Syrotuik J. Symptom reporting at the menopause. *Soc Sci Med* 1981;15:173–84

11. McKinlay J, McKinlay S, Brambilla D. Health status and utilization behavior associated with menopause. *Am J Epidemiol* 1987;125:110–21
12. Kammann R, Flett R. Affectometer 2: a scale to measure current level of general happiness. *Aust J Psychol* 1983;35:259–65
13. Dennerstein L, Dudley E, Burger H. Wellbeing and the menopausal transition. *J Psychosom Obstet Gynaecol* 1994;18:95–101
14. Kanner A, Coyne J, Schaefer C, *et al.* Comparison of two modes of stress measurement: daily hassles and uplifts versus major life events. *J Behav Med* 1981;4: 1–39
15. Dennerstein L, Lehert P, Burger H, *et al.* Mood and the menopausal transition. *J Nerv Mental Dis* 1999; 187:in press
16. Dennerstein L, Dudley E, Hopper J, *et al.* Sexuality, hormones and the menopausal transition. *Maturitas* 1997;26:83–93
17. McCoy N, Matyas J. Oral contraceptives and sexuality in university women. *Arch Sex Behav* 1996;25: 73–9
18. Dennerstein L, Lehert P, Burger H, *et al.* Factors affecting sexual functioning of women in the mid-life years. *Climacteric* 1999;2:in press
19. Bentler PM, Stein JA. Structural equation models in medical research. *Stat Methods Med Res* 1992;1: 159–81
20. Hoyle R. Introduction to special section: structural equation modelling in clinical research. *J Consult Clin Psychol* 1994;62:427–8
21. Dennerstein L, Lehert P, Burger H, *et al.* Biological and psychosocial factors affecting sexual functioning during the menopausal transition. In Bellino F, ed. *Biology of Menopause.* New York: Springer-Verlag, 1999:in press

Cancer diseases in the menopause: causes and prevention

8

I. R. Persson

INTRODUCTION

Cancers in organs that are regulated by ovarian hormones, i.e. the breast, ovary, endometrium, uterine cervix and possibly colon, impact on women's health in many countries. Because these cancers have been associated with hormone-related risk factors it is assumed that different types of sex steroids at different phases of life may affect the risk of their occurrence. Reproductive factors, the menopause itself and use of exogenous hormones may be important.

In this presentation, the burden of these cancers is described and their risk factors are reviewed. Particular emphasis is put on new findings in research that may improve the understanding of their etiology and on those that may have potential for prevention (primary and secondary).

BREAST CANCER

Burden

Breast cancer is the most common cancer in women worldwide, accounting for almost 800 000 cases per year[1]; it is also the leading cause of cancer deaths. The incidence varies among countries, the USA showing a cumulative incidence rate (in the mid-1980s, up to 75 years of age) of around 10%, as compared to Sweden (8%), Japan (4%) and China (2%)[2]. A stable increase in the incidence over time has been noted in several countries, particularly Japan during recent decades. Mortality has in most countries been fairly stable, except in Japan, where it has been rising.

A remarkable finding is the change in breast cancer incidence in migrants from low- to high-incidence countries, for instance from China to the USA[3]. Already in the second and third generations, women in the immigrant families seem to acquire the incidence of the native Americans. These observations demonstrate that environmental factors are crucial in the etiology of breast cancer.

Risk factors

The extensive literature on risk factors for breast cancer has been reviewed recently[4-6].

Genetic

A history of breast cancer in a first-degree relative, associated with a 2–3-fold increased risk of breast cancer, accounts for less than 10% of all breast cancers. Among those with such a family history, the high-penetrance, dominant, breast cancer genes BRCA1 and BRCA2 have been ascertained in less than a third[7].

Intrauterine exposures

Evidence for a new paradigm in breast cancer etiology was recently presented: that breast cancer risk is influenced by intrauterine exposures of the fetus[8,9]. Daughters of mothers developing pre-eclampsia during pregnancy – a condition associated with impaired placental function – experienced a substantially reduced risk of breast cancer during their lifetime[10]. Further, a high birth weight – reflecting intrauterine nutritional and hormonal exposures – has been positively associated with breast cancer risk[11] and with high-risk mammography patterns[12].

Endogenous hormones
Several risk factors have been established that pertain to variations in endogenous hormones at different phases of life[4].

Sex
Women have a 100-fold greater risk of developing breast cancer as compared with men.

Age
Breast cancer is infrequent before the age of 45; its incidence increases with age, reaching a maximum at about 65. An intriguing observation in the worldwide cancer statistics is the inflection of the incidence curve around age 50, i.e. the time of the menopause and decline of ovarian hormone production.

Age at menarche and menopause
An age at menarche of 12 years or earlier, as compared to 16 years or later, is associated with a 50–70% greater risk. Every 1-year increment in the age at menopause confers an approximately 3% increased risk[13]. Premature oophorectomy, performed before age 40, affords about a 50% reduced risk as compared to natural menopause.

Parity and age at first full-term pregnancy
To have given birth, relative to remaining nulliparous, is associated with a considerable protective effect. The magnitude of risk reduction is greater the earlier the first birth takes place. Each additional birth enhances the protective effect by some 15%[14]. A first full-term pregnancy actually gives rise to a *dual* effect: an initial risk increase during about 10–15 years after the birth and a subsequent long-term decrease. The net effect of a birth is usually protective; the later the first child is born, the more pronounced is the initial risk increase and the longer it takes before the protective effect occurs[15].

Stature
Tall stature is a risk factor for breast cancer. It is believed to reflect effects of nutritional status and the action of growth hormones during adolescence.

Body build
A high body mass index (BMI) is linked to a lowered risk in premenopausal women, but an increased risk in postmenopausal women. Obesity is believed to lower breast cancer risk in premenopausal women through an increase in anovulatory cycles (less progesterone production), and to elevate the risk in postmenopausal women through an enhanced production of estrogens in fat tissue. In some recent studies, a gain in weight has been associated with an increase in breast cancer risk[16].

Diet
Fat intake has long been assumed to be a risk factor, but studies have failed to find any evidence of a link in adult life[17]. Aspects of nutrition may be important during the adolescent period or intrauterine life – issues that are attracting increasing interest in research. There are indications that vegetables and fruit, olive oil and soy-based food may prevent breast cancer through antioxidant properties[17].

Alcohol intake
In several studies, regular intake of high amounts of alcohol has been associated with an excess risk, supposedly through elevation of endogenous estrogen levels[18].

Serum hormone levels
Improved laboratory assays have enabled more accurate measurements to be made of sex hormone levels in postmenopausal women. Both prospective cohort and retrospective case-control studies have shown a positive relationship between serum levels of estradiol, estrone and testosterone, and lowered levels of sex hormone binding globulin (SHBG), and postmenopausal breast cancer[19].

Physical exercise
Some studies have reported a decreased risk following rigorous physical exercise during adolescence

or during adult life. However, the evidence for this association is rather weak. Hypothesized mechanisms include a delay in age at menarche or reduced estrogen production by the ovaries[20,21].

Exogenous hormones

The use of exogenous hormones, both as combined oral contraceptives (COCs) in young women and for hormone replacement therapy (HRT) in postmenopausal women, has increased dramatically since the 1970s. Since these treatments entail long-term exposure to potent estrogens (often combined with progestins) in healthy women, there is concern that there may be adverse effects on breast cancer risk.

Combined oral contraceptives The original data from 50 epidemiological studies, including about 53 000 cases and 100 000 control subjects, were reanalyzed in a collaborative effort[22]. The key finding was a small (about 25%) increased risk of breast cancer for women under the age of 35, who had used COCs for 5 years or longer, predominantly for early-stage tumors. The association vanished 5 years after cessation of the treatment. The interpretation is not clear-cut, since the observed risk relationships may partly be explained by an earlier diagnosis of breast cancer in women taking COCs. These results, if valid, would translate into very minor effects in terms of absolute risk. For example, among 10 000 women treated with COCs for 5 years between the ages of 25 and 29, five new cases could be attributed to the exposure.

Hormone replacement therapy The data from about 50 studies including over 50 000 breast cancer cases and almost 100 000 control women were collaboratively reanalyzed[23]. Intake of replacement estrogens for 5 years or more was associated with about a 60% elevated risk, predominantly for early breast cancers. This risk relationship disappeared 5 years after treatment had been stopped. Further, the excess risk was verfied only in women with a normal or lean body build. The use of added progestins was infrequently reported, or information was not available in the source data. These results imply, in terms of absolute risk, that among 1000 women treated for 15 years, 12 new cases would be expected on account of this exposure.

Several studies have in recent years provided data on the effects of different estrogens, dosages and, importantly, their combinations with progestins. A duration-dependent risk increase after current or recent intake of both conjugated estrogens and estradiol compounds has been confirmed, with relative risk estimates ranging from 1.5 to 3 after 6–10 years of intake[19,24]. A growing number of studies have shown that added progestins do not seem to reduce or eliminate the excess risk associated with estrogen replacement. A recent Swedish study suggests that an adverse effect may persist long after discontinuation of treatment, and further that addition of progestins may enhance the risk above that for estrogens alone[24].

Data on the prognosis of breast cancer in women exposed to HRT are scarce and difficult to interpret, owing to a possible surveillance bias. There is support of the findings that breast cancers occurring after HRT are predominantly estrogen receptor-positive[25] and are associated with favorable charcteristics[26] and survival[27], and that there is little or no effect on mortality[28].

Prospects for prevention

Primary prevention

Prospects for prevention presuppose that the risk factors described above are causally related to breast cancer and that the factors can be effectively modified. Theoretically, it may be possible to modify aspects of lifestyle to prevent some breast cancer cases from occurring, e.g. to change diet in early life or during pregnancy, to maintain weight and avoid obesity in adult life, to reduce alcohol intake and to increase the level of physical exercise. A change in reproductive behavior towards earlier births and more children is not feasible. The use of HRT needs to be carefully considered, by weighing benefits against risks and by designing the safest possible treatment regimens.

Secondary prevention

Early detection and treatment may reduce the mortality due to breast cancer. Programs to teach breast self-examination have not proved to be efficient[29]. However, a mortality-reducing effect of mammography screening programs has been documented.

In Sweden, breast cancer mortality was reduced 30% in women participating in breast screening at ages 50–75 years and after 8 years of follow-up[30].

A recent study provides evidence that chemoprevention may be a possibility: treatment with anti-estrogens (tamoxifen) may lower the incidence of breast cancer in high-risk women[31].

ENDOMETRIAL CANCER

Burden

Cancer of the endometrium (corpus uteri) is the second most common gynecological cancer, with about 140 000 new cases per year in the world[1]. In Western countries, the cumulative incidence rates range from 1 to 2% (up to age 75), whereas figures in Asia are lower, for instance in China (0.2%). In Japan, both the incidence and the mortality are rising, whereas in most other countries mortality is declining. Endometrial cancer generally has a favorable clinical course, the 5-year average survival being about 75%[32].

Risk factors

It is established that estrogens cause endometrial cancer, the mechanism being an enhanced and long-standing proliferation of endometrial cells leading to a gradual development of the endometrium into hyperplasia and neoplasia. This is true for the majority of endometrial cancers, so-called type I, estrogen-related tumors[33]. The preponderance of risk factors reflects exposure to estrogens without an adequate opposition by progesterone[34].

Age

The incidence starts to increase at about 40 years of age, rising to a maximum at about 65–70 years. Interestingly, the rate of incidence increase becomes slower at the age of 50, i.e. about the time of the menopause.

Parity

A large number of studies have shown an inverse relationship between parity and risk, an effect attributed to high levels of placental progesterone during pregnancy. Nulliparity *per se* may be a risk factor, when associated with anovulatory infertility, i.e. exposure to unopposed estrogens[35].

Age at menopause

Like irregular menstrual cycles, a late menopause is a marker for a prolonged period of progesterone-unopposed estrogen exposure that gives rise to an increased risk.

Body build

Adult obesity is a consistently reported risk factor. It most importantly acts through an enhanced production of estrogens in the fat tissue of postmenopausal women.

Diabetes

Non-insulin-dependent diabetes mellitus is associated with an increased risk. This relationship is independent of the BMI (obesity), indicating that some other endocrine characteristic is operative, hypothetically elevated androgen and lowered SHBG levels[36].

Hypertension

Hypertension has been suggested to be an independent risk factor. However, data from recent studies indicate that it is rather part of a metabolic syndrome that is associated with endometrial cancer risk.

Cigarette smoking

The preponderance of evidence suggests that current cigarette smoking reduces endometrial cancer risk, the mechanism being an upregulation of estrogen metabolic liver enzymes resulting in reduced estrogen levels[37].

Endogenous estrogens

The polycystic ovary syndrome and estrogen-producing ovarian tumors, both entailing persistent production of unopposed estrogens, have been associated with an increased risk[37,38]. Further, high levels of estradiol, estrone and androstenedione in postmenopausal women have been associated with endometrial cancer risk[39].

Exogenous hormones

Combined oral contraceptives A remarkably consistent finding is the up to 40% reduced risk for endometrial cancer after a few years of COC intake, an effect persisting long after discontinuation of intake[40]. A recent study in women aged 50–74 years verified a protective effect, even decades after cessation of treatment[41]. The addition of a progestin during 3 out of 4 weeks is probably responsible for this remarkable effect.

Hormone replacement therapy A substantial duration-dependent increase in the risk is documented for women taking estrogens without progestins[34]. Numerous studies reported from the late 1970s show that the risk, pertaining predominantly to early and well-differentiated tumors, is increased about ten-fold after 10 years of intake of estrogens. Women developing tumors after HRT seem to have no change of survival.

Since the 1980s, progestins have increasingly been added to estrogens in order to protect the endometrium from development of hyperplasia and neoplasia. Different regimens have been used, e.g. cyclic (for 7–12 days of the cycle) or continuous. In a few recent studies, cyclic addition for less than 10 days was associated with a risk increase compared with non-users[42,43]. In a Swedish study there was evidence of a 60% excess risk also after addition for 10 days of a progestin, but a lowered risk compared to untreated women when the progestin had been added during all days of the treatment cycle[44]. Thus, progestins can counteract the carcinogenic effect of estrogens on the endometrium or even exert an absolute protective effect, depending on the number of days the progestins are added.

Tamoxifen
Tamoxifen has been classified as a carcinogen[45], owing to its effect in increasing the incidence of endometrial cancer[46]. The mechanism of action is proposed to be an agonistic estrogenic effect selectively in the endometrium.

Prevention

Modification of some risk factors may be possible. Avoiding obesity and ensuring treatment of anovulation with progestins could prevent some endometrial cancers from occurring. Further, one important benefit of oral contraceptive use is a long-lasting reduced risk for endometrial cancer. As for HRT, regimens for estrogen–progestin combinations could be designed so that risk is reduced.

There are no established methods for early detection that have been applied on a population level.

OVARIAN CANCER

Globally, ovarian cancer is the fifth most common cancer among women and the most frequent gynecological cancer, with about 165 000 cases per year worldwide[1]. Incidence rates are the highest in Scandinavia, with cumulative incidence rates up to 2%, intermediate in the USA and the lowest, but fastest increasing, in Japan[2]. Ovarian cancer is an important public health problem, since most of these cancers are diagnosed at an advanced stage, entailing as poor an average 5-year survival as 40% or less.

Reproductive risk factors

Hormone-related risk factors have recently been reviewed[47].

Menstruation
Several studies found a weak increase in risk with young age at menarche; others found no link. An increase for late age at menopause has been reported in retrospective studies, but was not verified in cohort studies. One popular hypothesis, although with weak evidence, is that the lifetime number of ovulations (from menarche to menopause) is related to ovarian cancer risk.

Parity and lactation
Preventive effects of a full-term pregnancy and prolonged lactation are documented. Parous women have a 30–70% lower risk as compared with nulliparous women. Lactation may confer a small

additional protective effect. Infertility, among women who never become pregnant, seems to be associated with an increased risk[48]. A late age at birth of a first child has been reported to confer a greater protective effect as compared with an early age[49], a finding, however, without confirmation in other studies.

Tubal ligation and hysterectomy

These procedures may, according to several studies, protect against ovarian cancer[47]. The mechanism is unclear; one theory suggests that the ovarian hormone production is compromised, another that ovulations are diminished and a third that retrograde blood flow is prevented.

Exogenous hormones

Combined oral contraceptives COCs confer a substantial and persistent reduction of ovarian cancer risk. Protection is observed after only a few years of intake, regardless of age at diagnosis. There are uncertainties regarding subtypes of tumors; prevention has not yet been clearly established for borderline or mucinous tumors. Further, the impact of modern low-dose COCs has not yet been studied. An overview of available studies reveals that 5 years of COC intake is associated with a 50% reduced risk, an effect persisting for at least 10 years after use has been stopped[50].

Hormone replacement therapy Replacement hormones may influence ovarian cancer risk, because of gonadotropin suppression or possibly because of direct hormonal effects. Nine epidemiological studies were evaluated in a recent meta-analysis[51]. Two of the studies showed a 70–80% increased risk of invasive cancer after about 10 years of estrogen intake[52,53], while the others showed a weaker (non-significant) positive effect, or no risk change. The meta-analysis yielded an estimate of about a 30% increased risk. These data, regarding replacement with estrogens alone, do not allow for a firm conclusion to be drawn about the effects of HRT on ovarian cancer risk. However, because of the newly arisen concern, more data from new studies are needed.

Infertility treatment

Hormonal regimens to induce ovulation in infertile women were introduced in the early 1970s. There is concern that hormonal infertility treatment may increase ovarian cancer risk. A pooled analysis of three studies conducted in the USA suggested a vastly increased risk for women exposed to 'fertility drugs', particularly if there was no subsequent birth[54]. The report was criticized but attracted much attention. One subsequent study, with a small number of ovarian tumors of mixed types, showed a small excess risk after clomiphene intake[55]. Another investigation of relatively young women who had received *in vitro* fertilization (IVF) treatments, found no effect on risk[56]. Lastly, a study from Canada[57] and one from Denmark[58] found no association. A crucial problem in these studies was the difficulty in separating the effects of infertility from those of the hormonal treatment.

Even though the latest reports give reassuring results, no firm conclusion can be drawn at present. Further, there are yet no meaningful data on the consequences of modern high-dose IVF regimens.

Etiological hypotheses

The etiology of ovarian cancer is still poorly understood. Risk factors observed in epidemiological studies have been considered compatible with two main hypotheses regarding mechanisms: the incessant ovulation and the gonadotropin theories. The former suggests that each ovulation traumatizes the ovarian epithelium and that the healing process entails increased cell division activity and an increased likelihood for entrapment of epithelial cells in the ovarian stroma that is rich in growth factors. The latter theory predicts that high levels of gonadotropins increase cancer risk by directly stimulating growth of the epithelium. Other, newer, hypotheses suggest that retrograde menstruations carry carcinogens to the ovary[59], that sex hormones exert direct effects on the ovarian epithelium to clear away premalignant cells[49] and that estrogens enhance while progesterone reduces epithelial proliferation[60].

Prevention

The most important preventive factor is childbearing, an aspect of lifestyle that may not be possible to modify. Use of COCs, clearly preventive at least for subtypes of ovarian cancer, may for this reason be positively advised. Recent research suggests that the type and content of HRT regimens may play a role in ovarian cancer risk; the safest possible regimens need to be investigated.

Screening to detect ovarian cancer at an early stage by use of tumor markers and ultrasound examinations is being evaluated[61]. There is no consensus whether such an activity can be regarded as cost effective. Prevention of ovarian cancer clearly remains a challenge.

CERVICAL CANCER

Burden

Cervical cancer is the most frequent gynecological cancer in the world, with some 370 000 new cases per year[1]. The highest rates are seen in developing countries, whereas in developed countries the burden has been decreasing substantially, in terms of both incidence and mortality. For countries that introduced screening programs early on, such as Sweden and Iceland[62], a particularly strong reduction in the incidence has been noted.

Risk factors

Sexual activity
Epidemiological studies have documented an adverse effect of sexual activity on cervical cancer risk, e.g. early age at onset of activity and high number of sexual partners.

Human papilloma virus infection
Sexual activity reflects the real causal agent, i.e. the human papilloma virus (HPV) of certain types that can cause transformation of squamous epithelial cells into premalignant lesions and eventually into malignant lesions[63].

Births
In some studies the number of births is related to cervical cancer risk. It is not clear, however, that this effect is independent from that of sexual activity.

Exogenous hormones

Combined oral contraceptives A few studies have reported that women taking COCs are at an increased risk of cervical cancer, even after sexual activity is taken into account[64]. It is assumed that contraceptive steroids may increase the susceptibility of the cervical epithelium to infection by HPV.

Hormone replacement therapy There is no evidence that replacement hormones affect cervical neoplasia risk.

Prevention

Primary prevention could most probably be accomplished by avoiding sexually transmitted HPV infections, through the use of barrier contraceptive methods (e.g. condoms, diaphragms). This has, however, not been clearly documented.

PAP-smear screening and removal of cervical intraepithelial neoplasia, as practiced in several countries, has been documented to reduce both incidence and mortality from cervical cancer[62].

COLON CANCERS

Burden

Cancer of the colon constitutes the second most frequent cancer in women worldwide, with over 380 000 reported cases per year[1]. The cumulative incidence rates vary among countries, with the highest rates in Japan (4.2%) and in the USA (3.1–6.7%)[2]. In most countries, a trend of an increasing incidence in recent decades is observed, particularly in Japan. Mortality, however, has generally been decreasing.

Risk factors

Genetic
The adenomatous polyposis (FAP) and non-polyposis colorectal cancer (HNPCC) syndromes predispose towards colon cancer. These syndromes, caused by inherited mutations in the

mismatch repair and the APC genes, account for less than 5% of all colon cancers[65].

Sex
The incidence of colon cancer is similar between men and women up to the age of about 50; at higher ages women have a lower incidence compared to men.

Nulliparity
Early studies showed an increased risk of colon cancer in nuns, but effects of parity have not been reproduced in subsequent studies.

Physical activity
Among both men and women, high levels of physical activity may decrease the risk of colon cancer by as much as 50%[66]. Physical activity has also been shown to reduce the risk of adenomatous polyps, suggesting an effect of physical activity in the early stages of the carcinogenous process[67]. Mechanisms for a protective effect include a decrease in gastrointestinal transit time, reduction of insulin levels and alteration of prostaglandin levels[65].

Obesity
In both men and women, obesity is associated with an increased risk of polyps and colon cancer[68]. One possible mechanism is an elevated level of insulin or of other growth factors associated with obesity.

Diet
Use over many years of multivitamin drugs and frequent ingestion of vegetables and fruit have seemed to reduce the risk of colon cancer by 30–50%[69,70]. Further, foods rich in fiber may afford protection, in addition to that of fruit and vegetables[71]. Suggested mechanisms of protection from fruit and vegetables include reduction of proliferation, antioxidation, induction of enzymes handling carcinogens and an increase in stool bulk with a decrease in transit time. High intake of red meat appears to increase the risk of colon cancer[72], possibly due to the presence of carcinogens in cooked meat and high concentrations of iron, generating free radicals[73].

Alcohol and tobacco use
The majority of studies have reported an association between alcohol intake and an increased risk of colon cancer[65]; in some studies a dose-response relationship was found. Long-term cigarette smoking may increase the risk of both colon cancer and colorectal adenoma[74]. However, this finding is not consistent among studies.

Hormone use
Use of replacement hormones may be beneficial, as indicated in a recent meta-analysis[75]. A 20% reduction in colon cancer risk was suggested for women who had ever taken HRT, the protective effect being the greatest with recent intake, whereas the effect of duration of intake was unclear. A lowered risk was also indicated for women taking COCs[76]. The hypothesis is that exogenous estrogens may influence colon cancer risk by altering bile acid production, DNA methylation and levels of insulin-like growth factor (IGF-1).

Prevention

The reported risk factors leave prospects for prevention. Suggested measures for primary prevention include changes in lifestyle factors towards increasing physical activity, consuming less red meat and alcohol, and more vitamins, vegetables, fruit and fiber and avoiding obesity. HRT may be protective but the present state of knowledge does not allow recommendations to be made.

There are tools – fecal blood detection and colonoscopy – for early detection of both adenomatous polyps and carcinomas[65], but the cost efficiency of screening needs to be evaluated.

It has been estimated that changes in lifestyle and population-based screening could accomplish a substantial reduction of colon cancers[65].

SUMMARY AND CONCLUSIONS

Cancers of the breast, endometrium, ovary, cervix and colon clearly have an important impact on women's health worldwide, in terms of their burden on incidence and mortality. Our understanding of the causes of these cancers is far from complete. However, the present state of knowledge does give clues on biological mechanisms and for continued research. At present, some prospects for prevention may be proposed. Changes in lifestyles regarding physical activity, diet and perhaps reproductive behavior, and also use of safe hormonal treatments, are possibilities for primary prevention. For secondary prevention, methods are available for screening of early lesions in the breast, uterine cervix and colon that may enable curative treatment and reduction of mortality. Urgent topics for research include the identification of risk factors acting early in life and of meaningful aspects of diet and lifestyle that can be modified, and finally the investigation of chemical agents to prevent breast cancer, for instance.

References

1. Parkin DM. The global burden of cancer. *Cancer Biol* 1998;8:219–35
2. Waterhouse J, Muir C, Correa P. Cancer incidence in five continents. *IARC Sci Publ* 1992;6:120
3. Yu H, Harris RE, Gao YT, Gao R, Wynder EL. Comparative epidemiology of cancers of the colon, rectum, prostate and breast in Shanghai, China versus the United States. *Int J Epidemiol* 1991;20:76–81
4. Lipworth L. Epidemiology of breast cancer. *Eur J Cancer Prev* 1995;4:7–30
5. Hulka BS, Liu ET, Lininger RA. Steroid hormones and risk of breast cancer. *Cancer* 1994;74:1111–24
6. Kelsey JL. A review of the epidemiology of human breast cancer. *Epidemiol Rev* 1979;1:74–109
7. Johannsson O, Ostermeyer EA, Håkansson S, *et al.* Founding BRCA1 mutations in hereditary breast and ovarian cancer in Southern Sweden. *Am J Hum Genet* 1996;58:441–50
8. Trichopoulos D. Hypothesis: does breast cancer originate *in utero*? *Lancet* 1990;335:939–40
9. Adami HO, Signorello LB, Trichopoulos D. Towards an understanding of breast cancer etiology. *Semin Cancer Biol* 1998;8:255–62
10. Ekbom A, Trichopoulos D, Adami HO, Hsieh CC, Lan SJ. Evidence of prenatal influences on breast cancer risk. *Lancet* 1992;340:1015–18
11. Michels KB, Trichopoulos D, Robins JM, *et al.* Birthweight as a risk factor for breast cancer. *Lancet* 1996;348:1542–6
12. Ekbom A, Thurfjell E, Hsieh CC, Trichopoulos D, Adami HO. Perinatal characteristics and adult mammographic patterns. *Int J Cancer* 1995;61: 177–80
13. Pike MC, Krailo MD, Henderson BE, Casagrande JT, Hoel DG. 'Hormonal' risk factors, 'breast tissue age' and the age-incidence of breast cancer. *Nature (London)* 1983;303:767–70
14. Magnusson CM, Persson IR, Baron JA, Ekbom A, Bergström R, Adami HO. The role of reproductive factors and use of oral contraceptives in the aetiology of breast cancer in women aged 50 to 74 years. *Int J Cancer* 1999;80:231–6
15. Lambe M, Hsieh C, Trichopoulos D, Ekbom A, Pavia M, Adami HO. Transient increase in the risk of breast cancer after giving birth. *N Engl J Med* 1994; 331:5–9
16. Magnusson C, Baron J, Persson I, *et al.* Body size in different periods of life and breast cancer risk in post-menopausal women. *Int J Cancer* 1998;76: 29–34
17. Hunter DJ, Willett WC. Diet, body size, and breast cancer. *Epidemiol Rev* 1993;15:110–32
18. Hankinson SE, Willett WC, Manson JE, *et al.* Alcohol, height, and adiposity in relation to estrogen and prolactin levels in postmenopausal women. *J Natl Cancer Inst* 1995;87:1297–302
19. Colditz GA. Relationship between estrogen levels, use of hormone replacement therapy, and breast cancer. *J Natl Cancer Inst* 1998;90:814–23
20. Petridou E, Syrigou E, Toupadaki N, Zavitsanos X, Willett W, Trichopoulos D. Determinants of age at menarche as early life predictors of breast cancer risk. *Int J Cancer* 1996;68:193–8
21. Kramer MM, Wells CL. Does physical activity reduce risk of estrogen-dependent cancer in women? *Med Sci Sports Exerc* 1996;28:322–34
22. Collaborative Group on Hormonal Factors in Breast Cancer. Breast cancer and hormonal contraceptives: collaborative reanalysis of individual data on 53 297 women with breast cancer and 100 239

women without breast cancer from 54 epidemiological studies. *Lancet* 1996;347:1713-27
23. Collaborative Group on Hormonal Factors in Breast Cancer. Breast cancer and hormone replacement therapy: collaborative reanalysis of data from 51 epidemiological studies of 52,705 women with breast cancer and 108,411 women without breast cancer. *Lancet* 1997;350:1047-59
24. Magnusson C, Baron JA, Correia N, Bergström R, Adami HO, Persson IR. Breast-cancer risk following long-term oestrogen and oestrogen-progestin replacement therapy. *Int J Cancer* 1999;81:339-44
25. Potter JD, Cerhan JR, Sellers TA, *et al.* Progesterone and estrogen receptors and mammary neoplasia in the Iowa Women's Health Study: how many kinds of breast cancer are there? *Cancer Epidemiol Biomarkers Prev* 1995;4:319-26
26. Magnusson C, Holmberg L, Nordén T, Lindgren A, Persson I. Prognostic characteristics in breast cancers after hormone replacement therapy. *Br Cancer Res Treat* 1996;38:325-39
27. Bergkvist L, Adami H-O, Persson I, Bergström R, Krusemo UB. Prognosis after breast cancer diagnosed in women treated with menopausal estrogens. *Am J Epidemiol* 1989;130:221-8
28. Yuen J, Persson I, Bergkvist L, Hoover R, Schairer C, Adami H-O. Hormone replacement therapy and breast cancer mortality in Swedish women: results after adjustment for 'healthy drug user effect'. *Cancer Causes Control* 1993;4:369-74
29. Thomas DB, Gao DL, Self SG, *et al.* General issues in breast cancer. Randomized trial of breast self-examination in Shanghai: methodology and preliminary results. *J Natl Cancer Inst* 1997;89: 355-65
30. Nyström L, Rutqvist LE, Wall S, *et al.* Breast cancer screening with mammography: overview of Swedish randomised trials. *Lancet* 1993;341:973-8
31. Fisher B, Costantino JP, Wickerham DL, *et al.* Tamoxifen for prevention of breast cancer: report of the National Surgical Adjuvant Breast and Bowel Project P-1 Study. *J Natl Cancer Inst* 1998;90: 1371-88
32. Coleman MP, Esteve J, Damiecki P, Arslan A, Renard H. Trends in cancer incidence and mortality. *IARC Sci Publ* 1993;121:1-806
33. Deligdisch L, Holinka CF. Endometrial carcinoma: two diseases? *Cancer Detect Prev* 1987;10:237-46
34. Grady D, Gebretsadik T, Kerlikowske K, Ernster V, Petitti D. Hormone replacement therapy and endometrial cancer risk: a meta-analysis. *Obstet Gynecol* 1995;85:304-13
35. Henderson BE, Casagrande JT, Pike MC, Mack T, Rosario I, Duke A. The epidemiology of endometrial cancer in young women. *Br J Cancer* 1983; 47:749-56
36. Kaaks R. Nutrition, hormones, and breast cancer: is insulin the missing link? *Cancer Causes Control* 1996;7:605-25
37. Grady D, Ernster V. Endometrial cancer. In *Cancer Epidemiology and Prevention*, 2nd edn. New York: Oxford University Press, 1996:1058-89
38. Björkholm E, Pettersson F. Granulosa-cell and theca-cell tumors. The clinical picture and long-term outcome for the Radiumhemmet series. *Acta Obstet Gynecol Scand* 1980;59:361-5
39. Sherman ME, Sturgeon S, Brinton LA, *et al.* Risk factors and hormone levels in patients with serous and endometrioid uterine carcinomas. *Mod Pathol* 1997;10:963-8
40. Hormonal contraception and post-menopausal hormonal therapy. *IARC Monographs on the Evaluation of Carcinogenic Risks to Humans*, Vol. 72. Lyon, France: IARC, 1999
41. Weiderpass E, Adami H, Baron J, Magnusson C, Lindgren A, Persson I. Use of oral contraceptives and endometrial cancer risk. *Cancer Causes Control* 1999;10:277-84
42. Beresford SA, Weiss NS, Voigt LF, McKnight B. Risk of endometrial cancer in relation to use of oestrogen combined with cyclic progestagen therapy in postmenopausal women. *Lancet* 1997; 349:458-61
43. Pike MC, Peters RK, Cozen W, *et al.* Estrogen-progestin replacement therapy and endometrial cancer. *J Natl Cancer Inst* 1997;89:1110-16
44. Weiderpass E, Adami H-O, Baron JA, *et al.* Risk of endometrial cancer following estrogen replacement with and without progestins. *J Natl Cancer Inst* 1999;91:1131-7
45. Some pharmaceutical drugs. Lyon, France, 13-20 February 1996. *IARC Monogr Eval Carcinog Risks Hum* 1996;66:35-445
46. Early Breast Cancer Trialists' Collaborative Group. Tamoxifen for early breast cancer: an overview of the randomised trials. *Lancet* 1998;351:1451-67
47. Riman T, Persson I, Nilsson S. Hormonal aspects of epithelial ovarian cancer: review of epidemiological evidence. *Clin Endocrinol (Oxf)* 1998;49: 695-707
48. Mosgaard BJ, Lidegaard O, Kjaer SK, Schou G, Andersen AN. Infertility, fertility drugs, and invasive ovarian cancer: a case-control study. *Fertil Steril* 1997;67:1005-12
49. Adami HO, Hsieh CC, Lambe M, *et al.* Parity, age at first childbirth, and risk of ovarian cancer. *Lancet* 1994;344:1250-4
50. Hankinson SE, Colditz GA, Hunter DJ, Spencer TL, Rosner B, Stampfer MJ. A quantitative assessment of oral contraceptive use and risk of ovarian cancer. *Obstet Gynecol* 1992;80:708-14
51. Garg PP, Kerlikowske K, Subak L, Grady D. Hormone replacement therapy and the risk of epithelial ovarian carcinoma: a meta-analysis. *Obstet Gynecol* 1998;92:472-9
52. Risch HA. Estrogen replacement therapy and risk of epithelial ovarian cancer. *Gynecol Oncol* 1996;63: 254-7

53. Rodriguez C, Calle EE, Coates RJ, Miracle-McMahill HL, Thun MJ, Heath CW Jr. Estrogen replacement therapy and fatal ovarian cancer. *Am J Epidemiol* 1995;141:828-35
54. Whittemore AS, Harris R, Itnyre J. Characteristics relating to ovarian cancer risk: collaborative analysis of 12 US case-control studies. IV. The pathogenesis of epithelial ovarian cancer. Collaborative Ovarian Cancer Group. *Am J Epidemiol* 1992;136: 1212-20
55. Rossing MA, Daling JR, Weiss NS, Moore DE, Self SG. Ovarian tumors in a cohort of infertile women. *N Engl J Med* 1994;331:771-6
56. Venn A, Watson L, Lumley J, Giles G, King C, Healy D. Breast and ovarian cancer incidence after infertility and *in vitro* fertilisation. *Lancet* 1995; 346:995-1000
57. Risch HA, Marrett LD, Howe GR. Parity, contraception, infertility, and the risk of epithelial ovarian cancer. *Am J Epidemiol* 1994;140:585-97
58. Mosgaard BJ, Lidegaard O, Kjaer SK, Schou G, Andersen AN. Infertility, fertility drugs, and invasive ovarian cancer: a case-control study. *Fertil Steril* 1997;67:1005-12
59. Cramer DW, Xu H. Epidemiologic evidence of uterine growth factors in the pathogenesis of ovarian cancer. *Ann Epidemiol* 1995;5:310-14
60. Risch HA. Hormonal etiology of epithelial ovarian cancer, with a hypothesis concerning the role of androgens and progesterone. *J Natl Cancer Inst* 1998;90:1774-86
61. Jacobs IJ, Skates SJ, MacDonald N, *et al.* Screening for ovarian cancer: a pilot randomised controlled trial. *Lancet* 1999;353:1207-10
62. Bergstrom R, Sparen P, Adami HO. Trends in cancer of the cervix uteri in Sweden following cytological screening. *Br J Cancer* 1999;81:159-66
63. Schoell WM, Janicek MF, Mirhashemi R. Epidemiology and biology of cervical cancer. *Semin Surg Oncol* 1999;16:203-11
64. La Vecchia C, Tavani A, Franceschi S, Parazzini F. Oral contraceptives and cancer. A review of the evidence. *Drug Saf* 1996;14:260-72
65. Harvard Report on Cancer Prevention. Volume 3: Prevention of colon cancer in the United States. *Cancer Causes Control* 1999;10:167-80
66. Colditz GA, Cannuscio CC, Frazier AL. Physical activity and reduced risk of colon cancer: implications for prevention. *Cancer Causes Control* 1997;8: 649-67
67. Kahn HS, Tatham LM, Thun MJ, Heath CW Jr. Risk factors for self-reported colon polyps. *J Gen Intern Med* 1998;13:303-10
68. Potter JD, Slattery ML, Bostick RM, Gapstur SM. Colon cancer: a review of the epidemiology. *Epidemiol Rev* 1993;15:499-545
69. Giovannucci E, Stampfer MJ, Colditz GA, *et al.* Multivitamin use, folate, and colon cancer in women in the Nurses' Health Study. *Ann Intern Med* 1998;129: 517-24
70. Thun M, Calle E, Namboordiri M, *et al.* Risk factors for fatal colon cancer in a large prospective study. *J Natl Cancer Inst* 1992;84:1491-500
71. Willett WC. Diet, nutrition and avoidable cancer. *Environ Health Perspect* 1995;103 (Suppl 8): 165-70
72. Giovannucci E, Willett WC. Dietary factors and risk of colon cancer. *Ann Med* 1994;26:443-52
73. Steinmetz KA, Potter JD. Vegetables, fruit, and cancer. I. Epidemiology. *Cancer Causes Control* 1991; 2:325-57
74. Giovannucci E, Martinez ME. Tobacco, colorectal cancer, and adenomas: a review of the evidence. *J Natl Cancer Inst* 1996;88:1717-30
75. Grodstein F, Stampfer MJ, Falkeborn M, Naessen T, Persson I. Postmenopausal hormone therapy and risk of cardiovascular disease and hip fracture in a cohort of Swedish women. *Epidemiology* 1999; 10:476-80
76. Martinez ME, Grodstein F, Giovannucci E, *et al.* A prospective study of reproductive factors, oral contraceptive use, and risk of colorectal cancer. *Cancer Epidemiol Biomarkers Prev* 1997;6:1-5

Aging for men

B. Lunenfeld

In times when the changes around us are accelerating, but our perceptions of these changes are lagging behind, it becomes of crucial importance to have a vision of the future. I will therefore make an attempt to review briefly in this paper some past and present data and, from the lessons learned, attempt to apply these to the most likely projections for the future.

Aging is a triumph, it is a victory of human will, endurance and technology[1]. However, as we near the millennium, new challenges are arising in relation to the lengthening lifespan. How do we use current and evolving technologies to impart a greater quality of life to this increasing time frame?

A rapidly growing and rapidly aging world population is a new feature in the history of mankind[2]. The human race entered the 19th century with a global population of 978 million, the 20th century with 1650 million and will enter the 21st century with a world-wide population of 6168 million. The estimates and projections of the United Nations (UN) indicate that, between 1900 and 2100, the world population will increase seven-fold, from 1.65 billion to 11.5 billion: an increase of almost ten billion people. This rapid increase in world population is despite the fact that effective family planning has significantly reduced fertility rates below the replacement level, and that the fertility rates in ten countries, including Italy, France and Germany, are today well below 1.6 (Table 1).

Due to the prolongation of life expectancy and the drastic reduction in fertility rate, it is projected that the elderly (over 65 years) will increase within the next 25 years by 82%, whereas the newborn population will increase only by 3%. The working age population will increase by only 46%. The UN projects (in its 1998 revision) that, by 2050, the proportion of persons above 60 years will exceed, for the first time, the proportion of children below 15 years, and 13 countries will have more than 10% of the oldest olδ (> 80 years old) in their population. Italy will be leading, with 14%.

Table 1 Total fertility rate per woman (1990–95) and population (1995) in millions in selected European countries. Reproduced with permission from reference 17

Country	*Total fertility rate*	*Population*
Italy	1.24	57.2
Spain	1.27	39.6
Germany	1.30	81.6
Slovenia	1.36	1.9
Greece	1.38	10.5
Austria	1.47	8.0
Romania	1.50	22.7
Portugal	1.52	9.8
Russian Federation	1.53	148.5
Bulgaria	1.53	8.5
Switzerland	1.53	7.2
Netherlands	1.59	15.5

The marked increase in the population of elderly in relation to the working age population will be compounded by a simultaneous decrease in the population of children, who will constitute the working age population of the next generation. Thus, a declining labor force will have to support an increasing number of elderly.

The 20th century has been marked by the triumph of prolonging life, and we have achieved an increase in life expectancy of more than 50% in the last 100 years. The development of antibiotics, vaccines, safer water, better sanitation and better personal hygiene has defeated most infectious diseases.

Life has been prolonged, and acute disease is no longer the major cause of death. Today, one dies from chronic disease, degenerative diseases, metastatic cancer, immunodeficiencies and other diseases that prolong disability, immobility and dependency, and make dying a long, painful and

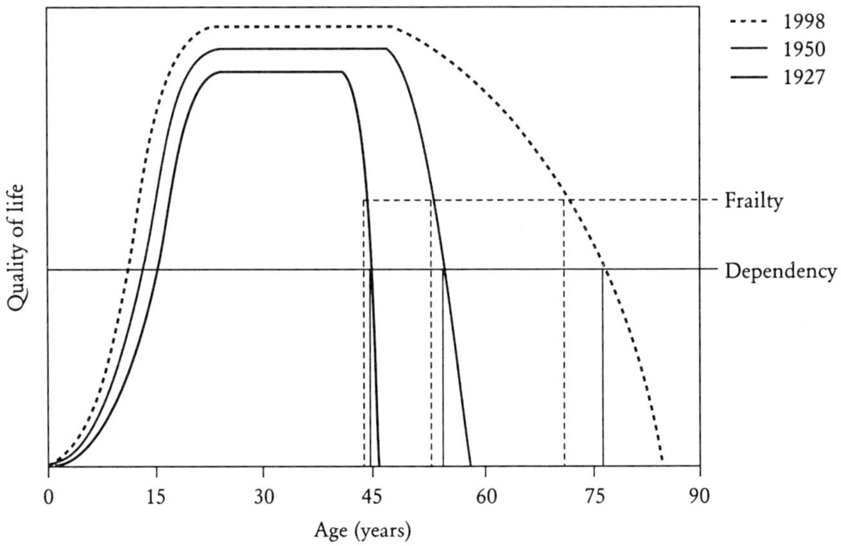

Figure 1 In 1927, the average lifespan was around 45 years and death resulted usually from acute disease. Hospitalization and/or dependency lasted for only days or, at most, weeks. In 1950, the average lifespan was about 58 years and hospitalization or dependency lasted for weeks or months. In 1999, the average lifespan is about 80 years and death results from cancer, degenerative diseases, organ failure or immune deficiencies. Hospitalization or dependency may last months or years

expensive procedure (Figure 1). Therefore, despite the enormous medical progress during the past few decades, 25% of life expectancy after the age of 65 years is spent with some disability, and the last years of life are accompanied by a further increase in incapacity and sickness.

Hence, we must take into account both 'life expectancy' and 'health expectancy' (Table 2). Health authorities should be encouraged to publish both these sets of data, as some already do. The cost of caring for the increasing population of senior citizens will become prohibitive, with the attendant socioeconomic consequences. To prudent health-care administrators, the establishment of preventive measures, rather than concentrating on interventive care, is an important strategic thrust in the overall management of the aging population. Frailty, disability and dependency will increase immensely the demands on the social and health services. The very high cost in relation to these services may strain to the limit the ability of health, social and even political infrastructures, not only of developing countries, but also of the most developed and industrialized nations.

The ability to permit men to age gracefully, maintain independent living, free of disability, for as long as possible is a crucial factor in aging with dignity and would, furthermore, reduce health service costs significantly. To achieve this objective, a holistic approach to the management of aging has to be adopted.

Table 2 Life expectancy (LE) versus health expectancy (HE) in selected countries

Country	*LE*	*HE*	*Difference*
United States	70.1	55.5	14.6
Canada	73.0	67.0	6.0
UK	71.8	58.7	13.1
France	70.7	61.9	8.8
Poland	67.0	60.0	7.0
China	66.6	61.6	5.0

The promotion of healthy aging and the prevention, or drastic reduction, of morbidity and disability of the elderly must assume a central role in the formulation of the health and social policies of many, if not all, countries in the next century. It must emphasize an all-encompassing lifelong approach to the aging process (Figure 2). Specific measures should include the promotion of a healthy lifestyle, including proper nutrition, appropriate exercise, avoidance of smoking and drug and alcohol abuse, social interactions to

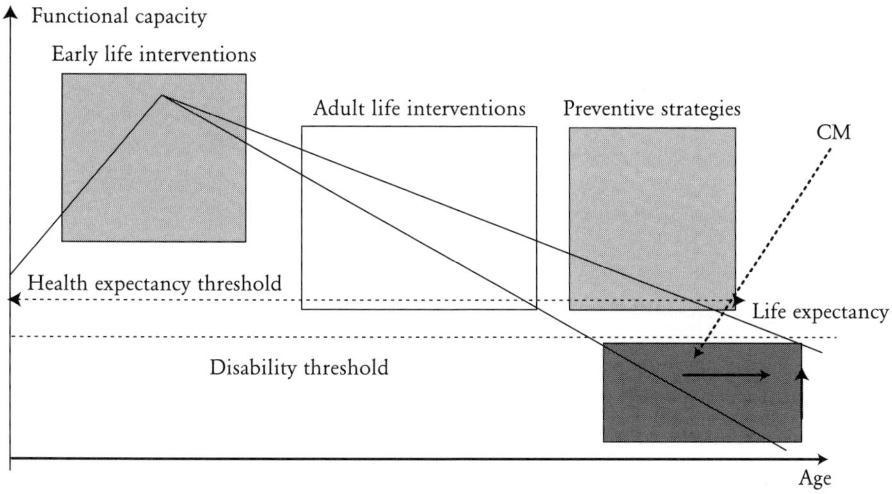

Figure 2 A life-course perspective for maintenance of highest possible level functional capacity and compression of morbidity (CM). Early life interventions should be aimed at maximizing functional capacity, bone mass and optimal body composition. They must include effective vaccination, promotion of a healthy lifestyle with outdoor activities, healthy nutrition and health and sex education. Adult life interventions should aim at maintaining maximal functional capacity and prevent acute diseases, including sexually transmitted diseases. Such interventions must include the promotion of a healthy lifestyle, including physical activity and the promotion of healthy dietary habits (prevention of alcohol abuse, promotion of a low-fat and high-fiber diet, as well as sufficient water, calcium and antioxidant intake, e.g. vitamins A, C and E (see Table 4)). It must encourage the prevention of smoking, since 90% of all lung cancers are attributable to cigarette smoking. Preventive strategies for men over 50 years should aim at maintaining functional capacity, delay frailty (disability threshold) and prevent dependency for as long as possible. These strategies must include the promotion of a healthy lifestyle, as described above. Obesity must be avoided and hypertension controlled. Preventive strategies must also encourage periodic comprehensive clinical screenings, including measurement of prostate-specific antigen and digital rectal examination for prostate and colorectal pathologies. Last, but not least, unsafe living environments should be eliminated or at least modified. Therapeutic interventions must start as soon as a pathological process is diagnosed and should include the control of hypertension, diabetes and osteoporosis, early interventions for benign prostate hypertrophy and urinary or fecal incontinence, hormone replacement therapy whenever hormone deficiencies are detected, and aim at maintaining, restoring or improving sexual function

maintain good mental health, and medical health care, including the control of chronic illnesses. If done effectively, it should result in a significant reduction in the health and social costs, reduce pain and suffering, increase the quality of life of the elderly, and enable them to remain productive and contribute to the well-being of society.

In contrast to the recent and much-needed attention on the social position and health status in women, the health concerns of men have been relatively neglected. Men continue to have higher morbidity and mortality rates for many of the important causes of mortality, and life expectancy for men is significantly shorter than that for women in most regions of the world[3]. The course of disease, response to disease and societal response to illness exhibit gender differences and often result in different treatments and different access to health care.

The major causes of morbidity and mortality all take effect over extended periods. Therefore, primary prevention strategies will be most effective when initiated at the earliest opportunity. Ischemic heart disease, hypertension and stroke, as well as lung cancer, are diseases to which primary prevention needs to be addressed. When problems are more prevalent at older ages, as with prostate and colorectal cancers and osteoporosis, early diagnostic tests, such as appropriate and periodic use of laboratory tests (e.g. prostate-specific antigen) and screening procedures, can play an important role in secondary prevention and self-care strategies[4].

A significant number of male-related health problems, such as changes in body constitution and fat distribution, muscle weakness, urinary incontinence, decay in cognitive functioning, reduction in well-being, depression and sexual dysfunction, could be detected and treated in their early stages if both physician and public awareness of these problems was more pervasive. This could effectively decrease morbidity, frailty and dependency, increase quality of life and reduce health service costs.

When discussing age-related problems, it is often difficult to separate and distinguish between the natural aging process, primarily genetically determined (which today cannot be changed), aging amplifiers, determined by environmental and developmental factors (which can be modified), and an acute or chronic illness or intercurrent diseases (which can be prevented, delayed or cured). It must not be forgotten that aging by itself is associated with reduced productivity and decreased general vigor ('frailty of the aged'), as well as an increased incidence of defined diseases. These include: cardiovascular diseases, malignant neoplasm, chronic obstructive pulmonary diseases, degenerative and metabolic diseases (arthritis, arthrosis, diabetes, osteoporosis, etc.) and visual and hearing loss, as well as various dementias (e.g. Alzheimer's disease), anxiety and mood disorders.

Depression is the most common functional mental disorder affecting aging males; it is underdiagnosed and undertreated. It has a high rate of recurrence and is associated with significantly increased mortality. Depression is closely linked in this group with physical illness, and altered presentation can make diagnosis difficult. Thorough holistic assessment and good communication skills are of utmost importance. Nurses and medical professionals can improve the mental health of these patients with therapeutic attitudes and actions. It must be remembered that about 90% of older men who attempt or complete suicide have depression either not diagnosed or inadequately treated.

However, the most important and drastic gender differences in aging are related to the reproductive organs. In contrast to the course of reproductive aging in women, with the rapid decline in sex hormones and expressed by the cessation of menses, men experience a slow and continuous decline of a large number of hormones, but do not show an irreversible arrest of reproductive capacity in old age[5].

In the aging male, endocrine changes and the decline in endocrine function involve:

(1) Reduced secretory output from the peripheral glands due to the sclerosis of blood vessels (in the interstitial tissue of Leydig cells, this process contributes, for example, to a large extent, to the decrease in gonadal androgens);

(2) Alterations in the central mechanism controlling the temporal organization of hormonal release. The heterogeneity in basal neuroendocrine function during the aging process, reported in the literature, is compounded by the fact that basal hormone levels are far from constant, but fluctuate considerably, due to the interaction of circadian rhythmicity, sleep and, for some of the hormones, intermittent pulsatile releases at different intervals. During aging, a number of morphological and neurochemical alterations have been found in the suprachiasmatic nuclei (the central circadian pacemaker) and are likely to be responsible for the dampened circadian hormonal and nonhormonal rhythms. These are, in part, responsible for the age-dependent decrease in the peripheral levels of testosterone, dehydroepiandrosterone (DHEA), growth hormone (GH), insulin-like growth factor-1 (IGF-1) and melatonin. In addition, sex hormone binding globulin (SHBG) increases with age, resulting in a further lowering of the concentrations of free biologically active androgens. Since, however, some Leydig cell function persists during aging, *stricu sensu* the andropause does not exist.

However, a growing body of literature supports the viewpoint that a true decrease in gonadal and adrenal bioavailable androgens[6,7], as well as of GH[8], develops in most aging men and results in 'partial endocrine deficiencies'. The partial endocrine deficiency syndrome of the aging male (PEDAM) may be associated with a broad spectrum of symptoms:

(1) A decrease in general well-being;

(2) A decrease in sexual pilosity;

(3) A decrease in libido;

(4) A decrease in cognitive function;

(5) A decrease in red blood cell volume;

(6) A decrease in muscle strength;

(7) Osteoporosis;

(8) A decrease in immunocompetence;

(9) An increase in fat mass and a change in fat contribution and localization;

(10) An increase in cardiovascular accidents.

Moreover, in aging men, melatonin secretion also decreases and the circadian periodicity of melatonin is gradually disrupted. Sleep in these older men is shallow and fragmented[9]. These alterations influence GH secretion in particular, which occurs with deeper stages of sleep (slow-wave sleep). In men, approximately 70% of the daily GH output occurs during early (slow-wave) sleep. During aging, slow-wave sleep and GH secretion decrease with the same chronology, raising the possibility that the peripheral effects of the hyposomatotropism of the elderly may partially reflect age-related alterations in sleep-wake homeostasis. While the association between sleep and GH release has been well documented, there is also evidence indicating that components of the somatotropic axis are involved in regulating sleep[10]. It has been shown that, in elderly men, the decrease in melatonin secretion and the circadian periodicity of melatonin were correlated with:

(1) Mood disorders;

(2) Decay in cognitive functions;

(3) Increase in sleep disorders;

(4) Regulation of platelet production, probably due to an inhibitory effect of melatonin on macrophage-mediated platelet destruction.

The secretion of GH and its tissue mediator, IGF-1, from the anterior pituitary declines with increasing age (somatopause). This observation, together with the changes in body composition associated with organic GH deficiency in adults, has led to the suggestion that the elderly without hypothalamic-pituitary disease are GH deficient and may benefit from GH therapy. However, it must be stressed that the impact of organic disease of the hypothalamic-pituitary axis in the elderly may result in a further reduction in GH secretion of up to 90%. This reduction in GH secretion is sufficient to cause a fall in the serum IGF-1 concentration, abnormal body composition and abnormal bone turnover, although bone mineral density is unaffected[11]. Older men are more sensitive to infections and sepsis, and find it more difficult to cope with sepsis. They respond poorly to healing and the repair of bone fractures. The administration of GH can attenuate the catabolic response to injury, surgery and sepsis.

In cases of endocrine deficiencies, traditional endocrinology aims to replace the missing hormone or hormones with substitutes. It has been demonstrated that interventions, such as hormone replacement therapies and use of antioxidant drugs, may favorably influence some of the pathological conditions in aging men, by preventing the preventable and delaying the inevitable.

A comprehensive medical, psychosocial and lifestyle history, a physical examination and laboratory testing are essential for the diagnosis and management of PEDAM. Acute, chronic or intercurrent diseases must be taken into consideration prior to initiating any hormonal substitution therapy. Hormone substitution should only be performed by physicians with basic knowledge and clinical experience in diagnosis, treatment and monitoring of endocrine deficiencies. Evidence is available that hormone replacement therapy (HRT) reduces cardiovascular disease. With the increase in lifespan, osteoporotic fractures are becoming more frequent in men. The sequelae of skeletal fractures diminish the quality of life, advance dependency and constitute an important public health problem. Hip fractures in men result in a higher mortality than in women. HRT, together with proper nutrition and physical activity targeted at specific muscle groups, may postpone the appearance of osteoporosis and delay or prevent bone fractures. In women, HRT was also shown to delay the onset of Alzheimer's

Table 3 Testosterone supplementation

(1)	Testosterone Depot - 250 mg/2-3 weeks (mixtures of testosterone propionate, isocaproate, decanoate, oroenanthate under development: undecanoate 1000 mg/8-10 weeks bucilate 1000 mg/12-16 weeks MENT 7α-methyl 19-nortestosterone (sustained-release subdermal implants)
(2)	Testosterone oral - undecanoate (160 mg daily) one tablet morning and noon and two in the evening (lymphatic absorption of this product requires it to be taken with meals) under development: sublingual testosterone cyclodextrin 2.5-5 mg twice daily
(3)	Testosterone transdermal - (testosterone in a proprietary, permeation-enhancing vehicle) 2.5-mg or 5-mg patches applied nightly to the back, abdomen, upper arms or thighs; 5 mg daily is comparable to a normal daily production rate
(4)	Testosterone transscrotal - consists of a film containing natural testosterone, 1 mg daily
(5)	Testosterone gels - applicable to the skin

disease. Such information is also urgently needed in men.

Secondary Leydig cell insufficiency in the aging man can often be reversed by stimulation with human chorionic gonadotropin (hCG). However, this kind of therapy is only recommended if the testosterone level doubles within 72 h following the injection of 5000 IU of hCG. In this situation, Leydig cell function can be temporarily restored by weekly injections of 5000 IU hCG. If testosterone levels do not double within 72 h following the injection of hCG, testosterone replacement therapy should be considered (Table 3). Patients with secondary partial androgen deficiency (PADAM) who are older than 40 years of age, receiving supplemental testosterone therapy, should have a clear indication for this therapy (history, physical examination, and laboratory assessment demonstrating a value of < 13 nmol/ml total testosterone, < 3 nmol/ml bioavailable testosterone and < 0.30 nmol/ml free testosterone). Testosterone therapy should also be considered for a trial period of 12 months in men with total testosterone < 15 nmol/l or bioavailable testosterone < 5 nmol/l if these levels coincide with complaints or physical evidence of androgen deficiency. Furthermore, testosterone replacement may be required in patients with a history of hepatitis, or liver cirrhosis with elevated levels of SHBG and clinical signs of androgen deficiency. Prior to the initiation of testosterone therapy, all patients should have a digital rectal examination and a serum prostate-specific antigen level measurement, which should be less than 3 ng/ml and should be repeated within 3 months of the initiation of therapy. If any of the following conditions apply, patients should continue with testosterone therapy and have a digital rectal examination and a prostate-specific antigen determination, lipid profile, hemoglobin and serum calcium at yearly intervals:

(1) Clinical history and physical examination show improvement (body composition, muscle mass and strength, sense of well-being and energy level, as well as an improvement in sexual function and libido);

(2) There is no history of adverse effects, particularly with regard to urinary obstructive symptoms, polycythemia (hematocrit > 42% and platelets < 600 000) and sleep apnea;

(3) No significant increase in prostate-specific antigen is found.

Testosterone administration should be stopped if prostate-specific antigen increases by 2.0 ng/ml at any time or if an increase of 0.75 ng/ml occurs over a 2-year period[4].

Replacement therapies for secondary DHEA deficiency are being developed. A 100-mg daily dose of DHEA for 6 months restored serum DHEA levels to those of young adults and serum DHEA sulfate (DHEAS) levels to those at or slightly above the young adult range[12]. Serum cortisol levels were unaltered and consequently the DHEAS/cortisol ratio was increased to pubertal (10 : 1) levels. Relative to baseline, DHEA administration also resulted in an elevation of serum IGF-1 levels in men (16 ± 6%; $p = 0.04$). Serum levels of insulin-like growth factor binding protein-1 (IGFBP-1) and IGFBP-3 were unaltered, body fat mass decreased 1.0 ± 0.4 kg (6.1 ± 2.6%; $p = 0.02$) and knee muscle strength (15.0 ± 3.3%; $p = 0.02$), as well as lumbar back strength (13.9 ± 5.4%; $p = 0.01$), increased.

Replacement therapy protocols for GH and melatonin deficiencies are currently under development. Within the next few years, standardized indications, effective products and treatment protocols will become available.

The administration of GH induces increases in both bone and lean body mass and a decrease in fatty tissue in elderly men with GH deficiency[13-15]. The dose of GH required to maintain serum IGF-1 levels in the normal range while minimizing side-effects in this group of patients, however, has not been fully assessed. Toogood and Shalet[16] demonstrated that the GH replacement dose in elderly subjects is considerably lower than that required by younger adults with GH deficiency. According to Janssen and colleagues[17], GH therapy at doses of 0.6 and 1.2 IU/day in male and female patients, respectively, is, in general, able to increase serum IGF-1 to the normal range after 12 weeks of treatment, without reaching supranormal levels of serum IGF-1. This dose could, therefore, be a starting dose in GH-deficient elderly patients. None of the low-dose GH-treated patients exhibited supranormal IGF-1 levels[16].

Hormone replacement therapy alone will not suffice to increase muscle strength, decrease fat mass and change the fat contribution and localization in aging men. Proper nutrition and physical exercise targeted at specific muscle groups is mandatory in order to obtain satisfactory results. Moreover, some authors demonstrated that resistance exercise training improved muscle strength and anabolism in older men, and these improvements were not enhanced when exercise was combined with daily GH administration[18].

It goes without saying that a healthy lifestyle with appropriate nutrition and a healthy and safe environment are critically important in preventing or reducing morbidity and disability. An aging male counselling session is not complete until detailed information is obtained on nutritional habits and daily food consumption. Individualized supplementation of antioxidants and vitamins will often be required in men over 50 years of age.

The impact of diet and specific food groups on aging and age-associated degenerative diseases has been widely recognized in recent years (Table 4). The modern concept of the free radical theory of aging takes as its basis a shift in the antioxidant/pro-oxidant balance that leads to increased oxidative stress, dysregulation of cellular function, and aging. In the context of this theory, antioxidants can influence the primary 'intrinsic' aging process, as well as several secondary age-associated pathological processes. Regarding the latter, several epidemiological and clinical studies have revealed potential roles for dietary antioxidants in the age-associated decline of immune function and the reduction of risk of morbidity and mortality from cancer and heart disease. Meydani and co-workers[19] reported that long-term supplementation with vitamin E enhances immune function in aged animals and elderly subjects. The addition of the trace element selenium (60–200 μg/day) to vitamin E is recommended, since this will significantly increase the antioxidant properties. Larry Clark from the University of Arizona claimed that this combination resulted in a significant reduction in prostate, colorectal and lung cancers. These and other observations indicate that, at present, the effects of dietary antioxidants are mainly demonstrated in connection with age-associated diseases in which oxidative stress appears to be intimately involved.

Table 4 Nutrition: low-calorie, low-fat, high-fiber, and vitamin- and mineral-rich diet

(1)	Drink at least 2 l of water per day
(2)	Eat lots of fruit and vegetables
(3)	Be sure you consume sufficient vitamins, especially vitamin C (500 mg), vitamin D (400 IU), vitamin E (200–600 IU), vitamin B complex and folic acid (25 mg) (vitamins C and E act as antioxidants)

Patients can be counselled to start their own 'anti-aging program' by getting more active, starting to exercise, and losing weight if obese. This will lead to tiredness, better sleep and consequently higher GH levels. Melatonin secretion will also rise, provided that the patient does not sleep in front of the television or with full lights. Eating only small portions or nothing at all before going to bed can also increase GH secretion.

Health professionals, educators and elderly men are becoming increasingly aware that libido, interest, capacity and sexual pleasure can remain throughout a lifetime. It was found that persistent interest in sexual activity results in positive mental and physical health benefits. Some men may become less sexually active with age. Reasons for decreased sexual activities include loss of libido (partially due to decreased androgen production), lack of a partner, chronic illness and/or various social and environmental factors, as well as erectile dysfunction. More than 100 million men worldwide are estimated to have some degree of erectile dysfunction. The Massachusetts Male Aging Study reported a combined prevalence of 52% for minimal, moderate and complete impotence in non-institutionalized 40–70-year-old men in the Boston area[20]. Erection is a neurovascular phenomenon under hormonal control and includes arterial dilatation, trabecular smooth muscle relaxation and activation of the corporeal veno-occlusive mechanism. Some of the major etiologies are hypertension, diabetes and heart disease (Table 5). Furthermore, genitourinary and colon surgery, as well as many drugs, particularly antihypertensive and psychotropic drugs, may cause various degrees of erectile dysfunction. When focusing on the maintenance of quality of life among aging men, efforts to maintain, restore or improve sexual function should not be neglected. Recent advances in basic and clinical research have led to the development of new treatment options for erectile dysfunction, including new pharmacological agents for intracavernosal, intraurethral and oral use (Table 6). The management of erectile dysfunction should only be performed following a proper evaluation of the patient and only by physicians with basic knowledge and clinical experience in the diagnosis and treatment of erectile dysfunction.

Men who are educated about the value of preventive health care in prolonging their lifespan, quality of life and their role as productive family members will be more likely to participate in health screening. To achieve this goal, it will be necessary to make available a group of trained medical professionals who can understand, guide, educate and manage the problems of the aging male. The International Society for the Study of the Aging Male (ISSAM) has delegated Parthenon Publishing to publish its official journal (*The Aging Male*), ISSAM Operations to assist in the standardization of protocols and products to be used in the quality of life management of aging men, and the ISSAM Academy to:

(1) Prepare, provide and assess the training curricula especially tailored for different medical specialties;

(2) Assist in the organization of training courses for 'men's health physicians';

(3) Certify such courses;

(4) Accredit those specialists who have qualified as 'men's health physicians'.

ISSAM Operations will assist and collaborate in the formation and medical management of clinics and/or health institutions that wish to include a men's health management program. ISSAM Operations will assist and collaborate with pension funds, insurance companies, and social and welfare institutions to help men to age in health and with dignity.

Table 5 Incidence of erectile dysfunction according to the Massachusetts Male Aging Study. From reference 20

Population	*New cases of erectile dysfunction/ 1000 men per year*
General	26.0
Hypertension	42.5
Diabetes	50.7
Heart disease	58.3

Table 6 Medical management of erectile dysfunction: the revolution!

1982: Virag®, the first injection
1986: Use of prostagladin E_1
1995: Caverject® on the market
1996: Muse® on the market
1998: Sildenafil on the market
Vasomax®

In development:
Oral phentolamine
Spontane® - oral apomorphine
Prostaglandin creams
New phosphodiesterase inhibitors of isoenzymes
New drug acting on different level of the erectile mechanism
Topical treatment
Gene (cell) therapy

Furthermore, there is a need to obtain the essential epidemiological data, to intensify basic and clinical research and to develop new and improved drugs for the prevention and treatment of the pathological changes related to aging. A holistic approach to this new challenge of the 21st century will necessitate a quantum leap in multidisciplinary and internationally co-ordinated research efforts, supported by new partnerships between industry and governments, philanthropic and international organizations. ISSAM, in collaboration with the World Health Organization (WHO), will attempt to co-ordinate such efforts.

ISSAM, in collaboration with WHO, will periodically organize a World Congress on the Aging Male, which will unite practitioners, experts and researchers of medical behavioral and social sciences, as well as providers of services and technologies for the aging population. This forum will provide an opportunity to exchange information, plan research activities, obtain funding and assist in the formulation of national health and social policies. ISSAM, in collaboration with its national affiliates, will periodically organize national and regional meetings and facilitate training courses.

It is my sincere hope that the next few years will enrich us with facts and clarify the state of our present knowledge to permit us to recognize some of the missing links and give us the tools and methodology to design and plan ways to understand the aging of men, help to improve their quality of life, prevent the preventable, and postpone and decrease the pain and suffering of the inevitable.

References

1. Lunenfeld B. Hormone replacement therapy in the aging male. *Aging Male* 1999;2:1-6
2. Diczfalusy E. An aging humankind: is our future behind us. *Aging Male* 1998;1:8-19
3. Lunenfeld B. Aging male. *Aging Male* 1998;1:1-7
4. Tremblay RR, Morales AJ. Canadian practice recommendations for screening monitoring and treating men affected by andropause or partial androgen deficiency. *Aging Male* 1998;1:213-18
5. Kaufman JM, Vermeulen A. Declining gonadal function in elderly men. *Baillieres Clin Endocrinol Metab* 1997;11:289-309
6. Deuschle M, Gotthardt U, Schweiger U, *et al.* With aging in humans the activity of the hypothalamus-pituitary-adrenal system increases and its diurnal amplitude flattens. *Life Sci* 1997;61:2239-46
7. Gooren LJG. Endocrine aspects of aging in the male. *Mol Cell Endocrinol* 1998;145:153-9
8. Holl R, Hartman M, Veldhuis J, Taylor W, Thorner M. Thirty-second sampling of plasma growth hormone in man. Correlation with sleep stages. *J Clin Endocrinol Metab* 1991;72:854-61
9. Copinschi G, Van Cauter E. Effects of ageing on modulation of hormonal secretion by sleep and circadian rhythmicity. *Horm Res* 1995;43:2412-20
10. Van Cauter E, Plat L, Copinschi G. Interrelations between sleep and the somatotropic axis. *Sleep* 1998; 21:553-66
11. Toogood AA, Shalet SM. Ageing and growth hormone status. *Baillieres Clin Endocrinol Metab* 1998; 12:281-96
12. Morales AJ, Haubrich RH, Hwang JY, Asakura H, Yen SS. The effect of six months treatment with a 100 mg daily dose of dehydroepiandrosterone (DHEA) on circulating sex steroids, body composition and muscle strength in age-advanced men and women. *Clin Endocrinol (Oxford)* 1998;49:421-32
13. Casanueva FF, Dieguez C. Interaction between body composition, leptin and growth hormone status. *Baillieres Clin Endocrinol Metab* 1998;12: 297-314
14. Rudman D, Feller AG, Cohn L, Shetty KR, Rudman IW, Draper MW. Effects of human growth hormone on body composition in elderly men. *Horm Res* 1999;36(Suppl 1):73-81
15. Goh VHH, Mu SC, Gao F, Lim LC. Changes in body composition and endocrine and metabolic functions in healthy elderly Chinese men, following growth hormone therapy. *Aging Male* 1999;1: 264-9

16. Toogood AA, Shalet SM. Growth hormone replacement therapy in the elderly with hypothalamic-pituitary disease: a dose-finding study. *J Clin Endocrinol Metab* 1999;84:131-6
17. Janssen YJ, Frolich M, Roelfsema F. A low starting dose of genotropin in growth hormone-deficient adults. *J Clin Endocrinol Metab*, 1997;82:129-35
18. Yarasheski KE, Zachwieja JJ, Campbell JA, Bier DM. Effect of growth hormone and resistance exercise on muscle growth and strength in older men. *Am J Physiol* 1995;268:E268-76
19. Meydani M, Lipman RD, Han SN, *et al.* The effect of a long-term dietary supplementation with antioxidants. *Ann NY Acad Sci* 1998;854:352-60
20. Feldman HA, Goldstein I, Hatzichristou DG, Krane RJ, McKinlay JB. Impotence and its medical psychological correlates; results of the Massachusetts Male Aging Study. *J Urol* 1994;151:54-61

Healthy aging: a gender perspective 10

M. F. Ramashala

The decade of the 1980s heralded a 'coming of age', with world-wide attention focused on population aging and its implications for societal development and the well-being of older persons.

Demographic data indicate that older people comprise the fastest-growing segment of the world population. Since the beginning of the 20th century there has been an eight-fold increase in older persons. This proliferation of older people is not unique to developed countries. Such demographic changes are occurring at various rates throughout the world. In fact, compared to the USA, many countries currently have or expect to experience in the next millennium an even greater percentage of persons aged 75 years and older. Not only is population aging universal, but it is unprecedented. Our generation is the first ever to confront such large numbers of very old people in the population. Prolonged lifespans into the extreme age groups generate large numbers of frail individuals, many of whom experience debilitating illnesses and/or periods of invalidism. However, the degree of incapacitation, vulnerability and powerlessness attributed to the chronic conditions of old age is largely dependent on the social context in which the elderly function and, therefore, the extent of dependency in old age is inseparably linked to such factors as economic, psychological, social and political structures and support systems[1].

Population aging has been facilitated by an admixture of increasing longevity, declining fertility and, in certain countries, immigration. The decline of the younger population during the 1960s contributed considerably to the abrupt and largely unanticipated demographic changes. In the USA, for example, birth rates fell steadily from 3.68 children per female in the 1950s to 1.8 children per female by the late 1970s. This sharp decrease in fertility, however, levelled off in the 1980s and 1990s[2].

During the first half of the 20th century, there were limited gains in life expectancy and these occurred mostly at the younger ages. Any progress was primarily due to better nutrition and public sanitation, the discovery of antibiotics, greater control over acute infectious diseases, and the reduction in the incidence of infant mortality[3]. Beginning in 1940, mortality declined significantly and, since 1970, improvements in longevity have occurred among the middle-aged and older populations. These dramatic changes are 'the legacy of longevity'[4] and its causes and consequences are linked to the health of the aging population. Increasing longevity is caused primarily by changes in lifestyle, social, economic and political environment, sanitation, nutrition and technology. These changes, in turn, affect the structure of social institutions dealing with older persons. Unfortunately, part of the legacy is that precipitous change is occurring in an atmosphere unprepared to cope.

Four trends characterize the older population:

(1) Increasing numbers;

(2) High proportions of elderly in the population;

(3) The proportion of the oldest old is growing most rapidly;

(4) The gender ratio indicates a growing feminization of the elderly.

Longevity has clearly increased between 1900 and 1985[5], with the greatest improvements in age-specific life expectancy among the old[6–8].

While the mandate for this paper is 'Healthy aging: a gender perspective', it is vital that it be placed in context. Kalache[9] noted that the 'most neglected of all developmental issues - and the surest in its progression - is population aging', further observing that this process has been taking place in most of the developed world for several years. Specific to developing countries, Kalache comments that the process of population aging has not captured the attention of the academic community or policy makers. This is largely due to the fact that other pressing problems make it difficult to focus on what is generally considered to be a phenomenon of the developed world. Numerous factors contribute to this relative neglect, among them a widely held fallacy that, in the developing world, the family structure continues to provide appropriate care for elders and that related problems are either minimal or non-existent. This dynamic process, usually referred to as the demographic transition, was first observed in post-industrial revolution European societies in the 19th century. By and large, it was the result of gradual improvements in living standards among most of the population in countries such as France and the UK. With limited contributions from medical technology, people benefited from better housing, public sanitation and improved nutritional status: mortality started to fall and subsequently fertility decreased. Aging is considered to be the long-term consequence of socioeconomic development. Most importantly, by the time a substantial proportion of the population in developed countries reached old age, many of the problems associated with classical underdevelopment had already been solved. In certain cases, resources were therefore potentially available to be diverted to an increasing elderly population. These were relatively affluent societies, with highly educated populations enjoying the best public services in the world. Yet population aging continues to be a significant challenge requiring (proactive and aggressive) societal responses on many fronts. If caring for their elderly remains a challenge for the rich countries that experienced a process of gradual aging over many decades, what then about aging in the developing world[9]? Some of the developed countries do not even have complete data on their aging population.

The demographic transition in many countries of the Third World is now taking place in a much shorter period of time. Unprecedented declines in mortality rates in countries throughout Latin America, Asia and, more recently, Africa are largely the result of the availability of effective treatment and/or the prevention of diseases previously responsible for huge numbers of premature deaths. However, the conditions that lead to these diseases in these countries still prevail and the morbidity they cause continues to be high. Population aging occurring in much of the Third World is not accompanied by real socioeconomic development. There is thus a cost for the failure to address the aging-related problems of any society.

Among the most pernicious and insidious consequences of aging, especially in youth-oriented societies, is the devaluation of the social status 'old'. Devaluation is so prevalent that elders are socialized to expect differential social and medical treatment as a consequence of being older. These expectations permeate not only the structure of social institutions and their participants' perceptions of the elderly, but also the self-concepts of elderly individuals. One emergent expectation is that being old implies being sick. Perhaps the most profound contribution to the 'old-equals-sick' assumption is that biological change through the course of life is an intrinsic property of the individual unaffected by the social context within which aging takes place[10]. This fallacy must be challenged – the aging process does not necessarily imply disease or illness.

The paucity of data on positive health and well-being inhibits our understanding of the health status of older people as a whole. While the majority of older people are in good health and lead full and active lives unhindered by illness or disability, one must admit that health is a major concern in later life. It is the most important factor in predicting life satisfaction[11], in contrast to those of younger age, where material well-being and the family are the most important sources of satisfaction and dissatisfaction. It is common knowledge that women live longer than men: on average, women live 5 years longer in the UK and 7 years longer in the USA. However, they experience substantially more disability than men, so that there is a smaller gender difference in the years of active life expectancy. The expectation of life at birth for women is 78 years in the USA and 77 years in the UK. Black men in the USA, however, have a particularly low expectation of life, 65 years. The gender difference in expectation of life narrows with advancing age to 4 years at the age of 65 in both the UK and the USA. Mortality in later life is lower in the USA than in the UK: at the age of 65 years, Americans can expect to live 2 years longer than the British, but black Americans have the same expectation of life as the British elderly. The mortality advantage of women over men is particularly striking among the young elderly. The higher death rates of men persist to the oldest ages, these being 28% higher for men than women over the age of 85 years. The substantial decline in the mortality rate of older people over the last 30 years has been greater for men than women and for the young elderly. These trends suggest that women's advantage in longevity is decreasing and, in the future, the numerical advantage of women over men in later life may diminish[12].

Following an analysis of causes of death in the USA, Verbrugge[13] concludes that 'Men and women die from fundamentally the same causes, even though their rates (of mortality) differ. In other words the pace of death differs much more than the reasons'. She goes on to show 'striking evidence of women's greater burden from non-fatal disease and men's from fatal disease'. In a study by Bearon[14] women over 65 years of age, ill-health was the most frequently mentioned source of dissatisfaction: 'Many older women voiced concern over non-specific health problems . . . and more specific problems, such as arthritis, knee problems, breathing problems, low blood count and vertigo, that interfere with daily tasks'.

Health is also the dominant concern in considering the future. When asked to think about 'What really matters' in their lives and to describe their wishes and hopes for the future, about three-quarters of the women surveyed referred to their health or that of their husband[14]. Many specifically mentioned concerns about their capacity to look after themselves, maintain independence and avoid becoming a burden on others. Good health was seen as necessary for avoiding dependence.

What, then, does 'healthy aging' mean? In this paper, I subscribe to the approach of Burnside[15]. Health in older women is considered from four perspectives of fitness:

(1) Physical;

(2) Intellectual;

(3) Social;

(4) Purposive.

Burnside emphasizes that it is not health *per se* that is so crucial in women's later lives, but rather their attitudes and their coping strategies to meet new situations, losses and crises. In addition, the responses of others, including medical professionals, are important in enabling older women to live productive lives in spite of adversity.

The term 'healthy aging' is probably a euphemism, since many older people do have varying degrees of health-related problems. The often-quoted World Health Organization's definition of health as 'a state of complete physical, mental and social well-being and not merely the absence of disease or infirmity'[16] rarely applies to the older age cohorts. However, if one views it from a conceptual perspective, it is especially relevant to defining the health of the elderly[17]. People of any age may have some degree of disease, but if they do not 'act' ill, they will describe themselves as being healthy[16]. It is possible that others may view older persons as healthy if they do not take on the sick role.

As early as 1959, the World Health Organization specifically defined health in older persons as best measured in function – degree of fitness rather than extent of pathology may be used as a measure of the amount of services the aged will require from the community. Focusing specifically on the issue of gender and aging, one must be realistic about the odds of healthy aging if the starting point is not health and health promotion beginning in childhood. Lifestyle changes focusing on good health must be the primary focus for everyone.

By the time women reach the age of 85 years or older, there are 220 women to every 100 men. Therefore, 'Does one need to ask if demography shapes, in part, the destiny of older women'[18] if the question of health is not addressed earlier in our lives?

Measuring health at any age is difficult, because there are so many types of measures to choose from. Two measures are considered here: a subjective measure (self-assessed health) and a measure of functional disability. Self-assessed health[19] is closely allied to feelings of well-being and quality of life[20]. Subjective health measures are important to consider, because self-reports of poor health have been found to be associated with early mortality[21,22] and with institutionalization, after controlling for other health and age variables[23].

In the British General Household Survey[24], respondents were asked whether their health had 'on the whole been good, fairly good or not good' over the last year. The proportion of older people who rated their health as 'good' declined with advancing age, but, even among the oldest age group, over a quarter of men and women rated their health as 'good'.

Gender differences in self-reported health are relatively modest and are less important than differences associated with class and financial resources. Nevertheless, in the British General Household Survey[24], older men consistently rated their health as better than women at each age (Figure 1). About 5% more men than women assessed their health as 'good' in age groups below 80. In the USA, gender differences in self-assessed health are smaller than in the UK (Table 1).

A recognition of health differences among those above the age of 65 years has led to the convention of subdividing this period on the basis of chronological age, defining the 'young elderly' as under 75 years of age and the 'old elderly' as over 75 years of age[27-29]. Although this distinction was originally made on the basis of health status, the age of 75 has become accepted uncritically as a concrete cutting point. The distinction between the 'young old' and the 'old old' is now routinely made on the basis not of health status but of chronological age[30]. A further age division is increasingly being drawn, marking off the 'oldest old' or the 'very elderly', defined as those over 85 years of age. Such distinctions are predicated on the assumption that chronological age is the fundamental determinant of health and other aspects of well-being in later life. However, such age-based divisions may simply represent a more refined ageism. Like gender, age should be treated as a sociological, not a biological, construct. For example, there is a need to examine the sociological correlates of poverty and ill-health within specific age–sex groups.

One of the objectives of this Congress is to facilitate the understanding of women's (and men's) experiences within their societal context and to construct non-sexist theories of human development and implications for healthy aging. Sexism and gender bias characterize, for example, psychological research and theory to the extent that unexamined assumptions about the sexes or untested distinctions based on gender enter into hypotheses, norms of adjustment, or coverage of the field[31].

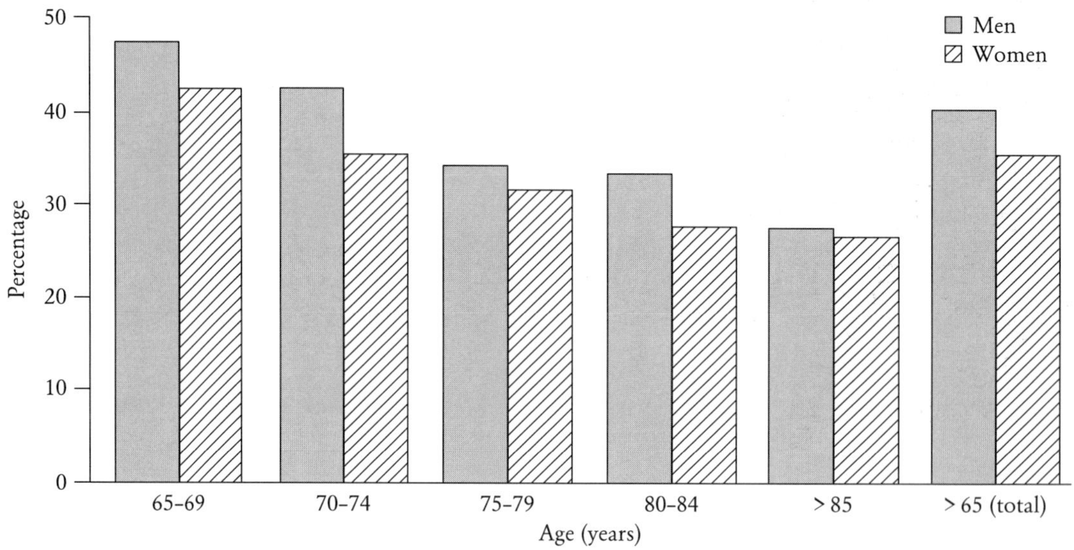

Figure 1 Percentage of elderly men and women reporting 'good health', by 5-year age groups. From reference 24

Table 1 Self-rated health status by age, gender and race in the USA. All values given are percentages. From references 25 and 26

	65–74 years of age		*75–84 years of age*		*> 85 years of age*	
	Men	*Women*	*Men*	*Women*	*Men*	*Women*
All (1986)						
Excellent/very good	40	37	33	35	41	36
Good	33	35	33	32	30	28
Fair/poor	27	28	34	33	29	35
Total	100	100	100	100	100	99*
Blacks (1983–84)						
Excellent/very good	26	24	28	25	24	22
Good	26	21	23	22	24	26
Fair/poor	47	55	48	51	49	50
Total	99*	100	99*	98*	97*	98*

*Figures do not sum to 100% in the original

However, I would like to deviate slightly and comment briefly on current research on women, especially at midlife, and implications for older women. Heilbrun[32] noted in her book, *Writing a Woman's Life*, that for too long we assumed all women had the same end, and that they were indeed all the same, and thus needed no place or voice in literature and history. Treating women the same also characterized research and theories on women. Traditionally, women were viewed not only as deficient in 'desirable' characteristics, but also as uninteresting to study because their lives were so predictable. This was particularly true for women at midlife, because it was believed that women's lives ended when they married and had children[33]. The only event left for them – menopause – in essence made women even less desirable to men and society (I will not comment on this because women's experiences with the menopause have been amply discussed throughout this Congress).

Today, as evident in several studies, women researchers are much more committed to understanding the diversity of women's lives and also the diversity of issues related to the life-cycle experience of the menopause. There is currently very little recognition of the heterogeneity of women's life experiences, not only across groups (culture, race and cohort), but also within groups, and hopefully there will be an increase in research of these variables within developing countries.

Suffice it to say, the major threat to women's health, particularly the health of aging women, is the persistence of myths and stereotypes about women, especially those associated with the gender processes discussed in various presentations during this Congress, and the resulting lack of knowledge about women's health as they age[34]. The homogeneity and invisibility that characterized earlier psychological theories and research on women also hold true for medical research. Foremost is the overemphasis on, and distortion of, the experience of the menopause.

Later life has become the subject of both media and political attention, especially in developed countries, not as a cause for celebration of societies' success in increasing the life expectancy of citizens, but primarily as a cause for concern. This characterization of later life as a societal problem reflects, I believe, ageist value judgements. In addition, since women form the majority of the elderly, ageism may also be based on sexist prejudice. Women form an increasing numerical majority as age advances. There are 25% more 'young elderly' women than men in, for example, the UK. This contrasts with the 'very elderly', where there are now three times more women than men over the age of 85 years. There are, however, significant variations across countries and cultures. These variations are evident in the developing countries. While chronological age cannot be the sole variable to be considered when examining the aging process, it is useful when examining differences in aging across societies and cultures[35]. An encumbered and different lifestyle inevitably affects the threshold of old age. Kalache[36] notes that, if a woman aged 50 living in a developing country has spent the whole of her life engaged in arduous physical labor, suffered malnourishment and experienced multiple pregnancies and lactating episodes, her aging process (and consequent health status) will be different from that of a woman who has had quite a different life experience. It is inevitable that, in a country such as Sierra Leone, where life expectancy is 34 years, the meaning of old age will be perceived differently from the meaning of old age in, for example, Japan, where life expectancy is 77 years[37].

Indeed, self-perceived status and notions of quality of life and functional capacity remain socioeconomically, as well as socioculturally, determined. Martin[38] reports that, in some Asian countries, local researchers define 'old age' at 50 years. Even in developed countries, there is considerable variability of attitudes and experiences among older people and their caregivers. Both attitudes and experiences are structured by class, gender, ethnicity, disability (or health status), religion, geography, age and household structure. These factors, therefore, must be considered in order to target resources to improve health in old age. Access to hormone replacement therapy, for example, is not a universal option. Much depends on these variables.

In developing countries, much debate is now focused on changes in age-specific death rates at older ages. A major current debate about social welfare concerns the costs incurred in maintaining older populations. Increasing survival at older ages has led in recent years to considerable debate about an extension in the number of years of 'disease-free life' (healthy aging) at older ages. This forms the core of the debate about the compression of morbidity, i.e. about whether an extension in life years will mean a qualitative, disease-free existence. Fries[39] believes that healthy aging is increasingly feasible, with specific health and social interventions to ensure a reduction in the number of years an elderly person lives in ill-health. According to Fries, a person could live disease-free and fully autonomous until natural death from biological aging. This implies a progressively rectangular survival curve as causes of premature mortality are removed, delaying the onset of chronic disease. The case presented by Fries has been much debated not only because it places a limit on the human lifespan at current levels (in developed countries), but also because it suggests that it is possible for death to be disease-free, which has implications for the degree of burden placed upon health care[35].

From a different perspective, however, Gruenberg[40] and Kramer[41], citing the 'failures of success' in later life, have argued that an extension of life essentially means a 'rising pandemic' of chronic disease, both physiological and psychological. An extension in the lifespan, according to this argument, would mean increasing the numbers of people surviving with chronic and progressive diseases, with particular implications for health and social services. But Manton[42], Kane and colleagues[43] and Lopez[44] suggest that, for a real appreciation of the personal and social impact of years added to overall life expectancy, there needs to be a much better understanding of the relationship between mortality and morbidity and, in particular, of the changing patterns of morbidity as one grows older.

Another perspective that follows from this debate suggests that future trends in mortality and the frequency, as well as the recurrence, of disease may be affected considerably by interventions that prevent or control disease onset[45]. This is based on the premise that patterns of mortality, morbidity and disability are subject to interventions and improvements. Therefore, strategies focusing on *primary prevention could have a considerable impact upon the future course and quality of survival*, particularly for older women.

Sen[35] comments that the various perspectives on the compression of morbidity have yet to be fully applied to the developing countries, owing, in part, to the uneven nature of the health transition. Suffice it to say, the data on health needs among aging populations in developing countries remain scant and whatever is available is based upon a handful of local and regional studies undertaken over the past decade. Varied definitions of old age make comparisons of the health status of older people within and between regions problematic. Despite methodological limitations and scarcity of data, available evidence from some developing countries reveals health trends among older populations that are similar to those of the developed world. These include:

(1) In the American region, an increasing incidence of chronic degenerative diseases[46];

(2) In Costa Rica, the same patterns of gender-related differences with advancing age in the ability to perform tasks of daily living[47];

(3) In Barbados, heart disease as the foremost cause of death among the elderly, with hypertension affecting 41% of persons over 65 years of age[48];

(4) In Malaysia, an increasing incidence of cardiovascular and cerebral diseases, malignancies and diseases affecting the locomotor system[49];

(5) Studies undertaken in India among the rural elderly, indicating growing levels of functional dependence and psychiatric morbidity[35].

It is reported that, although morbidity remains skewed towards infectious diseases, it is moving increasingly towards chronic degenerative diseases in most developing countries, with similar sex differentials in both morbidity and mortality.

The sex differential in survival means that women outlive men in nearly all the countries of the world and, therefore, predominate numerically in older populations[50]. In reality, women experience increased and longer periods of chronic health problems, due to non-fatal illnesses associated with the aging process and because of an accumulation of risk factors for these diseases. As pointed out previously, such factors are often associated with previous lifestyles, social, economic and environmental conditions, including occupational status.

Early in this paper, I asked the question 'What is healthy aging?' and, coming back to the topic at hand, I also confessed my belief in Burnside's[15] approach of four perspectives to the idea of fitness: physical, intellectual, social and purposive. According to Butler[51], there are four important categories of fitness that are essential to maintain as one ages. These are physical fitness, intellectual fitness (or fitness of the mind), social fitness and purposive fitness. These four categories provide a useful framework for professionals working with older women.

Physical fitness includes bodily strength, resilience and agility, attained by appropriate exercise[51]. This does not mean that those who are physically fit have been without disease. In fact, anecdotal data show that, for most of the women who cope with arthritis, hypertension, diabetes or cancer, for example, health has taken on a new (or even different) meaning. Women with chronic diseases often work vigorously at improving their health status, including following treatment regimens. They also learn to respond quickly to signals from their aging bodies. They do not sign up for high-impact aerobics, knowing that their aging arthritic knees will not respond favorably to step classes. Awareness of, and not succumbing to, their limitations is an important attribute of most of these women. The most healthy qualities of these older women are a healthy attitude and an amazing ability to cope, including the substitution of other activities for those that they are no longer able to do and/or participation in the same activities, but learning to do them in a different manner[15].

With regard to intellectual fitness, Birren[52] reports that '. . . evidence suggests that most older adults have not grown old sick, poor and lonely. Indeed, they are more concerned with opportunities for learning and experimenting with life than the young are prepared to believe'. Participation in 'Elder Hostel' programs in the USA, which provide intellectual stimulation, travel opportunities and socialization, is a good indication of older people's interest in maintaining intellectual fitness. In older women, however, stress may have some negative functional consequences on intellectual abilities. A study of older women by Sands[53] found that high levels of stress contributed to a decline in intellectual functioning. In the same study, a relationship was identified between intellectual functioning and specific stressful events. For example, changes in personal health or the health of a family member were positively correlated with decline in intellectual functioning. Work and intellectual stimulation can certainly help in coping with the stress caused by illnesses in later life.

Social fitness is defined as needing to accomplish 'forming and maintaining significant personal relationships that may be called upon in good times or in bad'[51]. There are a variety of ways in which older women work on social fitness. Some are very active in their churches (numerous examples in developing countries, among blacks in America, for example), while others are enrolled in different kinds of classes and acquire new friendships. Other women volunteer many hours to charitable work and maintain their social fitness because they feel they are making a contribution and that they are needed.

Finally, purposive fitness, which involves having feelings of self-esteem and control over one's life[51], is perhaps the most important anchor of healthy aging among women. There are numerous examples of incidents where family members take the initiative, especially concerning an older woman's decisions, which makes it difficult for her to maintain purposive fitness. Thus self-esteem is an important part of purpose fitness. As has been reported previously, it is closely associated with both physical health, functional abilities and an older woman's response to adversity. Self-esteem is diminished at times of illness, and interventions should be directed at helping the older person to improve functional abilities to enhance self-esteem.

While not all older women may fit into all of the four areas, there are those who have become the 'elite' and the 'privileged' elderly, as described by Birren. It is not health *per se*, defined in its more conservative sense, that is so important in women's later lives, but their 'attitude', the stance they take toward their own health problems, and their ability to cope, their finesse in meeting and adapting to new situations and crises, that produces healthy older women.

Finally, it is important to highlight a recent trend - the 'very old women'. Von Mehring[54] writes about the rising 'fourth age of life' - the population of great-grandparental age. These are the old old and some of them live in institutions and adapt well to their limitations[55]. They also find ways to live with amazing fortitude and resourcefulness[54] and 'they enlarge the possibilities and improve conditions for all women'[56]. In developing countries, these older women play an important part in role-modelling for families and communities. It is these women who are 'enlarging the possibilities' in spite of handicaps and hardships, and they deserve our attention[15]. Research is only now beginning to appear about old-old women, the women of the 'fourth age of life'.

The future of older women has been reviewed by some writers. Verbrugge[8], for example, writes that when 'comparing a women currently 75 years old with a woman that age in 2010, the future woman will probably feel better each day, have fewer disabilities, live longer and die more rapidly ... The chances are that an older woman will have a more comfortable and active life than her same-age peer today'. Even in developing countries, these women 'will reach older ages and have the opportunity to enjoy healthful old age'.

What are, then, the conditions that may enable older women to achieve the status to which Verbrugge and others refer? What strategies should be mobilized to ensure that this happens across the globe? Old age is not a time of inevitable decline. As stated earlier, most of the diseases that afflict older persons are the so-called lifestyle diseases - conditions such as lung cancer, diabetes and heart disease, which are strongly linked to risk factors such as cigarette smoking, poor nutrition, lack of regular exercise and chronic stress. Eighty per cent of older people suffer from one or more of these lifestyle diseases and chronic conditions and about half of all older persons are somewhat limited in their daily activities. Simple preventive measures can significantly reduce the negative impact that lifestyle diseases have on older adults. The American Surgeon General in *Healthy People*[57] suggested three powerful reasons for increasing disease prevention and health promotion activities for people of all ages:

(1) Prevention saves lives;

(2) Prevention improves quality of life;

(3) Prevention reduces health-care costs in the long run.

Examining these outcomes in relation to the older population, in general, suggests that health-promoting activities are critical. One striking feature of morbidity patterns, among non-white aged, for example, particularly with respect to males, is the high representation of health problems amenable to early detection and early treatment. Soldo and DaVita[58] report a considerable excess of older non-white male disease and death due to influenza, pneumonia and respiratory conditions such as bronchitis, emphysema and asthma. Non-white women, on the other hand, show higher mortality rates for diabetes. For many of these conditions, poor personal health care, inadequate or inappropriate diet, smoking and alcohol consumption are causal or exacerbating factors. Health education and preventive measures aimed at screening, early detection and lifestyle modification would go a long way toward reducing morbidity and mortality due to these conditions. The same applies to hypertension and related cardiovascular conditions[59].

From the preceding statements, the call for proactive strategies to achieve healthy aging is clearly compelling. Most citizens, irrespective of socioeconomic status, geography, race and ethnicity and environment, have visions of a 'quality of life' free of disease and disability. Earlier, I identified what I believe to be one of the objectives of this conference. I now suggest that there is another objective particularly specific to this presentation: to explore what is known about healthy living among older women, with particular emphasis on not only overcoming illness and adversity, but also on preventing illness and disease for the enjoyment of long, productive, personally fulfilling lives[60]. During this Congress, several presenters have provided helpful medical information for understanding the common illnesses and health problems afflicting women as they grow older and have offered prescriptions for dealing with the various associated complexities of diseases, structural changes and functional limitations. Concomitant feelings of powerlessness, low self-worth, isolation, stress and depression experienced by aging women with health problems have been the subject of many social scientists. Others have explored the demographics of aging, the importance of attitudes and definitions in shaping lives, the problems of discrimination, lack of financing and the inadequacy of health-care services for elderly women. The call for health-care reform, which incorporates health promotion and greater involvement of older women in shaping public policy, is loud and clear. Common themes emerge from works presented by a number of authors. How one defines 'health', for example, is critical in shaping one's response to health problems, illness, adversity or limitations. Health, most authors argue, is more than the absence of illness. Of the multiple changes that accompany the aging process, some are more troublesome than others. Some are physiological processes that occur normally in the course of aging (menopause, structural and sensory alterations). Some are diseases that require medical treatment (heart disease, cancer and diabetes). Some are conditions, syndromes or illnesses that do not have identified causation, known cures or even satisfactory treatment programs that are effective in reducing painful and annoying symptoms (sensory loss, arthritis, Alzheimer's disease, cancer and osteoporosis).

Burnside[15] differentiates between disease (a condition that impairs performance) and illness (an individual's perceptions and behaviors in response to the disease and the impact it has on one's life and the lives of significant others). Since no one is completely healthy - even in youth - it is imperative that the responses learned for coping with illness throughout life are effective, particularly for dealing with the higher incidence of illness that increases as one moves into the later years. Young and Garner[60] observe that 'To be the best one can be, should be a goal for all elderly women. Sometimes that means facing the reality of aging head on and not denying the aches and pains, nor diminishing the reality of impairment or disease when it occurs. Sometimes it means redefining oneself as an older person, developing a new sense of self-appreciation, "connectedness" and purpose in life, while legitimizing the inherent freedoms within, and providing new opportunities for their creative release'.

Jorgensen[61] challenges older women themselves to adopt health-promoting and healthy lifestyles that embrace nutrition, exercise, a positive attitude and the use of preventive screenings.

There are many unanswered questions about the differential care for women and men. Traditionally, it has been thought to be more socially acceptable for women than men to seek health services, which may explain the greater utilization of preventive health services in older age by women than men. However, it does not explain why women tend to have a greater incidence of, and more limitations from, chronic health problems than men or why men receive more procedures or why women are less likely than men to be referred for cardiac catheterizations, angioplasty or coronary bypass surgery for similar presenting symptoms. Neither does it explain why older women receive less adequate care for breast cancer than younger women or why male medical handling of the menopause in women is inadequate and inconsistent.

Roberto[62] reports on the frustrations women experience over inconsistent, conflicting information and confusing medical advice regarding treatment for problems of osteoporosis. Differing expert opinions, controversy and inconclusive evidence on the method, length and value of estrogen replacement therapy for the control of symptoms are also common experiences of women during the menopause.

For the majority of women, life will continue after the menopause for another 30, 40 or even 50 years. The challenge facing women as they enter the prime mid-years of the 50s is to prepare themselves for the future by becoming informed consumers and by taking an active role in making life and health-care decisions that will affect the quality of their lives in the long run.

Autonomy in decision-making promotes a sense of power and self-esteem that elderly women need in order to maintain their integrity during illness and times of adversity. Although the maximum health potential for aging women is individually defined, it is also related to multiple variables such as early health–promoting lifestyles, type of illness or impairment, one's education or knowledge about one's health, one's personal resources and coping skills, social support systems available in the form of caregivers, family, friends and community, and the degree of assistance needed.

Health-care providers, on the other hand, have an important responsibility in facilitating problem solving of elderly women in making their life changes and developing life and coping skills.

Elderly women today generally have an uncharted course for the future. Few norms are available to them and few examples of what constitutes successful aging are actually explicated. Research is desperately needed on all of the diseases that women commonly experience, on the needs of older women, the aging process in women and successful coping mechanisms for maintaining independence. Most of all, research is needed on the impact of health-promoting interventions, recognizing that individual health is influenced not only by voluntary personal lifestyle and behavior, but also by heredity and economics, and the social world in which we live.

Although Birren[52] was not writing about older women specifically, his prophetic words apply to the topic under discussion and can be applied to the future world of older people across the board. Increasingly, he says, there will emerge a positive model of growing old. It will probably begin with the increasing awareness of older persons who might be called the elite or accomplished (regardless of where they are and of their station in life). These are the people whom life refines and empowers (in whatever cultural, class and societal context). They move toward greater mastery of events and their adaptive strategies, both individually, collectively and in their communities, are such that they are increasingly strong and confident with the passage of years[52].

Of course, women still struggle in male-dominated societies. They deal with sexual harassment, lower wages, unpaid and unrecognized housework, and restrictions in personal advancement. Some of the most striking characteristics across cultures and societies are women's increasing poverty, increasing numbers of women who are single heads of households and increasing numbers of women who are caught in the grandparenting and adult parenting sandwich. Impoverished women, as we know, are a high-risk population, because they lack support or resources, experience undue stress and have reduced access to health services. Despite all this gloom, however, more and more women are defining and determining their own lives.

This appears to be particularly true of middle-aged women, whose creativity and generativity, in Heilbrun's[32] words, arise from their work and relationships with other women and not from the 'marriage plot' that has traditionally defined women's lives. LeGuin[63] remarks that becoming a 'Crone' when one turns 50 may mean becoming pregnant with oneself - at last.

I would like to end this paper on an upbeat note with a poem *After Sixty* by Zuckerman[64]:

> Everyone says the world is flat and finite
> on the other side of Sixty
> That I will fall clear off the edge
> into darkness
>
> That no one will hear me again or
> want to.
>
> But I am ready for the knife slicing into
> the future
> for the quest that explodes inside
> to join forces with the strong old women
> to throw everything away and begin again . . .
>
> . . . There are places on this planet
> where women past the menopause
> put on the tribal robes
> smoke pipes of wisdom, [and]
> - fly

References

1. Olson KL, ed. *The Graying of the World: Who Will Care for the Frail Elderly?* New York: The Haworth Press, 1994
2. Preston SH. Children and the elderly: divergent paths for America's dependents. *Demography* 1984; 4:435–57
3. Kayser-Jones JS. *Old, Alone and Neglected: Care for the Aged in Scotland and the United States.* Berkeley, CA: University of California Press, 1981
4. Stahl SM, ed. *The Legacy of Longevity: Health and Health Care in Later Life.* Newbury Park: Sage Publications, 1990
5. National Center for Health Statistics. *Health, United States, 1987.* DHHS Publication No. (PHS) 88-1232 Public Health Service. Washington DC: US Government Printing Office, 1988
6. Brody JA. Life expectancy and the health of older persons. *J Am Geriatr Soc* 1982;30:681–3
7. Fredman L, Haynes SG. An epidemiologic profile of the elderly. In Phillips HT, Gaylord SA, eds. *Aging and Public Health.* New York: Springer, 1985: 1–41
8. Verbrugge LM. An epidemiological profile of older women. In Haug MR, Ford AB, Sheafor M, eds. *The Physical and Mental Health of Aged Women.* New York: The Springer Publishing Co., 1985
9. Kalache A. Foreword. In Sen K, ed. *Aging: Debates on Demographic Transition and Social Policy.* London: Zed Books Ltd., 1994
10. Dannefer D. Adult development and social theory: a pragmatic reappraisal. *Am Sociol Rev* 1984;49: 100–16
11. Palmore EB, Kivett V. Change in life satisfactions: a longitudinal study of persons aged 46–70. *J Gerontol* 1977;32:311–16
12. Arber S, Ginn J. *Gender and Late Life: a Sociological Analysis of Resources and Constraints.* Newbury Park: Sage Publications, 1991
13. Verbrugge LM. The dynamics of population aging and health. In Lewis S, ed. *Aging and Health.* Michigan: Lewis, 1989:23–40
14. Bearon LB. No great expectations: the underpinnings of life satisfaction for older women. *Gerontology* 1989;29:227–84
15. Burnside I. Healthy older women. In Garner JD, Young AA, eds. *Women and Healthy Aging: Living Productively in Spite of It All.* New York: The Haworth Press, 1993:9–23
16. Birren JE, Zarit JM. Concepts of health, behaviour and aging. In Birren JE, Livingston J, eds. *Cognition, Stress and Aging.* Englewood Cliffs: Prentice-Hall, 1985:1–20
17. Schroot JJF. Current perspectives on aging, health and behavior. In Schroot JJF, Birren JE, Svanborg A, eds. *Health and Aging.* New York: Springer Publishing Co., 1988
18. Mercer SO, Garner JD. An international overview of aged women. In Garner JD, Mercer SO, eds. *Women as they Age: Challenge, Opportunity and Triumph.* New York: The Haworth Press, 1989: 13–45
19. Blaxter M. Self definition of health status and consultation rates in primary care. *Quart J Soc Affairs* 1985;1:131–71

20. Hughes M. Quality of Life. In Peace S, ed. *Research Social Gerontology*. London: Sage, 1990:46–58
21. Mossey JM, Shapiro E. Self-rated health: a predictor of mortality among the elderly. *Am J Pub Health* 1982;72:800–8
22. Welin L, Svardsudd K, Ander-Peciva S, *et al.* Prospective studies of social influences on mortality. *Lancet* 1985;1:915–18
23. Shapiro E, Tate R. Who is really at risk of institutionalization? *Gerontology* 1988;28:237–45
24. Arber S, Ginn J. *Gender and Later Life: a Sociological Analysis of Resources and Contraints*. London: Sage Publications, 1991:107–28
25. Verbrugge LM. Gender, aging and health. In Markides KS, ed. *Aging and Health: Perspectives on Gender, Race, Ethnicity, and Class*. Newbury Park, CA: Sage Publications, 1989:23–78
26. Jackson JJ, Perry C. Physical health conditions of middle-aged and aged blacks. In Markides KS, ed. *Aging and Health: Perspectives on Gender, Race, Ethnicity, and Class*. Newbury Park, CA: Sage Publications, 1989:111–76
27. Neugarten B. Age groups in American society and the rise of the 'young-old'. *Ann Am Acad Polit Soc Sci* 1974;415:187–98
28. Taylor R. The elderly as members of society: an examination of social differences in an elderly population. In Wells N, Freer C, eds. *The Aging Population: Burden or Challenge?* London: MacMillan, 1988:105–29
29. Wells N, Freer C, eds. *The Aging Population: Burden or Challenge?* London: MacMillan, 1988
30. Marshall V. Lessons for gerontology from healthy public policy initiatives. In Lewis S, ed. *Aging and Health*. Michigan: Lewis, 1989:319–29
31. McHugh MC, Koeske RD, Frieze IH. Issues to consider in conducting non-sexist psychology: a review with recommendations. *Am Psychol* 1986;41:879–90
32. Heilbrun CG. *Writing a Woman's Life*. New York: Balentine Books, 1988
33. Gilbert LA. Women at midlife: current theoretical perspectives and research. In Davis ND, Cole E, Rothblum ED, eds. *Faces of Women and Aging*. New York: The Haworth Press, 1993
34. Rodin J, Ickovics JR. Women's health: review and research agenda as we approach the 21st century. *Am Psychol* 1990;43:1018–34
35. Sen K, ed. *Ageing: Debates on Demographic Transition and Social Policy*. London: Zed Books Ltd., 1994
36. Kalache A. Aging in developing countries. In Pathy MSJ, ed. *Principles and Practice of Geriatric Medicine*, 2nd edn. Chichester: J Wiley, 1991
37. Veras R. *A survey of the health of elderly people in Rio de Janeiro, Brazil*. Unpublished PhD Thesis, University of London, 1992
38. Martin L. The status of South Asia's growing elderly population. *J Cross-Cultural Gerontol* 1990;5
39. Fries S. Aging, natural death and the compression of morbidity. *N Engl J Med* 1980;303:130–6
40. Gruenberg EM. The failure of success. *Milbank Memorial Fund Q/Health Soc* 1977;55:3–24
41. Kramer M. The rising pandemic of mental disorders and associated chronic diseases and disabilities. *Acta Psychiatr Scand* 1980;62(Suppl 285): 382–92
42. Manton KG. Changing concepts of morbidity and mortality in the elderly population. *Milbank Memorial Fund Q* 1982;60:183–244
43. Kane R, Evans GJ, MacFadyen D, eds. *Improving the Health of Older People: a World View*. Oxford: Oxford University Press, 1990
44. Lopez A. Some issues in the demography and epidemiology of aging populations. Presented at the *World Development Report Consultation on the Elderly*, Oslo, Norway, 1993
45. World Health Organization. *The Uses of Epidemiology in the Study of the Elderly*. Report of a WHO Scientific Group on the Epidemiology of Aging. Geneva: WHO, 1984
46. Pan American Health Organisation. *Toward the Well-being of the Elderly*. Scientific Publication 492. Washington, DC: PAHO, 1985
47. Kinsella K. *Aging in the Third World*. International Population Report Series No. 79. Washington, DC: US Department of Commerce, Bureau of the Census, 1988
48. Bureau of the Census. *Trend: Barbados*. Washington DC: US Department of Commerce, 1990
49. Andrews, GR, Esterman AJ, Braunack-Mayer AJ, Rungie CM. *Aging in the Western Pacific: a Four Country Study*. Western Pacific Region Research Report No. 1. Manila: WHO, 1986
50. Myers GC. Demographic aging and family support for older persons. In Kendig H, Hashimoto A, Coppard L, eds. *Family Support for the Elderly: an International Experience*. New York: Oxford University Press, 1992
51. Butler R. Foreword. In Birren JE, Deutchman DE, eds. *Guided Autobiography Groups: Exploring the Fabric of Life*. Baltimore, MD: The Johns Hopkins University Press, 1991
52. Birren JE. A gerontologist's overview. In Jarvik LF, ed. *Aging into the 21st Century*. New York: Gardner Press, 1978
53. Sands JO. The relationship of stressful life events to intellectual functioning in women over 65. *Int J Aging Hum Dev* 1981;14:11–22
54. Von Mehring O. Beyond the concept of successful aging: a transcultural and individual perspective. Presented at the *Southern Regional Educational Board Conference on Successful Aging - Going Beyond Illness*, Atlanta, GA, 1992
55. Wagnild G, & Young H. Resilience among older women. *Images* 1990;22:252–5

56. Thone RR. *Women and Aging: Celebrating Ourselves.* New York: The Haworth Press, 1992
57. Public Health Service. *Healthy People 2000: National Health Promotion and Disease Prevention Objectives.* DHHS Publication No. (PHS)91-50213. Washington DC: Government Printing Office, 1990
58. Soldo BJ, Davita C. *Profiles of the Black Aged.* Washington, DC: Georgetown University Center for Population Studies, 1977
59. Morrison JB. Physical health and the minority aged. In McNeely RL, Cohen JN, eds. *Aging In Minority Groups.* Beverly Hills: Sage Publications, 1983
60. Young AA, Garner JD. Women and healthy aging: conclusion. In Garner JD, Young AA, eds. *Women and Healthy Aging: Living Productively in Spite of It All.* New York: The Haworth Press, 1993:221-6
61. Jorgensen LAB. Public policy, health care and older women. In Garner JD, Young AA, eds. *Women and Healthy Aging: Living Productively in Spite of It All.* New York: The Haworth Press, 1993:201-20
62. Roberto KA. Osteoporosis and older women: productive lifestyle strategies. In Garner JD, Young AA, eds. *Women and Healthy Aging: Living Productively in Spite of It All.* New York: The Haworth Press, 1993
63. Leguin UK. *Dancing at the Edge of the World.* New York: Grove, 1989
64. Zuckerman M. After sixty. In Doress P, Siegal D, eds. *Ourselves Growing Older: Women Aging with Knowledge and Power.* New York: Simon and Schuster, 1988:405

The significance of the menopause in human life in the present and next centuries 11

T. Aso

GENERAL ASPECTS OF THE MENOPAUSE

As described in medical textbooks, the menopause has been defined as the transition from the reproductive to the non-reproductive period. Prior to the reproductive years, women pass through the stage of menarche and adolescence, during which they accumulate physical functions and mature mentally. However, a certain number of girls at this stage show an imbalance in systemic functions and a discrepancy between physical and mental development. As a result of these inadequacies, menstrual disorders and maladaptation symptoms are observed in some of these girls. Such findings are also commonly observed in perimenopausal women, who are also in a transitional period from one stage to another.

The reproductive aging process is essentially determined by the number of oocytes remaining in the ovaries. During this process, extremely accelerated oocyte depletion is observed in the premenopause, especially between 41 and 45 years of age. The observable changes in ovarian size and a decrease in steroidogenic capacity, as well as the deteriorating quality of the oocytes, are also essential events at this stage of reproductive life. As a consequence of diminishing ovarian function in the perimenopausal period, an imbalance in the hypothalamic-pituitary-ovarian axis is induced, and the sustained estrogen deficiency after the menopause increases the risk of a variety of disorders.

Increasing evidence shows that the alterations in the menopause are not solely the consequence of events during this stage, but they are greatly influenced by events that occurred during previous stages of life. At the same time, the changes in the menopause are closely linked to those in the elderly. Thus, it is essential to cover the entire sequence of events over the whole lifespan when we discuss the health care of menopausal women.

AGE AT THE MENOPAUSE

An early sign observed in the premenopausal period is the occurrence of irregular menstrual cycles. This is induced by the fluctuating estrogen production of the aging ovaries around the time of the menopause. An analysis of the menstrual status of Japanese women between the ages of 40 and 60 years revealed that a significant number of normally healthy women show irregular cycles at the age of 40. More than half of them reported cessation of menstruation at the age of 52 and all had become menopausal by the age of 57. In general, these results do not differ from the trends observed in other parts of the world[1].The results of retrospective surveys concerning age at the menopause during 1987–96 are shown in Figure 1. The menopausal ages of Japanese women born in the years 1901–10 were distributed almost symmetrically from the peak at 49–50 years of age. In the group of women born after 1921, the number of those reaching the menopause at an age higher than the 'peak age' increased gradually. This trend was more pronounced in recent years, even when the peak ages were the same as those in previous decades[2,3]. On the contrary, it has been widely recognized that the age at menarche has diminished in recent years. In fact, the age at menarche of Japanese women born in 1901–10 was 15.64 years, whereas that of women born in 1961–65 was 12.49[2]. Concerning the relationship between the ages at menarche and menopause, it has been suggested that a later age at menarche favors an earlier menopause[4]. However, the factors inducing such changes are not fully

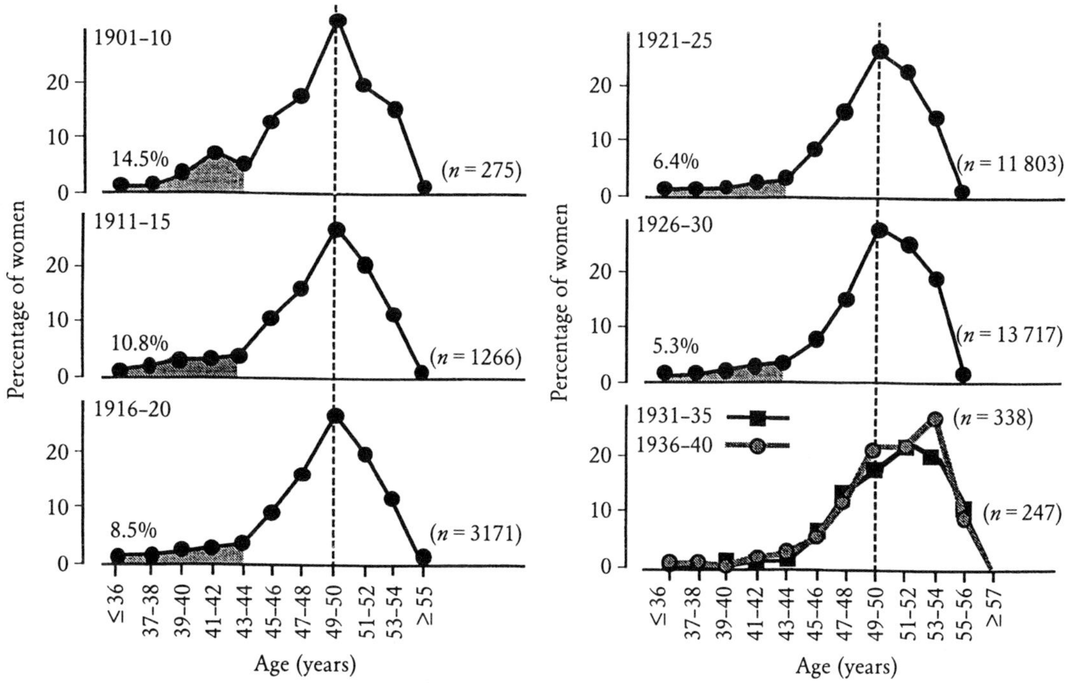

Figure 1 Distribution of the age at menopause of Japanese women born between 1901 and 1940

understood. It will be of great interest to evaluate the significance and impact of the suggested increase in menopausal age on women's reproductive life and the quality of life of the elderly in the next century.

CLIMACTERIC SYMPTOMS AND THEIR BACKGROUNDS

It was once assumed that the menopause was not only a universal event, but that its timing and physiological implications were universally the same. However, the accumulation of global information concerning the status of women during the menopause in different parts of the world has raised questions as to whether women experience the same menopausal symptoms, irrespective of where they live.

Characteristics of climacteric symptoms of Japanese women

To answer these questions, the influence of ethnic, cultural, socioeconomic and environmental factors on the events associated with the menopause have been extensively studied. A number of investigations have been conducted in particular countries or regions that show a great heterogeneity in socioeconomic and cultural backgrounds among women. In these investigations, some similarities and some differences in the status of menopausal women have been identified. In a previous report, it was concluded that the menopause seems to be associated with fewer and less severe symptoms in Asia compared to the West[5]. However, it should be borne in mind that this conclusion was drawn from the results of a survey using symptom evaluation scores developed for European women. One could therefore speculate that most previous studies might not have been able to identify clearly the symptoms of women living in non-Western countries. Even so, it is clear that menopausal Asian women experience to a lesser extent psychological and vasomotor complaints, including hot flushes, sweating, palpitations and dizziness. A recent survey conducted by our group involving more than 3200 healthy Japanese women between the ages of 45 and 60 years revealed that shoulder stiffness was the most common complaint (45%) and that the percentage of women who were disturbed by severe vasomotor symptoms was approximately 25%[3]. The results of a study analyzing the climacteric symptoms of women who had visited menopause clinics to obtain some medical care are illustrated in Figure 2. More than 80% complained of general fatigue and neck stiffness. Sweating, cold extremities, nervousness, feeling unstable, lumbago and irritability were observed in more than 65% of the subjects[6]. These results indicate that the major symptoms of Japanese menopausal women are less directly related to estrogen deficiency. Several factors have been suggested to explain the regional differences in climacteric symptoms. In particular, the beneficial influence of lifestyle, including dietary habits such as the high intake of soy products, has been indicated as one of the major benefits for Japanese women[7,8].

Factors influencing the climacteric symptoms of Japanese women

In order to specify the pattern of climacteric symptoms of Japanese women, their situation in the domestic and social environments should be also considered. It is usual in Japan for the long-term intimate relationship between parents and children to continue up to the time when the children leave home and become independent. Mothers devote most of their time and energy to the care and support of their children during the dependence period. In some cases, mothers are forced to sacrifice their own lives and hardly find extra time to look after themselves. At the time when mothers become free of taking care of their children, they are ready to enter the menopausal stage. Coincidentally, their husbands, who do not

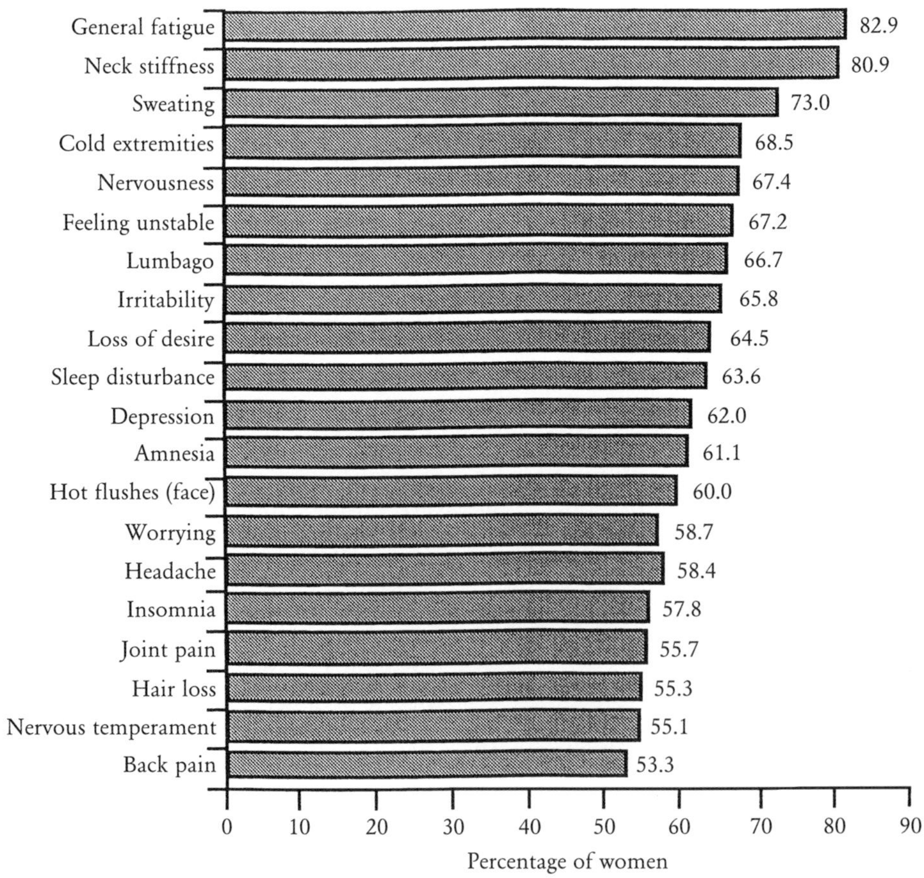

Figure 2 Incidence of climacteric symptoms in women visiting menopause clinics ($n = 445$)

make any active contributions to solving domestic problems, retire from their jobs. Hence, women at this age are then asked to take care of their husbands and, at the same time, their parents[9].

The average life expectancy of the Japanese has increased and is now one of the highest in the world. As illustrated in Figure 3, the life expectancy for males is 77.19 years and that for females is 83.82 years (1997 figures)[10]. At the same time, the proportion of elderly people in the total population continues to increase and it is predicted that the proportions will reach 20.0% and 24.1% in 2010 and 2040, respectively[11]. The same patterns of change can be seen in other advanced countries. This has resulted in the ratios of children to elderly decreasing tremendously, and further decreases will be observed in the next century. Such situations become a burden, both physically and psychologically, on families, especially on the wives tending the elderly if they need long-term care. As depicted in Figure 4, approximately 70% of long-term care for the bedridden elderly is provided by family relations, and the major providers are the daughters and daughters-in-law who are of menopausal age[12]. The chief factors causing stress for men and women are shown in Figure 5. For men, the stress from work is the most serious factor throughout their life. However, for women, the stress from childcare and education is the main factor up to the age of 40 years, and the stresses from family health and their own health and sickness obviously increase as they get closer to the age of menopause[13]. One can easily imagine that menopausal women under such stressful circumstances chiefly complain about psychological symptoms in addition to those induced by estrogen deficiency. Thus, it is obvious that the incidence and pattern of climacteric symptoms are also influenced by social factors relating to the aging society. In order to improve the quality of life of menopausal women, the establishment of long-term care for the elderly will be one of the essential issues in the aging society of the next century.

LIFESTYLE-RELATED DISEASES AND THE HEALTH-CARE SYSTEM

According to a survey of the causes of death in Japan, cancer is the leading cause of death, the

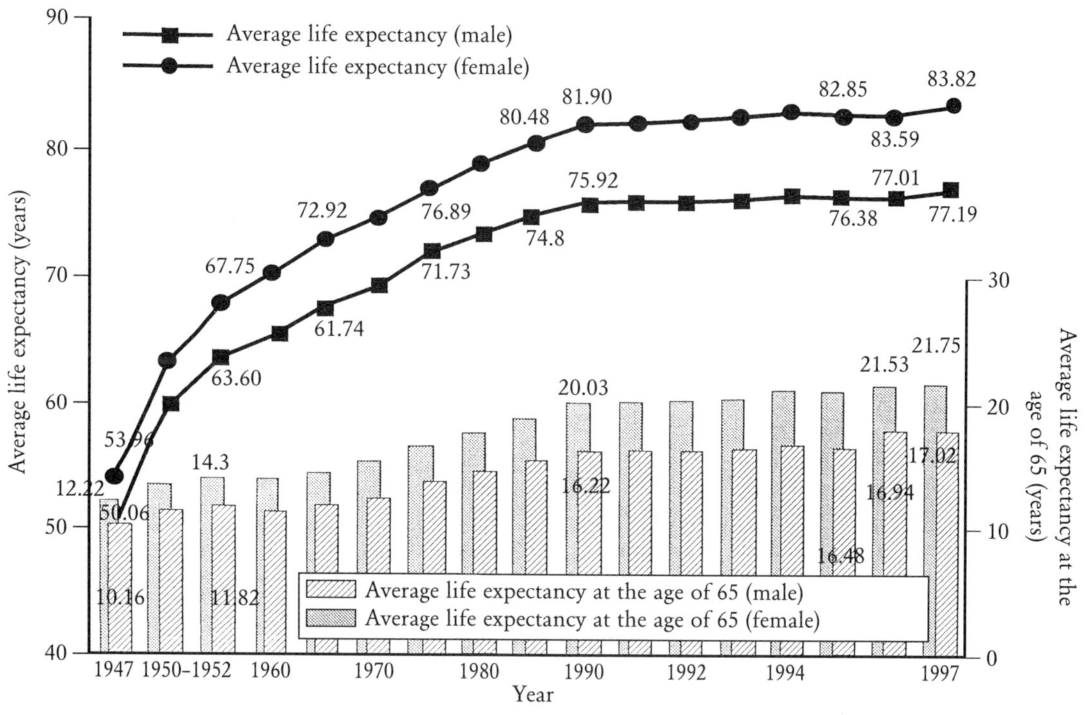

Figure 3 Changes in average life expectancy and that at the age of 65 years in Japan between 1947 and 1997

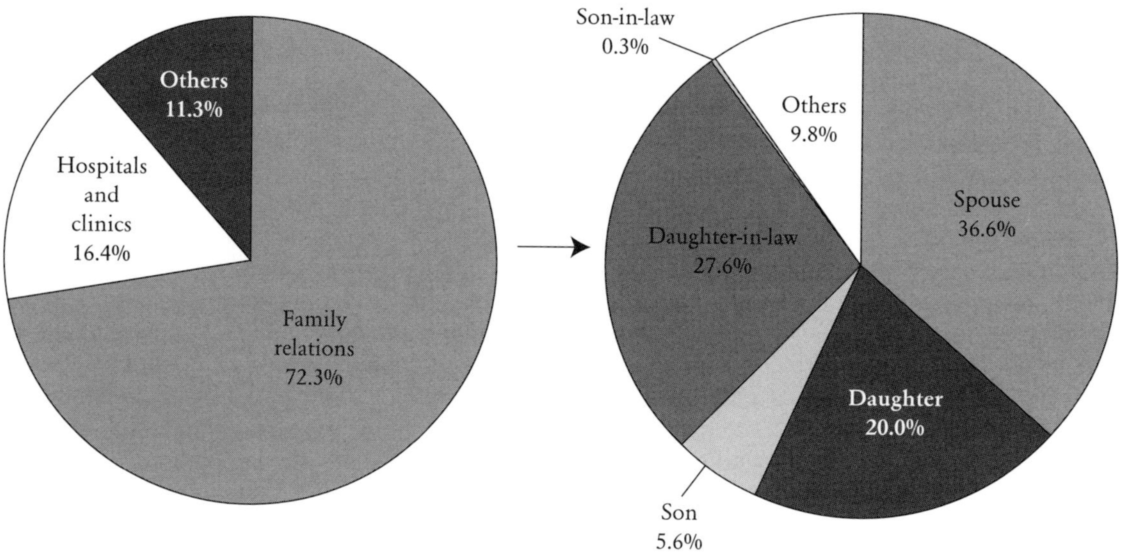

Figure 4 Long-term care providers for the bedridden elderly

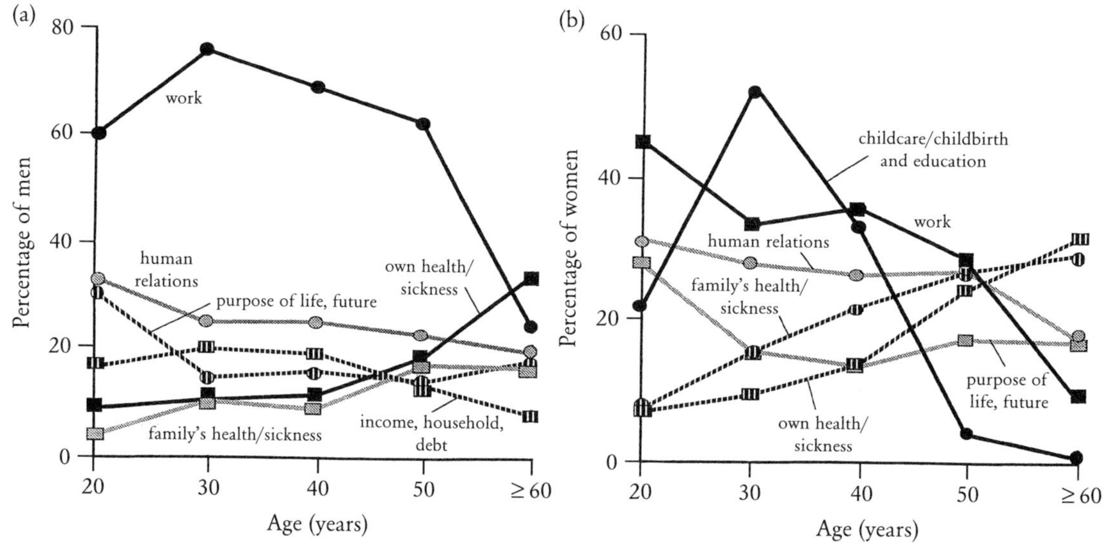

Figure 5 Factors causing stress in men (a) and women (b) in different age groups (multiple answers accepted)

second is cerebrovascular disease, and heart disease is the third[14]. This finding is common for all industrialized countries today. Epidemiological studies indicate that women in their reproductive years are protected from the risks of developing geriatric diseases mainly because of the beneficial effects of the ovarian hormone, estrogen, but once their estrogen levels decrease following the menopause, the risks increase. The accumulated information obtained from research in the natural sciences over the past few decades has broadened our knowledge of the biological actions of estrogen in the aging process. It has been shown that estrogen deficiency after the menopause increases the risk of disorders such as osteoporosis/fractures, hyperlipidemia/ischemic heart disease and dementia/Alzheimer's disease. Since the proportion of elderly will dramatically increase world-wide in the next century, there is an urgent need to establish a comprehensive health-care system providing preventive interventions for these disorders, which may develop into life-threatening conditions in the elderly.

In 1996, in the process of the establishment of such a comprehensive health-care system, the Council on Public Health of Japan introduced the concept of lifestyle-related diseases. The onset and prognosis of diseases are closely correlated with factors that can be categorized into three groups. The first group includes genetic factors such as aging; environmental factors, including pathogenic organisms, hazardous substances and stress, constitute the second group. Finally, lifestyle-related factors, such as eating and exercise habits, are classified as the third group. Based on this classification, the lifestyle-related diseases are defined as the diseases whose onset and development are directly related to dietary habits, lack of exercise, smoking, alcohol consumption, etc. Lack of exercise and impaired dietary habits, such as an excessive intake of animal fat and salt in unbalanced meals, are closely associated with the onset of obesity, hyperlipidemia and osteoporosis. These conditions eventually cause diabetes, circulatory diseases, fracture and colon cancer. It has been established that there is a causal relationship between smoking and lung cancer and between excessive alcohol consumption and liver cirrhosis. It goes without saying that the aim of introducing the concept of lifestyle-related diseases to the public is to emphasize the importance of people's lifestyle. Because basic habits are usually acquired during childhood, a long-term health-promotion program should be implemented from the early stages of life.

Since no apparent subjective signs appear in the initial phase of diseases such as atherosclerosis and osteoporosis, which are common among menopausal women, secondary prevention by carrying out health check-ups for the detection and early treatment of disease is important in addition to primary prevention. The introduction of health-promotion measures by combining primary and secondary prevention strategies resulted in a decrease in lost workdays due to long-term disease in one company (Figure 6). Furthermore, the number of people requiring medical treatment did not increase despite a rise in the average age of the employees[15].

To establish an optimal health-care system, there will be a need for a general awareness of the importance and effectiveness of holistic measures by society at large. It is promising that the support of such a system will enable elderly women of the

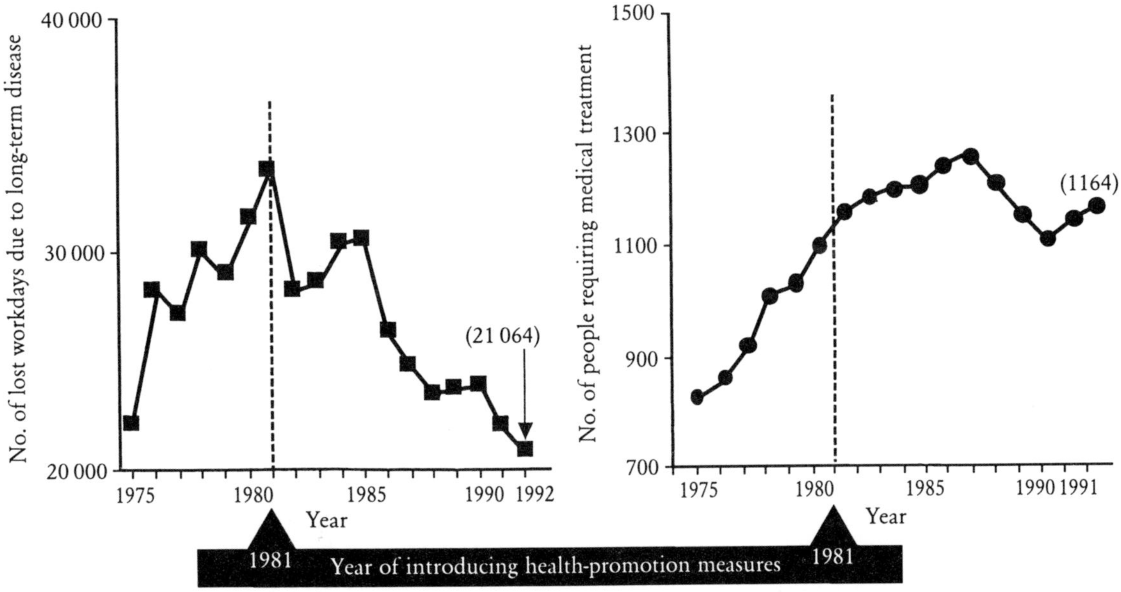

Figure 6 Effects of health-promotion measures on lost workdays and medical treatment requirements

next century to have a significantly improved quality of life during the period following the menopause.

CONCLUSION

This paper has discussed some specific issues of the menopause that require much attention as the 20th century draws to a close. The chronological and biological significance of the menopause has been clarified and there is much evidence to support the accumulated knowledge. The ongoing studies on the pathophysiological mechanisms involved in menopausal disorders will make a great contribution toward the better understanding of these processes and the development of medical interventions aiming to improve the quality of life in the menopause. On the other hand, the mental and societal significance of the menopause is influenced by various factors, which change in nature and quantity depending on the time and location of a particular society. Thus, it will be of great importance to keep re-evaluating the mental and social significance of the menopause in human life in order to progress toward a society for all ages in the next century.

References

1. Aso T. Demography of menopause and pattern of climacteric symptoms in the East Asian region. In Ratnam SS, Campana A, eds. *Proceedings of the 1st Consensus Meeting on Menopause in the East Asian Region*. Zeist, The Netherlands: Medical Forum International 1997:24–32
2. Kikuchi T. Interrelation between menopause age and frequency of ovulatory cycles in life. *Hokkaido Med J* 1987;62:469–75
3. The Study Group of Reproduction and Endocrinology. Annual report on the management of health care for the middle aged women. *Acta Obstet Gynecol Jpn* 1997;49:1019–43
4. Boulet MJ, Oddens BJ, Lehert P, *et al.* Climacteric and menopause in seven South-East Asian countries. *Maturitas* 1994;19:157–76
5. Payer L. International health report: menopause in various cultures. A portrait of the menopause. Carnforth, UK: Parthenon Publishing, 1991
6. The Study Group of Reproduction and Endocrinology. Annual report on the present status of HRT and its side effects in Japan. *Acta Obstet Gynecol Jpn* 1999;51:1193–204
7. Lock M. Contested meanings of the menopause. *Lancet* 1991;337:1270–2
8. Murkies AL, Limbard C, Strauss BJ, *et al.* Dietary flour supplementation decreases postmenopausal hot flushes: effect of soy and wheat. *Maturitas* 1995;21:189–95
9. Ministry of Health and Welfare. *Population Statistics 1992*
10. National Institute of Population and Social Research, Ministry of Health and Welfare. *Population Census of Japan*. Tokyo: Ministry of Health and Welfare, 1997
11. Management and Coordination Agency. *National Census 1995*
12. Statistics and Information Department, Minister's Secretariat, Ministry of Health and Welfare. *Comprehensive Survey of the Living Conditions of People on Health and Welfare*. Tokyo: Ministry of Health and Welfare, 1995
13. Health and Physical Strength Promotion Service Foundation. *Survey of Awareness on Health Promotion*, 1996
14. Statistics and Information Department, Minister's Secretariat, Ministry of Health and Welfare. *Vital Statistics 1995*. Tokyo: Ministry of Health and Welfare, 1995
15. Industrial Health Division, Ministry of Labor. *Guide on Health Promotion in the Work Place*. Tokyo: Ministry of Labor, 1995

Healthy aging in the 21st century 12

Khunying K. Limpaphayom

The menopause is regarded as a physiological change in which both ovaries permanently lose their reproductive function. Whereas some women undergo this transitional period without significant health problems, others suffer from progressive deterioration. The diversity in clinical manifestations and health consequences of the menopause has evoked various convictions in health perception. In the Thai society, the menopause is regarded by some humanistic groups, sociologists and health personnel as natural changes of life not requiring any particular treatment. On the other hand, some physicians consider menopausal endocrine disorders in need of immediate medical attention and therapy. Based on the latter notion, the menopause is regarded as a hormone deficiency state in need of hormone replacement therapy.

It has been widely accepted that the gene-environment interaction plays a pivotal role with regard to disease occurrence in a particular individual. In particular, genetic predisposition to menopausal deterioration, and environmental exposure including differential health-risk behaviors, probably determine the course of menopausal health in the short and the long term. Oriental philosophy has developed based on observational experience gathered over thousands of years in studying nature and the ways in which to comply with its rules. This long-standing concept has profoundly influenced the life-style and health behavior of Asian people, particularly Thai people. In the Thai society, a human being is perceived not only with regard to his/her physical and intellectual aspects, but is considered also from a spiritual perspective. This approach is fundamentally different from the occidental concept of systematic scientific thinking based on 'facts' requiring objective proof. Occidental medicine puts emphasis on mechanisms, for example the mental mechanism (psychology, psychodynamics), the biological mechanism (physiology, molecular mechanism), etc., all of which require in-depth research. This approach segregates modern medicine into myriads of specialties, in need of a specialist to focus on each particular issue of medical science. The way of thinking in oriental medicine is holistic. The human being is viewed from broad perspectives, in multidimensions of social, psychological and biocultural interaction. The original concept of occidental medicine stems from the treatment of diseases. Micro-organisms and carcinogens have been identified as causes of illness such as infectious diseases and cancer. Hence, human beings need medical weapons to combat these ailments, i.e. antibiotics, chemotherapeutic agents, hormones, etc. Nonetheless, occidental medicine is virtually effective in treating acute illness and trauma resulting from accidents. Oriental medicine emphasizes health promotion and prevention of disease occurrence. It emphasizes the way to live with nature and comply with natural rules to strengthen the defense system, and live healthily in a state of mental and physical balance. Illness is thought to be caused by a poor defense system or a health compromise. It is believed that causative agents, such as micro-organisms and carcinogens, exist in our surroundings, but what causes illness is the weakening of our health or protective system. Oriental medicine appears to be effective in prevention of chronic and non-communicable diseases such as mental stress, hypertension and coronary heart disease.

As is the case all around the world, life expectancy in the Thai population is increasing. This is probably due to better health care and increasing health awareness in the Thai society. It is projected that, by the year 2025, Thailand will have a total population of 76 million, of which 19.1% will constitute the older population (Table 1)[1]. Female life expectancy will increase from 71.8 years in 1995 to

78.7 years in 2025. However, the age at menopause has remained relatively stable throughout the past century. Thus, Thai females must spend one-third of their life in the menopausal period, as must all other women around the world (Figure 1)[2].

In developed countries, the causes of death have changed from communicable to non-communicable diseases. Thailand is one of the developing countries where health evolution has followed that in the developed nations. Health problems in some urban areas, which have adopted occidental culture and technology, have changed, revealing a similar trend. In 1996, the Ministry of Public Health[3] conducted a national survey of the health behavior of perimenopausal and postmenopausal Thai women ($n = 8300$). They found that the prevalence of hot flushes amounted to 15.8%, which is relatively low when compared with the prevalence in some European countries[4]. Most of the responders reported high prevalence of backaches, headaches, dizziness, forgetfulness, stiff joints or joint pain, and tiredness (Figure 2 and Table 2)[3].

Given that osteoporotic fractures are most common among the elderly, the influence of increasing life expectancy on the number and regional distribution of hip fractures will be dramatic. In 1998, the Asian Osteoporosis Study Group[5] reported that the prevalence of hip fractures in Thai females was 208 per 100 000 population, and the hip fracture rate was increasing, corresponding with age[6]. This figure is relatively low when compared with the prevalence in some occidental countries[7] (Figures 3–5). Recently,

Table 1 Population projection, Thailand

	1995	*2000*	*2025*
Population total (thousands)	58 791	61 909	76 042
Population female (thousands)	29 351	30 969	38 410
Sex ratio (per 100 males)	99.7	100.1	102
Life expectancy (years)			
male	66.3	65.1	73.2
female	71.8	71.6	78.7
Population 60 years + (% of total)	7.6	8.5	19.1
Diabetes prevalence (thousands)*	863	1017	1923
Annual growth rate (%)*, 1980–95			
all age groups	1.5		
65 years +	3.9		

*Data from reference 1

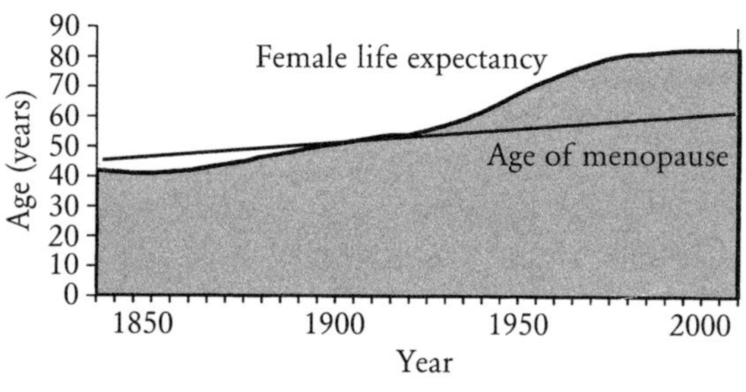

Figure 1 Female life expectancy

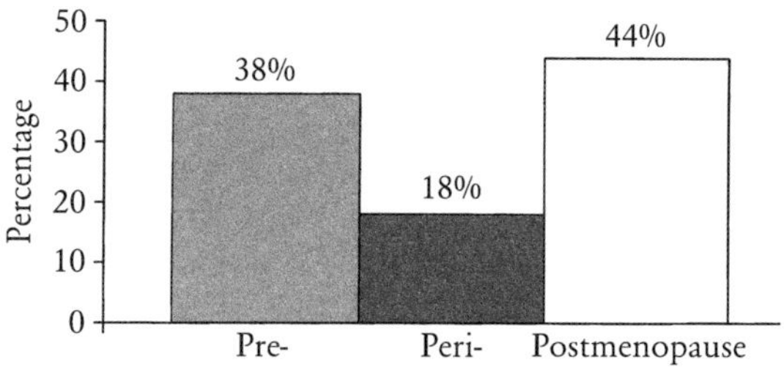

Figure 2 Distribution of pre-, peri- and postmenopausal women in Thailand. Data from reference 3

Table 2 Percentage of responders reporting bothersome symptoms during previous month ($n = 8300$). Data from reference 3

Symptoms	*Frequency*	*Percentage*
Backaches	1874	26.1
Headaches	1835	25.1
Dizziness	1806	24.7
Forgetfulness	1725	23.8
Aches or stiff joints	1630	22.5
Tiredness	1490	20.22
Muscle pain	1432	19.9
Irritability	1405	19.5
Insomnia	1159	16.0
Hot flushes	1167	15.8
Shortness of breath	1040	14.7
Pins and needles in hands and feet	1049	14.2
Uncontrolled urination	688	9.6

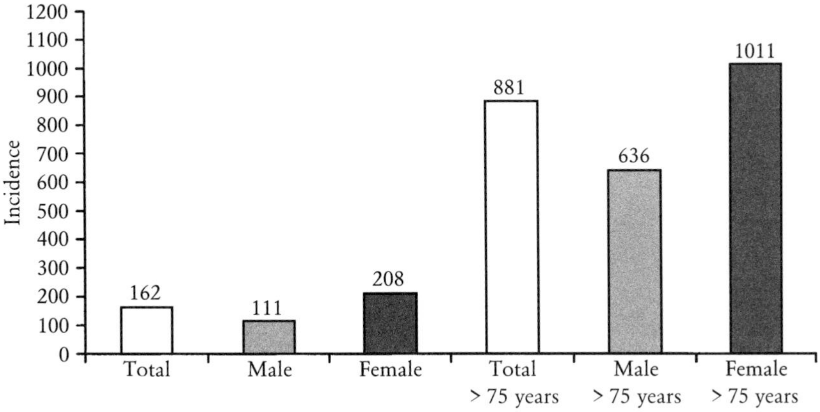

Figure 3 Hip fracture incidence (per 100 000) in Thailand according to sex. Data from reference 5

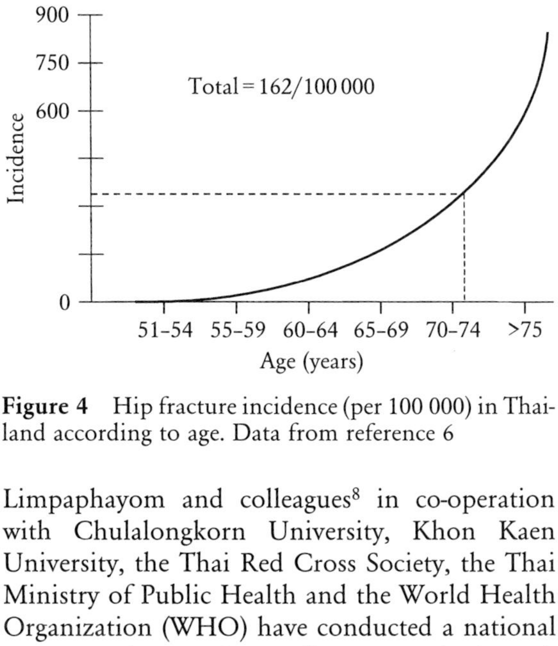

Figure 4 Hip fracture incidence (per 100 000) in Thailand according to age. Data from reference 6

Limpaphayom and colleagues[8] in co-operation with Chulalongkorn University, Khon Kaen University, the Thai Red Cross Society, the Thai Ministry of Public Health and the World Health Organization (WHO) have conducted a national survey on the prevalence of osteoporosis. According to the WHO[9], osteoporosis is defined as a level of bone mineral density (BMD) more than 2.5 standard deviations (SD) below the mean in young adults. With this cut-off value, it was found that, after adjustment for age redistribution, the prevalence of osteoporosis of the lumbar spine (L1–L4) and the femoral neck in postmenopausal Thai women was 19.75% and 13.6%, respectively (Figure 6). These figures are slightly lower than those reported from England and Wales[10].

The difference in the above frequencies is probably due to variations in the genetic background and life-style of people in various geographic locations, variations in life expectancy and the relative proportions of older populations. In addition, the applicability of WHO's criteria for osteoporosis in various communities, with their own reference database of BMD, might influence the dissimilarity in the reported prevalence of osteoporosis.

Thailand is located in a tropical zone with lots of sunshine all year round. In 1996, Chailurkit and colleagues[11] revealed a relationship between the concentration of serum levels of 25-OH-vitamin D and age. They found that serum 25-OH-vitamin D in Thai women is adequate and does not decrease with aging, as reported in some occidental countries located in areas less exposed to sunshine[12,13]. In 1994, Morrison and associates[14] showed the association of the vitamin D receptor gene with bone density. In 1997, Ongphiphadhanakul and co-workers[15] found that 78% of Thai people have the *bb* vitamin D receptor genotype, which is associated with higher calcium absorption than *Bb* and *BB*. In 1994, Komind and colleagues[16] conducted a survey of daily calcium consumption from dairy products by Thai people. They found that the average daily calcium intake was only 361 ± 168 mg. Interestingly, even though calcium consumption from dairy products in Thai growing adolescents is quite low, with a mean of 332.6 ± 305.7 mg/day, the peak BMD of young Thai adults is not different from that of Caucasians[17]. It is possible that Thai people receive calcium from a source other than dairy products, such as some traditional Thai food which is semi-

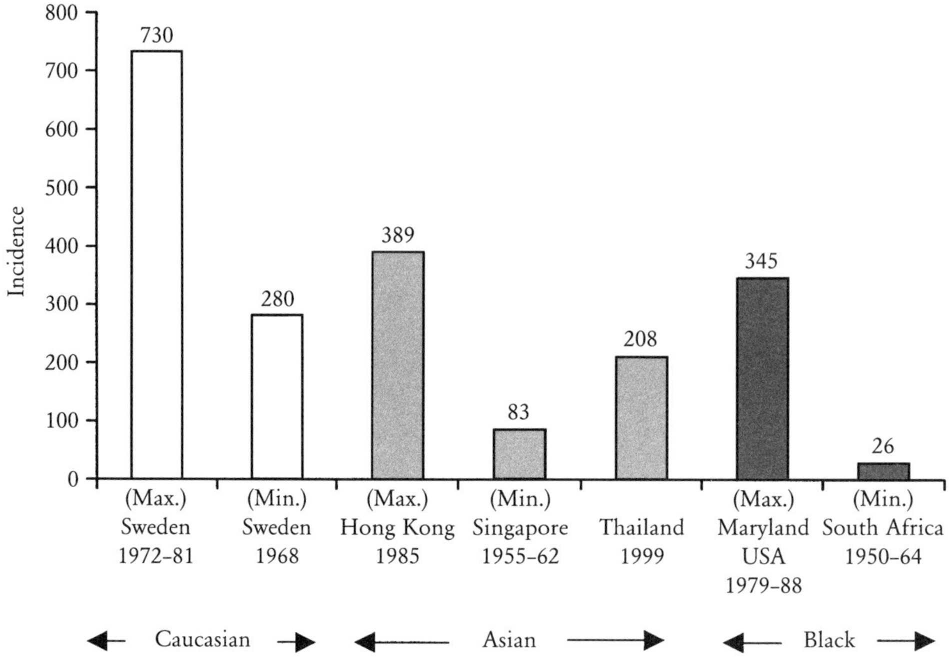

Figure 5 Age-adjusted rate of hip fracture per 100 000 population for females by ethnic group. Data from reference 7

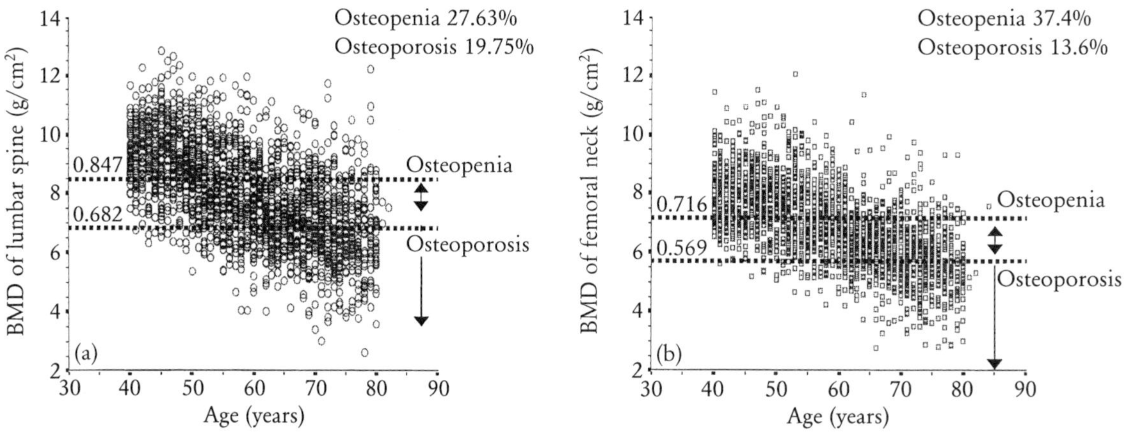

Figure 6 Age-adjusted prevalence of osteopenia and osteoporosis of (a) lumbar spine (L1–L4) and (b) femoral neck. BMD, bone mineral density. Data from reference 8

vegetarian. Other than the high prevalence of the *bb* vitamin D receptor genotype, the other possible explanation of the paradox of low calcium intake but low prevalence of osteoporosis might be the effect of sunshine, which stimulates vitamin D production by the skin and indirectly enhances calcium absorption by the gastrointestinal tract. This has been substantiated by the association of the serum 25-OH-vitamin D level with age, as discussed above[11].

Variations in ethnicity, genetic background, geographic location, life-style and sociocultural dimension should be taken into account when considering health promotion for aging women in different countries in the 21st century. It has been widely accepted that quality of life, not just prolongation of life, is the ultimate goal of global health policy. Living longer with a disability is unpleasant and implies suffering. Modern medicine with its scientific and analytical way of thinking has divided human beings into biological parts in need of further in-depth studies of their molecular mechanisms. The price paid by this approach is increasing specialization in health-care along with a decrease of holistic and spiritual attention. Recently, in Thailand, the biospiritual principle has emerged as an alternative medicine to offset the deficit of modern medicine. The biospiritual concept includes integrated medicine, macrobiotics, traditional exercise (based on oriental philosophy such as yoga, chiropractic, etc.) and the 'back to nature' concept. It also emphasizes the spiritual and mental aspect, and encourages positive thinking, mental gratitude, and cultural and communal sympathy sharing. These guidelines are barely accepted by the scientific community and even less by those in the modern medical arena. However, is it a phenomenon by which health-care seekers unintentionally communicate to the medical society the deficiencies of the modern health-care system?

Currently, an ongoing national study is being performed in Thailand to search for appropriate health behavior in the context of local culture and geography, to develop an alternative medicine for mid-life health promotion[18]. Hence, healthy aging in the 21st century should take into account the dimensions of biology, psychosociology, geography, culture-community, mind and nature. Should we reformulate our original concept of measuring quality of life by using the gross domestic product (GDP) as a standard? Might it be possible to use gross domestic happiness (GDH) as our superior standard in the upcoming century?

References

1. World Health Organization. *The World Health Report 1997. Conquering Suffering, Enriching Humanity*. Geneva: WHO, 1997
2. Cope E. Physical changes associated with the postmenopausal years. In Campbell S, ed. *The Management of the Menopause and Post-Menopausal Years*. Baltimore, MD: University Park Press, 1976:33
3. Department of Health. *The National Study of Health Behaviors of Pre and Postmenopausal Thai Women*. Bangkok: Ministry of Public Health, 1996
4. Oldenhave A. Hot flushes and their relation to other symptoms: results from the third Ede Study in The Netherlands. Presented at the *International Menopause Society World Congress on the Menopause*, Sweden, 1990:abstr 093
5. Asian Osteoporosis Study Group. Incidence of hip fracture in Chiang Mai, Thailand. Presented at the *Annual Meeting of The Royal College of Orthopedics of Thailand*, November 1999
6. Bunyarajtavej N, Rajatanavin R, Suriyawongpaisarn P. Study of epidemiology of fracture neck of femur in Thailand. 1998;in press
7. Villa MC, Melson L. Ethnicity and skeletal health, In Marcus R, ed. *Osteoporosis*. Boston: Blackwell Scientific Publications, 1994:125–45
8. Limpaphayom K, Taechakraichana N, Bunyavejchevin S. Chulalongkorn University in co-operation with Thai Red Cross Society, Ministry of Public Health, World Health Organization, 1999
9. World Health Organization. *Assessment of fracture risk and its application to screening for postmenopausal osteoporosis*. Technical Report Series. Geneva: WHO, 1994
10. Kanis JA, Melton LJ III, Christiansen C, Johnston CC, Knaltaev N. The diagnosis of osteoporosis. *J Bone Miner Res* 1994;9:1137–40
11. Chailurkit L, Rajatanavin R, Teerarungsikul K, Ongphiphadhanakul B, Puavilai G. Serum vitamin D, parathyroid hormone and biochemical markers of bone turnover in normal Thai subjects. *J Med Assoc Thai* 1996;79:499–503
12. McKenna MJ, Freaney R, Meade A, Muldowney FP. Hypovitaminosis D and elevated serum alkaline phosphatase in elderly Irish people. *Am J Clin Nutr* 1985;41:101–9
13. Lawson DEM, Paul AA, Black AE, Cole TJ, Mandal AR, Davie M. Relative contributions of diet and sunlight to vitamin D state in the elderly. *Br Med J* 1979;2:303–5

14. Morrison NA, Qi JC, Tokita A, *et al.* Prediction of bone density from vitamin D receptor alleles. *Nature (London)* 1994;367:284-7
15. Ongphiphadhanakul B, Rajatanavin R, Chanprasertyothin S, *et al.* Vitamin D receptor gene polymorphism is associated with urinary calcium excretion but not with bone mineral density in postmenopausal women. *J Endocrinol Invest* 1997; 10:592-6
16. Komind S, Piaseu N, Pattamakorn V, *et al.* Calcium status and factors relating to bone mineral content in normal Thais living in Bangkok. Program of the *10th Annual Academic Meeting of the Royal College of Physicians of Thailand*, Chomtien, 1994:61
17. Suthutvoravut U, Charoenkiatkul S, Mahachoklertwattana P, *et al.* Determinants of bone mineral density in children aged 9-18 years. Program of the *11th Annual Meeting of the Endocrine Society of Thailand*, Bangkok, 1988:29
18. Chirawatkul S, *et al.* supported by Health System Research Institute. *The Development of Alternative Medicine for Midlife Health Promotion 1999-2001*

Menopause in the aging society 13

M. Birkhäuser

DEMOGRAPHIC ASPECTS

Today, most women reach menopausal age. The percentage of women over the age of 50 years has increased constantly since the beginning of the century. In the developed world, women spend one-third of their life after the menopause. For example, in Switzerland, the percentage of women over 50 years of age of the total female population has tripled since the turn of the century and the mean life expectancy has increased from 50 to 81.7 years[1]. At the turn of the last century, the increase in life expectancy was mainly due to a reduction in postpartum mortality, to better nutrition and to better hygienic conditions. Today, modern medicine, including hormone replacement therapy (HRT), is the main cause of the prolongation of life in women[2-4]. The demographic evolution is characterized by a marked decrease in the younger generation between 20 and 40 years of age and an increase in the elderly over 70. This trend is particularly marked in women. To remain demographically equilibrated, developed countries must ensure that the active part of their total population remains stable. To reach this goal, they have to increase the birth rate per couple or accept the immigration of young people from other regions. The actual demographic crisis can be compared to other critical periods of cultural and political change such as the Renaissance, the industrial revolution or the contraceptive revolution. A rupture in the former equilibrium between the generations has marked all these periods. Furthermore, they have been marked by the end of a stable system of values and the necessity to find new values has marked all these periods. These periods are characterized by a deficit of ethical values and guidelines. One of the consequences is a decreasing respect for elderly people in our aging society.

SOCIOECONOMIC ASPECTS

Such a demographic evolution has direct economic consequences. If a new economic balance between the generations is not found, there will be a dangerous dependency of an increasing number of professionally inactive elderly on an underfinanced social-security and health-care system. This uncomfortable and problematic projection to the next 50 years can only be corrected if the prolongation of life is accompanied by a frank amelioration of the quality of life after the menopause. The prolongation of life is not an aim in itself, but has to be paralleled by measures to guarantee long-lasting good health, independence and autonomy of the elderly. For women, one of the basic conditions for a better quality of life is the availability of an efficient health-care system guaranteeing the availability of HRT.

A new contract between the generations has to be established. It will necessarily imply a flexible age of retirement. To finance the social-security system, a low fixed age of retirement cannot be maintained for economic reasons. The alternative would be a variant of Orwell's *1984*. This social challenge has to be solved by politicians without dogmatism. It will be the most important political task of the next millennium.

MEDICAL ASPECTS IN THE AGING WOMAN

Aging is not a disease, but can be associated with decreasing physical and intellectual capacities and with increasing disability and discomfort. The menopause, which is not a disease either, may lead to a diminished quality of life and to an increased risk of osteoporosis and coronary heart disease. The occurrence of the menopause, as well as of the previous progressive subfertility and infertility, is the perfect time for a woman's primary care physician or her gynecologist to assess her overall health and the need for health-maintenance measures, which may include HRT. Age at the menopause and at the preceding reproductive changes, such as the beginning of subfertility and infertility, is likely to be predetermined by the processes of atresia and follicle depletion. This process is influenced by lifestyle factors, such as smoking, and possibly by the use of oral contraceptives[5]. However, genetic factors and events during intrauterine life may play a more important role in the age-dependent decrease of female fertility[6] than was earlier estimated. The role of the primary health-care provider and the gynecologist is twofold: to guarantee an optimal quality of life, as well as physical integrity and mobility, by the prevention of diseases of the bone, the cardiovascular system and the central nervous system.

The climacteric syndrome

Peri- and postmenopausal vasomotor symptoms and consequential insomnia can seriously affect the overall quality of life. Results obtained from controlled clinical studies indicate that estrogen replacement therapy (ERT) or HRT substantially improve a woman's quality of life[7] (Table 1). A good quality of life is decisive and reflects the way a woman feels and functions. Women scheduled to undergo surgical menopause are particularly concerned by estrogen deprivation[8]. New data suggest that estrogen–androgen replacement therapy provides additional relief in the presence of persistent or severe vasomotor symptoms resistant to the usual estrogen–progestogen combinations.

Table 1 Quality of life after the menopause: influence of hormone replacement therapy. From reference 33

Result after 6 months of treatment compared to basal levels before therapy	*Estradiol (transdermal) (TTS 100) (n = 240)**		*Symptomatic treatment (n = 239)†*	
	n	%	*n*	%
Very good	128	56.9	39	18.2
Good	78	34.7	70	32.7
Acceptable	18	8.0	74	34.6
Bad	1	0.4	31	14.5

*225 completed the study; †224 completed the study

There is a generally recognized close association between lifestyle and health. Assessing the impact of a condition on the quality of life is particularly relevant in symptomatic conditions such as the ones encountered in the climacteric period. A range of measurement tools are available for monitoring how climacteric symptoms affect patients with regard to their well-being, sleep disturbance, other somatic symptoms, cognitive function and sexual functioning. Only standard and well-validated measurement tools should be used, such as those suggested recently[7]. Much is still to be learned about the reciprocal influences of lifestyle, HRT choices and quality of life. The most relevant factors influencing a woman's quality of life during the menopausal transition appear to be her previous emotional and physical health, her social situation, her experience of stressful life events (particularly bereavements and separations), as well as her beliefs about the menopause. There are considerable cultural differences in the reporting of vasomotor symptoms, which may be explained by the meaning ascribed to them and the value of older women in societies, as well as possible dietary, lifestyle and genetic differences. Those who seek medical help for menopausal problems tend to report more physical and psychological problems in general. They are more likely to be under stress and to hold particular beliefs about the menopause. These personal and social issues need to be addressed in their own right and should not be automatically attributed to the menopause[9].

Prevention of osteoporosis

Osteoporosis is a systemic skeletal disease characterized by a low bone mass and microarchitectural deterioration of the bone tissue, with a consequent increase in bone fragility and susceptibility to fracture. The World Health Organization defines osteoporosis in women in relation to bone mass or density. In osteoporosis, the bone density has a value below –2.5 SD of the healthy premenopausal population.

HRT (or ERT in hysterectomized women) is still the measure of choice to prevent osteoporosis and related fractures after the menopause. The route of administration is not important if an adequate dose of estrogen is used[10]. Some progestogens may be helpful to preserve bone mass. Low-dose estrogen administration is also effective in elderly women with osteoporosis. In the elderly, pre-existing fractures may significantly influence the prognosis of the disease and should be included in the diagnostic and prognostic assessments.

The challenge in osteoporosis prevention will be to determine the minimal doses needed in each age group to pass from global to individual preventive care and to define the strategy for elderly people. There will be an important role for alternatives to classical HRT, such as tibolone, selective estrogen receptor modulators (SERMs) or bisphosphonates, in the prevention and management of osteoporosis. Optimal non-HRT treatment strategies in osteoporosis prevention depend on age, nutritional status[11] and physical activity. Women (and men) at all ages should have an adequate intake of calcium and vitamin D. In the elderly, strategies aimed at preventing falls or the impact of falls have to be defined.

Aging of the skin and connective tissues

In postmenopausal estrogen-deficient women, collagen synthesis decreases and the skin becomes progressively thinner and wrinkled. HRT has a positive effect on collagen content and skin thickness. It can retard the process of skin wrinkling. Estrogens and HRT may therefore prevent or mitigate the clinical consequences of decreased collagen synthesis such as atrophy of the skin (including hair loss)[12,13], dry eyes (sicca syndrome)[14] and joint pain. The importance of these beneficial estrogen effects, often wrongly called 'cosmetic', is largely underestimated and may significantly improve self-image and self-esteem and enhance well-being.

Urogenital aging

Urogenital aging, the most prevalent clinical consequence of later postmenopause, affects at least 50% of postmenopausal women. For different reasons, including shame, the importance of urogenital symptoms due to estrogen deficiency is underrated. Urogenital symptoms can lead to pain at intercourse and/or micturition, to incontinence and to sexual problems, and can significantly diminish the quality of life. ERT and HRT positively influence urogenital aging[15]. Estrogens seem to alleviate urge incontinence and other urogenital problems related to atrophy. Recurrent lower urinary tract infections may be reduced. However, placebo-controlled studies are scarce.

In the elderly, the long-term use of low-dose estrogens effectively mitigates nycturia and irritable bladder and reduces lower urinary tract infections. Although the menopause is often considered a risk factor for urinary incontinence, epidemiological studies have generally not found an increase in the prevalence of incontinence in menopausal patients[16]. The role of estrogens in the management of postmenopausal urinary disorders has to be considered as an adjunct to other methods of treatment such as surgery, physiotherapy and drugs[15,17].

Cardiovascular risk

Coronary heart disease is the major cause of death in women in the developed world. After the menopause, the female risk of cardiovascular death progressively approaches the male risk. Most women do not know that the most dangerous killer after the menopause is not breast cancer, but coronary heart disease: about ten times more women die from a heart attack than from breast cancer[2]. Although cardiovascular mortality is decreasing, morbidity and health-care costs are increasing. Interventions to reduce the risk of coronary heart disease by correcting abnormalities of known cardiovascular risk factors in postmenopausal women are warranted both in public health and for the individual.

Women with estrogen deficiency exhibit many metabolic features of the insulin resistance syndrome. Insulin resistance may contribute to their increased risk for coronary heart diseases. HRT may correct many of these metabolic alterations, both directly and indirectly, to benefit the cardiovascular system. Although observational studies can be subjected to bias due to both selection and compliance with treatment, a large number of differently designed epidemiological studies have uniformly suggested that ERT and HRT protects against coronary heart disease[2-4,18,19]. There is sufficient epidemiological evidence to merit the consideration of HRT for primary prevention in women[20]. Randomized clinical trials still need to be performed. Depending on the type and the dosage, a progestogen might produce unwanted effects. However, data available today do not suggest that progestogens given in low therapeutic doses impede the beneficial cardiovascular effects of estrogen[21,22]. The benefits of HRT are likely to be seen with the oral as well as the non-oral administration of estrogens.

The recently published HERS study[23] questioned the value of secondary prevention by HRT. During the first 2 years of the trial, the relative risk increased slightly, mainly because of a higher incidence of thromboembolic events. However, the long-term effect seems to be beneficial. These results lead to the conclusion that it does not seem appropriate to start HRT as a routine in a patient who never took estrogens before her heart attack, but that it is not necessary to stop well-tolerated HRT after a myocardial infarction. In the presence of a given indication, the transdermal route should be preferred.

Estrogen deficiency and the central nervous system

Estrogen and progesterone receptors are widely distributed in the human brain and mediate genomic action. In addition, estrogens and progestogens display non-genomic effects. Estrogens stimulate the outgrowth of neuronal processes and synaptic connections, with positive effects on neuronal size, number, connectivity, volume and plasticity. Androgens and progesterone produce many effects in the nervous system. Alterations in the circulating levels of androgens play an important role in the psychological and sexual changes that occur after the menopause[24]. However, primary mental disorders are not primarily caused by a deficiency of sex hormones. Therefore, estrogens cannot currently be employed as causative primary therapy for mental disorders in the postmenopause. Other factors, such as psychosocial and environmental conditions, may contribute to the pathogenesis of psychological disorders in menopausal women[9].

There is evidence to suggest that HRT positively influences alertness, cognitive function, affective and sexual behaviors, memory, motor activity, pain perception and well-being in general[25] (Table 2). Thus, HRT has a clinically evident mental tonic effect. It is a more physiological substitute for tranquillizers and antidepressants, which are still used too often to treat the climacteric syndrome. Dementia of the Alzheimer's type has become a major health problem. Some epidemiological studies have shown a reduction in the incidence of Alzheimer's disease in postmenopausal women treated with HRT. However, other trials did not confirm these findings. Further studies are needed.

Sexuality after the menopause

Although androgens are secreted by the ovary before and to a lesser degree after the menopause, they are rarely substituted. There has never been a healthier, better-educated, better-informed and wealthier generation of older women than that of today. There is no doubt that a positively lived sexuality can help to improve the quality of life[26]. However, difficulties in defining, reporting and sampling the sexual experience of older women have limited the information available today. The effects of short-term estrogen therapy in improving psychological symptoms, maintaining vaginal lubrication, decreasing vaginal atrophy and increasing pelvic blood flow in postmenopausal women is well known. However, some patients require more than estrogen alone to improve

Table 2 Comparison of the quality of life in two postmenopausal groups (group 1 with hormone replacement therapy (HRT) and group 2 without HRT) with a premenopausal control population. The greatest improvements were observed in anxiety, vitality, self-control, sleep quality, general well-being, social isolation and sexuality. From reference 25

Group	*Life quality score*
Without HRT	87
With HRT	105
Controls	105

psychological dysfunction, decreased sexual desire or other sexual problems associated with the menopause. Some authors postulate that postmenopausal androgen deficiency should be treated by androgen administration[27,28]. Although there is no statistical relationship between testosterone levels and libido after the menopause, clinical experience demonstrates that testosterone can be beneficial in patients with a loss of libido when estrogens alone have no effect. Results from clinical studies show that HRT with estrogens plus androgens provides a greater improvement in psychological (e.g. lack of concentration, depression and fatigue) and sexual (e.g. decreased libido and inability to have an orgasm) symptoms than does estrogen alone in naturally and surgically menopausal women[24]. In spite of these findings, androgen administration is still rarely used in postmenopausal women. Dehydroepiandrosterone, a common precursor of estrogens and androgens, could become of practical importance in hormonal substitution in females and males. Unfortunately, solid short- and long-term studies are lacking. However, it has to be stressed that a loss of libido can be due to other causes, such as stress or partner problems, and not only to hormonal deficiency.

The recent discovery of human pheromones might open up some HRT-independent sexual options for maturing women. Both the adrenal and the ovarian sources of estrogens, androgens and progesterone show age-related changes that alter a woman's capacity to attract sexual attention through both her physical appearance and condition and her pheromonal excretions[29]. Pheromones are not yet available for clinical use.

Amelioration of acceptance

Although epidemiological data strongly suggest that HRT induces a significant improvement in the quality of life for postmenopausal women, the majority do not choose HRT[30]. The development of regimens with substantially better acceptance did not greatly change their attitude, although today, oral and transdermal as well as sequential and continuous-combined regimens are available. Surveys generally reveal that only a small proportion of postmenopausal women use HRT[31]. In Belgium, just 14% of postmenopausal women use HRT[30]. However, no regimen or any mode of administration has proven superior with regard to patient compliance if we do not take into account some national and cultural particulars[31]. In several cultures, women do not accept uterine bleeding after the cessation of ovarian function. As long as the occurrence of uterine bleeding is linked to any HRT regimen in non-hysterectomized women, adherence will remain low. Therefore, new molecules, such as tibolone or raloxifene, are highly interesting. Adherence to HRT can only be ameliorated by better individualization and better information. Determination of the optimum dose, best molecules, time of initiation and duration of therapy needs further study, particularly in the elderly[32].

The second important challenge for the future is the amelioration of nutrition in the geriatric population. Nutrition plays a significant modulating role in the aging process and is an important component in the health care of the elderly. The dynamic interrelationships of nutrition and aging emerge as highly important aspects of modern medicine[11].

CONCLUSIONS

Both the demographic and the social evolution are strongly linked to the solutions medicine can offer to menopausal women in our aging society. The medical target is to guarantee optimal health care to maintain our elderly population autonomous and independent. This challenge cannot be solved without a deep understanding of the medical possibilities and limits by health-care officials, politicians and economists.

The main points postulated in the 1990s are still fully valid[9,34]. Their fulfilment is the basic challenge to the medical community: the medical community has to provide balanced information about the menopause and aging to women and their families. The community has to be ready to discuss attitudes towards the menopause and reassure overly pessimistic beliefs. Furthermore, the medical community has to organize health-promotion sessions focusing upon diet, exercise and smoking: these factors are associated with both general and personal health and social issues met by women during midlife[9]. HRT must be offered, be discussed and be used in given indications.

To reach these goals, the following conditions have to be fulfilled:

(1) Standardization of the terminology;

(2) Better education of doctors and paramedics;

(3) Availability of support groups for menopausal women;

(4) More specific medical counselling;

(5) Improved menopausal center organization to meet women's individual needs;

(6) Access to HRT for women in low socioeconomic conditions.

In our aging society, the quality of life of elderly and very old women will largely depend on the ability of society to cope with the economic, social and medical challenges of the menopause.

References

1. Schweiz. Jarbuch für Statistik 1999, *www.adm*.ch
2. Grodstein F, Stampfer MJ, Colditz GA, *et al.* Postmenopausal hormone therapy and mortality. *N Engl J Med* 1997;336:1769–75
3. Grady D, Rubin SM, Petitti DB, *et al.* Hormone therapy to prevent disease and prolong life in postmenopausal women. *Ann Intern Med* 1992;117: 1016–37
4. Henderson BE, Paganini-Hill A, Ross RK. Decreased mortality in users of estrogen replacement therapy. *Arch Intern Med* 1991;151:75–8
5. Zichella L. The importance of life style after menopause. *Int J Fertil Menopausal Stud* 1995;40:9–15
6. te Velde ER, Dorland M, Broekmans FJ. Age at menopause as a marker of reproductive ageing. *Maturitas* 1998;30:119–25
7. Wiklund I. Methods of assessing the impact of climacteric complaints on quality of life. *Maturitas* 1998;29:41–50
8. Bachmann GA. Vasomotor flushes in menopausal women. *Am J Obstet Gynecol* 1999;180:312–16
9. Hunter MS. Predictors of menopausal symptoms: psychosocial aspects. *Baillières Clin Endocrinol Metab* 1993;7:33–45
10. Lippuner K, Haenggi W, Birkhaeuser MH, Casez JP, Jaegar P. Prevention of postmenopausal bone loss using tibolone or conventional peroral or transdermal hormone replacement therapy with 17beta-estradiol and dydrogesterone. *J Bone Miner Res* 1997;12:806–12
11. Young EA. Nutrition, aging, and the aged. *Med Clin North Am* 1983;67:295–313
12. Pierard GE, Letawe C, Dowlati A, Pierard-Franchimont C. Effect of hormone replacement therapy for menopause on the mechanical properties of skin. *J Am Geriatr Soc* 1995;43:662–5
13. Brincat M, Kabalan S, Studd JW, Moniz CF, de Trafford J, Montgomery J. A study of the relationship of skin content, skin thickness, and bone mass in postmenopausal women. *Obstet Gynecol* 1987;70:840–5
14. Sator MO, Joura EA, Golaszewski T, *et al.* Treatment of menopausal keratoconjunctivitis sicca with topical estradiol. *Br J Obstet Gynaecol* 1998;105: 100–2
15. Cardozo LD, Keleher CJ. Sex hormones, the menopause and urinary problems. *Gynecol Endocrinol* 1995;9:75–84
16. Thom DH, Brown JS. Reproductive and hormonal risk factors for urinary incontinence in later life: a review of the clinical and epidemiologic literature. *J Am Geriatr Soc* 1998;146:1411–17
17. Notelovitz M. Urogenital aging: solutions in clinical practice. *Int J Gynaecol Obstet* 1997;59:S35–9
18. Grodstein F, Stampfer MJ. Estrogen for women at varying risk of coronary disease. *Maturitas* 1998; 30:19–26
19. Stampfer MJ, Colditz GA. Estrogen replacement therapy and coronary heart disease: a quantitative assessment of the epidemiologic evidence. *Prev Med* 1991;20:47–63
20. Rosano GM, Sarrel PM, Poole-Wilson PA, Collins P. Beneficial effect of oestrogen on exercise-induced myocardial ischaemia in women with coronary artery disease. *Lancet* 1993;342:133–6
21. Haenggi W, Lippuner K, Riesen W, Jaeger Ph, Birkhäuser MH. Long-term influence of different hormone replacement regimens on serum lipids and lipoprotein(a): a randomised study. *Br J Obstet Gynaecol* 1997;104:708–17
22. PEPI Trial Writing Group. Effects of estrogen or estrogen/progestin regimes on heart disease risk

factors in postmenopausal women: the Postmenopausal Estrogen/Progestin Interventions (PEPI) Trial. *J Am Med Assoc* 1995;273:199-208
23. Hulley S, Grady D, Bush T, *et al.* for the Heart and Estrogen/Progestin Replacement Study (HERS) Research Group. Randomized trial of estrogen plus progestin for secondary prevention of coronary heart disease in postmenopausal women. *J Am Med Assoc* 1998;280:605-13
24. Sarrel PM. Psychosexual effects of menopause: role of androgens. *Am J Obstet Gynecol* 1999;180:319-24
25. Wiklund I, Karlberg J, Mattsson LA. Quality of life of postmenopausal women on a regimen of transdermal estradiol therapy. *Am J Obstet Gynecol* 1993; 168:824-30
26. Roughan PA, Kaiser FE, Morley JE. Sexuality and the older woman. *Clin Geriatr Med* 1993;9:87-106
27. Bachmann GA. Androgen cotherapy in menopause: evolving benefits and challenges. *Am J Obstet Gynecol* 1999;180:308-11
28. Warnock JK, Bundren JC, Morris DW. Female hypoactive sexual desire disorder due to androgen deficiency: clinical and psychometric issues. *Psychopharmacol Bull* 1997;33:761-6
29. Cutler WB, Genovese-Stone E. Wellness in women after 40 years of age: the role of sex hormones and pheromones. *Dis Mon* 1998;44:421-546
30. Rozenberg S, Vandromme J, Kroll M, Pastijn A, Liebens F. Compliance to hormone replacement therapy. *Int J Fertil Menopausal Stud* 1995;40(Suppl 1):23-32
31. Dören M, Schneider HPG. The impact of different HRT regimens on compliance. *Int J Fertil Menopausal Stud* 1996;41:29-39
32. Miller KL. Hormone replacement therapy in the elderly. *Clin Obstet Gynecol* 1996;39:912-32
33. Limouzin-Lamothe MA, Mairon N, Joyce CR, Le Gal M. Quality of life after menopause: influence of hormonal replacement therapy. *Am J Obstet Gynecol* 1994;170:618-24
34. Birkhäuser M, ed. European Menopause Society. European consensus development conference on menopause. *Hum Reprod* 1996;11:975-9

The climacteric in Latin America: actual state and future trends 14

N. O. Siseles, A. P. Gutiérrez and F. C. Sayegh

HEALTH FOR ALL, AND WOMEN IN MIDLIFE

The name Alma-Ata has become synonymous with one of the great public health movements in history: the search for health equity, as a goal stated by the World Health Organization (WHO) in 1978[1]. Item IV of Alma-Ata's declaration emphasizes the fact that it is the people's right and duty to take part, both individually and collectively, in the planning and implementation of their own health care.

In Latin American countries, the meaning conveyed by the 'health for all' premise is adapted to women in midlife.

The difficulties that middle-aged women meet in the Americas are an extension of those confronting younger women, but yet another burden is added because of the stage they have reached in their lives. Nevertheless, women have also acquired resources of wisdom and ability, which will enable them to manage in a physical and social environment that is, on the whole, a hostile one. This environment has, in fact, often been disregarded.

The grounds for the advancement of health are established in WHO's principles, which advocate health for all: adding life to years rather than years to life. So far, emphasis has been laid on the duration of life, with little or no concern about the quality of life[2].

EPIDEMIOLOGY OF AGING

Today we are witnessing the fastest rate of world population growth in the whole of human history. Still, in the case of Latin America, growth is heterogeneous and differs widely across the various countries of the region.

Over the past three decades, the region has experienced significant improvements in matters of health. One indicator of such improvements is the increase in life expectancy from birth, which is higher in the case of women: this was 53.5 years in 1950, it will have reached 72.4 years by the year 2000 and it will go up to 81.1 years by 2050[3].

Our countries, which are less prepared to cope with a rapidly aging population, are likely to be faced with the impending danger of having to come to grips with the problem in the near future. Women make up the majority of the aged population, both in developed and developing countries of the region[4].

DEMOGRAPHIC TRANSITION

The notion of demographic transition aptly describes the consequences of changes in the population's fertility and mortality patterns. This frame of reference describes the transition from a poor growth stage (resulting from a combination of high fertility rates and equally high death rates) to another, also poor growth stage, which is due to a combination of low fertility and low death rates. In between these two stages, a decrease in mortality followed by a decrease in fertility has given rise to the century's rapid population growth[5].

As a consequence of the above, the most remarkable fact in the most recent decades becomes apparent, namely, population aging. This phenomenon has occurred everywhere in Latin America[6]; compared to the way it occurred in industrialized countries, in Latin America it came about in a much shorter period of time and it has seldom been possible to foresee its consequences. There are wide differences between countries and, inside each particular country, there are also differences between urban and rural areas, as well as among social classes and ethnic groups[7].

The dramatic change in the pyramid population structure of Latin America over the past 30 years reflects the changes in each age group within the population. Over this period in both sexes, the base of the pyramid has shrunk, while both the middle and the top have widened. It is at the top where we find the oldest population group. This enables us to make a projection about 2020[8,9] (Figure 1).

On the whole, the population of Latin America may be said to be young. Some countries, such as Bolivia and Haiti, are at an incipient demographic transition stage, with high fertility and death rates[8], or else at a moderate demographic transition stage, as is the case with El Salvador, Guatemala, Honduras, Nicaragua and Paraguay. The birth rates in these countries have increased while mortality is moderate, a combination which results in a naturally high growth rate, about 3% per year.

Cuba, Uruguay, Argentina and Chile rank among the less young countries. They are in an advanced demographic transition stage; in other words, they are moving towards a middle-aged population with less growth on account of low birth rates and low-to-moderate death rates, which implies a naturally low growth rate of about 1% per year.

Countries such as Brazil, Colombia, Costa Rica, Ecuador, Mexico, Panama, Peru, the Dominican Republic and Venezuela are in a demographic transition process, with moderate birth rates and moderate-to-low mortality, which result in a naturally moderate growth rate, about 2% per year[7].

The rapid increase in the postmenopausal population, especially in countries going through an advanced demographic transition stage, has brought ever more increasing demands on social welfare systems; at the same time, it has increased poverty issues among the older part of the population.

Aging, and its impact on the quality of life of the Latin American female population, poses a dramatic socioeconomic challenge. In this respect, demographic changes have played a significant role in the so-called epidemiological transition.

EPIDEMIOLOGICAL TRANSITION

By epidemiological transition, we mean a change from a morbid structure, with predominant intestinal infections and respiratory diseases affecting the whole of the population from very early childhood, to another structure marked by cardiovascular diseases, cancer and stroke, which mainly affect elderly adults[7]. On studying the main causes of death, it can be seen that there is an epidemiological transition in most countries of the region[10].

MORBIDITY AND MORTALITY IN MIDDLE-AGED AND ELDERLY WOMEN

Despite longer life expectancy, there is no concomitant growth in life expectancy free from disability. Consequently, there are more middle-aged and

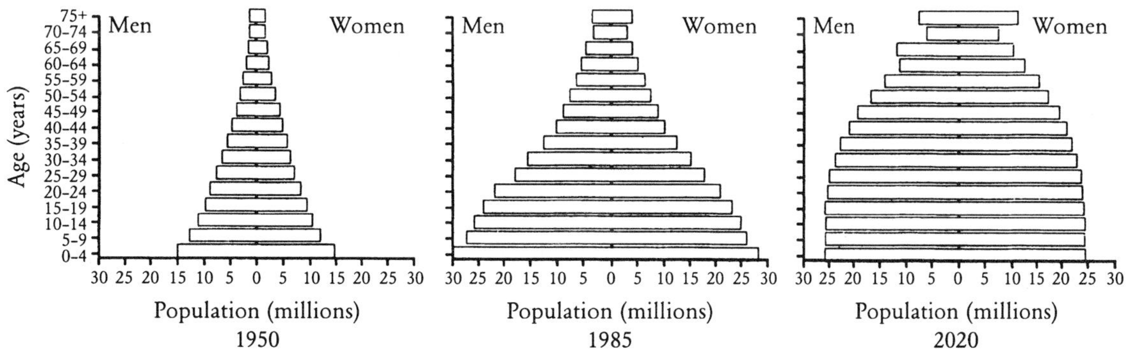

Figure 1 Demographic transition in Latin America. Evolution of the population (1950–2020) from references 8 and 9

elderly women suffering from disabilities; this is a personal tragedy where independence is lost, with a subsequent impoverishment of the quality of life. Thus, society is confronted with the problem of providing suitable health and prevention services to these women amidst a threatening economic environment[11].

The women in this group have lived under strain throughout their lives; they have been subjected to malnutrition, had too many children born after pregnancies separated by very short intervals, and had a double or triple workload. These factors often cause Latin American women to age prematurely.

Even though the order varies from one country to another, the five main causes of death for Latin American women above 65 years of age are cardiovascular disease, cancer, stroke, diabetes and infections.

Cardiovascular disease

By the year 2000, the number of deaths caused by cardiovascular disease in Latin America is estimated to be 1 000 000, which amounts to almost 50% of the deaths caused by non-transmissible diseases[12].

As regards its female population, Argentina has the highest rate of premature deaths resulting from cardiovascular diseases. While it is true that there is a downward trend for cardiovascular diseases, it is also true that few countries have succeeded in reducing them.

There is no available information about the prevalence of the main risk factors for this disease in our region. The CARMEN project (Action for the Multifactorial Reduction of non-Transmissible Diseases), where Chile represents our region, shows that sedentariness and heavy smoking have a much higher prevalence in Chile than they do in Canada. It shows, too, that hypertension, sedentariness and obesity are more frequently found in the lower strata of society[13].

Cancer

The prevalence of different tumors varies in the different Latin American countries. In the more industrialized countries, there has been a significant decrease in cervical cancer. As living conditions improve, its incidence may well go down, for it is poorly educated women that have more seriously advanced tumors[14].

Deaths resulting from breast cancer are lower in Latin America than in industrialized countries; however, some of the data point to a fast increase in deaths from this disease.

In Argentina, breast cancer in women between 45 and 63 years of age yields an annual death rate of 53.3 per 100 000 women. This figure has remained relatively stable since 1980. Moreover, it is in the richer provinces that mortality is higher, a fact that highlights the importance of environmental factors in the etiology of this kind of cancer[15].

As in Argentina, more women die of breast cancer than of cervical cancer in Chile, Cuba and Uruguay[16] (Table 1).

Stroke

Most premature deaths caused by stroke are to be found in Brazil, Argentina and Colombia. In the past few years, death rates associated with this disease have decreased significantly, though not in Cuba, El Salvador and Venezuela[16].

Diabetes

The incidence of diabetes in elderly Latin American women has increased, particularly in developing countries. This is correlated with an

Table 1 Death rates from breast and cervical cancer (per 100 000 women) in women aged 45–64 years in some Latin American countries (1994). From reference 16

Country	*Breast cancer death rate*	*Cervical cancer death rate*
Argentina	54.3	10.9
Chile	31.7	27.1
Colombia	25.0	27.5
Costa Rica	33.8	32.4
Cuba	43.1	12.9
Mexico	24.3	34.8
Venezuela	30.6	27.8
Uruguay	74.0	13.4

increase in *obesity*[14]. Morbidity through diabetes has high-impact effects, which is not the case with other causes of death.

Infections

The primary causes of death among the indigenous population of Latin America are infectious diseases, parasitic diseases, and diseases acquired from arthropod vectors[17].

The incidence and prevalence of tuberculosis and other infectious diseases, including malaria and Chagas-Mazza disease, have been gradually yet steadily decreasing in the region. However, rural and indigenous populations show a higher incidence than the national mean average[18,19].

These diseases, most of which can be handled through adequate prevention, are a consequence of malnutrition, unhealthy living conditions and a poor supply of basic utilities.

Further causes of morbidity in middle-aged Latin American women are arthrosis and osteoporosis, both of which appear as signs of premature aging. The former is due to the excessive physical exertion that these women cannot avoid if they are to support themselves and their families, whereas the latter stems from an endemic, nutritional calcium deficiency. There is virtually no data about either the incidence or the prevalence of osteoporosis in Latin America. Among the few existing studies, one, carried out in Argentina, reported that the incidence rate of proximal hip fracture affected 233.4 women per 100 000 inhabitants in a population group over 50 years old. Another study, conducted in Chile, found a prevalence of 110 hip fractures per 100 000 women. We lack accurate information about other risk factors threatening Latin American women; moreover, we do not know whether a dark skin and suitable exposure to sunlight - both protective factors - could compensate for nutritional deficiencies[20].

Mental diseases deserve special consideration because of their striking impact. Although they are not to be found among the five main causes of death, their onset is likely to be a consequence of women having suffered 60 or more years of social subjection, multiple tasks, double or triple working hours, responsibility devoid of authority, continual assistance to others and chronic diseases[4].

Studies about the prevalence of Alzheimer's disease in Latin America show that, among people, particularly women, aged 60 years or more, 8.4–19.7% may suffer from dementia or show some cognitive deficiency[5].

SOCIOECONOMIC CONTEXT OF WOMEN IN MIDLIFE

All over Latin America, women are responsible for reproduction and assistance to others. However, the circumstances surrounding these duties are often out of their control. When this happens in less-developed countries, there arise problems of malnutrition and its sequelae. A large number of adult women in Latin America suffer from anemia caused by nutritional deficiency; the long-term effect of this may be deleterious as regards both productivity and overall health. In the more developed countries of the region, women give birth to fewer children, but malnutrition is still present, disguised as obesity[5].

Multiple deliveries, together with the genetic and gynecological-obstetric alterations resulting from them, lead to the risk of high death rates in mothers. As women advance in years, we have to think of the shape of a 'J'; that is, after 35 years of age, the older the woman, the higher the risk[21].

The burden of having to assist several generations results in women being driven from their role of carers into the role of individuals in need of care, without a transitional period in between. Living together with the family is mostly a cultural phenomenon; in almost every Latin American country, there is a solid tradition of family support[4].

Table 2 summarizes some of the most important socioeconomic factors, as well as their consequences, which affect middle-aged Latin American women.

LATIN AMERICAN WOMEN'S PERCEPTION OF THE MENOPAUSE

In Latin American women, the experience of the menopause is determined by a combination of biological and cultural factors[22]. There are wide, sociological-based differences across countries

Table 2 Socioeconomic factors and their consequences affecting middle-aged women in Latin America

Factors	*Consequences*
Malnutrition	anemia, obesity
Multiple deliveries and aging mothers	genetic and gyneco-obstetric alterations
Large families	role of carer to several generations
Prevalence of extreme poverty and poor schooling	higher vulnerability: low adaptability to rapidly changing societies, poor health, lack of information

and, in one same country, there are differences between urban and rural areas, social sectors and ethnic groups. Women living in rural areas are supposed to be clearly aware of the changes that they are undergoing, but they must keep silent about them because there is a lack of space where they can be discussed. The kind of life these women have led has prevented them from taking good care of their bodies, let alone the sort of sophisticated care in which well-off women can indulge. Different social sectors are affected by different pathologies and diseases. Reaching the menopause with excessive obesity or crippling varicose veins results from a lack of economic means that prevents these women from choosing their food wisely; it is also a consequence of working on their feet for long hours without the possibility of taking a break.

Few studies have been carried out in the region. A survey in Montevideo, Uruguay, revealed the mass media to be the largest source of information about the menopause: nearly 50% of the women interviewed never consulted a physician on this issue. Their major concern was the long-term risk of diseases such as osteoporosis and stroke. They attributed a beneficial effect to hormone replacement therapy (HRT) in terms of an improved quality of life, but they also believed that it had a negative effect (hormones are fattening)[23].

Anthropological research carried out in Havanna, Cuba, found that women going out to a job while also doing household chores show a low incidence of menopausal symptoms, especially those related to emotional frailness and diminished libido. Moreover, this study found that menopausal symptoms appeared more frequently whenever there was some family/couple dysfunction[24].

In 1986, Barnett[25] studied a group of Peruvian women and noted that acceptance of, and adjustment to, the menopause were dependent on the woman's satisfaction with her main role in life. Two main roles stood out: that of the mother and that of the worker. Mothers whose children had not fulfilled their expectations experienced more difficulties during the menopause, whereas working women, whose satisfaction depended not only on their children but also on their own behavior in life, responded better[25].

ACTUAL STATE OF HRT IN LATIN AMERICA

HRT prevalence in Latin America is quite low, but it is increasing steadily. In 1990, only 2.8% of women received HRT; in 1998, the percentage rose to 5.6%, and this is projected to reach 9.6% of the postmenopausal female population by the year 2000[26]. This acceptance rate varies in the different countries of the region included in this study, as can be seen in Figure 2.

The most usual methods of HRT treatment are oral, followed by patches, injections and gel. The majority of women who use HRT in Latin America belong to the upper classes, where the prevalence of HRT use is 18%, but the wide distribution of HRT by laboratories and competition among them have enabled middle-class women to access this therapy. Thus, in middle-class women, HRT use has increased from 4.2% in 1994 to 7.8% today[26].

According to the International Marketing Service, the foreseen increase in the use of HRT will be higher in Latin America than in the rest of the world, rising from 16.1 million units in 1994 to 37.5 million units in the year 2000, which means a growth of 133% over the period[26].

FUTURE TRENDS

Women in the 45–59-year age range constitute a population subgroup about which little is known from a demographic point of view. The reason

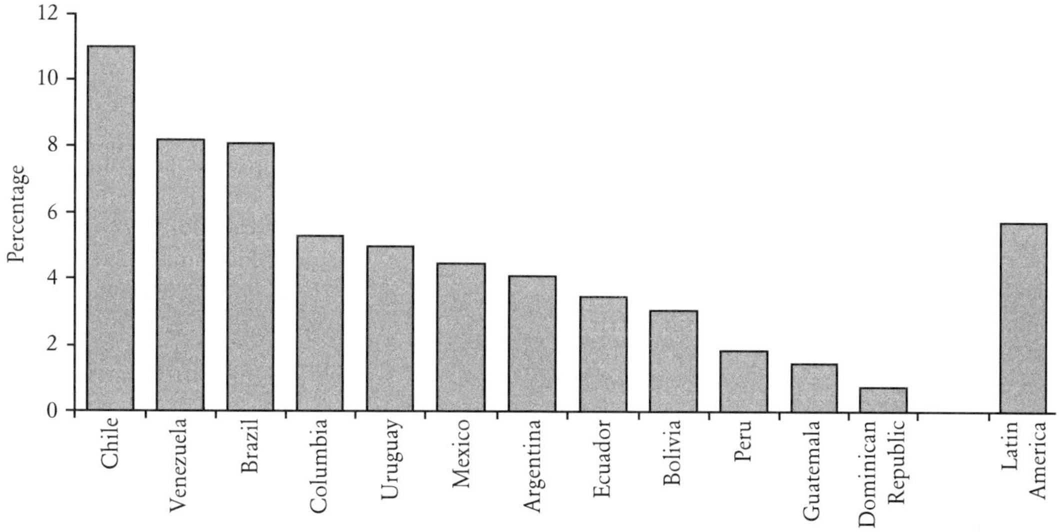

Figure 2 Acceptance rate of hormone replacement therapy in Latin American countries (1998). From International Marketing Service countries

for this lies in the fact that they are rendered invisible, as it were, among women in their reproductive years (15–49 years old) and elderly women (over 60 years old). On the whole, women in their 50s have remained outside every health study and are not addressed by any specific program[24].

The Pennell report states that only a small percentage of scientific advances in the field of medicine accounts for health improvement in the 20th century, since, in fact, the better quality of life and better working conditions are the main reasons for the increase in life expectancy[27].

It is essential to put into practice an integral approach to women, assessing them from a biological and social standpoint. In order to do so, we should reform health policies and offer opportunities and new programs promoting the said approach, while fostering development in the region.

Governmental bodies, professionals involved in health areas, pharmaceutical industries and women themselves can together maintain and improve the health of women in midlife by means of various strategies aimed at reducing morbidity and mortality at this time of life.

Climacteric societies should make the following recommendations to governmental bodies:

(1) Research should be carried out into the possibilities of improving women's health from menopause onwards;

(2) Climacteric women should be granted equal rights and be included in health policies in the planning of health services;

(3) The potential cost to governments, stemming from avoidable deaths and disabilities, should be evaluated;

(4) Primary and secondary prevention strategies against stroke and osteoporosis should be outlined by means of campaigns aimed at changing unhealthy hygienic and dietary habits;

(5) Screening programs should be put into practice with a view to detecting genital and breast cancer in their very early stages;

(6) Educational materials should be devised so as to help middle-aged women know more about their own health.

We physicians should achieve awareness of the following:

(1) Undergraduate curricula should be expanded so that a wider knowledge of their future professional life in relation to the age group in

question can be achieved. Furthermore, a continual medical update should be encouraged so that graduate physicians may resort to the latest findings.

(2) Clinical studies researching middle-aged women, elderly women and women in ethnic minorities should be carried out.

(3) The multidisciplinary nature of health should be emphasized, integrating both sociological and biological aspects in the fields of assistance and research.

(4) A satisfying patient–doctor relationship should be worked out. This will ensure that women have a clear understanding of their choices and will enable them to talk about what they choose when it comes to making decisions about treatment for seeking a better quality of life. This will result in easy, suitable, convenient courses of treatment (individual choice of treatment).

(5) Helping women to make correct decisions about their health and the care it requires, as well as fostering awareness about the need to restructure their way of living and to find alternative ways towards self-fulfilment (proactive co-management).

(6) Periodic assessments should be carried out in order to monitor the chosen treatment, particularly in the early stages.

In order to improve women's compliance with HRT use, pharmaceutical industries should:

(1) Carry out further research into and development of new molecules with negligible side-effects;

(2) Develop new therapies, bearing in mind the profile of the target population, in order to meet the new needs of the demographic transition in Latin America;

(3) Adjust product costs so that their products are more accessible to the low-income female population in Latin American countries;

(4) Reach agreements with scientific societies and universities so as to promote long-term effectiveness and security studies;

(5) Aid governmental drug regulation organizations, such as the Food and Drug Administration and Administración Nacional de Medicamentos y Tecnologia (ANMAT), by providing them with more accurate information and thereby increasing compliance.

It would be desirable for women to look upon midlife as a time of change and to seek early advice about the steps they could take for their well-being. A healthier lifestyle can be achieved by the following:

(1) Undertaking more physical exercise and giving up unhealthy habits;

(2) Developing personal skills and abilities;

(3) Playing an active part in their own health care;

(4) Interacting with health services.

CONCLUSIONS

Rather than viewing the aging of their population as a problem, countries should take a pride in their increased lifespan. Healthy aging is an accomplishment of civilized, advanced nations.

Women's longevity appears to be a marked biological advantage; yet, in Latin America, it is frequently blurred by the social and cultural disadvantages confronting women. The explanation for ordinary physical and psychosocial problems afflicting women in midlife can usually be found in their living conditions.

It must be clearly understood that no egalitarian health policies can be developed unless the needs, contributions, opportunities and risks of both sexes are borne in mind; middle-age requires attention along these lines. Latin America lacks personalized attention programs for climacteric women, let alone programs including gender as a category for epidemiological analysis.

Societies should behave with solidarity and support the transcendental type of change that is required. Without social commitment, there is no political commitment on the part of the governments, and fragmentary attempts at improving the condition of women, particularly that of middle-aged women, end in failure.

Nevertheless, a higher level of acceptance would not suffice to improve the standard of living, as this depends upon the quality of integral medical care. This should undergo some changes. Prevention is important and economic and cultural barriers must be overcome so that all women have access to information. This is not easy, but it appears to be the most suitable way forward if we wish to achieve health for all at the dawn of the new century.

References

1. World Health Organization. *From Alma Ata to the Year 2000: Reflections at the Midpoint.* Geneva: WHO, 1988:9-12
2. Pan American Health Organization, Regional Office for Europe. *Targets for Health for All.* Copenhagen: Euro, 1985. In Anzola Perez E, ed. *Elderly Care, a Challenge in the 1990s.* Washington, DC: PAHO, 1996;546:453-71
3. Diczfalusy E. La humanidad que envejece: ¿estaremos adelantándonos a nuestro futuro?. *Ginecol Reprod* 1998;6:122-33
4. Sennott-Miller L. Older women in the Americas: problems and potential. In *Gender, Women and Health in the Americas.* Washington, DC: PAHO, 1993;541:104-11
5. Pan American Health Organization. Health of the elderly. In *Health in the Américas.* Washington, DC: PAHO, 1998;569:82-7
6. Medina Lois E. Epidemiology of aging in Latin America. In Gonzalez Campos O, Arteaga Urzúa E, Contreras Castro P, eds. *Menopausia y Longevidad. Perspectiva Clínica y Epidemiológica en Latinoamérica.* Santiago de Chile: Ediciones Sociedad Chilena de Climaterio, 1998:41-8
7. Valdés T, Gomariz E. *Mujeres Latinoamericanas en Cifras.* Chile: Instituto de la mujer, Ministerio de Asuntos Sociales de España y Facultad Latinoamericana de Ciencias Sociales (FLACSO), 1995
8. Kinsella K. Dimensiones demográficas y de salud en América Latina y el Caribe. In Anzola Perez E, ed. *Elderly Care, a Challenge in the 1990s.* Washington, DC: PAHO, 1996;546:3-15
9. Lavín Acevedo P. Aging population and menopause. In Gonzalez Campos O, Arteaga Urzúa E, Contreras Castro P, eds. *Menopausia y Patologías Asociadas.* Santiago de Chile: Ediciones Sociedad Chilena de Climaterio, 1998:71-83
10. Pan American Health Organization. Health situation trends. In *Health in the Americas.* Washington, DC: PAHO, 1998;569:7-64
11. Utian WH. Determining the role of long-term hormone therapy after menopause in the context of primary preventive health care for women. *Menopause* 1996;3:65-70
12. Beer V, Bisig B, Cutiwiller F, *et al.* Social class gradients in years of potential life lost in Switzerland. *Soc Sci Med* 1993;37:1011-18
13. CARMEN Project. *Report and Recommendations on the Progress of the CARMEN Project in Chile.* Washington, DC: PAHO, 1997
14. Corral F, Cueva P, Yepez J, *et al. Limited Education as a Risk Factor in Cervical Cancer.* Washington, DC: PAHO, 1996;30:322-9
15. Matos E. *Atlas of Cancer Mortality in Argentina 1989-1992.* Comité Argentino de Coordinación Programa Latinoamericano Contra el Cáncer (CONICET). Buenos Aires, 1997
16. Pan American Health Organization. Diseases or health impairments. In *Health in the Americas.* Washington, DC: PAHO, 1998;569:106-220
17. National Center for Health Statistics. Contraloría General de la República de Panamá, Dirección de Estadística y Censo. *Panamá en Cifras, años 1989-1993.* Panamá: Dirección de Estadística y Censo, 1994. In Health in indigenous population. *Health in the Americas.* Washington, DC: PAHO, 1998;569:95-101
18. Pan American Health Organization. *Strategy analysis report of Health for All for the Year 2000. III. Evaluation: Paraguay.* Paraguay, 1997. In Health of indigenous population. *Health in the Americas.* Washington, DC: PAHO, 1998;569:95-101
19. Pan American Health Organization. Health initiative of the indigenous people. Reports on analysis of the situation of the indigenous people of Perú. Washington, DC: PAHO, 1997
20. Mosquera M, Maurel D, Pavón S, *et al.* Incidence and risk factors associated with fractures of the proximal femur due to osteoporosis. *Pan Am J Public Health* 1998;4:211-19

21. Secretaría de Políticas de Salud y Regulación Sanitaria. Ministerio de Salud y Acción Social de la Nación Argentina, 1995
22. World Health Organization Scientific Group on Research on the Menopause in the 1990s. Menopause symptoms and treatment. In *Research on the Menopause in the 1990s*. Geneva: WHO, 1996; 866: 24-32
23. Sociedad Uruguaya de Endocrinología Ginecológica y Menopausia. *Hormone Replacement Therapy Compliance. Final Report*. Montevideo, Uruguay, 1997
24. Artiles Visbal L, Manzano Ovies B, Sarduy M, *et al.* Gender impact in the climacterium. Presented at the *Seminario Internacional Climaterio y Menopausia, CIMEQ '99*, La Habana, Cuba, 1999
25. Barnett EA. Perceptions of menopause: importance of role satisfaction in a Peruvian town. California, Stanford University, 1986. In Sennott- Miller L, ed. Health and socioeconomic situation of midlife and elderly women in Latin America and the Caribbean. In *Midlife and Elderly Women in Latin America and the Caribbean*. Washington, DC: PAHO, 1990:3-130
26. Parra Armendáriz M. Menopause in Chile and Latin America. In Gonzalez Campos O, Arteaga Urzúa E, Contreras Castro P, eds. *Menopausia y Patologías Asociadas*. Santiago de Chile: Ediciones Sociedad Chilena de Climaterio, 1998:85-91
27. Fritchie Dame Rennie. *The Pennel Report on Women's Health*. Manchester: University of Manchester, 1997

Menopause and six chronic conditions of aging: the Study of Women's Health Across the Nation (SWAN)

15

S. S. Sherman, R. E. Goldstein, S. L. Crawford, M. Ory and J. M. Guralnik

INTRODUCTION

The National Institute on Aging (NIA), which is part of the National Institutes of Health, has been at the forefront of the national effort to understand the processes of aging and to maximize the healthy, active, productive years of later life. Established in 1974, the NIA's mission has been to support biomedical, social and behavioral research and research training aimed at, first, understanding the etiology of age-related processes, conditions, diseases and disabilities and, second, improving their diagnosis, treatment and prevention. The NIA has an active research program on the menopause, which is part of a comprehensive, multidisciplinary program on aging that explores physiological, cognitive, social, behavioral and demographic domains. Approaches range from those used in basic biology, to epidemiological investigations to identify risk factors and markers that predict ongoing pathophysiology or susceptibility to disease, to sociocultural and psychosocial perspectives, to small- and large-scale intervention studies to reduce the development of age-related conditions and diseases.

Clarification is urgently needed on the significance of the menopause in healthy aging or on its role in the etiology of chronic diseases/disorders of old age such as cardiovascular disease, osteoporosis, urinary incontinence and Alzheimer's disease. Not surprisingly, considerable controversy exists over the scope of the physiological changes surrounding the menopause or presenting later in life that are attributable to reduced ovarian function *per se*. The menopause is a universal phenomenon. However, the manifestations of the menopause are not. Cross-cultural research demonstrates considerable variability between populations in symptom presentation and associated psychosocial and physiological sequelae. Future success in preventing and managing diseases and disorders that impact on women, particularly during midlife and old age, will require a substantially improved knowledge base to differentiate the contribution of 'hormone deficiency' *per se* from that of aging. Such distinctions are critical in identifying those women whose conditions are largely the result of ovarian hormone insufficiency and who will benefit from hormone replacement therapy (HRT), from those women whose disorders are due to extra-ovarian factors and who may experience more of the risk side of the risk/benefit equation. Such advances can do much to clarify ambiguities in the presentation of age-related disease, improve diagnosis and treatment, and ultimately reduce health-care costs.

To address the need for broader, more reliable information on the menopause, in 1994, seven clinical sites, a co-ordinating center and a central laboratory were funded in response to the NIA initiative *Menopause and Health in Aging Women*[1]. This request for applications was designed to generate collaborative observational studies characterizing 'the chronology of the biological and psychosocial antecedents and sequelae of the menopausal transition and the effect of this transition on subsequent health and risk factors for age-related disease'. The funded study, the Study of Women's Health Across the Nation (SWAN), uses a co-operative agreement mechanism and is supported by the NIA, the National Institute for Nursing Research, the Office of Research on Women's Health (ORWH), the National Institute of Mental Health, the National Center for

Alternative and Complementary Medicine and the Office of AIDS Research.

In characterizing the psychosocial aspects, the biological processes and the sequelae of the pre- to peri- to postmenopausal transition, SWAN is collecting data on changing menstrual cycle characteristics, markers of hypothalamic-pituitary-ovarian function, symptoms, health and social characteristics, race/ethnicity, reproductive history, current sexuality, risk factors for diabetes, osteoporosis, hypertension and cardiovascular disease, and medications (including estrogen use). Additional research objectives include monitoring changes in bone mass, body composition and psychiatric and psychosocial aspects.

SWAN was designed in two phases: an initial cross-sectional survey and a prospective cohort study[2]. All seven SWAN clinical field sites completed recruitment for the cohort by 31 December 1997. Two annual follow-ups were completed and a third started during the first 5-year funding cycle that ended on 31 May 1999. SWAN has recently been renewed for a second 5-year funding cycle, and, at the end of SWAN II, a baseline plus five annual follow-up visits will have been completed on the cohort.

To gain insight into the potential roles of aging versus menopausal status on the development of the chronic diseases of aging, we evaluated the associations of aging and menopausal status, as well as that of ethnicity, with six chronic conditions of aging: high blood pressure, diabetes, heart attack or angina, arthritis, osteoporosis and cancer. Analyses were conducted using cross-sectional data obtained during a telephone survey that was administered to determine eligibility for participation in the SWAN longitudinal cohort.

METHODS

A detailed description of the design of SWAN is provided in reference 2. To summarize briefly, different community-based sampling strategies were conducted in Boston, Chicago, Detroit, Los Angeles, Newark NJ, Oakland CA and Pittsburgh. Established lists of populations were used at some sites and random-digit dialling combined with a 'snowball' approach at other sites to sample women representative of a definable and racially/ethnically diverse community. Each site recruited Caucasian women and women from one other racial/ethnic group, which gave a total of five racial/ethnic groups across the seven sites. A telephone interview was conducted with women aged 40–55 years, who spoke English or a designated other language, resided in the appropriate geographic area, self-identified, at least partially, with one of the site's target racial/ethnic groups, and who gave verbal consent. This interview served the dual purposes of identifying women eligible for SWAN's cohort study and providing cross-sectional data regarding the menopause and health from a community-based sample of middle-aged women. A total of 15 615 subjects completed an interview relevant for this study: 7772 Caucasians, 4383 African-Americans, 651 Chinese, 1955 Hispanics and 854 Japanese. The analyses reported here omitted data from subjects who were pregnant or breastfeeding, or who reported 12 or more months of amenorrhea not due to the menopause, as well as women of unknown or mixed race/ethnicity.

The outcome variables in this analysis were six chronic diseases or conditions: high blood pressure, diabetes, heart attack or angina, arthritis, osteoporosis and cancer (other than skin cancer). Participants were asked whether 'a doctor, nurse practitioner or other health-care provider' had ever diagnosed them with any of these diseases. Our primary predictor of interest was menopausal status, which was determined using the answers to three questions regarding bleeding patterns and past gynecological surgery. Women who had undergone a hysterectomy or who had both ovaries removed were classified as 'surgically menopausal'. 'Postmenopausal women' were those who had not had a menstrual period in the past 12 months (and who were not pregnant or breastfeeding, had not undergone radiation or chemotherapy, or had not experienced severe weight loss). Women who had bled in the past 12 months, but not in the past 3 months, were considered to be 'late perimenopausal'. Women who had bled in the past 3 months, but whose periods had become less predictable over the past 12 months, were considered to be 'early perimenopausal'. Women who had bled in the past 3 months and whose periods were predictable were considered to be

Table 1 Distribution of study population characteristics by race/ethnicity

Characteristics	*African-American*	*Hispanic*	*Chinese*	*Japanese*	*Caucasian*	*Total*
Age (mean (SD), years)	47.3 (4.3)	46.8 (4.4)	46.2 (3.9)	47.0 (4.3)	47.1 (4.4)	47.06 (4.3)
BMI (mean (SD), kg/m^2)	30.0 (6.9)	27.0 (5.5)	22.9 (3.6)	22.9 (3.7)	26.4 (6.2)	27.16 (6.5)
Menopausal status (*n* (%))						
premenopausal	1030 (24.1)	638 (33.7)	294 (46.1)	370 (44.5)	2183 (28.8)	4515 (29.7)
early perimenopausal	1018 (23.8)	398 (21.0)	158 (24.8)	183 (22.0)	1805 (23.8)	3562 (23.4)
late perimenopausal	169 (4.0)	78 (4.1)	19 (3.0)	30 (3.6)	317 (4.2)	613 (4.0)
postmenopausal	557 (13.0)	363 (19.2)	77 (12.1)	94 (11.3)	1131 (14.9)	2222 (14.6)
surgical	1361 (31.8)	342 (18.0)	37 (5.8)	83 (10.0)	1325 (17.5)	3148 (20.7)
pre-/perimenopausal HRT user	144 (3.4)	77 (4.1)	53 (8.3)	72 (8.7)	813 (10.7)	1159 (7.6)
Paying for basics (*n* (%))						
very hard	538 (12.6)	569 (30.0)	36 (5.6)	25 (3.0)	597 (7.9)	1765 (11.6)
somewhat hard	1532 (35.8)	887 (46.7)	170 (26.7)	216 (25.8)	2168 (28.5)	4973 (32.6)
not very hard	2213 (51.7)	444 (23.4)	432 (67.7)	595 (71.2)	4836 (63.6)	8520 (55.8)
Education (*n* (%))						
below high school	364 (8.5)	676 (35.6)	109 (16.9)	5 (0.6)	350 (4.6)	1504 (9.9)
high school	1193 (30.0)	517 (27.2)	111 (17.2)	163 (19.4)	2009 (26.4)	3993 (26.2)
some college	1686 (39.5)	427 (22.5)	147 (22.8)	304 (36.2)	2249 (29.6)	4813 (31.6)
college	495 (11.6)	208 (10.9)	165 (25.6)	253 (30.2)	1403 (18.5)	2524 (16.5)
graduate degree	527 (12.4)	73 (3.8)	113 (17.5)	114 (13.6)	1595 (21.0)	2422 (15.9)
Smoking (*n* (%))						
never	2096 (48.8)	1241 (65.3)	545 (93.6)	581 (69.3)	3486 (45.8)	7949 (52.2)
past only	981 (22.8)	333 (17.5)	24 (4.1)	171 (20.4)	2280 (29.9)	3789 (24.9)
current	1218 (28.4)	328 (17.3)	13 (2.2)	86 (10.3)	1848 (24.3)	3493 (22.9)

BMI, body mass index; HRT, hormone replacement therapy

'premenopausal'. Because the use of HRT affects bleeding patterns, a user's underlying menopausal status is unobservable; thus, women with bleeding in the past 12 months who used HRT were considered as a separate status group.

Other covariates included ethnicity, age, body mass index (BMI), smoking and an indication of socioeconomic status based on educational level and difficulty in paying for basic necessities. Women in the SWAN cohort self-identified as one of five ethnicities: African-American, Caucasian, Chinese, Hispanic or Japanese. Age and BMI were fit as continuous variables. Ability to pay for basic needs was categorized as not very hard, somewhat hard or very hard. Education was classified into five levels: below 12th-grade education; 12th-grade (high-school diploma or General Education Development (GED)); some college education or training after high school; college degree; and graduate education. Participants were categorized by smoking status as current smokers, past smokers or those who never smoked.

Statistical analyses

We first evaluated the prevalence of each condition by ethnicity and menopausal status and conducted pair-wise tests of differences. Subsequently, we fit multivariate logistic regression models for each of the six chronic conditions in order to adjust these comparisons for the covariates described in the preceding section.

RESULTS

Characteristics of the cross-sectional sample are shown in Table 1. Mean ages ranged from 46.2 years in the Chinese women to 47.3 years in the African-American women, while mean values for BMI ranged from 22.9 in the Chinese and Japanese women to 30.0 in the African-American women. As seen in Table 2, premenopausal women comprised 29.7% of our sample. A total of 23.4% of our sample were early perimenopausal and 4% were late perimenopausal. Women who had had a natural menopause made up 14.6% of our sample and those with a surgical menopause constituted 20.7%. The remaining 7.6% of our sample were HRT users. Table 2 shows that about one-quarter of our sample (24.8%) reported having received a diagnosis of high blood pressure and 22.6% reported a diagnosis of arthritis. The other chronic conditions were less prevalent, with 6.5% reporting diabetes, 3.7% reporting cancer (other than skin cancer), 2.9% reporting having had a heart attack or angina, and 2.5% reporting osteoporosis.

The frequency of each chronic disease differed significantly by menopausal status (p value from overall χ^2 test < 0.0001 for each condition), increasing with advancing menopausal status. The frequencies of all conditions were profoundly different in surgically menopausal women - at least double those reported by premenopausal women. Tests for pair-wise differences show that, for each outcome, most menopausal groups were significantly different ($p < 0.05$) from the premenopausal women. The exceptions were late perimenopausal women with cancer and HRT users with diabetes, heart attack/angina or cancer. Even after adjusting for all covariates (data not shown), surgically menopausal women were more likely than premenopausal women to have been diagnosed with each chronic condition. Compared to the premenopausal reference group, naturally postmenopausal women were significantly more likely to have been diagnosed with every condition except high blood pressure. Early and late perimenopausal women were more likely to report arthritis. Early perimenopausal women were also somewhat more likely to report osteoporosis, heart attack or angina, and cancer.

The frequency of chronic disease reporting also differed significantly ($p < 0.0001$) by race/ethnicity (Table 3). Reported history of chronic conditions was significantly different ($p < 0.05$) in each of the four racial/ethnic groups compared to the Caucasian group for every outcome, except for osteoporosis in Hispanics and diabetes in Japanese and Chinese. After adjusting for the other covariates (data not shown), African-Americans were more likely than Caucasians to report a diagnosis of high blood pressure, diabetes, and heart attack or angina. However, they were less likely than Caucasians to report osteoporosis and cancer. In Hispanic women, only cancer diagnoses remained significantly different when compared to Caucasians. Chinese-Americans were more likely to have had diabetes and less likely to have had arthritis than Caucasians. In Japanese-Americans, only lower arthritis reporting was significantly different when compared to Caucasians.

Table 2 Chronic conditions by menopausal status

	Number (and %) reporting each condition by menopausal status						
Chronic condition	*Premenopausal* ($n = 4515$; 29.7%)	*Early perimenopausal* ($n = 3562$; 23.4%)	*Late perimenopausal* ($n = 613$; 4.0%)	*Postmenopausal* ($n = 2222$; 14.6%)	*Surgical* ($n = 3148$; 20.7%)	*HRT user* ($n = 1159$; 7.6%)	*Total* ($n = 15\,219$)
High blood pressure	807 (17.9)	780 (21.9)	171 (27.9)	619 (27.9)	1135 (36.1)	256 (22.1)	3768 (24.8)
Diabetes	194 (4.3)	198 (5.6)	48 (7.8)	186 (8.4)	308 (9.8)	50 (4.3)*	984 (6.5)
Heart attack/ angina	49 (1.1)	74 (2.1)	14 (2.3)	91 (4.1)	193 (6.1)	14 (1.2)*	435 (2.9)
Arthritis	599 (13.3)	714 (20.0)	159 (25.9)	651 (29.3)	1080 (34.3)	230 (19.8)	3433 (22.6)
Osteoporosis	40 (0.9)	58 (1.6)	13 (2.1)	103 (4.6)	141 (4.5)	33 (2.8)	388 (2.5)
Cancer	67 (1.5)	84 (2.4)	15 (2.4)*	79 (3.6)	303 (9.6)	20 (1.7)*	568 (3.7)

For each chronic condition, the p value from the $\chi 2$ test for differences by status was < 0.0001. An asterisk (*) indicates that a group was not significantly different from premenopausal women for this outcome ($p < 0.05$)

Table 3 Chronic conditions by ethnicity

	Number (and %) reporting a condition within each racial/ethnic group					
Chronic condition	*African-American* (n = 4302; 28.0%)	*Hispanic* (n = 1908; 12.5%)	*Chinese* (n = 645; 4.2%)	*Japanese* (n = 840; 5.5%)	*Caucasian* (n = 7625; 49.8%)	*Total* (n = 15 320)
High blood pressure	1707 (39.7)	408 (21.4)	78 (12.1)	118 (14.0)	1481 (19.4)	3792 (24.8)
Diabetes	476 (11.1)	120 (6.3)	28 (4.3)*	30 (3.6)*	341 (4.5)	995 (6.5)
Heart attack/ angina	185 (4.3)	67 (3.5)	6 (0.9)	4 (0.5)	176 (2.3)	438 (2.9)
Arthritis	1235 (28.7)	460 (24.1)	55 (8.5)	76 (9.0)	1619 (21.2)	3445 (22.5)
Osteoporosis	96 (2.2)	63 (3.3)*	5 (0.8)	9 (1.1)	218 (2.9)	391 (2.6)
Cancer	156 (3.6)	27 (1.4)	15 (2.3)	23 (2.7)	349 (4.6)	570 (3.7)

For each chronic condition, the p value from the χ^2 test for differences by ethnicity was < 0.0001. An asterisk (*) indicates that a group was not significantly different from Caucasians for this outcome ($p < 0.05$)

CONCLUSIONS

In this large cross-sectional survey of women from diverse racial/ethnic backgrounds, menopausal status appears to be an important predictor in the reporting of key chronic conditions and diseases of aging. Compared to premenopausal women, postmenopausal women were substantially more likely to have received a diagnosis of high blood pressure, diabetes, heart attack/angina, arthritis, osteoporosis and cancer, even after adjustment for the effects of age, BMI and other potential confounders. The differences were most striking in surgically menopausal women. Race/ethnicity also played a significant role in the reporting of these age-related conditions and diseases. The limited number of questions asked during the survey and the cross-sectional design of this study limit the interpretation of temporal sequence and inferences on potential causation (e.g. the role of smoking or BMI in the pathogenesis of cardiovascular disease, etc.). Longitudinal follow-up of the SWAN cohort and their transitions from pre- to peri- to postmenopause will provide much-needed answers on the separate roles of the menopause and aging, as well as that of race/ethnicity, in the pathophysiology of the chronic diseases of aging.

ACKNOWLEDGEMENTS

This work was funded by the National Institute on Aging, the National Institute for Nursing Research and the NIH Office of Research on Women's Health; grant numbers: U01 AG12505, U01 AG12531, U01 AG12535, U01 AG12539, U01 AG12546, U01 AG12553, U01 AG12554, U01 NR04061, U01 AG12495.

References

1. National Institutes of Health. *Menopause and Health in Aging Women*. RFA: AG-94-002. NIH Guide, 1993;22 (no. 32)
2. Sowers MF, Crawford S, Sternfeld B, *et al.* SWAN: a multi-center, multi-ethnic, community-based cohort study of women and the menopausal transition. In Lobo R, Marcus R, Kelsey J, eds. *Menopause*. New York: Academic Press, 2000:175–88 (accepted for publication)

Role of reproductive health in the quality of life of women in the menopause 16

B. Xiao and Q. S. Ge

INTRODUCTION

Population aging is a problem not only in the developed countries but globally. With the rapid decline of total fertility rate in some regions of developing countries, aging of the population is now becoming a serious concern for the area of population and development. In the approaching 21st century, China faces a new challenge with the aging of the population. In the past decade, particularly in the past 5 years, China has made great advances in population and development. According to the State Statistical Bureau, the crude birth rate from 1993 to 1997 declined from 18.09 to 16.57 per thousand, the crude death rate from 6.64 to 6.51 per thousand and the natural rate of increase declined from 11.45 to 10.06 per thousand. The total fertility rate has declined to under two children per woman in the 1990s[1]. With the rapid decline of total fertility rate, the aging population in the 1990s is rapidly increasing, and is almost double that in the 1960s. The latest statistics indicate that, at the end of 1998, China's population had reached 1.248 billion, with the number of people over 65 years of age reaching 83.75 million or 6.7% of the total population. Experts estimate that, in the year 2000, the number of people over 60 years of age will exceed 129 million or 10.15% of the total[2]. With this change in age structure of the population it is a great concern of the government in social and economic development to meet the needs of the elderly, among whom almost 55% are women over 50 years of age. Women in the peri- or postmenopausal period are facing new problems concerning their quality of life.

Following the International Conference of Population Development and the Fourth World Conference on Women, the reproductive health of women has been one of the major concerns of the government, and family planning and maternal and child health care were the priorities in the reproductive health-care program. In 1997, a total of 3180 maternal and child health-care institutions had been set up. The maternal mortality rate had dropped to 63.6 per 100 000 live births, compared with 94.7 in 1990. Family planning and maternal and child health care not only decreased the maternal mortality, but also significantly reduced the morbidity due to bleeding, anemia, infection and other obstetric complications, thereby leading to a much healthier life after the menopause. Average life expectancy for women increased from 70.6 years in 1990 to 73.2 in 1997[3]. In the early 1950s, the heavy burden of giving birth to and bringing up a large number of children resulted in a miserable life for a woman in her old age, in addition to the obstetric complications and gynecological diseases. Changes in family planning strategies have focused on client-oriented quality of care. Improvements in maternal and child health care and the family planning program in the 1970s have produced a great impact on the reproductive health of women who are now of menopausal age.

NATURAL MENOPAUSAL AGE AND THE INFLUENCING FACTORS

The age of natural menopause in women is considered a health indicator[4,5]. In 1990, an epidemiological survey of 5134 women aged 40–65 years was conducted in the Beijing area. Of these women, 54.1% were postmenopausal; 93.8% of the women were in natural menopause, 5.4% were menopausal following hysterectomy and 0.8% were menopausal due to drug or radiation treatment. The mean age of natural menopause was 48.4 ± 3.8 years and premature menopause, before the age of

40 years, occurred in 3.1% of the women. It was also interesting to find that, in their early years, their mean age at menarche was 14.8 years and, on average, they had had 3.3 pregnancies and 2.5 children. A total of 79.8% of them had adopted various methods of contraception, mainly intrauterine devices, condoms and oral contraceptive pills. The average marriage age was 22.3 years. The percentages of married, divorced, widowed and unmarried women were 90.5%, 1.3%, 7.4% and 0.8%, respectively. Only 16.7% and 0.5% of the women smoked or drank alcohol, respectively. There are many factors that affect the natural menopause: menorrhagia, the use of oral contraceptive pills, obesity and high parity are the main factors. Smoking and accidental events in life may cause a premature menopause. The use of contraception, fewer pregnancies, low divorce and widow rates, and less smoking and drinking when the women were younger have brought them a healthy and happy life, both physically and mentally in the menopause.

MENOPAUSAL SYMPTOMS

Menopausal symptoms, such as irritability, night sweats or flushing, appeared in most menopausal women, but varied greatly in frequency and severity. The symptoms were affected by several factors, such as accidental events in life, higher education level, late age at menopause, tubal ligation, premenopausal irregular menstruation and marital status. One or two menopausal symptoms occurred in 60% of the women in this survey, and only 10–20% complained of serious symptoms, compared to Western countries where the number may be as high as 80% (Table 1)[4].

Although menopausal symptoms may not be harmful to women's physical health, serious symptoms will affect harmony in family life and efficiency at work. Prevention and treatment of menopausal symptoms are essential to the quality of life.

Table 1 Menopausal symptoms among 5143 women aged 40–65 years. From reference 4

Symptom	*Number with symptom*	*% with symptom*
Irritability	2396	46.6
Sweating	1913	37.2
Flushing	1888	36.7
Palpitations	1780	34.6
Backache	1758	34.2
Fatigue	1691	32.9
Insomnia	1684	32.7
Dizziness	1556	30.3
Joint pain	1404	27.3
Headache	1301	25.3
Numbness	1101	21.4
Expression	1065	20.7
Soreness	874	17.0
Dry vagina	532	10.3

CERVICAL CANCER

The health benefits of fewer births during reproductive age can be expected to lead to a healthier life in the menopause. In addition to the relief from the household burden, the relief from the social economic stress of bringing up a large number of children and the relief from obstetric and gynecological diseases related to pregnancy and birth also contribute to the quality of life in the menopause. Many institutions and factories conduct regular cancer screenings for women workers. An overall check-up and treatment for cervicitis in the Beijing area was established in 1977. From 1977 to 1993, more than 79% of the married women in Beijing (over 3.5 million) had received medical check-ups. The incidence of cervical cancer was reduced from 46.4/100 000 women in 1977 to 2.23/100 000 in 1992[6]. In studies of cervical cancer with a previous obstetric history it was found that the main risk factor for cervical cancer is a higher number of pregnancies (odds ratio 4.04). Younger age at the first pregnancy is another risk factor[7]. Family programs advocating fewer and later births are beneficial in the prevention of cervical diseases.

OSTEOPOROSIS AND FRACTURE

Age and menopause are the two important factors contributing to bone loss, owing to deprivation of estrogens. Osteoporosis and fractures are the most frequent diseases encountered in the menopause. In a study of 172 women in natural menopause, the loss of bone mineral content (BMC) from its peak value during reproductive age through menopause to the age of 75 years was 31.1% of the total, with an annual loss of 0.89% for the radius. The loss of BMC of the lumbar vertebrae was even more marked, being 59.7% of the total, with an annual loss of 1.41%. On average, the BMC in the menopause is only 34.8% of the normal peak value[8]. An acceleration of bone loss began in the perimenopausal period and the annual loss of BMC in women with irregular menstruation was almost three times higher than in those with normal menstruation. Table 2 presents the bone loss in relation to age and menstruation status.

The prevalence of fracture among the naturally menopausal women was 12.8%. The average BMC of the radius in fracture and non-fracture patients was not significantly different, whereas the average BMC of the lumbar vertebrae in fracture patients was significantly lower that that in the non-fracture patients, being 97.9 ± 23.6 mg/cm and 122.2 ± 28.1 mg/cm, respectively. The fracture rate was much lower than that reported in Western countries, where, among women over 70 years of age, at least 50% had had one fracture. The difference could be due to the higher BMC peak during reproductive age, the higher calcium content of the Chinese compared to the Western diet, or possibly a higher physical activity rate in daily life. A healthy diet and increased physical activity during reproductive age are essential for women to prepare for a good quality of life in the menopause.

CARDIOVASCULAR DISEASE

Cardiovascular diseases increase in women with advancing age[9]. In a survey of 2245 menopausal women, cardiovascular disease was present in 17.2%[10]. Changes in serum lipids after the menopause suggest a relationship with estrogen deprivation. Total serum cholesterol and triglyceride concentrations increase and high-density lipoprotein (HDL) cholesterol decreases. Changes in serum lipids predispose to cardiovascular diseases. Due to ethnic variability, the incidence of cardiovascular diseases is much lower than that in Western countries. Differences in diet as well as smoking and drinking habits could be causes, but there are not enough studies on lipids, cholesterol and cardiovascular diseases among Chinese menopausal women for definite conclusions to be drawn.

Table 2 Reduction in bone density in relation to menstrual status and age. From reference 8

	Total (annual) percentage bone density reduction	
	41–45-year-old women	*46–50-year-old women*
Radius		
Normal menses	2.8 (0.56)	9.4 (0.94)
Premenopause	8.1 (1.63)	9.5 (0.95)
Postmenopause	11.8 (2.36)	11.7 (1.17)
Lumbar vertebrae		
Normal menses	6.4 (0.64)	7.7 (0.51)
Premenopause	23.6 (2.36)	25.1 (1.67)
Postmenopause	29.1 (2.91)	33.1 (2.21)

HORMONE REPLACEMENT THERAPY

The use of hormone replacement therapy (HRT) to relieve vasomotor symptoms, reduce bone loss and prevent cardiovascular diseases is very popular in Western countries[11]. It is estimated that about one-third of menopausal women receive HRT, but in China HRT is limited only to urban professional women in some large cities. In the Beijing survey, less than 1% of perimenopausal women were using HRT. Lack of knowledge of the benefits of HRT for protecting against sclerosis of the blood vessels, osteoporosis, damage of brain cells and disturbances of lipid metabolism is the main reason for the non-popularity of HRT. The other reason is the misleading concept of a carcinogenic effect of estrogens on the endometrium. The correct use of HRT plays an important role in the prevention and treatment of diseases connected with the menopause. Based on their clinical experiences, the Peking Union Medical School Hospital recommend the use of the lowest effective dose, for example reducing the dose of tibolone to one-half or one-quarter of the original dose (2.5 mg per day) or reducing the dose of Premarin® from 2.5 mg to 0.625 mg or 0.3 mg per day. A 3-year follow-up study confirmed that postmenopausal women using one-half or one-quarter of the original dose of tibolone showed an increase in bone density, a decrease in triglycerides and no stimulation of the endometrium. It was also found that daily continuous use of combined estrogen and progestogen had a better suppressive effect on the endometrium than estrogen and progestogen used cyclically[12-14]. It is essential to treat every patient individually according to her symptoms and the underlying pathogenic causes, in order to obtain a better therapeutic effect.

Recently, HRT with a progestogen supplement has become more acceptable in menopausal women, as it prevents hyperplasia of the endometrium and bleeding after treatment with estrogen alone. Various preparations have been developed so that they can be used for longer durations and more conveniently, such as the dermal patches of estradiol and the levonorgestrel-releasing system[15-18]. A 3-year follow-up study on the use of the levonorgestrel-releasing intrauterine system in combination with estrogen in 25 women showed that 79% were amenorrheic and the others had spotting for 1–2 days monthly. The endometrial thickness was 2 mm and no signs of proliferation were observed. The levonorgestrel-releasing intrauterine system has been used for the treatment of menorrhagia in perimenopausal women, with good results regarding contraceptive effect and the reduction of bleeding. Further expanded studies are needed in China to give a better evaluation of its use in combination with estrogen preparations for menopausal women.

SOCIAL ASPECT OF REPRODUCTIVE HEALTH CARE FOR MENOPAUSAL WOMEN

While good reproductive health care is essential to the quality of life of menopausal women, there are other basic requirements leading to a healthy life. In China, by culture and tradition, support in old age usually falls on sons of the family. With the decline of family size, old age support becomes the responsibility of government, community and family members. A harmonious family relationship constitutes a very important component to the quality of life, particularly in rural areas. Along with the decline of the total fertility rate to below 2, the rapid aging of the population in Shanghai is particularly acute. To solve the problem of medical care for elderly people, the Shanghai government has, since the 1980s, established 30 nursing centers for the elderly with 2680 beds[19]. Nevertheless, it is not sufficient for the large number of people over 60 years of age, which has reached 2.34 million. In Shanghai, it is planned to build ten more nursing centers with standard facilities. Furthermore, in one of the industrial districts where many retired workers live, 20 million yuan is to be spent on building a 400-bed hospital for aging people.

We can conclude that quality of life in the menopause depends on psychosocial and economic welfare, family relationships, and mental and physical health care, which require an integrated reproductive health-care program throughout the woman's whole life span.

ACKNOWLEDGEMENTS

The support and collaboration from Schering AG in our studies on the menopause and the support for our participation at the 9th Congress of the Menopausal Society are sincerely acknowledged.

References

1. Anonymous. Follow up on ICPD and meet challenge of new century. *China Population Today* 1999;16:4–6
2. Anonymous. Population aging. *China Population Today* 1999;16:23–5
3. Li BK, Zhang WF. Trend of population aging in China and the strategy. *China Population Today* 1998;15:2–4
4. Xu L, Zhao H, Ge QS. Epidemiology of perimenopause. *J Reprod Med* 1993;2:23–7

5. Chen JH, Ho SC. The age at natural menopause and the frequency of climacteric symptoms in Chinese women. *J Reprod Med* 1997;6(Suppl):14–21
6. Fengyan L. Gynecologic checkup for cancer prevention and women's health. In Maternal Health Care Society of China Preventive Medical Association, ed. *Proceedings of Panel on Women's Health and Development at the NGO Forum of the Fourth World Conference on Women*, Beijing, China, 30 August–8 September. Beijing: People's Health Publishing House, 1995:96–7
7. Wu JQ, Dong ZL, Pang JY, Duan G. The case controlled study of risk factors of cervical cancer. *Reprod Contracept* 1997;17:166–70
8. Lin SQ, Zhang T, He FF, Xu L, Gu CX, Yu W, Ge QS. Clinical significance of changes in cortical and trabecular bone density after menopause. *J Reprod Med* 1994;3(Suppl 1):42–56
9. Xiao B. Reproductive health in the People's Republic of China. *Adv Contracept* 1996;12:257–63
10. Yuceng B. Menopausal women and their health. In Maternal Health Care Society of China Preventive Medical Association, ed. *Proceedings of Panel on Women's Health and Development at the NGO Forum of the Fourth World Conference on Women*, Beijing, China, 30 August–8 September. Beijing: People's Health Publishing House, 1995:21–2
11. Segal SJ. Women's health issues beyond the reproductive years. *South South Newslett* 1997;7:4–6
12. Ge QS. Postmenopausal hormone replacement therapy. *J Reprod Med* 1993;2:195–8
13. Lin SQ. Hormone replacement therapy improves postmenopausal quality of life. *J Reprod Med* 1996; 5:120–3
14. Ge QS. New trends in postmenopausal hormone replacement therapy. *J Reprod Med* 1998;7:67–70
15. Andersson K, Mattsson L-A, Rybo G, Stadberg E. Intrauterine release of levonorgestrel – a new way of adding progestogens in hormone replacement therapy. *Obstet Gynecol* 1992;79:963–7
16. Suhonen SP, Holmstrom T, Lahteenmaki P. Three-year follow-up of the use of a levonorgestrel-releasing intrauterine system in hormone replacement therapy. *Acta Obstet Gynecol Scand* 1997;76: 145–50
17. Suhonen SP, Holmstrom T, Allonen HO, Lahteenmaki P. Intrauterine and subdermal progestin administration in postmenopausal hormone replacement therapy. *Fertil Steril* 1995;63:336–42
18. Suhonen SP, Allonen HO, Lahteenmaki P. Sustained-release estradiol implants and a levonorgestrel-releasing intrauterine device in hormone replacement therapy. *Am J Obstet Gynecol* 1995;172: 662–7
19. Anonymous. New concept of nursing care of the elderly. *Newslett Population Inf* 1999;8:5–7

Quality of life for changing health: perimenopause among Japanese in Japan and the USA

17

A. Noji

INTRODUCTION

This is the first time that the World Congress on the Menopause has been held in Japan or elsewhere in Asia. This study focuses on the quality of life of Japanese women in the menopausal period, and attempts to answer the following three questions:

(1) What are the factors influencing quality of life in the menopausal period?

(2) How should we evaluate quality of life in the menopause?

(3) How can we improve quality of life in the menopause?

There are two Japanese governmental strategies for assisting the aging society in the year 2000. The first is independent support. A new law on nursing care insurance will go into effect in the year 2000. The second strategy is the prevention of lifestyle-related disease. 'Healthy Japan 21' is a national mandate modelled on 'Healthy People 2000' in the USA. This focus on aging, while positive in general, fails to consider women's health and aspects of menopausal health care.

The national health insurance system operates on a fee-for-service basis in Japan. Due to the sharp rise in medical costs in recent years, more attention is being paid to prevention and health promotion. However, medical funding is not appropriate for prevention.

Women's health is not an area of specialization in nursing, health and medical sciences. There are few medical facilities in the country where there is a menopause clinic. Currently, about 1.5% of women between 45 and 54 years of age receive hormone replacement therapy.

WHAT ARE THE FACTORS INFLUENCING THE QUALITY OF LIFE OF JAPANESE PEOPLE?

The World Health Organization (WHO) began studying quality of life in 1991[1]. Quality of life is defined by WHO as 'the individual's perceptions of their position in life in the context of the culture and value systems in which they live and in relation to their goals, expectations, standards, and concerns'. Quality of life, as studied by WHO, consists of six domains and 29 subcategories (Table 1).

Table 1 Six domains and subcategories of quality of life according to the World Health Organization

Domain 1: Physical domain
Pain and discomfort
Energy and fatigue
Sexual activity, etc.
Domain 2: Psychological domain
Work capacity
Thinking, memory and concentration
Self-esteem, etc.
Domain 3: Level of independence
Mobility
Activities of daily living
Dependence on medical substances and medical aids, etc.
Domain 4: Social relationships
Personal relationship
Practical social support
Activities as provider/supporter
Domain 5: Environment
Physical safety and security
Home environment
Work satisfaction, etc.
Domain 6: Spirituality/religion/personal beliefs

Tazaki and Noji participated in the international project in which the universal quality of life questionnaire was developed, by overseeing all project data collection in Japan. The results from the focus group sessions[2] we conducted showed that 'family' and 'purpose of life' should be added to the subcategories to measure Japanese quality of life[3].

THE QUALITY OF LIFE QUESTIONNAIRE FOR THE MENOPAUSE IN JAPANESE WOMEN

The quality of life questionnaire for the menopause in Japanese women was developed by Sugiyama and Tanaka[4]. This questionnaire measures the concept of quality of life as a subjective health view of physical, mental and social dimensions, and possesses verified validity and reliability. There are four components and 38 questions (Table 2). The components are physical health concerns, mental health concerns, life satisfaction, and social participation and support. In this study, we used this tool to evaluate quality of life.

HOW CAN WE IMPROVE QUALITY OF LIFE IN THE MENOPAUSE?

System development and methods

At the menopause clinic of Tokyo Medical and Dental University, we have developed an education system of systematic life modification support. This system is based on a 'precede/proceed' model[5] and consists of assessment, planning, implementation and evaluation, targeting quality of life as the final goal.

Figure 1 shows the flow chart of this system. The first step is a screening by a physician. The second step is an assessment, including a questionnaire, physical measurements and observations, as well as a measurement of each individual's health needs.

We introduced the social learning theory and offered personal counselling sessions and group sessions to the subjects for planning and implementation. The clients decided which daily habits and in which areas they wanted to improve, based on the results of their own assessment data and with the advice of co-medical staff. Supportive counselling was offered that put the client at the center of the educational process and empowered her.

Table 2 Quality of life questionnaire for the menopause in Japanese women. From reference 4

Component of questionnaire	*Number of questions/ points score*
Physical health concerns	9 questions, score 27 points
Mental health concerns	12 questions, score 36 points
Life satisfaction	5 questions, score 15 points
Social participation, support	12 questions, score 16 points

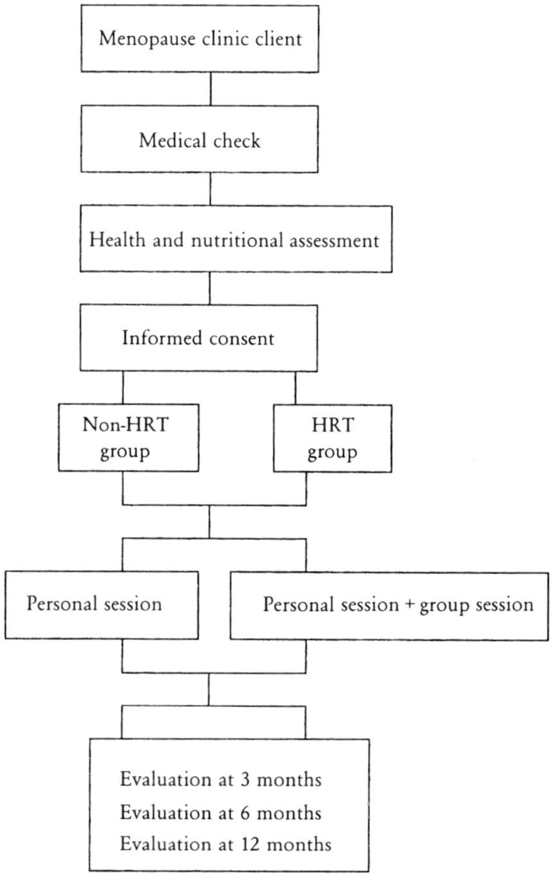

Figure 1 Flow chart of the health promotion system

Group sessions were set up to address subject areas including nutrition, fitness, rest and stress reduction, mental health, and medical management of women's health problems. The group sessions were held in small groups of about ten clients to encourage participation from all group members.

Program evaluation was conducted at four intervals: before intervention, and 3 months, 6 months and 1 year after intervention.

Results

The subjects were 229 patients who were seen in the menopause clinic of the Obstetrics and Gynecology Department of Tokyo Medical and Dental University Hospital.

The results of a baseline survey showed that patients who came to the menopause clinic had an average age of 55.0 ± 6.5 years. Sixty-six per cent of these had an average age of menopause of 49.2 ± 4.2 years.

Forty-three patients participated in the series of evaluations after having undergone 3 months of the program. We divided the subjects into four groups and examined the effectiveness of the program (Table3). The groups were divided into those who took hormone replacement therapy (the HRT group) and those who did not (the non-HRT group). These groups were further divided into those who had participated only in the personal session (the PS group) and those who had participated in both the personal and group sessions (the PS + GS group). No significant differences were detected among the four subgroups in terms of attributes, such as blood test results, prior to the intervention.

Table 3 Number of subjects and mean age of patients in each of the four study groups

	Non-HRT patients		*HRT patients*	
	PS	*PS + GS*	*PS*	*PS + GS*
Subjects (*n*)	10	8	14	11
Mean age (years)	55.4	52.9	53.7	54.0

HRT, hormone replacement therapy; PS, personal session; GS, group session

After all the subjects had completed 3 months of intervention, we compared their body fat and total cholesterol. Body fat tended to decrease in all groups after the health education program. There was a tendency, however, for upper arm circumference to increase after the health education program. Total cholesterol in the blood decreased significantly in all four groups after intervention.

The results in terms of quality of life points are shown in Figure 2. A significant improvement in awareness of mental health was seen in the PS + GS group, whether or not HRT was used. The same tendency for quality of life points to increase in the PS + GS group after the health education program was seen in the area of participation in society.

Our results showed that, after 3 months, whether hormone replacement therapy was used or not, group sessions with personal sessions resulted in a modification of health-related behavior and notably improved the awareness of mental health in quality of life. This shows the importance of the health promotion model[6–8] and group work in health promotion programs aimed at improving quality of life.

IMAGES OF MENOPAUSE

The purpose of studying images of the menopause was to explore the factors influencing the quality of life, affected by different types of social systems and social norms, in the menopausal period.

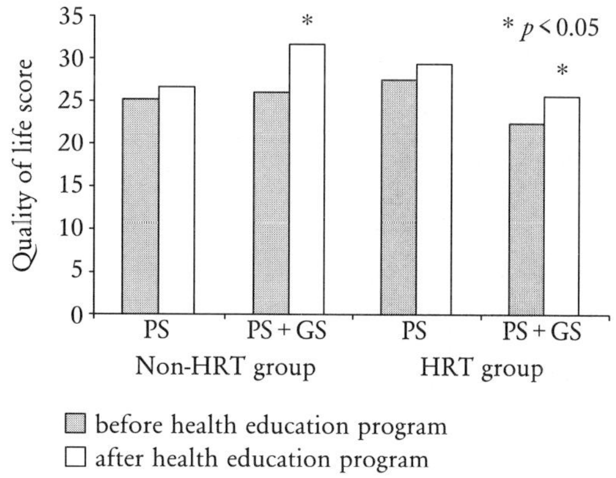

Figure 2 Quality of life score for mental health concerns. HRT, hormone replacement therapy; PS, personal session; GS, group session

The method used semi-structured interviews, and participants were asked to take photographs that symbolically captured their image of the menopause. Participants took photographs of what menopause looks like.

The participants were Japanese women who lived in Japan and Japanese women who had been living in the USA for more than 15 years. They ranged in age from 45 to 60 years old.

The images captured on the photographs were compared. In both groups, certain themes were repeatedly captured on the photographs, including the aging process and death, nutritional supplements and complementary therapies, and future projects. On the other hand, the groups differed in the degree to which their photographs captured images representing positive decision-making in preparing for their deaths.

The photograph of a US respondent and the photograph of a Japanese respondent (Figures 3 and 4) both suggest that the respondents perceive the younger generation as having a bright future.

In contrast, the next two photographs (Figures 5 and 6) contain images of death and dying: a dead tree and a setting sun. However, the respondent who took the photograph of the tree said that this dead tree has strong energy inside and the respondent who took the photograph of the setting sun said it was beautiful and would rise the next morning.

Figures 7 and 8 show photographs of nutritional supplements and complementary therapies. These respondents were seeking methods by which to manage their uncomfortable minor everyday symptoms.

Figures 9 and 10 show photographs representing future projects. One is of a computer, while the other is of a care worker's training school. Both

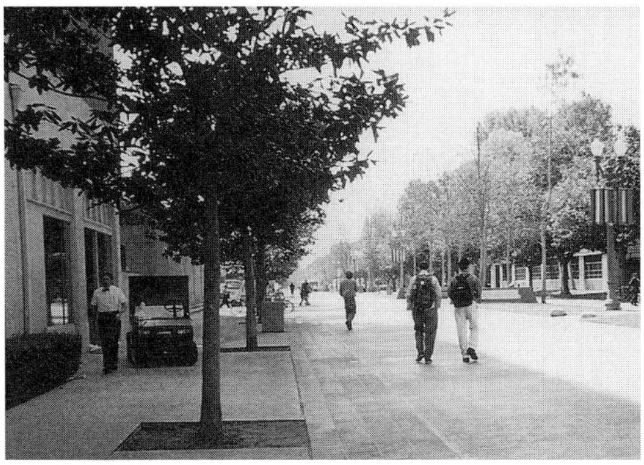

Figure 3

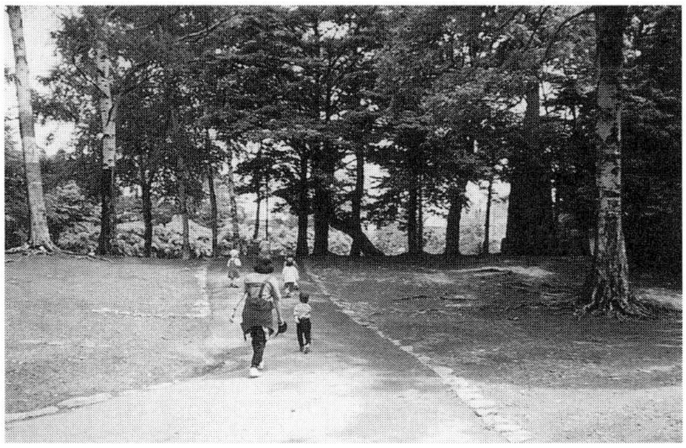

Figure 4

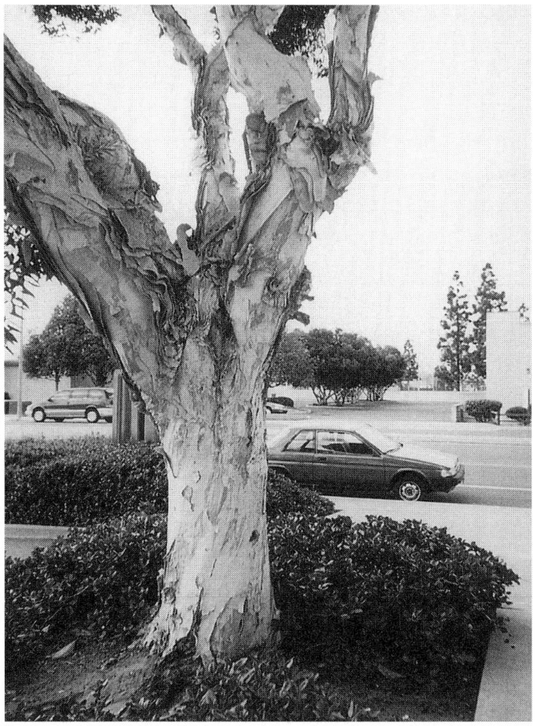

Figure 5

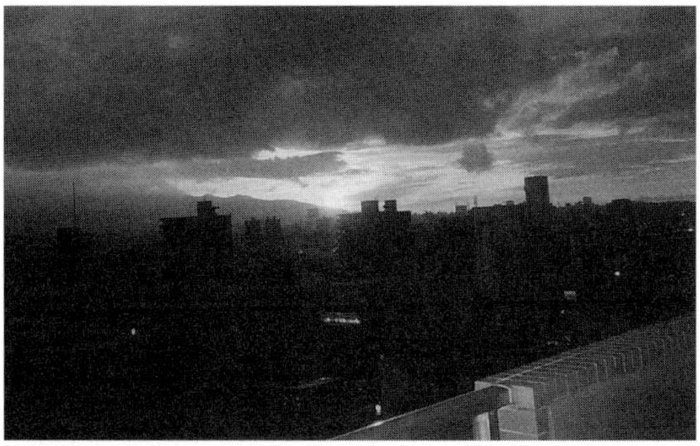

Figure 6

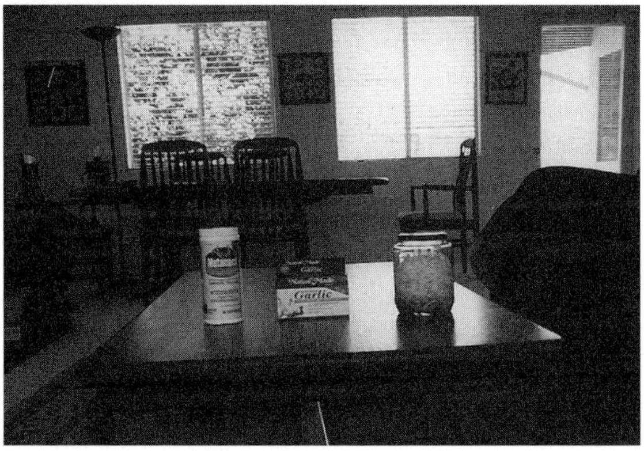

Figure 7

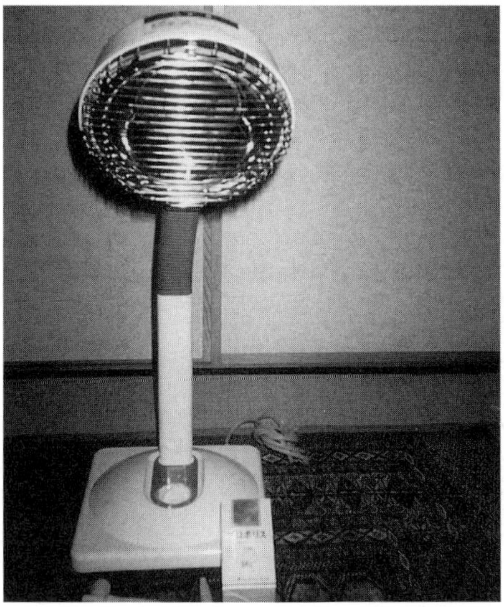

Figure 8

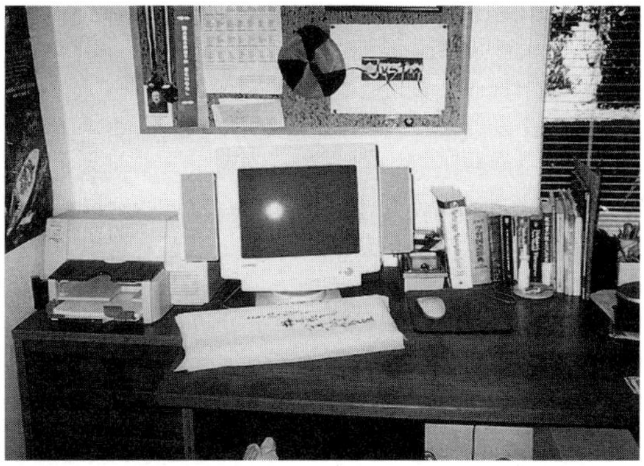

Figure 9

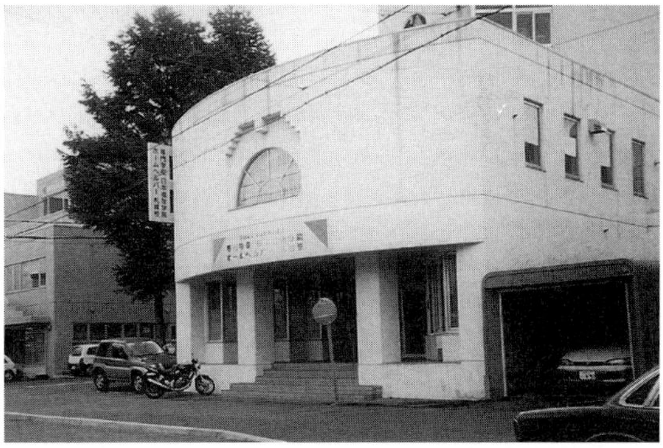

Figure 10

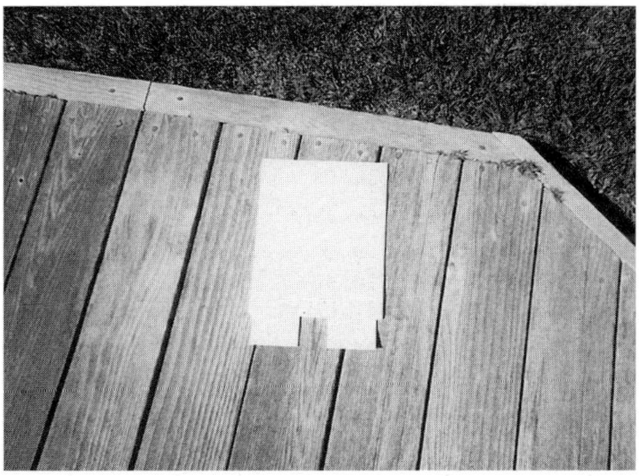

Figure 11

photographs capture the importance of social interaction to the respondents and their desire to have a purpose in life.

The theme of the next photograph (Figure 11) can be interpreted as signifying processes for designing one's own life. This picture was taken by a Japanese woman living in the USA. She took a draft of her living trust that she had made during the menopausal period. This process was exceedingly difficult for her, because the trust included the words 'upon her death', which frightened her. However, after developing the living trust, she felt relieved. She said that the Japanese resist thinking about death.

It appears from the results of the interviews and focus groups that striving for autonomy and independence brings about conflict and frustration for menopausal women in Japan[9]. This qualitative finding is in accordance with the finding reported in the Tokyo Medical and Dental University Study.

On the other hand, in US society, individualism and individual responsibility is embraced as a social norm. The woman who took the picture shown in Figure 11 was affected by this American social norm and took an action that would have been difficult in traditional Japanese culture.

CONCLUSION

Family relationships in Japan have a strong impact on the factors influencing the quality of life in the menopausal period. Therefore, striving for autonomy and independence brings about conflict and frustration for menopausal women in Japan.

The improvement of the quality of life of menopausal women requires a supportive approach to advocate the autonomous decision-making process. Systematic lifestyle modification support that focuses on empowerment can improve the quality of life of menopausal women.

Comprehensive and interdisciplinary efforts need to be made to further refine the menopausal health-care system to improve the quality of life in the menopause for both older and younger generations.

References

1. World Health Organization. *World Health Organization Report of the WHO Meeting on the Assessment of Quality of Life in Health Care.* (MNH/PSF/91.4). Geneva: WHO, 1991
2. Krueger RA. *Focus Groups*, 2nd edn. California: SAG Publications, Inc., 1994
3. Tazaki M, Noji A, Nakane Y. WHO/Quality Of Life. *Diagn Treat* 1995;83:135–50
4. Sugiyama M, Tanaka H. *A Study on Quality of Life in Menopause and Nutrition Deficiency.* Grant in Aid for scientific research (C). Tokyo: Ministry of Education, 1996
5. Green LW, Kreuter MW. *Health Promotion Planning*, 2nd edn. California: Mayfield Publishing Company, 1991
6. Woods NF, Mitchell S. Anticipating menopause: observations from the Seattle Midlife Women's Health Study. *Menopause* 1999;6:167–73
7. Woods NF, Saver B, Taylor T. Attitudes toward menopause and hormone therapy among women with access to health care. *Menopause* 1998;5:178–88
8. Hautman MA. Changing womanhood: perimenopause among Filipino-Americans. *J Obstet Gynecol Neonat Nurs* 1996;25:667–73
9. Morley P. *The Mountain is Moving: Japanese Women's Lives.* British Colombia: UBC Press, 1995

The use of hormones and psychopharmacy: women's views

18

G. V. Miranda, S. Miranda and A. F. Camargos

INTRODUCTION

Quality of life assessment is becoming an important measure in understanding the impact and success of health-care interventions in people's lives. An improvement in the quality of life has been accepted as the ultimate goal of health care and is therefore a crucial subject of investigation for health authorities[1]. The cleft between health and illness remains in domains such as mental health and aging, and the quality-of-life concept may be suitable for bridging it. There are several advantages of the quality-of-life concept:

(1) It is accepted by all players in the health-care field: patients, family members, professionals, health politicians, administrators and, recently, industry;

(2) It is a positive and therefore optimistic concept, corresponding to positive health, rather than to illness and disabilities;

(3) It is related to self-help, consumer initiatives and 'empowerment';

(4) It is scientifically based and can be measured both subjectively and objectively[2].

Provision of women's health is influenced by the resources available, political expectations, professional community, individual needs and demand by users. Therefore, defining quality standards of care has to take such complexity into consideration.

Most developing countries are integrating mental health with primary health care by using the community approach to treat a great number of patients. Gynecologists, as women's primary-care physicians, must be prepared to deal with women's mental-health issues.

Depression is a serious problem affecting more than 17% of the population. Epidemiological transcultural studies found that depression occurs twice as often in women as in men[3].

Psychological symptoms can occur some years before the menopause in vulnerable women. It has been shown that the brain has receptors for estrogens and progesterone in the limbic system and the hypothalamus[4].

Studd and colleagues[5] and other authors have reported a higher incidence of depressive symptoms in women seeking treatment in climacteric clinics. However, Pearce and co-workers[6] concluded that this incidence is the same when the study includes women from the general population or from menopause clinics. Many clinicians believe that the menopause may cause a form of depression that is easily alleviated by hormone replacement therapy (HRT). The administration of estrogens to depressed peri- and post-menopausal women quickly improved mood and well-being[7].

Women who have major depression at the menopause are likely to have had prior depressive episodes, postpartum affective syndromes or premenstrual dysphoric disorder. The menopause seems to be a time of increased risk for the expression of affective disorders in these women. Some should be treated with antidepressants and be seen by a psychiatrist[8]. Numerous etiologies, particularly related to neurotransmitter and neuroendocrine changes secondary to hypoestrogenism, are suggested.

Despite the documented benefits of HRT, the number of women using it is still relatively low and varies widely from country to country and from region to region[9,10]. The presence of menopausal symptoms (physical, neurovegetative and/or psychological) is frequently associated with stress factors that occur during this period, most of which are evaluated by quality-of-life measurement instruments.

There is no quality-of-life measurement instrument that has obtained scientific community consensus for use during the menopause. Some questionnaires do not take into account important areas and symptoms that affect women's quality of life. Physical and/or psychological symptoms, sexual disturbances, and cultural and religious aspects must be focused and balanced to have a consistent transcultural evaluation of women's quality of life. The World Health Organization has been trying to develop an instrument, but it does not have specificity for the climacteric phase. Observing how physical symptoms and psychological suffering disrupt climacteric women's lives, we chose to analyze depression, antidepressant use and hormone use at Belo Horizonte, Brazil.

OBJECTIVE

The purposes of our study were, first, to evaluate social adjustment, the incidence of depression, and HRT, anti-anxiety and antidepressant pill use by climacteric women, and, second, to obtain information from women in order to understand how to approach, relate to and medically attend pre-, peri- and postmenopausal patients.

METHODS

The study took place at Belo Horizonte, the third most populated Brazilian city (3 200 000 people). Women constitute 52% of the population and 25% are climacteric.

Study 1

Two groups of women were studied:

(1) Climacteric women who sought treatment from the climacteric clinic at the Federal University of Minas Gerais. A total of 45 women were randomly selected (44.4% were 45–49 years of age, 44.4% were 50–59 years of age and 11.2% were 60–65 years of age).

(2) Climacteric women from the community. A total of 42 women were randomly selected (50.0% were 45–49 years of age, 40.5% were 50–59 years of age and 9.5% were 60–65 years of age).

First, all women were interviewed by a trained staff using the standard questionnaire of the climacteric clinic and the Montgomery and Asberg Depression Scale (MADRS). The results were classified as absent/mild, moderate, severe and very severe. Exclusion criteria included women who had been using HRT, antidepressants or benzodiazepines in the past 6 months.

Second, using a standard questionnaire and answering the Self-Adjustment Social Scale (SAS), 95 peri- and postmenopausal women were interviewed by the same staff. Work, leisure, family, marital status, sex, relationship with children, family unit and income were analyzed.

Study 2

Quantitative survey research took place at Belo Horizonte. A structured and standardized questionnaire was answered by a randomized sample of women aged 45–65 years. Women were either pre-, peri- or postmenopausal and belonged to the A/B and C/D/E social classes, according to the Brazilian Association of Market Research Institutes. They were interviewed by trained staff (to ensure standardization, interviewers were trained together), using a standard, semi-structured questionnaire, and by a dynamic group discussion, mediated by the same expert (12 women each). Six debate groups, formed according to the criteria described below, informally discussed the menopause so that participants were able to express themselves, give their point of view about the subject and the use of hormones, sleeping pills and antidepressants, thus providing a different way of analyzing quality of life during the climacteric phase. A total of 300 interviews generated results:

(1) From a group of women from Belo Horizonte aged 45–65 years old;

(2) From groups of women aged 45–55 and 56–65 years old;

(3) From groups of women of the A/B and C/D/E social classes;

(4) Concerning social economic variables (age, educational background, income).

RESULTS

Study 1

We noticed that 73.3% of women attending the climacteric clinic had absent or mild scores in the MADRS; 20.0% had moderate scores and 6.7% had severe scores. In comparison, 85.7% of the community women had absent or mild scores, 9.5% had moderate scores and 4.8% had severe scores. The χ^2 test evaluated only the absent/mild score incidence in both groups. Similarity in this incidence was observed (Figure 1).

We noticed that 89.6% of perimenopausal women had absent/mild scores, 8.3% had moderate scores and 2.1% had severe scores. In the postmenopausal groups, 66.7% had absent/mild scores, 23.1% had moderate scores and 10.2% had severe scores. The χ^2 test was performed and we found that absent/mild depression was significantly higher ($p = 0.018$) in the perimenopause group. Hence, postmenopausal women have a higher incidence of moderate or severe depression in this population (Figure 2).

The Social Adjustment Scale showed differences between groups. With regard to leisure, perimenopausal women, both attending the climacteric clinic and in the community, seemed to be more adjusted than postmenopausal women ($p < 0.001$) (Figure 3).

Women in the peri- and postmenopause had similar SAS scores with regard to family, marital status, relationship with children, family unit, work and income. With regard to sexual adjustment, women from the community had a better score than those attending the climacteric clinic ($p = 0.01$), but there was no difference between climacteric phases (Figure 4).

Study 2

A total of 35% of women reported HRT use: 16% reported previous use and 19% were current users. Of the women with basic schooling, 14% were on HRT, compared to 26% of university graduates (Figure 5). Figure 6 shows the association between hormone use and social class.

Antidepressants were found to be currently used by 4% of women, never used by 80% of women and used in the past by 9% of women.

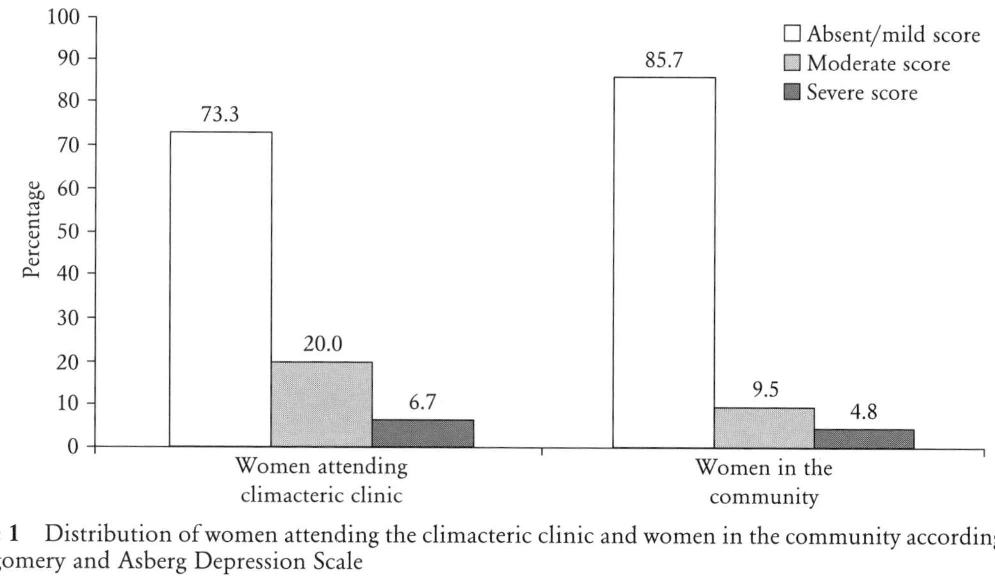

Figure 1 Distribution of women attending the climacteric clinic and women in the community according to the Montgomery and Asberg Depression Scale

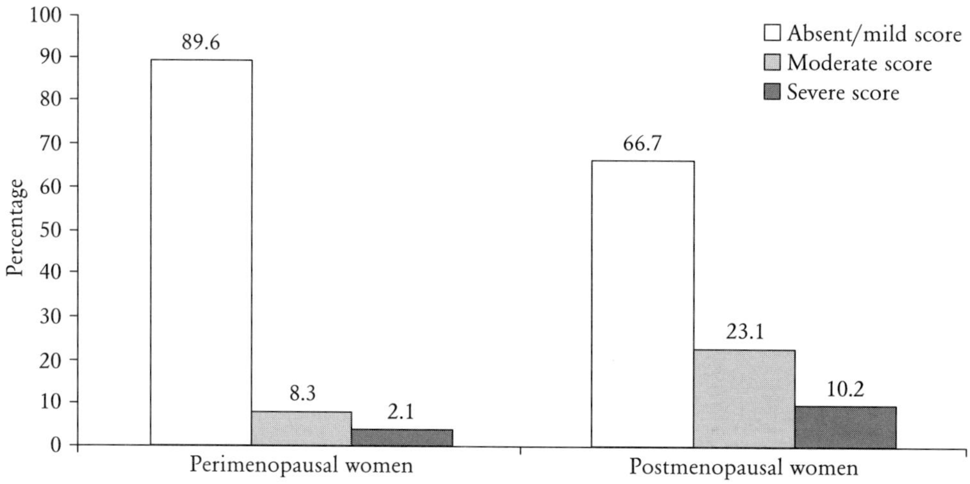

Figure 2 Distribution of perimenopausal and postmenopausal women according to the Montgomery and Asberg Depression Scale

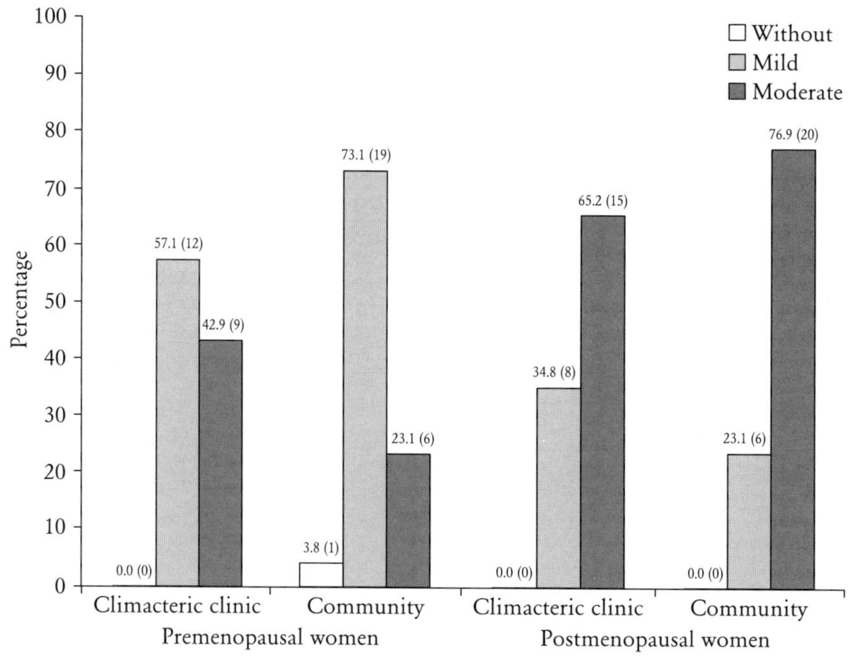

Figure 3 Leisure adaptation problems of climacteric women

The starting ages of antidepressant use in past and current users are shown in Figure 7. The distribution of antidepressant prescribers is shown in Figure 8.

The way women go through the menopause – their anxieties and expectations – is quite individual. Frequently it is a lonely experience and an experience that is not shared. Some findings are listed below:

'My children don't understand me. Nobody knows what is inside us, it is very difficult . . .' (Social group D, 45–50 years old.)

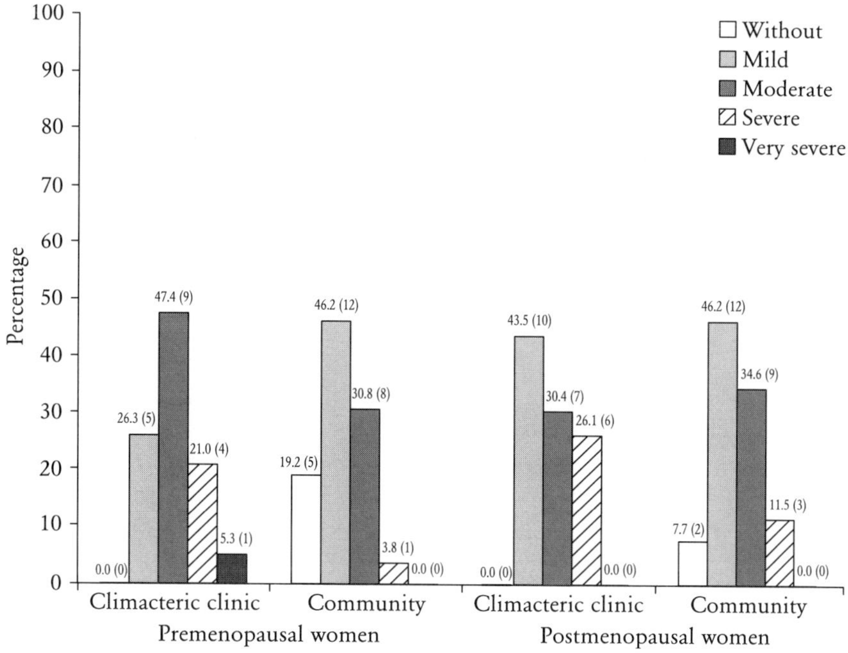

Figure 4 Sex adaptation problems of climacteric women

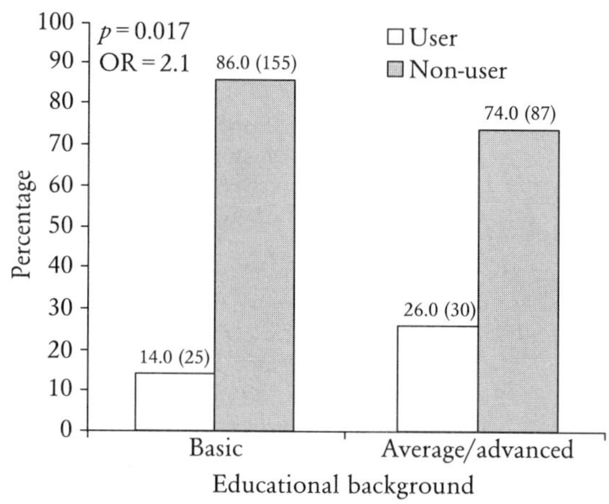

Figure 5 Hormone use and educational background

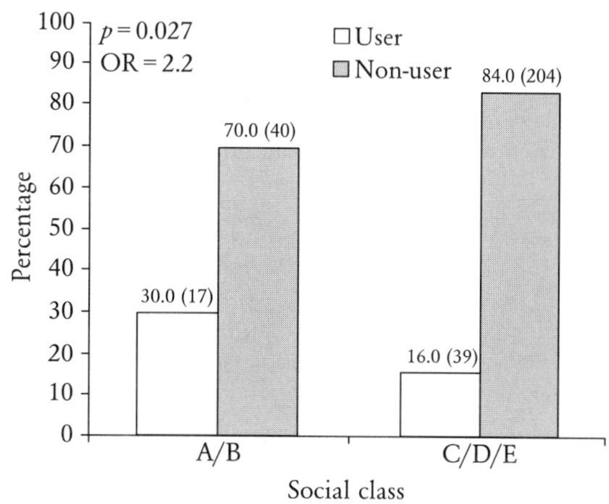

Figure 6 Hormone use and social class

'I know that the menopause almost kills us. So, I think that hormones were great for me. The hormones that were given to me were excellent. I began to take them and became better; it makes life much better. There are also other ways to come.' (Social class A/B, 55–65 years old.)

'I would like to know if it [insomnia, depression] is from the menopause. Because there must be a remedy for us.' (Social class D, 55–65 years old.)

Because of hot flushes, reactions and strange behavior, women at this stage of life do not trust their 'mental health'. They lie down on the floor, take off their clothes, stay close to the wall when going to bed, don't take off their clothes when they take a shower. They feel like screaming, they want

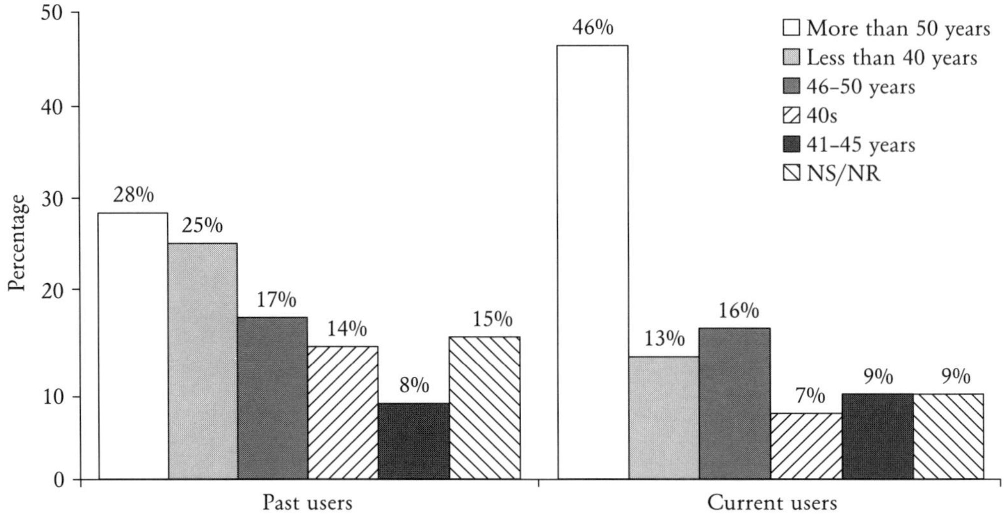

Figure 7 Starting age of antidepressant use

to be far away from their husband and feel uncomfortable in public places. The following are the experiences of some women:

'Suddenly sweating, really perspiring, and I really menstruated, a continuous bleeding, . . . and I feel hot flushes.' (Social group A/B, 55–65 years old.)

'I couldn't keep my shoes on, and if I had my shoes on, I had to put my feet on the cold floor . . . then I said I had forgotten; I had turned 40 years old.' (Social group D, 55–65 years old.)

'It's the hot climate, I think that's why. Because hot flushes make us nervous, sometimes I feel I'm going to become mad.' (Social group D, 55–65 years old.)

Menopause is almost law. It is associated with decadency, loss of vitality, old age and death. The following statements were made by some of the women in this study:

'To say that I am in menopause is to be old.' (Social group C, 45–50 years old.)

'At this phase, every little thing you feel, you think you're going to die.' (Social group C, 45–50 years old.)

'My fear was so great . . . that once I went to confession because I thought it was a sin to be afraid of death.' (Social group C, 45–50 years old.)

'We feel lonely; because we are old, nobody wants us.' (Social group C, 45–50 years old.)

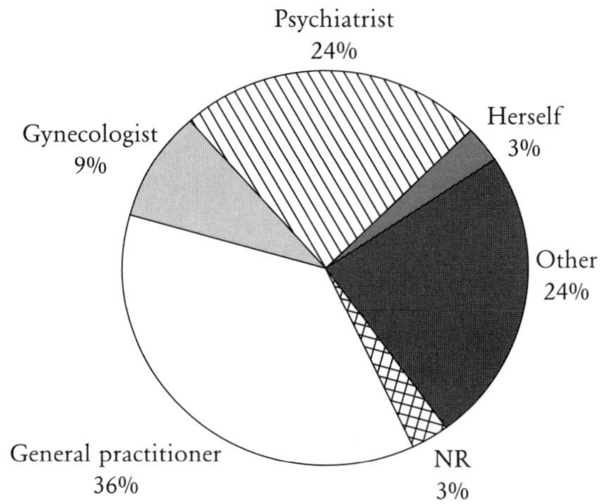

Figure 8 Distribution of antidepressant prescribers

'I'm sure I'm going down hill.' (Social group C, 45–50 years old.)

'When we speak of the menopause, we consider old age.' (Social group C, 55–65 years old.)

Generally, the menopause coincides with important changes. For example, children go away, sickness may occur, parents become more dependent, parents die and there are instabilities at work and in married life. The experiences of some women are listed below:

'It was loneliness, necessity. I didn't have anybody: my daughter got married, my son used to go out with his girlfriend and I was left alone.' (Social group C, 45-50 years old.)

'I was already 46 and I couldn't put up with anything . . . then I asked to be fired.' (Social group C, 45-50 years old.)

'We become nervous and tense. Everything has high weight. I'm nervous with everything. Anything my husbund says, I feel like I have a lump in my throat.' (Social group C, 45-50 years old.)

'Menopause produces intensity, but there are also problems at work. I have to go to my room constantly or go out.' (Social group A/B, 55-65 years old.)

Considering sexuality, there are various reactions where new elements (thoughts, desires, wishes, doubts, fantasies, complaints and expectations) are introduced. Women in the premenopause are afraid of losing their desire, whereas those in the perimenopause are afraid of an increase in desire. No matter which phase they are in, the most frequent topics of conversation are loneliness, how distant the partner is, lack of affection, love, care, concern and sex, loss of desire and doubts about their own sexuality. The following statements were made by women in this study:

'If I had a really nice husband, I would have sex.' (Social group D, 55-65 years old.)

'I felt uncomfortable and lost the interest for that . . . afterwards, I didn't have any interest at all - dry vagina, sometimes cracked, I really felt uncomfortable.' (Social group A/B, 55-65 years old.)

'I had less sexual appetite, but it doesn't disturb me anymore.' (Social group A/B, 55-65 years old.)

'I know that I have arrived at the menopause and old age; I don't think I have any more sexuality.' (Social group A/B, 45-50 years old.)

'Today, I feel more like a woman than before. Some time ago, I didn't miss having sex . . . right now, I have an appetite for sex.' (Social group C/D, 45-50 years old.)

'I think everybody, all organisms, need sex.' (Social group D, 45-50 years old.)

Experience and information concerning hormones vary quite a lot. There are meaningful differences between the perceptions among women of high average income and women of low income. Women of high average income are relatively much more well-informed, have more experience and understand better the role hormones play. Some findings are listed below:

'Replacement makes you feel better. It's for the hormone we've lost. This replacement makes our body work as before.' (Social group A/B, 55-65 years old.)

'Hormones prevent cancer, old age and osteoporosis.' (Social group A/B, 55-65 years old.)

'When hot flushes come, hormones solve the problem.' (Social group A/B, 55-65 years old.)

'I began to take hormones and my headache went away, so I continued with them.' (Social group A/B, 55-65 years old.)

Women of low average income have very little information, their experience tends to be more ephemeral and they know very little about the role of hormones and their effect. For example:

'I don't take them . . . I don't want to have either a beard or a mustache.' (Social group D, 55-65 years old.)

'I also don't take any kind of pill for the menopause . . . but I like home-made tea very much.' (Social group D, 55-65 years old.)

'I have never heard of these pills.' (Social group D, 55-65 years old.)

'I've heard hormones are to keep skin and nails healthy.' (Social group D, 55-65 years old.)

'Hormones kill us.' (Social group D, 55-65 years old.)

'I don't need to take hormones. Women at my age, 54 years old, don't have to take anything.' (Social group D, 55-65 years old.)

Most women in the menopause feel that their husband, children, friends and even society don't understand them. The menopause is considered to be a prejudice of old age, decadency and bad humor. Women that live a happy life and have a good sexual life go through the menopause in a much easier way. Statements made by women in this study included:

'If, during the menopause, women don't have love and care from their husband and a lot of support of others, she will go crazy, she will die . . .' (Social group C, 55-65 years old.)

'I tell my husband and he laughs at me. I say: "I'm feeling hot". . . he laughs and says: "It's the menopause".' (Social group C, 55-65 years old.)

'I'm glad I have a partner, because I wouldn't be able to carry the iron bar by myself.' (Social group D, 55–65 years old.)

One woman said:

'I think that every woman likes to be loved.' (Social group D, 55–65 years old.)

CONCLUSIONS

Study 1

Sex and leisure are aspects that revealed more adaptation problems; in contrast, family, family unity, relationship with children, marital status, work and income did not show any statistical differences.

Study 2

HRT use was higher in better socioeconomic classes and more educated women. The study did not show a significant association between antidepressant use and social class, educational background and type of care (private or public). Most women started using antidepressants after the age of 45 years. Climacteric experience, level of information and self-perception varied significantly according to socioeconomic class.

Women's views of the menopause are changing for the better, but there is a lack of information on HRT, especially in the low-income population.

ACKNOWLEDGEMENTS

This study has been sponsored by The John and Catherine MacArthur Foundation and United Nations Population Fund (UNFPA).

References

1. Sartorius N. Improving quality of life is the main purpose of health care. *Curr Opin Psychiatry* 1999; 12(Suppl 1):429
2. Katschnig H. Mental illness vs. mental health vs. quality of life. *Curr Opin Psychiatry* 1999;12(Suppl 1):429
3. Kessler RC, McGonagle KA, Zhao S, *et al.* Lifetime and 12-month prevalence of DSM-III-R psychiatric disorders in the United States; results from the National Comorbidity Survey. *Arch Gen Psychiatry* 1994;51:8–19
4. Shekhar S, Dhanesh K. QOL assessment in community psychiatry training. *Curr Opin Psychiatry* 1999; 12(Suppl 1):427
5. Studd J, Watson N, Montgomery J. Depression and menopause. *Br Med J* 1990;300:1653
6. Pearce J, Hawton K, Blake F. Psychological and sexual symptoms associated with the menopause and the effects of hormone replacement therapy. *Br J Psychiatry* 1995;167:163–7
7. Kopera H, Utian W. 25 years of hormone replacement therapy. *Maturitas* 1990;12(Special Issue):159
8. Pearlstein TB. Hormones and depression: what are the facts about premenstrual syndrome, menopause, and hormone replacement therapy? *Am J Obstet Gynecol* 1995;173:646
9. Mattsson LA, Stadberg E, Milsom I. Management of hormone replacement therapy; the Swedish experience. *Eur J Obstet Gynecol Reprod Biol* 1996; 64(Suppl 1):S3
10. Oddens BJ, Boujet MJ, Lehert P, Visser AP. A study on the use of medication for climacteric complaints in Western Europe – II. *Maturitas* 1994;19:1

Determinants and quantification of quality of life after the menopause: the Utian Menopause Quality of Life score

19

W. H. Utian, J. W. Janata, S. A. Kingsberg and L. D. Patrick

INTRODUCTION

Clinical use over many years of an unvalidated Utian Menopause Quality of Life scale of postmenopausal women confirmed the need for and value of such an instrument. Widespread usage, however, mandated that the construct 'quality of life' be more clearly articulated and that the scale be updated, tested and validated.

Quality of life during the climacteric years is an issue that has important implications for both women and the health professionals who provide medical care to them. How a woman perceives her quality of life depends on many factors and affects all aspects of her functioning as well as her satisfaction with the health care she receives. A patient's perceptions of her quality of life may be critical to her adherence to her prescribed plan of health care. If a patient believes a treatment will decrease distress or will decrease distress in the future she may be more likely to adhere to that treatment regimen[1]. Similarly, if a treatment prescribed by a physician causes distressing side-effects or if a patient worries that the treatment will harm her in some way, as in the case of hormone replacement therapy (HRT) possibly increasing the risk of breast cancer, the patient may be less likely to comply with the plan of care[2]. It would therefore be beneficial for health-care providers to be able to measure this perception accurately and incorporate it into a woman's care plan in order to meet her health-care needs.

Perceived quality of life is difficult to define and measure, because there is no universal agreement on what it is and how it can be quantified. Objective measurements of health status do not describe the patient's own sense of overall life satisfaction. Quality of life may be defined as a reflection of a person's beliefs about functioning and achievement in various aspects of life. From a behavioral perspective, it can be viewed as a spectrum that ranges from perceived distress at one end to the absence of distress and a sense of well-being at the other. From a medical perspective, quality of life is defined in the domains of physical and psychological functioning[1]. 'Health-related' quality of life can be conceptualized as patients' perception of their physical, cognitive and mental health as well as their social circumstances[3].

Traditionally, medicine has used concrete biomedical measurements to assess quality of life. Although these outcome measures are essential to determining a patient's health status, they are not the whole picture and do not always accurately reflect the patient's global sense of well-being. Many factors must be examined when assessing quality of life including somatic, psychological and cognitive symptoms, sexual functioning and social/life circumstances.

Somatic symptoms usually have a significant impact on perceived quality of life and it is very important that any quality of life assessment accurately identifies and measures somatic symptoms. When treating menopausal women, most physicians use some type of menopause symptom checklist to identify and evaluate symptoms and severity. Research over the past decade or so has determined that there are very few symptoms related to the menopause[4-7]. Vasomotor symptoms (hot flushes, excessive sweating) and vaginal dryness are the only symptoms to be consistently related to the menopause status. Most menopausal checklists include other somatic symptoms that patients perceive to be related to the menopause.

This information is important to the care of these patients, because it can affect treatment choices and patient compliance with prescribed therapy.

Psychological symptoms (depression, mood swings, irritability and anxiety) remain incorporated into descriptions of the menopause for both the lay public and clinicians. However, over the past three decades the relationship between mood disorders and the menopause has been extensively researched, but is still unclear. The most widely accepted belief is that there is no specific relationship between natural menopause and mood syndromes. This does not preclude the fact that psychological disorders may simultaneously occur during the climacteric, and therefore identification of these must be included in any quality of life assessment. The tool used to identify psychological symptoms or depression in the menopausal woman should be easy to administer and provide reliable results.

Life circumstances also play an important role in perceived quality of life. Even if all other areas in a woman's life are optimum, an external event can dramatically affect her perception of overall life satisfaction. To fail to include an assessment of stressful life events in any quality of life measurement could result in an inaccurate determination of perceived quality of life.

The objectives of our study were:

(1) To articulate the concept of quality of life in the perimenopause more fully;

(2) To understand the factor structure underlying quality of life in the perimenopausal population;

(3) To establish a psychometric foundation for the development of a validated quality of life scale.

METHOD

Initially, a pool of questions was developed by four senior clinicians with expertise in the psychological and medical aspects of the menopause. The questions were written to tap a broad array of topics relevant to quality of life and well-being. The questions were arbitrarily written in either a positive or a negative direction. For example, either 'I am able' or 'I am unable . . . to control things in my life that are important to me'. Questions were to be rated by the degree to which the subject agreed with the statement, as it applied to them within the past month. Each question was answered using a five-point Likert scale, with '1' defined as 'not true of me' and '5' defined as 'very true of me'.

Subsequently, the investigators arranged a focus group session involving eight menopausal women who had been previous study participants. These women were given the questions in scale format to review and discuss with a moderator. None of the investigators was present. As a result, 40 questions were selected for inclusion in the pool of items to be studied.

These 40 items, with an equal number of positively and negatively worded questions, constituted the content of a questionnaire that was completed by a new set of subjects. The study population comprised literate, English-speaking women who were between the ages of 45 and 65 years old. A total of 327 women, recruited from obstetrics/gynecological practices and hospital employees in 12 communities in the East and Midwest USA, completed the survey.

RESULTS

Data collected on the quality of life instrument were subjected first to a correlation analysis to determine intercorrelations between individual items as a component of an exploratory factor analysis. The assumption was that quality of life subsumes several correlated domains. For example, physical and sexual domains are assumed to be somewhat correlated. Therefore, the exploratory factor analysis first employed principal components analysis, followed by a factor analytic method that used a promax rotation. With the use of an eigenvalue minimum of 2.0, and the demand that individual items showed a correlation of at least 0.40 with the factors, four factors emerged, with 24 items retained of the original 40. Exemplars of each factor are shown in Table 1. Factor 1 includes items that emphasize occupational vitality. Factor 2 includes physical health and health control items. Factor 3 contains sex and romance items and factor 4 reflects emotional quality of life.

Table 1 Exemplars of items included in the four factors

Factor 1
Occupational quality of life
'I feel challenged by my work'
'I believe my work benefits society'

Factor 2
Health quality of life
'My diet is not nutritionally sound'
'Routinely, I engage in active exercise three or more times each week'
'I feel physically well'

Factor 3
Sexual quality of life
'I am content with my romantic life'
'I am content with the frequency of my sexual interactions with a partner'

Factor 4
Emotional quality of life
'My mood is generally depressed'
'I consider my life stimulating'
'Most of the things that happen to me are out of my control'

Following initial factor extraction, the pool of items was subjected to Cronbach's alpha analysis to ensure that each item contributed positively to the factor on which it loaded. The Cronbach's alpha correlation for the 24-item scale as a whole was 0.834. The Cronbach's alpha analysis led to the elimination of only one item.

DISCUSSION

The factor analysis demonstrated the presence of four contributory, correlated factors that underlie the quality of life construct in this sample. Among the many quality of life measures currently used, most are symptom inventories or scores relating to specific life phases or diseases. Although important and useful information is provided by these measures, they are narrow in range and focus, providing only one dimension of what in this study suggests is a multidimensional construct. A review of the general medical literature on quality of life suggests that individual measures tend to focus either on symptom lists, the *impact* of symptoms of a particular disease on health status, or on general well-being. One of the most salient criticisms of quality of life research and assessment tools is that they remain vague in conceptualization and are defined differently across medical specialties. On a conceptual level, many published studies consider quality of life to be the same as presence/absence of symptoms and use measures that are simply symptom checklists. Others consider quality of life to be completely subjective and global, with little consideration of an individual's physical status. For example, those studying quality of life in cancer patients may consider quality of life as it relates to choosing whether to continue chemotherapy or not, while those studying a physician's career choices may consider quality of life as it relates to perceived autonomy and success.

Guyatt and colleagues[8] reviewed how quality of life was measured in clinical trials and offered a taxonomy of quality of life measures. They determined that measures were either generic and included health profiles and utility measurements, or specific instruments that focused on specific aspects of health status (e.g. menopause). They concluded that there were strengths and weaknesses to both approaches that and each situation must be carefully considered. Our views regarding quality of life assessment complement this perspective. While health status is a domain that may be critical to an individual's quality of life, it is our belief that the multidimensional construct of quality of life is actually independent of health status. Rather, it is a subjective appraisal of life satisfaction. For example, one person may objectively be experiencing debilitating and/or painful symptoms but perceive their life as having excellent quality, while another person may be symptom free but perceive their life to have poor quality. Therefore, the construct of quality of life may more accurately refer to a 'sense of well-being' that is impacted by the experience of symptoms but not solely determined by them.

With regard to menopause-specific quality of life assessment, most measures are primarily symptom inventories and few have credible psychometric properties. The Blatt/Kupperman Index[9] is the most notable example of this. It remains widely used, yet has been discredited[10]. In response to the paucity of valid measures in menopause research, Greene[11] developed a reliable and valid assessment tool. However, as stated by the author himself, it is 'intended specifically to be a brief and standard measure of core climacteric symptoms'. Therefore, this scale is limited in its focus. Most of the other menopause-specific quality of life measures are also symptom focused, rendering the impact of the menopause on quality of life indeterminable.

During this development/validation process it became apparent that a quality of life instrument should be used together with a symptom score instrument. The Greene score seemed ideal because it is precise and validated[10,11]. It is generally accepted that vasomotor symptoms may induce stress or psychological discomfort and that this can increase the severity of symptoms[12]. A combination of the Utian Menopause Quality of Life (UMQOL) score and a symptom score would seem ideal to capture both a woman's sense of the quality of her life and its somatic context.

References

1. Kingsberg SK. Maintaining and evaluating quality of life after menopause. *Female Patient* 1996;May (Suppl):19–24
2. Mansfield PK, Voda AM. Hormone use among middle-aged women: results of a three-year study. *Menopause* 1994;1:99–108
3. Wiklund I, Karlberg J. Evaluation of quality of life in clinical trials: selecting quality-of-life measures. *Controlled Clin Trials* 1991;12(Suppl):204S–16S
4. Holte A, Mikkelson A. Psychosocial determinants of climacteric complaints. *Maturitas* 1991;13: 205–15
5. Kaufert PA, Gilbert P, Hassard T. Researching the symptoms of menopause: an exercise in methodology. *Maturitas* 1988;10:117–31
6. Utian WH. The true clinical features of postmenopause and oophorectomy, and their response to oestrogen therapy. *S Afr Med J* 1972;46:732–7
7. Hunter MS, Battersky R, Whitehead M. Relationship between psychosocial symptoms, somatic complaints and menopausal status. *Maturitas* 1986;8:217–28
8. Guyatt GH, Veldhuyzen Van Zanten SJO, Feeney DH, Patrick DL. Measuring quality of life in clinical trials: a taxonomy and review. *Can Med Assoc J* 1989;140:1441–8
9. Kupperman HS, Blatt MHG, Wiesbaden H, Filler W. Comparative clinical evaluation of estrogenic preparations by menopausal and amenorrheal indices. *J Clin Endocrinol* 1953;13:688–703
10. Greene JG. A factor analytic study of climacteric symptoms. *J Psychol Res* 1976;20:425–30
11. Greene JG. Constructing a standard climacteric scale. *Maturitas* 1998;29:25–31
12. Olderhave A, Jazmann LJB, Haspels AA, *et al.* Impact of climacteric on well being. *Am J Obstet Gynecol* 1993;168:772–80

The menopause and ovarian cell death 20

A. Amsterdam, K. Hosokawa, R. Gold, Y. Yoshida, R. Sasson, Y. Jung, F. Kotsuji and B. Almog

INTRODUCTION

One of the most significant events on entering the menopause is the loss of ovarian function in producing the steroid sex hormones estradiol and progesterone. The use of hormone replacement therapy (HRT) around the time of the menopause will relieve menopausal symptoms, but whether, in particular in long-term treatment, it may lead to a substantial increase or decrease in cancer, cardiovascular disease or osteoporosis is still under debate[1]. On average, the balance between the risks and the benefits is not overwhelming in either direction. For many women, the benefits of long-term HRT use will outweigh the risks, while for others, the risks outweigh the benefits. The use of HRT has to be tailored to meet the needs and desires of the individuals, and alternative strategies to maintain ovarian function in aging women must be sought. In this review, we outline two possibilities to improve the quality of life of aged women by delaying the menopause, first, by attenuation of ovarian follicular cell death and, second, by implantation of young ovarian tissue into aging women. Although the potential of these two applications is evident, considerable intensive and extensive research must be conducted before application to human beings can be considered.

CHARACTERISTICS OF OVARIAN CELL DEATH

Ovarian cell death is an essential process for the homeostasis of ovarian function in human and other mammalian species. It ensures the selection of the dominant follicle and the demise of excessive follicles[2-4]. This process in turn minimizes the possibility of multiple embryo development during pregnancy and assures the development of few, but healthy, embryos. Degeneration of the old corpora lutea in each estrous/menstrual cycle by programmed cell death is essential to maintain the normal cyclicity of ovarian steroidogenesis. Since about half a million follicle-enclosed oocytes are present after birth in the human female, and very few survive in postmenopausal women, apoptosis must play a key role in entering the menopause[5]. Therefore, we studied ovarian cell death both in the human and in rodents[6-8].

Although there are multiple pathways that can determine cell death or survival, crosstalk among endocrine, paracrine and autocrine factors, as well as among proto-oncogenes, tumor suppressor genes, survival genes and death genes, plays an important role in determining the fate of ovarian somatic and germ cells[5,9]. The establishment of immortalized rat[10] and human[11] steroidogenic granulosa cell lines, as well as the investigation of pure populations of primary granulosa cells[6-8], allows systematic study of the mechanisms that control steroidogenesis and apoptosis of granulosa cells (Figures 1 and 2). These cells are the most abundant somatic follicular cells. Moreover, crosstalk between *p53* and extracellular matrix components such as laminin, fibronectin and basic fibroblast growth factor, between cyclic adenosine monophosphate- and *p53*-generated signals and between steroid hormones and *Bcl-2* can explain some of the fine tuning that controls ovarian steroidogenesis and apoptosis[12]. Further studies of the mechanisms of ovarian cell death in perimenopausal women will lead to a better understanding of the processes involved and permit the formulation of novel strategies for the treatment and delaying of entry into the menopause.

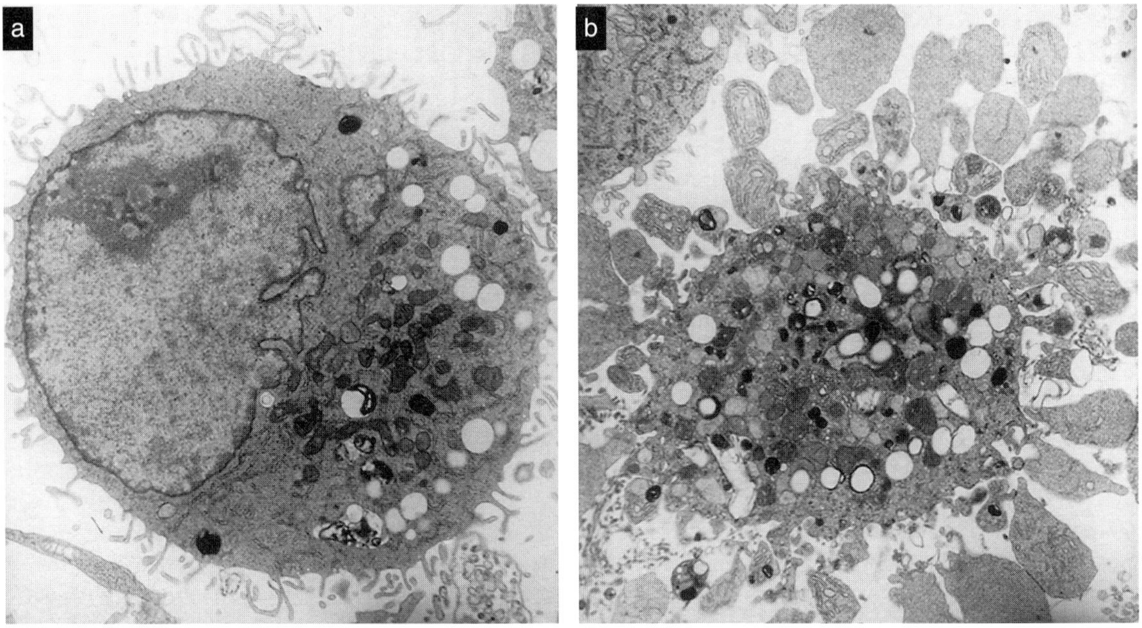

Figure 1 (a) Normal appearance of a steroidogenic human granulosa cell loaded with mitochondria and covered with microvilli. (b) Human granulosa cells stimulated to undergo apoptosis by the tumor suppressor gene *p53*. Electron microscope pictures × 5000. Note the intensive blebbing of the cytoplasm, characteristic of apoptosis (see reference 11 for details)

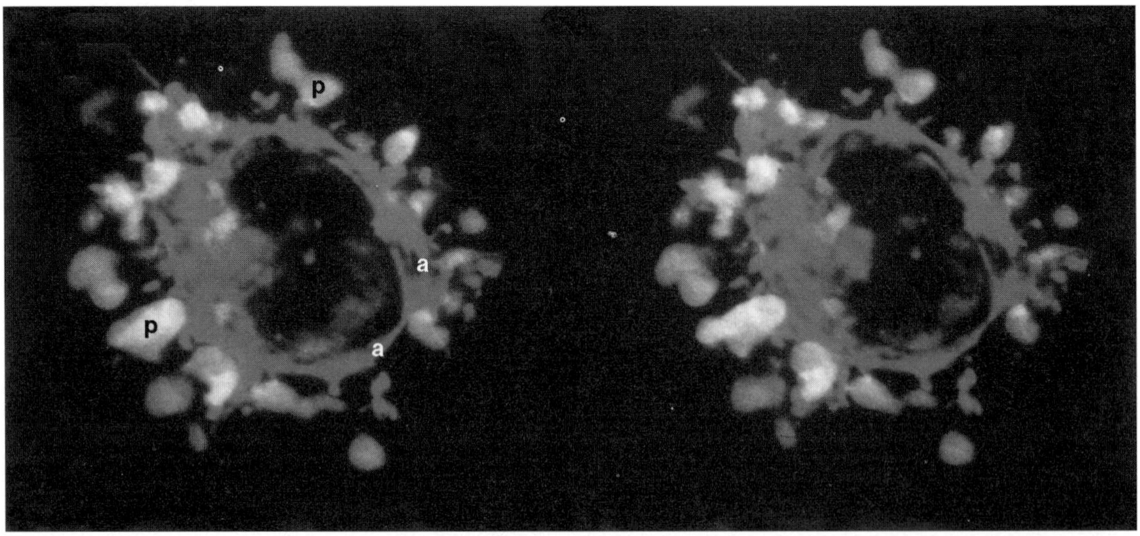

Figure 2 Apoptotic granulosa cell visualized with the aid of a confocal laser microscope (× 2500). The two opposing images (left and right) are tilted at 5° one against the other to demonstrate the intracellular organization in three dimensions. Note that the apoptotic blebs loaded with intracellular protease (proteasome) (p) and the actin (a) cytoskeleton acquire a ring shape (see reference 15 for details)

SURVIVAL GENES AND DEATH GENES WHICH CONTROL OVARIAN CELL DEATH

One of the strategies to attenuate ovarian cell death is to characterize genes whose activation leads to cell death and to find a way to suppress their expression to negate their activity by activation of survival genes.

Bax, which is known as a death gene upon activation, plays an important role in the induction of ovarian cell death (apoptosis). Interestingly, it was reported that, in *Bax* knock-out mice (*Bax* –/–), the ovarian lifespan is dramatically extended[9]. Young adult *Bax*-deficient mice possess three times the number of primordial follicles in their ovarian reserve than their wild-type sisters, and this surfeit of follicles is maintained in advanced chronological age, such that 20-22-month-old female *Bax*-deficient mice possess hundreds of follicles at all developmental stages and exhibit ovarian steroid-driven uterine hypertrophy. These observations contrast with the ovarian and uterine atrophy seen in aged wild-type female mice. Aged *Bax*-deficient female mice fail to become pregnant when housed with young adult males; however, metaphase-II oocytes can be retrieved from the ovaries of aged *Bax*-deficient females following superovulation with exogenous gonadotropins, and some oocytes are competent for *in vitro* fertilization and early embryogenesis. This would suggest that, by attenuation of *Bax* expression and apoptosis, one may save or extend some of the characteristic functions of the ovary in a fertile female.

Bcl-2 is a survival gene that plays an important role in preventing ovarian cell death. We have found recently that leptin, the cytokine that is involved in the control of obesity, can effectively reduce apoptosis in ovarian follicles (B. Almog *et al.* unpublished data). We discovered that the effect of leptin is mainly due to the upregulation of *Bcl-2*, which can already be observed 1 week after immature rats have been injected with leptin. The massive depletion of follicle-enclosed oocytes by apoptosis seems to be a major event in approaching and entering the menopause in women. In a recent study, we observed massive apoptosis in corpora lutea of women in the perimenopausal period (K. Hosakawa *et al.* unpublished data).

It was recently discovered that the expression of *Mcl-1*, an antiapoptotic *Bcl-2* member expressed in ovarian follicles, is transiently increased by gonadotropins. This may result in a shift in the balance of ovarian anti- and proapoptotic *Bcl-2* family proteins to favor survival and rescue follicles from atresia. The induction of *Mcl-1* along with other antiapoptotic genes, such as inhibitors of apoptotic proteins, may therefore represent a molecular basis for the suppression of follicular apoptosis and atresia by gonadotropins[13].

The loss of ovarian function, which results in a dramatic decrease in estrogen and progesterone production, is one of the most characteristic features of the menopause and controls entry into it. Estrogen has been demonstrated in numerous reports to attenuate osteoporosis and to prevent cardiovascular disease[1]. The main strategy today is HRT, in which estrogen is taken to prevent the above diseases. In view of the advanced knowledge of how to control programmed cell death in experimental animals, we suggest further exploring the possibility that attenuation of the expression of ovarian death genes, or alternatively upregulation of the expression of survival genes, may prolong ovarian function and delay the menopause.

This strategy cannot apply at the present time, because much more information needs to be obtained from experimental animals regarding how to achieve control of the essential genes for life and death in the ovary with minimal side-effects. Furthermore, the proper means to achieve this goal need to be found without elevating the risk for cancer in the ovary and other target organs.

CRYOPRESERVATION OF IMMATURE HUMAN OVARIAN TISSUE

Recent attempts at the cryopreservation of small pieces of ovarian tissue, including the immature follicle, have been made[14]. This approach was developed so that patients could protect their fertility by banking ovarian tisuse before undergoing potentially sterilizing therapy for cancer. More speculatively, if ovarian tissue banking becomes a proven effective method, young healthy women may request the storage of ovarian biopsy samples to maintain their reproductive options and the balance of sex hormones in middle life when oocyte fertility is declining and menstrual irregularity is increasing. The implantation of young ovarian tissue in perimenopausal women may therefore be another strategy in the prolongation of the fertile period and delaying the menopause. Although cryotechnology is not perfect, the major question is how and when precisely to use the tissue most effectively after thawing. At present, ovarian tissue cryopreservation is still at the experimental stage, but it holds the promise of valuable applications, including delay of the menopause[14].

In conclusion, it seems that the most effective way to increase the quality of life of menopausal women today is HRT. As for future goals, increasing the quality of life of aging women may be achieved by delaying the menopause. These goals may be accomplished either by the attenuation of ovarian cell death or by the renewal of ovarian function by implanting young ovarian tissue in the perimenopausal period.

ACKNOWLEDGEMENTS

We thank Ms Vivienne Laufer for excellent technical assistance. This paper was supported by research grants from the Kugler Foundation, Mr and Mrs Leonard B. Drell, Mr and Mrs Jordan Nerenberg and from the Israeli Academy of Science. Professor A. Amsterdam is the incumbent of the Joyce and Ben B. Eisenberg Professorial Chair in Molecular Endocrinology and Cancer Research.

References

1. Grant C, Gray A, Paoletti R, *et al.* Hormone replacement therapy. *Lancet* 1999;354:152–5
2. Amsterdam A, Selvaraj N. Control of differentiation, transformation and apoptosis in granulosa cells by oncogenes, oncoviruses and tumor suppressor genes. *Endocr Rev* 1997;18:435–61
3. Amsterdam A, Dantes A, Selvaraj N, Aharoni D. Apoptosis in steroidogenic cells: structure-function analysis. *Steroids* 1997;62:207–11
4. Amsterdam A, Keren-Tal I, Aharoni D. Cross-talk between cAMP and p53-generated signals in induction of differentiation and apoptosis in steroidogenic granulosa cells. *Steroids* 1996;61:252–6
5. Amsterdam A, Gold RS, Hosokawa K, *et al.* Cross talk among multiple signaling pathways controlling ovarian cell death. *Trends Endocrinol* 1999;10:255–62
6. Breckwoldt M, Selvaraj N, Aharoni D, *et al.* Expression of Ad4-BP/cytochrome P450 side chain cleavage enzyme and induction of cell death in long term cultures of human granulosa cells. *Mol Hum Reprod* 1996;2:391–400
7. Aharoni D, Dantes A, Oren M, Amsterdam A. c-AMP mediated signals as determinants for apoptosis in primary granulosa cells. *Exp Cell Res* 1995;218:271–82
8. Aharoni D, Meiri I, Atzmon R, Vlodavsky I, Amsterdam A. Differential effect of components of the extracellular matrix on differentiation and apoptosis. *Curr Biol* 1997;7:43–51
9. Perez IG, Robles R, Knudson CM, Flaws AJ, Korsmeyer SJ, Tilly JL. Prolongation of ovarian lifespan into advanced chronological age by Bax-deficiency. *Nat Genet* 1999;21:200–3
10. Keren-Tal I, Suh BS, Dantes A, Oren M, Amsterdam A. Involvement of p53 expression in cAMP mediated apoptosis in immortalized granulosa cells. *Exp Cell Res* 1995;218:283–96
11. Hosokawa K, Dantes A, Schere-Levy C, *et al.* Induction of Ad4BP/SF-1, StAR and cytochrome P450scc enzyme system expression in newly established human granulosa cell lines. *Endocrinology* 1998;139: 4679–87
12. Hosokawa K, Aharoni D, Dantes A, *et al.* Modulation of Mdm2 expression and p53-induced apoptosis in immortalized human ovarian granulosa cells. *Endocrinology* 1998;139:4688–700
13. Leo CP, Hsu SY, Chun SY, Bae HW, Hsueh AJW. Characterization of the antiapoptotic Bcl-2 family member myeloid cell leukemia-1 (Mcl-1) and the stimulation of its message by gonadotropins in the rat ovary. *Endocrinology* 1999;140:5469–77
14. Oktay K, Newton H, Aubard Y, Salha O, Gosden RG. Cryopreservation of immature human oocytes and ovarian tissue: an emerging technology? *Fertil Steril* 1998;69:1–7
15. Pitzer F, Dantes A, Fuchs T, Baumeister W, Amsterdam A. Removal of proteasomes from the nucleus and their accumulation in apoptotic blebs during programmed cell death. *FEBS Lett* 1996;394: 46–50

Estrogen replacement therapy: an endocrinologist's perspective

21

H. G. Burger

The levels of the major estrogen, estradiol, are well preserved with reproductive aging until the onset of the menopausal transition, a phase in a woman's life marked by features which indicate that the menopause is approaching. During that transition, hormone levels may fluctuate very widely and may begin to give rise to symptoms. The concentrations of estradiol fall by about 90% across the time when the final menses are experienced, although the lowest levels are not usually reached until 1–3 years later.

Interestingly, despite that very marked fall in estradiol, the impact of the menopause varies from one individual to another in the same community and among women in different communities and in different countries. From community surveys, it can be concluded that the impact of the menopause is generally not very great for the majority of women, but it is very great for a minority.

Estrogen supplementation may be used for both short-term symptom control and for the long-term prevention of a number of diseases which are believed to result directly or indirectly from the menopause. Short-term symptom control may be required for hot flushes, the symptoms that follow from lower genital tract atrophy such as difficulty with intercourse or urinary symptoms, sleep disturbances and mood disturbances. Although prospective controlled trials such as the Postmenopausal Estrogen/Progestin Interventions (PEPI) study[1] do not substantiate a specific response of mood disturbances to hormone therapy, anecdotal clinical evidence indicates that these do frequently respond.

For long-term disease prevention, a number of indications for systemic hormone therapy are generally accepted. Apart from the preservation of postmenopausal quality of life, however, none of them is really rigorously established. The general consensus view of the established indications includes reduction in the risk of osteoporotic fracture, treatment of established osteoporosis and reduction in the risks of atherosclerotic cardiovascular disease, particularly myocardial infarction.

In the context of discussing the balance between benefit and risk for hormone therapy, it must be noted that cardiovascular disease is by far the most important cause of morbidity and mortality in most societies and that, in particular over age 64, it is far more prevalent than breast cancer. Potential benefits in reduction of cardiovascular risk weigh heavily in such a benefit/risk analysis.

It is also important in the context of such considerations that the strength of the evidence available should be reviewed. The most powerful evidence regarding the benefit or risk of a therapy is the prospective randomized controlled clinical trial, of which there are very few in the area of hormone therapy. A lower level of evidence is provided by observational epidemiological studies. Studies may follow one of two major designs: the cohort study, in which groups of women are followed up longitudinally for the occurrence of certain diseases and the rates of occurrence of those diseases in users of hormone therapy are compared with the rates in non-users; a weaker design, the case–control study, in which cases of a certain disease are compared with controls for their use of hormone therapy. The majority of evidence regarding benefit and risk of hormone therapy is based on such observational studies.

Osteoporosis is a major cause of morbidity and mortality, and health expenditure world-wide. Its prevalence varies very greatly. It is estimated to affect about 75 million women in the United States, Europe and Japan. About one in three postmenopausal women will suffer from the consequences of this disease, the majority being elderly, and it has been estimated that in the United States there are about 1.3 million fractures per year, with a cost to the health-care system of $10 billion. The particularly significant fracture is hip fracture, which may result in a 12–20% 1-year mortality rate, and frequently leads the individual woman to lose her independence.

Estrogen deficiency increases bone remodelling and leads to bone loss. Estrogen administration reverses that process, the mechanisms involved becoming increasingly established. The effect ceases when therapy is ceased. Many believe that most benefit is seen when treatment is initiated within 5 years of the menopause, although there is no consensus on when treatment should be initiated nor on how long it should be continued. No controlled clinical trials have shown a reduction in hip fracture. Only a small number of placebo-controlled trials have shown actual reductions in fractures such as vertebral fractures. Critical reviews of this area have appeared recently[2,3].

The dose of estrogen given is important, while the route by which it is given is probably not. The effects of progestins are variable, with some, such as norethisterone, reported as showing synergism with estrogen in effects on bone mineral density.

Cardiovascular disease is generally regarded as a major area of interest in terms of hormone therapy. Australian 1993 female mortality data showed that almost half of all deaths were due to cardiovascular disease, 47.5%, with 23.8% being from coronary heart disease. In contrast, breast cancer accounted for 4.7% of deaths, in other words, about one-fifth of the coronary heart disease mortality rate. The mortality for breast cancer, when it is compared to the mortality for heart disease, will vary as a function of the age group in which that comparison is made.

For coronary heart disease, randomized controlled clinical trials of hormone therapy for primary prevention are being performed, but will not be reported until 2007. None at the moment can be used as a rigorous basis for determining whether postmenopausal hormone therapy really reduces the risk of heart disease. The general consensus from observational epidemiological data is that estrogens substantially (by 35–50%) reduce coronary disease risk in those without established heart disease.

Estrogen administration has both acute and chronic effects in both human and animal studies that are consistent with having such a protective effect and, despite figures to the contrary, it appears from the major, more recently published studies that progestins do not exert a great influence on the apparent effect of estrogen. The mechanisms are very large in number and include favorable effects on serum lipids as well as a large variety of direct effects on the blood vasculature[4].

In secondary prevention, in women who have already had a heart attack or who have clear evidence clinically of coronary artery disease, a number of observational studies again show an even greater risk reduction, up to 80% for subsequent disease or death. One important prospective secondary prevention study has been reported[5]. Unexpectedly, this showed that there was no statistically significant difference in coronary events in women treated with combined continuous hormone therapy or with placebo. In fact, there was an increase in coronary events in the first year of therapy, with apparent protection observed in the third and fourth years.

There are currently some *possible* indications for hormone therapy. One which has arisen in the more recent past is the possibility of reducing the risks of and even treating Alzheimer's disease[6].

A number of studies suggest that there may be a reduction in the risk of colon cancer and in some forms of arthritis. Although there are very few data, estrogens may also be beneficial in a number of the complications particularly related to macrovascular disease in diabetes.

The long-term risks of hormone therapy are widely discussed. Unopposed estrogen substantially increases the risk of endometrial cancer and that increased risk is largely abolished by concomitant progestin use. There is some question about whether that abolition is complete or only semi-complete[7].

We know that, regarding breast cancer, the ever use or short-term use of estrogens has been reported not to be associated with an increased risk. Long-term use in a number of studies has been suggested to be associated with an increased relative risk, in the order of 30% increase or perhaps even a little more, although there are questions about surveillance bias and the possibility of withholding estrogens from those at increased risk, which may confound that data. The effect of added progestins is unclear. There is the possibility from current data that breast cancer may be a little more common than heart disease in the 50–65 age group and, therefore, that is an age group in which we, perhaps, need to be particularly careful. Most women, however, are likely to benefit in heart disease prevention at what is probably a small risk.

The most important analysis of potential risk of breast cancer from hormone therapy was published late in 1997[8], and suggests that in European or American populations, 5 years of hormone therapy between the ages of 50 and 70 years will lead to two extra cases of breast cancer per 1000 women treated (above a baseline of 45). Ten years of therapy will give rise to six extra, and 15–20 years, 12 extra - an absolute risk increase of 1.2%. It must be emphasized that all these data are also based on observational epidemiological studies.

'Established' contraindications to hormone therapy would include a history of breast and endometrial cancer, liver disease and venous thromboembolism. In some of the older publications, established heart disease was also a contraindication. Undiagnosed vaginal bleeding and pregnancy are universally regarded as contraindications.

In terms of women with a history of breast cancer, there remains great controversy. A recent review[9] suggested that hormone therapy does not appear to have a pronounced adverse effect on cancer outcome, although the number of patients studied and the data are still very few. It will be important to determine whether women with a past history of breast cancer should be denied hormone therapy when that is indicated for other reasons. A thorough discussion of the issue can be found in the proceedings of a consensus conference[10].

With regard to liver disease, a recent review[11] suggested that hormone therapy should be considered in all women with chronic liver disease who are postmenopausal, have primary or secondary amenorrhea, or have had an oophorectomy. Those with primary biliary cirrhosis, sclerosing cholangitis, alcohol or tobacco use, or who are taking long-term steroids for autoimmune hepatitis are especially at risk of osteoporosis and ought to be treated with estrogens.

With regard to venous thromboembolism, three observational studies published in late 1996 found an association between hormone therapy and venous thromboembolism, although that would only confer an extra risk of about one in 5000 women per year. Five other studies found no association. In a review[12], the conclusion was that all of these studies have methodological problems that preclude definitive conclusions about the association, and that the biological plausibility of the association was not convincing. It is noteworthy, however, that in the secondary prevention study referred to above, with a randomized controlled design[5], there was a three-fold increase in venous thromboembolic risk in women treated with hormone therapy.

To summarize, it can be concluded that, for women without significant risk factors for heart disease, osteoporosis and Alzheimer's disease, the indications for hormone therapy are equivocal. For those with significant risks of heart disease or osteoporosis, the benefits very considerably outweigh the risks. Currently stated contraindications should be viewed with scepticism and most may not be valid. Finally, ongoing clinical trials should hopefully provide helpful guidelines. Other options must always be considered for management, including life-style advice, avoidance of smoking, dietary measures, exercise, lipid-lowering agents and bisphosphonates.

A recent review addresses many of the above issues[13].

References

1. Greendale GA, Reboussin BA, Hogan P, *et al.* Symptom relief and side effects of postmenopausal hormones: results from the Postmenopausal Estrogen/Progestin Interventions Trial. *Obstet Gynecol* 1998;92:982–8
2. O'Connell D, Robertson J, Henry D, Gillespie W. A systematic review of the skeletal effects of estrogen therapy in postmenopausal women. II. An assessment of treatment effects. *Climacteric* 1998;1:112–23
3. Henry D, Robertson J, O'Connell D, Gillespie W. A systematic review of the skeletal effects of estrogen therapy in postmenopausal women. I. An assessment of the quality of randomized trials published between 1977 and 1995. *Climacteric* 1998;1:92–111
4. Mendelsohn ME, Karas RH. The protective effects of estrogen on the cardiovascular system. *N Engl J Med* 1999;340:1801–11
5. Hulley S, Grady D, Bush T, *et al.* Randomized trial of estrogen plus progestin for secondary prevention of coronary heart disease in postmenopausal women. *J Am Med Assoc* 1998;280:605–13
6. Yaffe K, Sawaya G, Lieberberg I, Grady D. Estrogen therapy in postmenopausal women. Effects on cognitive function and dementia. *J Am Med Assoc* 1998;279:688–95
7. Beresford SAA, Weiss NS, Voigt LF, McKnight B. Risk of endometrial cancer in relation to use of oestrogen combined with cyclic progestogen therapy in postmenopausal women. *Lancet* 1977; 349:458–61
8. Collaborative Group on Hormonal Factors in Breast Cancer. Breast cancer and hormone replacement therapy: collaborative reanalysis of data from 51 epidemiological studies of 52 705 women with breast cancer and 108 411 without breast cancer. *Lancet* 1997;350:1047–59
9. Vassilopoulou-Sellin R, Theriault R, Klein MJ. Estrogen replacement therapy in women with prior diagnosis and treatment of breast cancer. *Gynecol Oncol* 1997;65:89–93
10. Santen R, Pritchard K, Burger HG, eds. The consensus conference on treatment of estrogen deficiency symptoms in women surviving breast cancer. *Obstet Gynecol Surv* 1998;53(Suppl 10):S1–83
11. O'Donohue J, Williams R. Hormone replacement therapy in women with liver disease. *Br J Obstet Gynaecol* 1977;104:1–3
12. Douketis JD, Ginsberg JS, Holbrook A, *et al.* A re-evaluation of the risk for venous thromboembolism with the use of oral contraceptives and hormone replacement therapy. *Arch Intern Med* 1997;157:1522–30
13. Clinical Synthesis Panel on HRT. Hormone replacement therapy. *Lancet* 1999;354:152–5

Morphological changes in reproductive organs during the aging process in perimenopausal women

22

P. M. Motta and S. Makabe

INTRODUCTION

Considering that the lifespan of women today is rapidly increasing, and that the structural and functional changes of the reproductive organs are a result of the lack of estrogens after the menopause, the study of such alterations is of great importance because of the hormonal and pathological implications.

To our knowledge, only a few microscopic investigations have been performed on the woman's reproductive system during the menopause[1-5]. In recent studies, the three-dimensional ultrastructural view obtained from transmission and scanning electron microscopic results, often enriched by artificially colored images[6,7], further emphasized the microdynamic aspects of these structures[7-10]. The aim of this paper is to summarize the most important morphofunctional features of the woman's reproductive organs, as viewed by high-resolution three-dimensional microanatomical methods.

MATERIALS AND METHODS

For this study, biopsies of the ovary, Fallopian tube and uterus, including the cervix and upper vagina, from women in the perimenopausal period (45–55 years of age) were employed. The fragments were obtained during surgery or endoscopic diagnostic procedures with the consent of the patients. The samples, which were not affected by any specific diseases, were fixed in 2.5% glutaraldehyde in 0.1 mol/l phosphate-buffered saline for at least 48 h. All the specimens were postfixed in 1% osmium tetroxide in 15 mol/l buffer solution and dehydrated in a graduated ethanol series. Finally, each sample was divided into two parts: one was used for scanning electron microscopy, while the other was embedded in Araldite™ for transmission electron microscopy.

Scanning electron microscopy

The specimens were dried using a critical-point dryer with CO_2, mounted on aluminium stubs, coated with 3 nm of platinum in an iron coater and then observed with a Hitachi S-4500 (Tokyo, Japan) scanning electron microscope.

Transmission electron microscopy

Ultra-thin sections were cut with an ultramicrotome, mounted onto copper grids, stained with uranyl acetate and lead citrate in Reynolds' solution and then observed with a Zeiss M 10 (Jena/Oberkochen, Germany) transmission electron microscope.

RESULTS AND DISCUSSION

Ovary

The volume of the ovary in menopause was drastically reduced to one-half to two-thirds and showed a number of wide atrophic areas with respect to the normal ovary in fertile age. A decrease in its superficial papillae and crypts was noted (Figure 1). In some zones, the superficial epithelium was very flattened and fragile, with clear signs of apoptosis and necrosis, and tended to slough off, exposing the subjacent tunica albuginea. The ovarian cortex and medulla were occupied by a dense stroma rich in collagen fibers and many scars (residual corpora albicantia). With aging, characteristic changes were noted within the walls of blood vessels, which showed a thickened tunica intima, probably due to the influence of low estrogen levels[11,12].

Fallopian tube and uterus

A low active endometrium was the most common aspect in the peri- and postmenopausal periods. In fact, the endometrium appeared to be very thin. Its epithelial layer showed rare mitotic figures. Organelles and glycogen deposits within the cells were very scarce. Another characteristic feature of the endometrium was a progressive deciliation of its epithelial layer (Figure 2). In fact, in some areas this epithelium consisted of tall and/or extremely flattened polyhedral-shaped cells. The apical surface of these cells showed few microvilli and mostly atypical microplicae (Figure 3), which were curiously rather similar to those found on the squamous surface cells of the ectocervix (Figure 4). Generally, the epithelium of the Fallopian tube

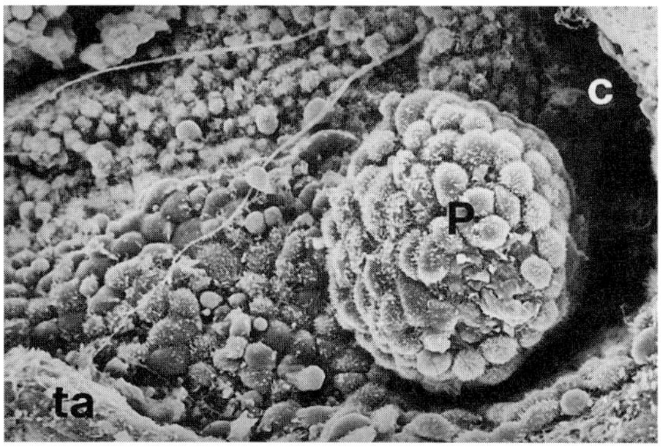

Figure 1 Menopausal ovary from a woman aged 53 years. The ovarian superficial epithelium completely covers some crypts (c) and papillae (P). Some areas with occasional loss of the surface epithelium can be seen showing subjacent connective tissue of the tunica albuginea (ta). Scanning electron microscopy, × 300

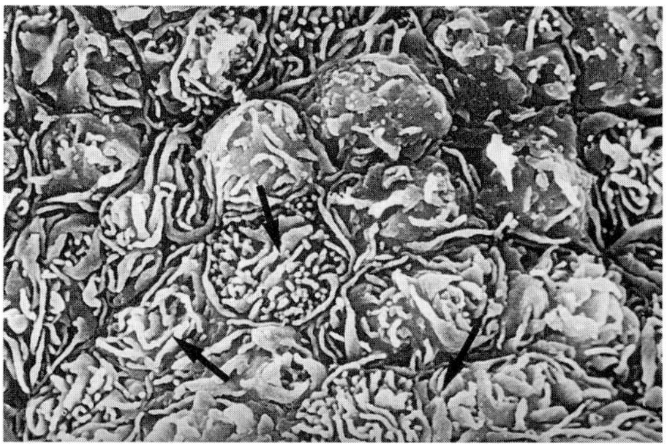

Figure 3 Endometrium from a woman aged 52 years. The epithelial cells of this area of the endometrium are flattened and their apical surface shows many characteristic microplicae (arrows). They curiously resemble the squamous cells of the ectocervix (see Figure 4). Scanning electron microscopy, × 4200

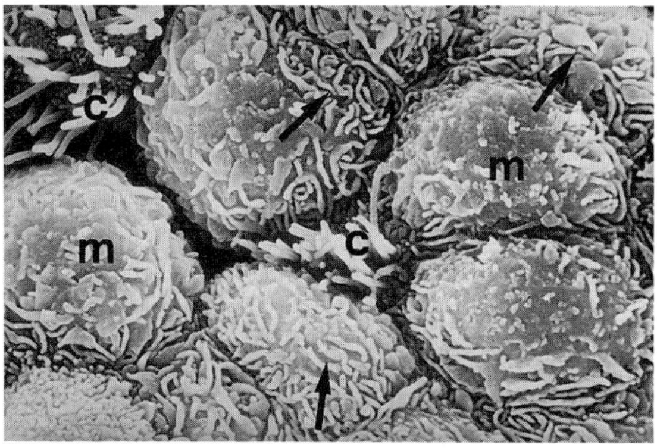

Figure 2 Endometrium from a woman aged 52 years. The epithelium has a few ciliated cells (c) and numerous microvillous cells (m). Some of these reveal irregularly shaped microplicae (arrows). Scanning electron microscopy, × 6500

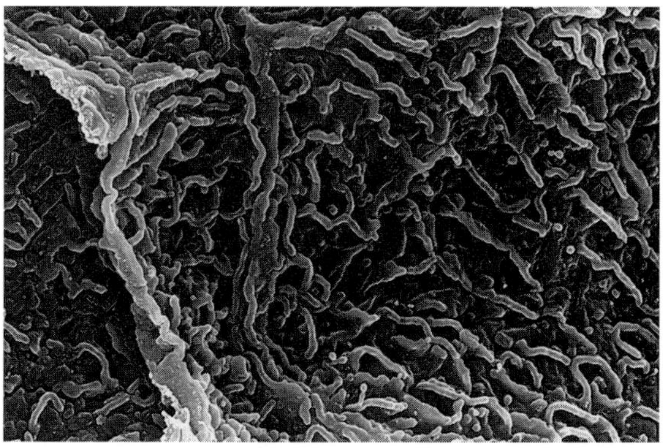

Figure 4 Ectocervix from a woman aged 53 years. The squamous cell borders become irregular and their surface shows thin and rare microplicae, along with altered microvilli. Scanning electron microscopy, × 38 000

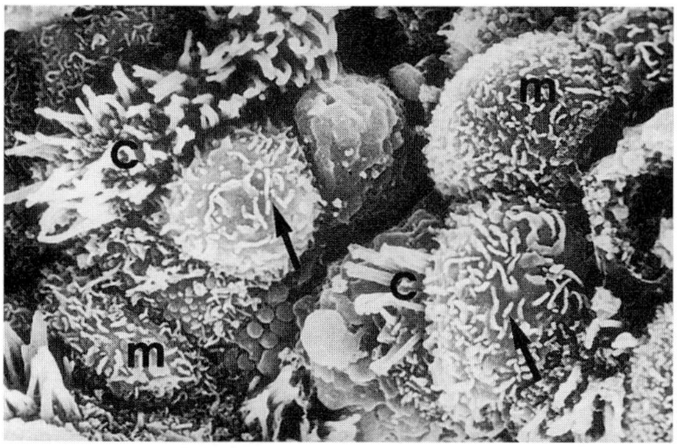

Figure 5 Fallopian tube ampulla from a woman aged 49 years. The epithelial cells of the mucosa reveal a few ciliated cells (c). Other cells show only scarce and short microvilli (m), with an increasing number of irregularly shaped microplicae (arrows). Scanning electron microscopy, × 4200

also revealed a drastic deciliation (Figure 5). In the postmenopause, some fimbriae showed apoptotic and/or necrotic desquamative epithelial cells, and this resulted in an exposed basal lamina and a stroma rich in collagenous fibers. At the same time, the epithelium of the tubal ampulla consisted of dome-shaped cells showing scarce and short cilia, along with numerous microvilli. Microplicae were also commonly found in the epithelial cells of the Fallopian tubes at the menopause (Figure 5).

Ectocervix and vagina

The covering epithelium was smoother and thinner in these mucosal regions of postmenopausal samples when compared to those belonging to fertile women. Furthermore, it showed an increasing desquamation of apoptotic and necrotic surface cells (Figure 4). Similar aspects were found in the upper zones of the vaginal epithelium, where most of the surface cells showed shallow and simple microplicae.

CONCLUSIONS

In the light of the above three-dimensional results, it is likely that the ultrastructural changes of a woman's reproductive system are caused by the lack of estrogens after the menopause. Furthermore, this new integrated three-dimensional microscopic approach offers the possibility of evaluating in great detail dynamic events that cannot be seen with other bidimensional techniques. In this way, normal and eventual pathological aspects can easily be correlated, offering solid parameters for helpful clinical evaluations to the histopathologist and gynecologist.

References

1. Ferenczy A, Richart RM. *Female Reproductive System: Dynamics of Scanning and Transmission Electron Microscopy*. New York: John Wiley and Sons, 1974
2. Ludwig H, Metzer H. *The Human Female Reproductive Tract. A Scanning Electron Microscopic Atlas*. Berlin: Springer-Verlag, 1976
3. Hafez ESE, Kenemans P, eds. *Atlas of Human Reproduction*. Lancaster, UK: MTP Press, 1982
4. Mestwerdt W. Function and structure of postmenopausal ovaries. *Med Klin* 1976;71:96-103
5. Crow J, Amso NN, Lewis J, *et al*. Morphology and ultrastructure of Fallopian tube epithelia at different stages of the menstrual cycle and menopause. *Hum Reprod* 1994;9:2224-33
6. Motta PM, Nottola SAR. Colored scanning electron microscopic pictures in teaching anatomy. In Motta PM, ed. *Cells and Tissues: a Three-dimensional Approach by Modern Techniques in Microscopy*. New York: Alan R Liss, 1989:629-34
7. Motta PM, Makabe S, Naguro T, *et al*. The beauty of menopause. A colorful microworld of images. In Limpaphayom K, ed. *Proceedings of 1st Asian-European Congress on the Menopause*. Bologna: Monduzzi Editore, 1998:89-93
8. Motta PM, Makabe S, Naguro T, *et al*. Morphodynamics of the female reproductive organs in menopause: a 3-D microanatomical approach. In Birkhaüser MH, Rozenbaum H, eds. *Proceedings of*

IV European Congress on Menopause, Vienna. Paris: Editions ESKA, 1997:27–32

9. Makabe S, Naguro T, Motta PM. Three dimensional features of female reproductive organs in menopause by ODO method and field emission scanning electron microscopy. *Menopause Rev* 1997; 2:52
10. Makabe S, Motta PM, Naguro T, *et al.* Microanatomy of the female reproductive organs in postmenopause by scanning electron microscopy. *Climacteric* 1998;1:63–71
11. Shimada T, Morita T, Nagai K, *et al.* Morphological changes in spiral artery of the mammalian ovary with age. *Horm Res* 1993;39(Suppl):9–15
12. Motta PM, Makabe S. The evolution of the ageing ovary. The Solvay Lecture. *J Br Menopause Soc* 1999;5 (Suppl 3):4–7

Xerostomia and other oral problems in the menopause

23

T. Fujibayashi

INTRODUCTION

This paper is a review article on some oral problems arising in women in the menopause, with some emphasis on sex steroid hormones. Xerostomia (Figure 1) is one of the most frequent symptoms associated with Sjögren's syndrome, which involves not only exocrine glands in the mucosal surfaces of the body, such as the eye, mouth, nose, laryngotracheal tissues and genital tract, but also internal organs such as the lungs, pancreas, gastrointestinal tract, kidneys and liver. This disease sometimes also involves the proliferation of monoclonal B lymphocytes.

DESIGN AND METHODS

A review study of Sjögren's syndrome was performed using 823 cases, including the controls. These cases were registered in the Japanese Medical Society for Sjögren's Syndrome. The number of patients with Sjögren's syndrome was 482, including 256 cases of primary Sjögren's syndrome (showing sicca complex alone) and 226 cases of secondary Sjögren's syndrome, where the disease was accompanied by other autoimmune diseases. Oral manifestations and functions involving the salivary glands were studied by evaluating subjective oral symptoms, objective oral symptoms,

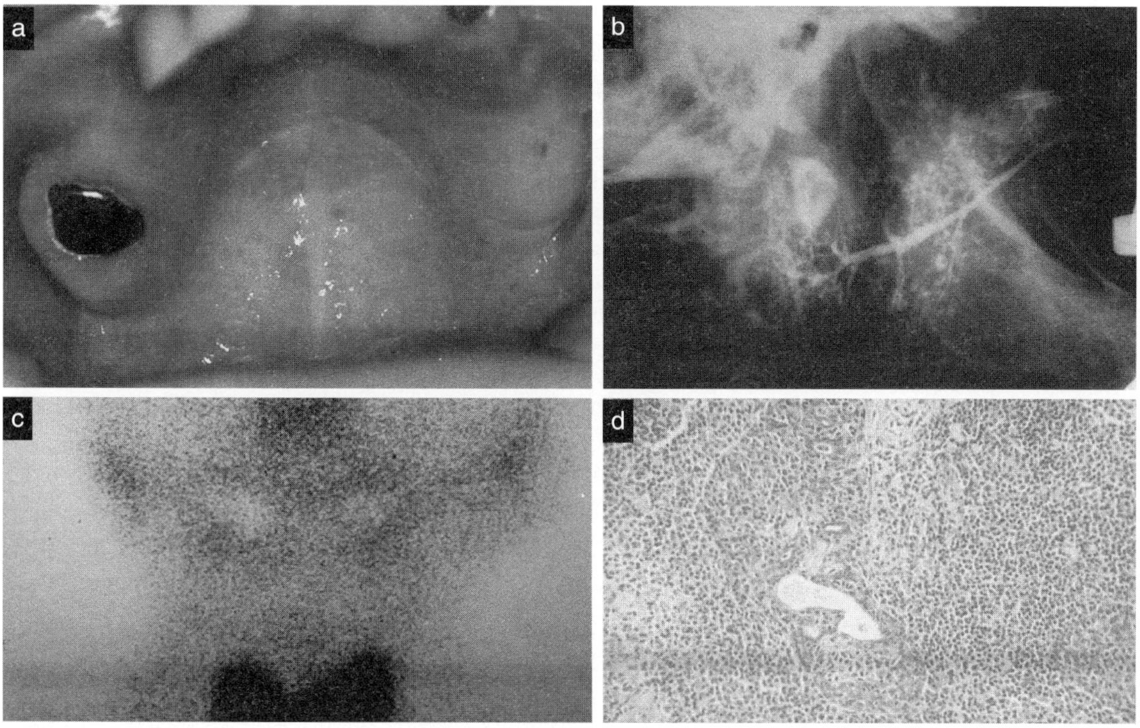

Figure 1 Xerostomia in Sjögren's syndrome. (a) Oral manifestations showing dry mouth; (b) sialography of the parotid gland showing globular pattern of change (stage II); (c) salivary gland scintigraphy showing decreased accumulation and secretion; (d) histopathology of the labial salivary gland showing strong lymphocyte infiltration

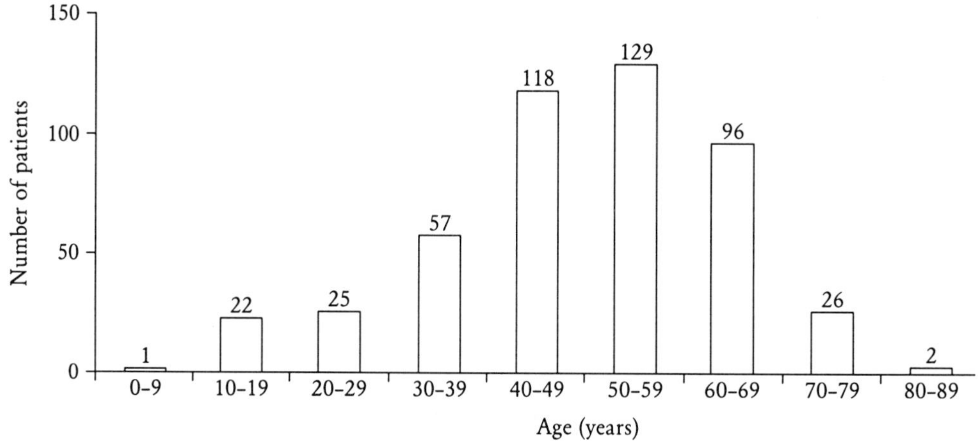

Figure 2 Age distribution of patients with Sjögren's syndrome

sialometry, salivary scintigraphy, parotid sialography and histopathological examinations of minor salivary glands taken by lip biopsy. The sex steroid influence on autoimmune disease, with special emphasis on the influence of estrogen on Sjögren's syndrome, was reviewed by looking at studies of animal models for Sjögren's syndrome.

RESULTS

Over 90% of the patient group were female. More than half of the patients were over 50 years old. The highest incidence of Sjögren's syndrome was observed in the sixth decade, followed by the fifth and seventh decades of life (Figure 2).

The disease is manifested orally by various degrees of dry mouth, including glossitis, cheilitis and mucositis, owing to hyposalivation. Dental caries and periodontal disease are common, and candidal infection is also rather frequent. Most of the patients complain to some degree of subjective oral symptoms.

Sialometry, carried out by chewing gum test, showed that 75% of the patients had a salivary flow rate of less than 10 ml/10 min, and this hyposalivation was a little more frequent in primary Sjögren's syndrome than in secondary Sjögren's syndrome patients. Salivary gland scintigraphy is a useful image tool for evaluating salivary gland function, and 89.2% of the patients showed various degrees of abnormality by quantitative analysis of the time-activity curve. Parotid sialography is a classical but still effective image analysis, and specificity in the diagnosis of Sjögren's syndrome is high when the patient shows a globular, cavitary or destructive pattern of change. A total of 41.9% of patients showed a globular pattern of change (Stage II), 11.6% showed a cavitary pattern of change (Stage III) and 10.5% showed a destructive pattern of change (Stage IV). Histopathology of minor salivary glands taken by lip biopsy showed periductal infiltration of lymphoid cells in Sjögren's syndrome. The focal accumulation of more than 50 lymphoid cells was counted as one focus. This focus score increased with the advancement of the disease. Figure 3 illustrates the incidence of cases showing each grade of lymphoid cell infiltration measured by Chisholm and Mason's grading system[1]. Seventy-eight per cent of the patients also had eye involvement, with keratoconjunctivitis sicca being found in both primary and secondary Sjögren's syndrome patients. Accompanying autoimmune diseases in secondary Sjögren's syndrome patients were rheumatoid arthritis (found in 45% of secondary patients), followed by systemic lupus erythematosus (found in 25% of patients), progressive systemic sclerosis (found in 14% of patients) and others (Figure 4).

Autoantibodies were frequently detected in the peripheral blood. Anti-SS-A/Ro antibody was present in 68.6% of primary Sjögren's syndrome patients and in 66.0% of secondary Sjögren's syndrome patients (Figure 5). Anti-SS-B/La antibody was observed less frequently, but the incidence in primary Sjögren's syndrome patients (25.7%) was a

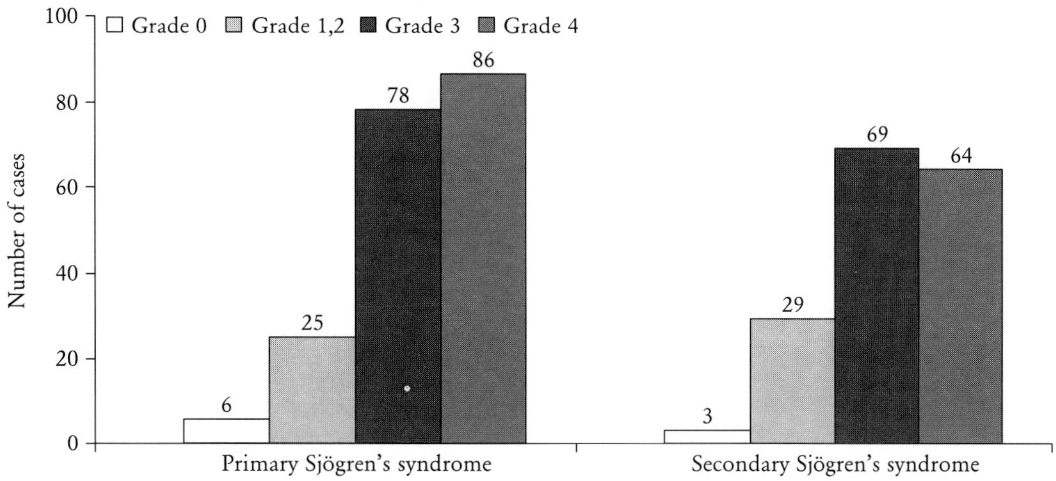

Figure 3 Histopathology of the minor salivary gland

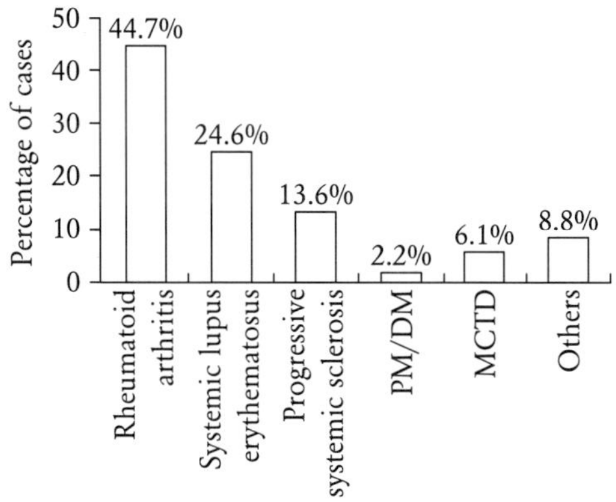

Figure 4 Accompanying autoimmune diseases in secondary Sjögren's syndrome. PM/DM, polymyositis and/or dermatomyositis; MCTD, mixed connective tissue disease

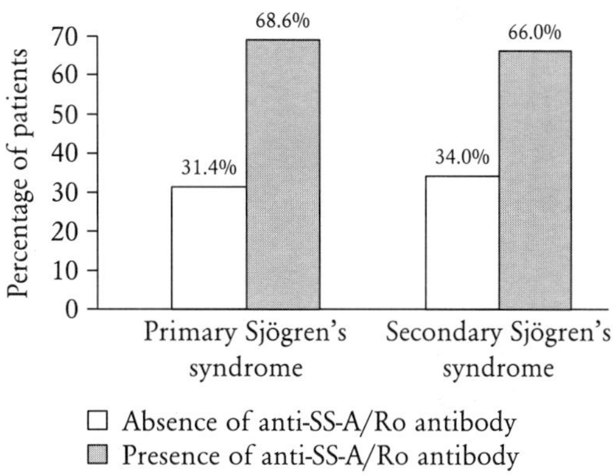

Figure 5 Prevalence of the anti-SS-A/Ro antibody in primary and secondary Sjögren's syndrome patients

little higher than that in secondary Sjögren's syndrome patients (15.9%).

Many studies on the immunological analysis of Sjögren's syndrome patients indicate that the subset of T cells infiltrating glandular tissues consists mainly of CD4-positive cells in the initial phase. These cells are gradually replaced by B cells showing polyclonal activation and proliferation with autoantibody production. Then they may go to oligoclonal, and sometimes monoclonal, proliferation in the third phase.

Estrogen receptor mRNA and/or protein has been identified in premature B lymphocytes, thymocytes, CD8 T cells, memory T cells, peripheral blood mononuclear cells, splenic lymphocytes and lymphokine-activated killer cells, but has not been detected in mature B cells[2]. Thus, estrogen may exert a direct action on immune cells. Progesterone receptor mRNA and/or protein in specific lymphocytes or their subsets has not been clearly identified.

The following mouse strains have been used as animal models for Sjögren's syndrome: NZB/NZW F1, MRL/lpr, SJL/J and NOD,NFS/sld. According to these animal model studies, estrogens appear to be involved in the etiology, progression and amplification of Sjögren's syndrome by enhancing polyclonal B-cell activation in MRL/lpr[3] and normal mice[4]. In contrast, chronic estrogen treatment improved

T-cell-mediated focal sialadenitis in the same MRL/lpr mice[5]. Therefore, the effect of estrogen in the Sjögren's syndrome mouse model is rather controversial. Androgens appear to provide a protective influence in Sjögren's syndrome. Testosterone administration to female MRL/lpr mice[6] and NZB/NZW F1 mice[7] produced a big suppression of lymphoid cell accumulation in the lacrimal gland. However, recent work on NFS/sld mice by Ishimaru and colleagues[8] provides another view on the role of estrogen in the pathogenesis of Sjögren's syndrome. These NFS/sld mutant mice[9] manifested glandular organ-specific autoimmune lesions after thymectomy at 3 days and then ovariectomy at 4 weeks after birth. The histology at 8 weeks of age showed an apparent accumulation of lymphocytes in the glandular tissues of estrogen-deficient thymectomized and ovariectomized mice. These lymphocytes mainly consisted of CD4-positive T cells. The administration of estrogen between 4 and 8 weeks of age resulted in a decrease in cellular infiltration in glandular tissues, and this finding suggests a protective effect of estrogen in this mouse model. The administration of testosterone instead of estrogen showed a similar effect in the submandibular and sublingual glands, but did not show this effect in the parotid and lacrimal gland. Analysis of serum autoantibody production compared with organ-specific autoantigen showed an intense band of anti-120-kd α-fodrin[10] autoantibody in sera from thymectomized and ovariectomized mice compared with mice that had undergone thymectomy alone, using the Western blotting method. A significant increase in apoptosis in the ductal epithelium of the salivary gland was observed in thymectomized and ovariectomized mice by TUNEL assay. Interferon-induced Fas expression in cultured salivary gland cells was clearly reduced by estrogen *in vitro*.

Therefore, in this NFS/sld mouse model, autoimmune salivary and lacrimal lesions developed in ovariectomized and hence estrogen-deficient mice, and these lesions were reduced by estrogen administration. This may suggest a protective action of estrogen in Sjögren's syndrome.

CONCLUSION

Xerostomia associated with Sjögren's syndrome is one of the frequent oral problems for women in the menopause. Sjögren's syndrome has a strong predominance in middle-aged or elderly females. Estrogens may be involved in the progression and modulation of the disease. However, the role of estrogens in the pathogenesis and/or background of the disease is rather controversial in animal models. Further studies of this relationship will lead to a better understanding of this disease.

References

1. Chisholm DM, Mason DK. Labial salivary gland biopsy in Sjögren's disease. *J Clin Pathol* 1968;21: 656–60
2. Sullivan DA. Sex hormones and Sjögren's syndrome. *J Rheumatol* 1997;24(Suppl 50):17–32
3. Carlsten H, Tarkowski A, Holmdahl R, Nilsson LA. Oestrogen is a potent disease accelerator in prone MRL lpr/lpr mice. *Clin Exp Immunol* 1990;80: 467–73
4. Ahmed SA, Aufdemorte TB, Chen JR, Montoya AI, Olive D, Talal N. Estrogen induces the development of autoantibodies and promotes salivary gland lymphoid infiltrates in normal mice. *J Autoimmun* 1989;2:543–52
5. Carlsten H, Nilsson N, Jonsson R, Backman K, Holmdahl R, Tarkowski A. Estrogen accelerates immune complex glomerulonephritis but ameliorates T cell-mediated vasculitis and sialoadenitis in autoimmune MRL lpr/lpr mice. *Cell Immunol* 1992;144:190–202
6. Ariga H, Edwards J, Sullivan DA. Androgen control of autoimmune expression in lacrimal glands of MRL/Mp-lpr/lpr mice. *Clin Immunol Immunopathol* 1989;53:499–508

7. Vendramini AC, Soo CH, Sullivan DA. Testosterone-induced suppression of autoimmune disease in lacrimal tissue of a mouse model (NZB/NZW F1) of Sjögren's syndrome. *Invest Ophthalmol Vis Sci* 1991;32:3002-6
8. Ishimaru N, Saegusa K, Yanagi K, Haneji N, Saito I, Hayashi Y. Estrogen deficiency accelerates autoimmune exocrinopathy in murine Sjögren's syndrome through Fas-mediated apoptosis. *Am J Pathol* 1999;155:173-81
9. Haneji N, Hamano H, Yanagi K, Hayashi Y. A new animal model for primary Sjögren's syndrome in NFS/sld mice. *J Immunol* 1994;153:2769-77
10. Haneji N, Nakamura T, Takio KH, *et al.* Identification of alpha-fodrin as a candidate autoantigen in primary Sjögren's syndrome. *Science* 1997;276:604-7

Connective tissue changes in the menopause and with hormone replacement therapy 24

M. Brincat, R. Galea and Y. Muscat Baron

INTRODUCTION

Collagen is the major protein component of most connective tissues of vertebrates. In mammals it constitutes about 25–35% of their total protein. It is present in virtually every animal tissue, providing an extracellular framework for all metazoan animals. It is a highly conserved, evolutionarily ancient family of molecules.

Type I collagen, which constitutes 90% of the total collagen in the body, is the most important[1]. It is predominant in skin and bone. Skin contains in addition an amount of the very similar type III collagen.

Bone and skin are the two organs that together contain some 80% of all the connective tissues found in the human body. Both show a deterioration with estrogen deficiency. This deterioration can be prevented and even reversed with appropriate and adequate estrogen replacement[2-5].

BONE

The collagens are mainly type I collagen with type V making up a minor component. The non-collagen proteins include plasma proteins, proteoglycans, osteocalcin, osteopontin, osteonectin and bone sialoprotein. Collagens make up the greatest proportion, as they constitute approximately 35% of dry defatted bone mass. The organic matrix of bone acts rather like internal girders, and confers on bone its tensile strength. It has been suggested that it is a decline in this organic matrix that is the primary pathological event leading to osteoporosis[6,7].

Bone loss is age related in both sexes, but in women there is an acceleration in the rate of bone loss following the menopause. It has been shown[8] that by the age of 70 years women lose up to 50% of their bone mass, while a man would be expected to lose only 25% by the age of 90.

The relationship between age, bone mass and skin thickness was investigated in a study on postmenopausal women. This consisted of a biophysical study that looked at differences in various bone density measurements and in skin thickness. Bone was measured using a dual energy X-ray absorptiometer (between lumbar vertebrae 2 and 4, at the femur neck and at Ward's triangle) and skin thickness was measured using high-frequency (22 MHz) ultrasound. Skin thickness correlates with the collagen content in the skin. These measurements were carried out in a group of untreated postmenopausal women and a group of untreated postmenopausal women who had sustained an osteoporotic fracture. The results showed that the skin thickness and bone density parameters were much lower in women who had sustained osteoporotic fractures compared to controls (Figure 1).

Women with fractures had mean bone mass values that were some 20% below the mean values of controls. Skin thickness varied within a narrower range (mean difference 4%) but significant differences between controls and women who had sustained an osteoporotic fracture were also consistently noted. When the skin thickness measurements were combined with bone density parameters the accuracy of predicting an osteoporotic fracture increased, as shown in Figure 2[9].

The effect of estrogen on osteoblasts (bone-forming cells) may be a direct effect or it may rely on an alteration of the coupling phenomenon of bone formation and bone resorption[10].

Estrogen replacement affects osteoporosis in two ways: it can prevent it or it can correct it once it has occurred. It has been postulated that estrogen

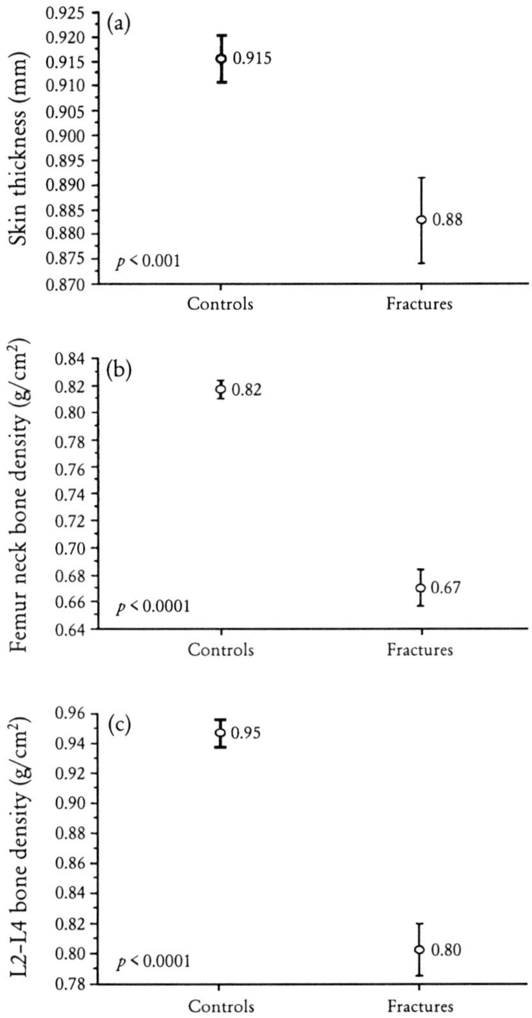

Figure 1 Mean skin thickness (a), femur neck bone density (b) and L2–L4 bone density (c) in 411 untreated postmenopausal women as controls and 119 untreated postmenopausal women who had suffered an osteoporotic bone fracture

replacement therapy leads to an increase in bone mass by increasing the collagen levels in bone. Indeed, the observation that women on estrogen replacement therapy had a higher dermal skin collagen content than those who were not on estrogen replacement therapy had led to the idea that a similar increase in bone collagen content in women on estrogen replacement therapy occurred. Possibly this increase in collagen content leads to an increase in bone strength and thus a diminution of osteoporotic fractures. When estrogen treatment is started in the menopausal period and continued into later life the best result for bone density is obtained. However, if estrogen therapy is initiated later in life, there are also benefits[11].

In order to look at the collagen changes occurring with estrogen therapy, our group undertook another study[12]. This study was a biophysical/biochemical study between a group of untreated postmenopausal women and a group of women who were on estrogen replacement therapy. Apart from having the same bone density and skin thickness measurements as in the previous study (mentioned above), the women in this study also had collagen marker estimations.

In this study we looked at the excretion of procollagen IC end-terminal peptides (PCICP), a marker for bone formation, and pyridinium crosslinks, a marker for bone resorption.

When the untreated postmenopausal controls were compared with women who had been on hormone replacement therapy, the latter showed a drastic decrease in osteoclastic activity (pyridinium crosslink excretion). The mean decrease was 27.2%. There was also a decrease in bone formation, osteoblastic activity (PCICP) being decreased by a mean of 11.3%. All these differences ($p < 0.001$) indicated that bone remodelling had readjusted in patients on estrogen replacement therapy. The women in this study who were taking hormone replacement therapy had only been on this treatment for a short time (mean 6 months). This may imply that changes occur rapidly. It is interesting to note that, according to the above calculations based on bone collagen markers, a mean positive change of 15.9% occurred in bone remodelling in women on estrogen replacement therapy. This value is of the same order as the mean percentage change in bone mass of the same women, measured using the biophysical method. This showed a mean positive change at the L2–L4 region of 16.1%[12] (Figure 3).

This could indicate that these markers are indeed sensitive and can be used in monitoring postmenopausal bone loss as well as accurately titrating the response to treatment, both when such treatment is prophylactic and when it is used therapeutically in the management of established osteoporosis. The excretion of pyridinium crosslinks of collagen in the first morning void urine

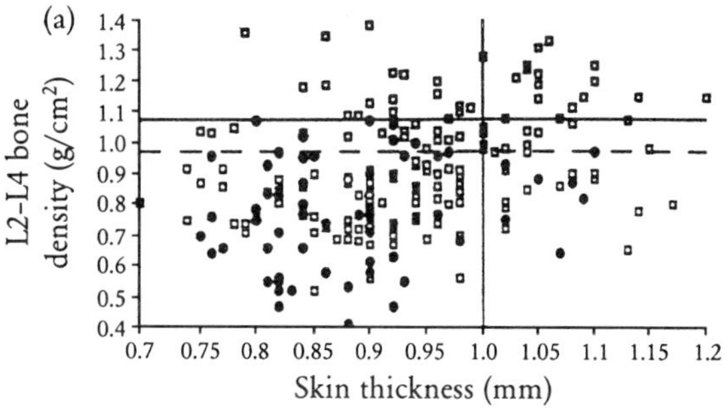

	Sensitivity	Accuracy
Skin thickness	91.8%	38.7%
L2-L4	100.0%	39.6%
Box L2-L4	91.8%	50.1%

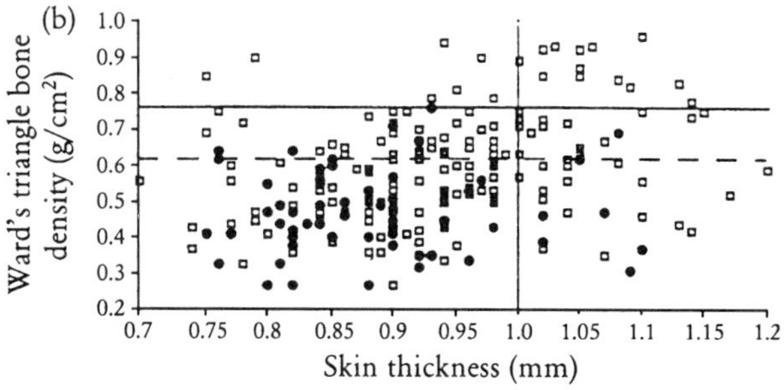

	Sensitivity	Accuracy
Skin thickness	91.7%	39.2%
Ward's triangle	100.0%	50.9%
Box Ward's triangle	91.7%	59.1%

Figure 2 Bone density at L2-L4 vertebrae (a) and at Ward's triangle (b) plotted against skin thickness in 411 untreated postmenopausal women as controls (squares) and 129 untreated postmenopausal women who had suffered an osteoporotic bone fracture (circles). The accuracy of combining skin thickness measurements with bone density parameters in predicting bone fractures is shown

sample showed some intraindividual variation[13] and this may be a limitation of its usefulness. Some authors[14] claim that the intact amino-terminal propeptide of type I procollagen, a protein set free from the other end on the same procollagen molecule, is a more dynamic marker for bone metabolism than PCICP (the carboxyl-terminal propeptide of type I procollagen). It can therefore be recommended according to these authors that it be used as a marker reflecting the effect of estrogen on bone collagen formation during estrogen replacement therapy. Increasing evidence is now available[15] that collagen markers can become a useful tool in predicting osteoporosis and fracture risks, in addition to bone mineral density measurements alone.

It remains to be shown how soon after treatment these collagen markers will change, although crosslink excretion has been shown characteristically to decrease after 6 months of treatment.

SKIN

The skin is one of the largest organs in the body, containing a sizeable proportion of total body collagen. This organ is composed of a population of cells of diverse embryonic origin that, under normal conditions, exist side by side in complete harmony, forming a complex mosaic.

Atrophy of the dermis after the menopause is due to a decrease in the dermal skin collagen content. The amounts of hydroxyproline and glycosylated hydroxylysine[16,17] in type I collagen and of immature and reducible crosslinks decrease with age[18]. To what extent these changes are fundamental to the aging process is still unknown. This decrease is not only arrested but reversed by hormone replacement therapy[19]. There is now strong evidence, as seen from the National Health and Nutrition Examination Survey[3], that estrogen use prevents dry skin and skin wrinkling, thus extending the potential benefits of postmenopausal estrogen therapy to include protection against selected age- and menopause-associated dermatological

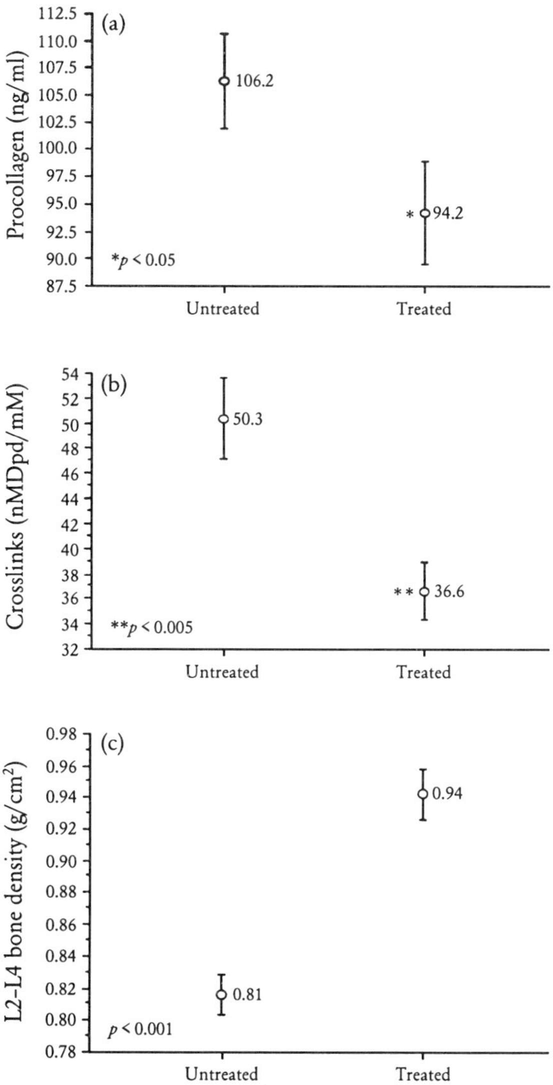

Figure 3 (a) Mean procollagen value in 92 untreated postmenopausal women and 68 postmenopausal women on hormone replacement therapy. An 11.3% difference in bone formation was seen in treated women compared with untreated women. (b) Mean value of pyridinium crosslinks in 129 untreated and 76 treated women. A 27.2% difference in bone resorption was seen in treated women compared with untreated women. (c) Mean bone density measured at the L2–L4 vertebrae in 140 untreated women and 83 treated women. A 16.1% difference in bone density was seen in treated women compared with untreated women

conditions. Estrogens have in fact been shown to enhance the dermal content of water, glycosaminoglycans (GAGs) and collagen. Both estrogen and androgen receptors have been identified on dermal fibroblasts[20].

Estrogen could increase the rate of collagen production[21] by altering the degree of polymerization of GAGs. Estrogens increase hydroscopic qualities[22], probably through the enhanced synthesis of dermal hyaluronic acid[23]. Collagenous fibrils were found to be less fragmented in the dermis of women treated with estrogens[24].

Studies have been carried out on skin changes in various connective-tissue and endocrine disorders. Black[25] and Shuster and colleagues[26] looked at the relationship between skin thickness and skin collagen in women with systemic sclerosis, osteoporosis of mixed etiology and hirsutism and found a good correlation between the two parameters. In a small study, Black[25] demonstrated changes in the collagen content and thickness of the skin in women with osteoporosis (mixed etiology) treated with androgens, when compared to women with osteoporosis who had not been on this treatment. Shuster and co-workers[26] found an increase in skin collagen in women with hirsutism, but the increase was not statistically significant. Reports on the skin collagen changes with age are conflicting. Shuster and Bottoms[27,28] showed that the best way of expressing skin collagen content was by measuring the collagen content of a skin biopsy of 1 mm^2 of skin surface. This method takes into account the possibility of changes in the total mass of the dermis. They reported a reduction in total skin collagen with age, but this was not confirmed by Reed and Hall[29]. Shuster and Black[30] found that the amount of collagen present in skin was at all ages higher in males than in females. Hall and associates[19] confirmed that skin collagen content was higher in males than in females but once again could not confirm a significant decline of skin collagen with age.

With increasing age past the menopause, the skin tends to get thinner and this is reversed with adequate estrogen replacement therapy[6]. This was first noted by Albright and co-workers[31] in 1940. They reported that old women with osteoporotic fractures had a higher incidence of thin skin. McConkey and colleagues[32] also showed that osteoporosis was more common in women with transparent skin than in women with thick opaque skin.

The dermal skin itself, composed as it is of connective tissue including the predominant protein collagen as well as elastin (small amounts) and GAGs, also has more than one variable that is affected by estrogen lack or its replacement. In work in the rat, for example[23], castrated rats that were given estrogens had a 70% increase in their GAG content in 2 weeks. Similar increases in women would lead to skin thickness increases that far outstrip what would be expected from collagen content increases alone.

Most of the studies have measured the thickness of the dermis, since this is the layer that is mainly composed of connective tissue. Subcutaneous tissue is an added variable. Studies using Harpenden's calipers, which also include subcutaneous fat, have been conflicting[33,34]. Ultrasound can be used to measure skin thickness. Ultrasound examination has been used by dermatologists when assessing dermal malignancies. Good reproducibility has been obtained by using high-frequency (22 MHz) ultrasound to determine the thickness of the skin, excluding the subcutaneous tissues. Various studies have now shown that skin thickness increases with estrogen replacement therapy. Skin changes and bone changes with estrogen at the menopause are linked[6,7].

In animals, estrogens appear to alter the vascularization of the skin[35] and a change in the connective tissue of the dermis occurs, as is reflected by increased mucopolysaccharide incorporation, hydroxyproline turnover and alterations in ground substance. In addition to the increased dermal turnover of hyaluronic acid, the dermal water content is enhanced with estradiol therapy[23]. Rauramo and Punnonen[36] observed that oral estrogen therapy in castrated women caused thickening of the epidermis for 3 months, and that this persisted for 6 months.

Punnonen[37], using two different strengths of estrogen in castrated women, showed a statistically significant thickening of the epidermis after 3 months with both strengths, but this thickness persisted only with the lower dose. A third of patients on the higher dose started showing significant thinning of the epidermis, possibly because the treatment was too strong, therefore exerting a corticosteroid effect. Other authors were also able to show beneficial skin changes, using both topical estradiol[7,38] and estradiol implants[6]. Topical estradiol gel has also been shown to increase skin collagen content, as measured by skin hydroxyproline content. Skin blister fluids were assayed and an increase of both procollagen I carboxyl terminal propeptide (PICP) and procollagen I N-terminal propeptide (PINP) characterized the gel.

In comparing a group of patients who had been treated with estradiol and testosterone implants from 2 to 10 years with a group of untreated postmenopausal women, it was shown that the treated group had a highly significantly greater skin collagen content than the untreated group. An optimum skin collagen level was obtained after 2 years of treatment with an optimum estrogen regimen. Levels that are too high or too low give lower levels of collagen[39]. The same conclusions were also reported in relation to the epidermis[40].

The decline in skin collagen content after the menopause occurs at a much more rapid rate in the initial postmenopausal years than in the later years. Some 30% of skin collagen is lost in the first 5 years after the menopause[39], with an average decline of 2.1% per postmenopausal year over a period of 20 years. The increase in skin collagen content after 6 months of sex hormone therapy depends on the collagen content at the start of treatment[39]. In women with a low skin collagen content, estrogens are initially of therapeutic and later of prophylactic value, while in those with mild loss of collagen content in the early menopausal years estrogens are of prophylactic value only. Therefore, a deficiency in skin collagen can be corrected but not overcorrected.

Skin collagen content has been shown to have a strong correlation with skin dermal thickness measured radiologically[39]. With the use of 100 mg subcutaneous estradiol implants, significant increases in skin thickness and metacarpal index occurred over a 1-year period. Most of the increase occurred in the first 6 months.

Brincat and Castelo-Branco and their colleagues[38,39,41,42] have shown that, following the menopause, skin collagen content and skin thickness are higher in women on estrogen replacement therapy compared to age-matched women on no treatment. Prospective studies have shown that skin thickness, skin collagen and bone mass increase in postmenopausal women who start estrogen replacement therapy. Estrogen has been shown to reduce collagen turnover and improve collagen quality[41,43]. When postmenopausal women were treated with topical estrogens[4] it was found that, after treatment for 6 months, the elasticity and firmness of the skin had markedly improved and the wrinkle depth and pore sizes had decreased by 61–100%. Furthermore, the skin moisture was also increased and the measurement of wrinkles, using skin profilometry, revealed significant, or even highly significant, decreases of wrinkles. On immunohistochemistry of the same subjects, significant increases of type III collagen labelling were combined with increased numbers of collagen fibers at the end of the treatment period. This was also confirmed by Creidi and colleagues in their study[44]. The mechanical properties of the skin have been shown to be improved with estrogen replacement therapy in other studies[45].

Brincat and co-workers[6,46,47] found significant correlations between the skin (dermal) collagen, skin thickness (measured radiologically) and metacarpal index, both in postmenopausal women who had been on estrogen replacement therapy and in untreated postmenopausal women. The common factor was the connective tissue present in all three sites. These findings were irrespective of the woman's age, number of years since the menopause, original skin thickness or metacarpal index.

Attempts to identify a value of skin thickness that could be used as a threshold in screening for menopausal osteoporosis have been under way for some time[48].

CAROTID ARTERIES

The cardioprotective effect of hormone replacement therapy has been proven over the years[49]. This has been attributed to the favorable serum lipoprotein profile brought about by this treatment in postmenopausal women[50]. Only 20–25% reduction in coronary artery plaque formation, however, can thus be accounted for[51]; other mechanisms of cardioprotection are therefore present. One such mechanism could be due to postmenopausal connective tissue changes that mimic those in skin and bone. Using high-frequency ultrasound, our group looked at the differences in the layers of one of the major blood vessels, the carotid artery. One study investigated differences in the externa, the media and the intima of the carotid artery in two groups of postmenopausal women on estrogen replacement therapy and an untreated group. The results showed that the media, the layer containing the greatest amount of collagen, was thicker in the estrogen-treated group than in the

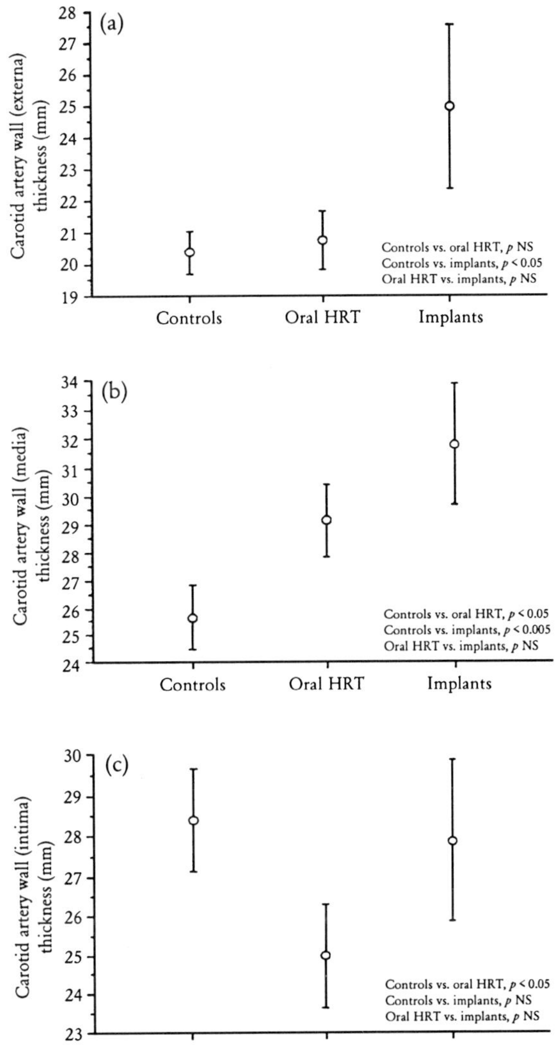

Figure 4 Mean ± SE of carotid artery wall externa (a), media (b) and intima (c) thickness in 51 untreated postmenopausal women as controls, 46 postmenopausal women on oral hormone replacement therapy (HRT) and 32 postmenopausal women on estradiol implants

untreated group. The intima of the untreated group was also shown to be significantly thicker than that of the treated group (Figure 4). This signifies that there was less atherosclerotic plaque in the treated than in the untreated group. However, in women on a higher dose of estrogen, such as in estradiol implants, the intima was as thick as in the untreated group. This was postulated as being due to the collagen portion of the intima following the media and increasing in size at the expense of thinning of the athersclerotic plaque[52,53]. It is postulated that these changes are brought about by estrogens. If these arterial changes induced by hormone replacement therapy also occur in the coronary arteries (and some suggestion of this has been made) then these may partially explain the cardioprotective effect this treatment has in postmenopausal women.

Early evidence suggests that selective estrogen receptor modulators (SERMs) do the same. Raloxifene has been shown to have the same effect on estrogen markers as estrogens.

CONCLUSION

Sex steroids play a vital role in the integrity of the connective tissues of an individual, and this constitutes yet another strong argument for long-term hormone (or SERMs) replacement therapy.

References

1. Murry RK, Keeley FW. The extracellular matrix. In Murray RK, Granner DK, Mayes PA, Rodwell VW, eds. *Harper's Biochemistry*, 24th edn. London: Appleton & Lange, 1996:667–85
2. Punnonen R, Vilska S, Rauramo L. Skinfold thickness and long-term post-menopausal hormone therapy. *Maturitas* 1984;5:259–62
3. Dunn LB, Damesyn M, Moore AA, Reuben DB, Greendale GA. Does estrogen prevent skin aging? Results from the First National Health and Nutrition Examination Survey (NHANESI). *Arch Dermatol* 1997;133:339–42
4. Schmidt JB, Binder M, Demschik G, Bieglmayer C, Reiner A. Treatment of skin aging with topical estrogens. *Int J Dermatol* 1996;35:669–74
5. The Writing Group for the PEPI trial. Effects of hormone therapy on bone mineral density: results from the postmenopausal estrogen/progestin interventions (PEPI) trial. *J Am Med Assoc* 1996;276: 1389–96
6. Brincat M, Moniz CF, Kabalan S, *et al.* Decline in skin collagen content and metacarpal index after the menopause and its prevention with sex hormone replacement. *Br J Obstet Gynaecol* 1987;94: 126–9
7. Brincat M, Kabalan S, Studd JWW, *et al.* A study of the relationship of skin collagen content, skin thickness and bone mass in the postmenopausal woman. *Obstet Gynecol* 1987;70:840–5
8. Gordan GS. Prevention of bone loss and fractures in women. *Maturitas* 1984;6:225–42
9. Brincat M, Galea R, Muscat Baron Y. Keynote Lecture, Italian Menopause Society, Rome, 1994
10. Väänänen HK, Härkönen PL. Estrogen and bone metabolism. *Maturitas* 1996;23(Suppl):S65–9
11. Schneider DL, Barrett Connor EL, Morton DJ. Timing of postmenopausal estrogen for optimal bone mineral density. The Rancho Bernardo Study. *J Am Med Assoc* 1997;277:543–7
12. Brincat M, Galea R, Muscat Baron Y, Xuereb A. Changes in bone collagen markers and in bone density in hormone treated and untreated postmenopausal women. *Maturitas* 1997;27:171–7
13. Ginty F, Flynn A, Cashman K. Inter and intraindividual variations in urinary excretion of pyridinium crosslinks of collagen in healthy young adults. *Eur J Clin Nutr* 1998;52:71–3
14. Suvanto Luukkonen E, Risteli L, Sundström H, Penttinen J, Kauppila A, Risteli J. Comparison of three serum assays for bone collagen formation during postmenopausal estrogen-progestin therapy. *Clin Chim Acta* 1997;266:105–16
15. Melton LJ 3rd, Khosla S, Atkinson EJ, O'Fallon WM, Riggs BL. Relationship of bone turnover to bone density and fractures. *J Bone Miner Res* 1997; 12:1083–91
16. Barnes MJ, Constable BJ, Morton LF, *et al.* Age-related variations in hydroxylation of lysine and proline on collagen. *Biochem J* 1974;139:461–8
17. Murai A, Miyahara T, Shiozawa S. Age-related variations in glycosylation of hydroxyproline in

human and rat skin collagens. *Biochim Biophys Acta* 1975;404:345–8

18. Risteli J, Kivirikko KI. Intracellular enzymes of collagen biosynthesis in rat liver as a function of age and in hepatic injury induced by dimethylnitrosamine: changes in prolyl hydroxylase, lysyl hydroxylase, collagen galactosyltransferase and collagen glucosyltransferase activities. *Biochem J* 1976;158:361–7
19. Hall DA, Reed FB, Noki G, Vince JD. The relative effects of age and corticosteroid therapy on the collagen profiles of dermis from subjects with rheumatoid arthritis. *Age Ageing* 1974;3:15–22
20. Stumpf WE, Sur M, Joshi SE. Estrogen target cells in the skin. *Experimentia* 1976;30:196
21. Boucek RJ, Noble NL, Woessner JF Jr. Properties of fibroblasts. In Page IH, ed. *Connective Tissue Thrombosis and Atherosclerosis.* New York: Academic Press, 1959:193–211
22. Danforth DN, Vies A, Breen M, Weinstein HG, Buckingham JC, Manalo P. The effect of pregnancy and labour on the human cervix: changes in collagen, glycoproteins and glucosaminoglycans. *Am J Obstet Gynecol* 1971;120:641–51
23. Grosman N, Hindberg E, Schen J. The effect of oestrogenic treatment on the acid mucopolysaccharide pattern in skin of mice. *Acta Pharmacol Toxicol* 1971;30:458–64
24. Goldzieher MA. The effects of oestrogens on the senile skin. *J Gerontol* 1946;1:196
25. Black MM. A modified radiographic method for measuring skin thickness. *Br J Dermatol* 1969;1:661
26. Shuster J, Black MM, McVitie E. The influence of age and sex on skin thickness, skin collagen and density. *Br J Dermatol* 1975;93:639
27. Shuster S, Bottoms E. Senile degeneration of skin collagen. *Clin Sci* 1963;25:487–91
28. Shuster S, Bottoms E. Effect of ultraviolet light on skin collagen. *Mature* 1963;199:192–3
29. Reed VB, Hall DA. In Frische R, Hartmann F, eds. *Connective Tissues - Biochemistry and Pathophysiology.* Berlin: Spinger Verlag, 1974:290
30. Shuster S, Black MM, Bottoms E. Skin collagen and thickness in women with hirsuties. *Br Med J* 1970;4: 738, 770
31. Albright F, Bloomberg E, Smith PH. Postmenopausal osteoprosis. *Trans Assoc Am Phys* 1940;55: 298–305
32. McConkey B, Fraser GR, Bligh AS, Whitely M. Transparent skin and osteoporosis. *Lancet* 1963;1: 693–5
33. Varila E, Rantala I, Ikarinem A, *et al.* The effect of topical oestriol on skin collagen of postmenopausal women. *Br J Obstet Gynaecol* 1995;102:985–9
34. Tan CY, Stratham B, Marks R, Payne PA. Skin thickness measurements by pulsed ultrasound: its reproducibility, validation and variability. *Br J Dermatol* 1994;96:1392–4
35. Goodrich SM, Wood JE. The effect of oestradiol 17β on peripheral venous distensibility and velocity of venous blood flow. *Am J Obstet Gynecol* 1966;96:407–12
36. Rauramo L, Punnonen R. Wirking einer oralen estrogentherapie mit oestriolsuccinat auf die haut hastierter. *Frauen Haut Gerchluts Kr* 1969;44:463–70
37. Punnonen R. Effect of castration and peroral therapy on skin. *Acta Obstet Gynecol Scand* 1973;21(Suppl):1–4
38. Brincat M, Moniz CJ, Studd JWW, *et al.* Long term effects of the menopause and sex hormones on skin thickness. *Br J Obstet Gynaecol* 1985;92:256–9
39. Brincat M, Moniz CF, Studd JWW, *et al.* Sex hormones and skin collagen content in postmenopausal women. *Br Med J* 1983;287:1337–8
40. Shahrad P, Marks RA. Pharmacological effect of oestrone on human epidermis. *Br J Dermatol* 1977;97:383–6
41. Castelo-Barcia C, Pons F, Gratacos E, Fortuny A, Panrell JA, Gonzalez Merlo J. Relationship between skin collagen and bone changes during ageing. *Maturitas* 1994;18:199–206
42. Castelo-Branco C, Duran M, Gonzalez-Merlo J. Skin collagen changes related to age and hormone replacement therapy. *Maturitas* 1992;15:113–19
43. Holland EFN, Studd JWW, Mansell JP, Leather AT, Bailey AJ. Changes in collagen composition and cross-links in bone and skin of osteoporotic postmenopausal women treated with percutaneous estradiol implants. *Obstet Gynecol* 1994;83:180–3
44. Creidi P, Faivre B, Agache P, Richard E, Haudiquet V, Sauvanet JP. Effect of a conjugated oestrogen (Premarin) cream on ageing facial skin. A comparative study with a placebo cream. *Maturitas* 1994;19: 211–23
45. Pierard GE, Letawe L, Dowlati A, Pierard-Franchimant L. Effect of hormone replacement therapy for menopause on the mechanical properties of skin. *J Am Soc* 1995;43:662–4
46. Brincat M, Studd JWW, Moniz CF, Parsons V, Darby AJ. Skin thickness and skin collagen mimic an index of osteoporosis in the postmenopausal woman. In Christiansen C, *et al.*, eds. *Osteoporosis,* vol 1. *Proceedings of the Copenhagen International Symposium on Osteoporosis,* 1984:353–5
47. Brincat M, Studd JWW, Moniz CF, Parsons V, Darby AJ. Skin thickness measurement. A simple screening method for determining patients at risk of postmenopausal osteoporosis. In Christiansen C, *et al.*, eds. *Osteoporosis,* vol 1. *Proceedings of the Copenhagen International Symposium on Osteoporosis,* 1984:323–6
48. Brincat M, Galea R, Muscat Baron Y. A screening model for osteoporosis using dermal skin thickness and bone densitometry. In Wren BG, ed. *Progress in Management of the Menopause.* Carnforth, UK: Parthenon Publishing, 1997:175–8

49. Stampfer MJ, Colditz GA, Willem WC, *et al.* Postmenopausal oestrogen therapy and cardiovascular disease. Ten year follow-up from The Nurses' Health Study. *N Engl J Med* 1991;325:756–62
50. PEPI Trial Writing Group. Effects of estrogen and estrogen/progesterone regimens on heart disease risk factors in postmenopausal women. The Postmenopausal Estrogen/Progestogen Intervention (PEPI) trial. *J Am Med Assoc* 1995;273:199–208
51. Adams MR, Kaplan JR, Mauck SB. Inhibition of coronary artery atherosclerosis by 17β-estradiol in ovariectomised monkeys: lack of an effect of added progesterone. *Atherosclerosis* 1990;10:1051–7
52. Muscat Baron Y, Brincat M, Galea R. Carotid artery wall thickness in women treated with hormone replacement therapy. *Maturitas* 1997;27:47–53
53. Muscat Baron Y, Galea R, Brincat M. Carotid artery wall changes in estrogen treated and untreated postmenopausal women. *Obstet Gynecol* 1998;91: 982–6

Estrogen regulates lymphopoiesis 25

P. W. Kincade, K. L. Medina, K. J. Payne, K.-S. Tudor, M. I. Rossi and T. Kouro

INTRODUCTION

Sex steroids are known to influence many biological systems and a serendipitous observation allowed us to implicate them in a vital process known as B lymphopoiesis. This term refers to the daily production of hundreds of billions of B lymphocytes within the bone marrow. B cells represent the antibody-forming arm of the immune system and, while many of them have extremely long lifespans, most of the newly formed lymphocytes survive for only a few days. We found that pregnancy and elevated sex steroids shut down this process in mice, while it increased with hormone deficiency. Most of our subsequent studies focused on the molecular and cellular mechanisms behind these responses. The experiments revealed significant gaps in our basic understanding of how B cells are made, and especially with respect to very early events. Progress in that area is now providing an improved differentiation model and an appreciation of critical, hormone-sensitive stages. Humans are exposed to many sex steroids and related compounds, in addition to the endogenous hormones that fluctuate with age. It is therefore essential to learn if development of the humoral immune system in man is influenced by these compounds. We have been developing procedures for exploring this important question and recently found that B-lymphocyte production is depressed in pregnant women. This important observation can now be expanded to include studies of normal aging, hormone replacement and other types of endocrine therapy.

THE INITIAL DISCOVERY

Bone marrow represents a highly specialized blood-cell factory and, in adults, new B cells are exclusively produced in that site. For some years, our laboratory has been identifying molecules within the bone marrow that contribute to the lymphopoietic microenvironment. For example, we determined that the vascular cell adhesive molecule (VCAM)-1 present on stromal cells was recognized by the very late activation (VLA)-4 integrin expressed by lymphocyte precursors, accounting for physical interactions between these two cell types[1]. B-cell precursors derive signals for their survival, proliferation and differentiation from stromal cells. Indeed, they quickly die when separated from their supportive influence[2]. A complicated series of experiments was designed to assess the importance of these two cell adhesion molecules in the formation of bone marrow during embryonic life. The emphasis of our studies suddenly shifted when we found that there were very few B-cell precursors within the marrow of pregnant mice.

Subsequent experiments established that B lymphopoiesis progressively declined during pregnancy and that the rate of recovery postpartum was influenced by lactation[3]. We suspected that hormonal fluctuations might be linked to the events within the bone marrow, but acknowledged that it would be impossible to experimentally simulate pregnancy. Pre-B-cell numbers selectively declined when mice were treated with either of three forms of estrogen and, while progesterone was without influence when used alone, it augmented the responsiveness to estrogen[4].

SEX STEROIDS AS STEADY-STATE REGULATORS

While these observations were interesting within the context of pregnancy and hormone therapy, there is reason to believe that sex steroids control the daily output of new lymphocytes from the bone marrow. Castration is known to increase the size of the thymus, an organ responsible for the production of the other major class of lymphocytes, T cells. We and others found that castration increased pre-B-cell numbers within the marrow of mice. The same situation was found in hypogonadal mice that were unable to produce sex steroids, and pre-B-cell numbers returned to normal when these mutant animals were given estrogen[5]. Testosterone may also be involved in the steady-state regulation of bone marrow, because B lymphopoiesis was augmented in androgen receptor-deficient Tfm mice[6]. Thus, the production of new B cells increases as systemic levels of sex steroids fall below normal and, reciprocally, decreases when hormone levels are high.

AN IMPROVED DIFFERENTIATION MODEL

Rare multipotential hematopoietic stem cells represent the source of all blood cells, and their immediate progeny are usually referred to as 'progenitors'. 'Committed progenitors' are cells that can proliferate substantially and give rise to mature cells of one or, at best, a few lineages. Multicolor flow cytometry and other procedures that exploit cell surface properties have been extensively used to identify and isolate stem cells and committed progenitors. As progenitors become more specialized, there is selective expression of genes and markers that typify a particular lineage. For example, transcripts for globin genes are only present in erythroid cells, and immunoglobulin genes are selectively expressed in B-lineage cells. Combinations of receptors displayed on the cell surface also change in accordance with lineage commitment and maturation. In principle, a 'family tree' can be constructed, showing the properties of cells at each stage in the various pathways of blood-cell formation.

We injected mice with estrogen and monitored many changes in populations of B-cell precursors, but the results were confusing when considered within the context of popular differentiation models. For example, cells that were supposed to represent a given stage in the pathway increased in number, while cells thought to precede or follow that step declined. In addition, we documented the accumulation of cells in the marrow of estrogen-treated mice that had very unusual characteristics[7]. This difficulty inspired attempts to use new combinations of monoclonal antibodies and procedures to resolve early differentiation steps. The resulting model provides a much better basis for documenting estrogen-induced changes and suggests that the hormone regulates critical early events. For example, we found that most early 'pro-B' cells in the bone marrow express the α-chain of the interleukin-7 receptor, a moderate level of the c-kit transmembrane tyrosine kinase-type receptor and the nuclear terminal deoxynucleotidyl transferase (TdT) enzyme[8,9]. They can be further distinguished from more differentiated precursors by the absence of markers associated with erythroid, myeloid and lymphoid blood-cell lineages. Cells with these properties decline within the marrow of estrogen-treated animals (Medina and colleagues, manuscript in preparation). This work is helping to identify key hormone-sensitive control points within the bone marrow of mice and parallel attempts to resolve analogous populations of blood-cell precursors within humans.

POTENTIAL MECHANISMS AND TARGET TISSUES

Other investigators demonstrated functional androgen and estrogen receptors in stromal cells, so this component of bone marrow represents one potential target for estrogen action[10]. Estrogen slowed the production of lymphocytes in co-cultures established with lymphocyte precursors and stromal cells, but had little influence when added directly to cytokine-dependent pre-B cells[11]. There also appeared to be inhibitory substances in the conditioned medium of estrogen-pulsed stromal cells. More recent culture experiments have involved much earlier lymphocyte precursors, because of the findings in estrogen-treated mice. It still seems that stromal cells must be present to observe the whole spectrum of estrogen-induced changes. However, some of them take place when highly purified precursors are cultured with recombinant cytokines rather than stromal cells. Thus, our tentative conclusions are that estrogen causes stromal cells to produce some substance(s) that suppresses B lymphopoiesis. However, lymphocyte precursors also represent direct targets of hormone action and it will be important to identify genes for transcription factors or other critical molecules that are estrogen-regulated.

AGE-RELATED CHANGES IN BONE MARROW AND THYMUS

The thymus decreases in size with age and, until recently, was thought to be non-functional in adult humans. However, it has been found that the organ not only retains the ability to make T lymphocytes, but probably does so to some degree in aged individuals[12]. Similarly, the marrow from 90-year-old humans contains B-cell precursors and our unpublished observations suggest they are actively proliferating[13,14] (also Rossi and colleagues, manuscript in preparation). The proportion of fat within the marrow changes as a function of age, such that it is difficult to calculate absolute values for an individual and determine what is typical for a given age. It would be extremely useful to have procedures for determining how many newly formed B cells leave the bone marrow and we have now devised such an assay for human peripheral blood (Medina and colleagues, manuscript in preparation). Interestingly, absolute numbers of such immature cells decline 70% during pregnancy. This key observation will inspire considerable effort to learn the extent to which the process is sex steroid-dependent.

IMPLICATIONS FOR NORMAL AGING AND HORMONE USE

Rodent studies suggest that the size and activity of lymphopoietic tissues decline with age[15]. Until recently, there were no procedures for determining normal values for humans, so we have little idea of sex differences or how these processes change during puberty and the menopause. Such baseline values might be extremely useful indicators of the side-effects of hormone replacement and cancer chemotherapy.

Mature lymphocytes that have previously participated in immune responses have the ability to survive and proliferate extensively in many parts of the body. As long as such 'memory' cells represent a large number of antibody specificities, the immune system remains effective. However, antibody responses become progressively restricted and less protective with age[16], and newly formed B cells from the bone marrow may make a significant contribution. Again, it is important to devise procedures for evaluating the activity of the marrow in humans.

Recent animal studies suggest there could be some interesting relationships between pre-B-cell numbers within the bone marrow and bone density[17,18]. Forced expansion of pre-B cells effectively causes osteoclastosis and it is now known that osteoprotegerin, an important stimulus for osteoclast differentiation, is expressed by lymphocytes. Therefore, information obtained about the formation of the humoral immune system may have implications for understanding bone physiology. Estrogen, tamoxifen and recently developed selective estrogen receptor modifiers (SERMs) could influence bone density in part via their effects on B lymphopoiesis.

There are many other important questions regarding the normal events that occur within the bone marrow. For example, most of our experiments with mice involve the manipulation of systemic hormone levels and there is no information available about concentrations of sex steroids within the marrow. The brain and thymus represent other important organs that are markedly influenced by steroids and responsive to circulating hormone levels. It is becoming clear that those tissues have the capacity to locally synthesize, and possibly also to degrade, steroid hormones[19,20]. Animal models will continue to be valuable as we explore these fundamental issues.

ACKNOWLEDGEMENTS

Our studies are supported by Grants AI-20069 and AI-33085 from the National Institutes of Health. P.W.K. holds the William H. and Rita Bell Chair in biomedical research.

References

1. Miyake K, Medina K, Ishihara K, *et al.* A VCAM-like adhesion molecule on murine bone marrow stromal cells mediates binding of lymphocyte precursors in culture. *J Cell Biol* 1991;114:557-65
2. Borghesi LA, Smithson G, Kincade PW. Stromal cell modulation of negative regulatory signals that influence apoptosis and proliferation of B lineage lymphocytes. *J Immunol* 1997;159:4171-9
3. Medina KL, Smithson G, Kincade PW. Suppression of B lymphopoiesis during normal pregnancy. *J Exp Med* 1993;178:1507-15
4. Medina KL, Kincade PW. Pregnancy-related steroids are potential negative regulators of B lymphopoiesis. *Proc Natl Acad Sci USA* 1994;91: 5382-6
5. Smithson G, Beamer WG, Shultz, *et al.* Increased B lymphopoiesis in genetically sex steroid-deficient hypogonadal (*hpg*) mice. *J Exp Med* 1994;180:717-20
6. Smithson G, Couse JF, Lubahn DB, *et al.* The role of estrogen receptors and androgen receptors in sex steroid regulation of B lymphopoiesis. *J Immunol* 1998;161:27-34
7. Medina KL, Strasser A, Kincade PW. Estrogen influences the differentiation, proliferation and survival of early B lineage precursors. Submitted 1999
8. Payne KJ, Medina KL, Kincade PW. Loss of c-kit accompanies B-lineage commitment and acquisition of CD45R by most murine B-lymphocyte precursors. *Blood* 1999;94:1-12
9. Tudor K-S RS, Payne KJ, Yamashita Y, *et al.* Functional assessment of precursors from murine bone marrow suggests a sequence of early B-lineage differentiation events. Submitted 1999
10. Bellido T, Girasole G, Passeri G, *et al.* Demonstration of estrogen and vitamin D receptors in bone marrow-derived stromal cells: up-regulation of the estrogen receptor by 1,25-dihydroxyvitamin-D_3. *Endocrinology* 1993;133:553-62
11. Smithson G, Medina K, Ponting I, *et al.* Estrogen suppresses stromal cell-dependent lymphopoiesis in culture. *J Immunol* 1995;155:3409-17
12. Jamieson BD, Douek DC, Killian S, *et al.* Generation of functional thymocytes in the human adult. *Immunity* 1999;10:569-75
13. Ghia P, Ten Boekel E, Sanz E, *et al.* Ordering of human bone marrow B lymphocyte precursors by single-cell polymerase chain reaction analyses of the rearrangement status of the immunoglobulin H and L chain gene loci. *J Exp Med* 1996;184: 2217-29
14. Nunez C, Nishimoto N, Gartland GL, *et al.* B cells are generated throughout life in humans. *J Immunol* 1996;156:866-72
15. Kline GH, Hayden TA, Klinman NR. B cell maintenance in aged mice reflects both increased B cell longevity and decreased B cell generation. *J Immunol* 1999;162:3342-9
16. Song H, Price PW, Cerny J. Age-related changes in antibody repertoire: contribution from T cells. *Immunol Rev* 1997;160:55-62
17. Miyaura C, Onoe Y, Inada M, *et al.* Increased B-lymphopoiesis by interleukin 7 induces bone loss in mice with intact ovarian function: similarity to estrogen deficiency. *Proc Natl Acad Sci USA* 1997; 94:9360-5
18. Burgess TL, Qian YX, Kaufman S, *et al.* The ligand for osteoprotegerin (OPGL) directly activates mature osteoclasts. *J Cell Biol* 1999;145:527-38
19. Mellon SH, Deschepper CF. Neurosteroid biosynthesis: genes for adrenal steroidogenic enzymes are expressed in the brain. *Brain Res* 1993;629: 283-92
20. Vacchio MS, Papadopoulos V, Ashwell JD. Steroid production in the thymus: implications for thymocyte selection. *J Exp Med* 1994;179:1835-46

Eye and ear as target organs for sex hormones 26

M. O. Sator and J. C. Huber

At the end of the 19th century, Eugen Steinach observed changes in the skin, hair, nails and even eyes of hormonally treated rats[1]. These changes led to the first description of a hormonal impact on the so-called extragenital target organs. Regarding the problem of the climacteric syndrome, some typical symptoms include hot flushes and sleep disturbances, but there are also a number of complaints which are not ascribed to the climacteric syndrome but which nevertheless respond well to hormonal treatment.

More recently, gynecological endocrinologists have found connections between sex hormones and eye problems in females, especially in the postmenopause, such as dry eyes and high intraocular pressure[2,3]. Keratoconjunctivitis sicca is a common disease in postmenopausal women, affecting them significantly more often than men of the same age group[4]. Also, the incidence of primary open-angle glaucoma is much higher in men than in women under 50 years of age[5]. These differences between the sexes become less pronounced after this age, which leads to the idea of a relationship between the occurrence of intraocular pressure and keratoconjunctivitis sicca, and a reduction of estrogen and progestin in postmenopausal women.

KERATOCONJUNCTIVITIS SICCA

Keratoconjunctivitis sicca manifests itself mainly through a feeling of dryness and foreign-body sensation in the conjunctival region. One possible reason for its occurrence is the reduction in endogenous estrogen during the menopause. It has already been shown that the eye is a locus of action of female sex hormones[6]. To date, therapy for keratoconjunctivitis sicca has mainly focused on the local application of tear substitutes and vitamin A preparations[7].

However, these therapeutic approaches do not produce substantial benefit as they treat only the symptom of the eye feeling dry. The importance of sex steroids for the integrity of the conjunctiva has previously been shown[8]. Therapeutic methods should concentrate on the preservation or restoration of cell integrity rather than on a mere substitution of tear fluid. To investigate the effect of 17β-estradiol ophthalmic drops in comparison with a traditional tear substitute in postmenopausal women with keratoconjunctivitis sicca, a randomized prospective trial was carried out on 84 postmenopausal women suffering from keratoconjunctivitis sicca and needing hormone replacement therapy (HRT) general climacteric symptoms[9]. The women were randomized into two groups and were given 17β-estradiol eye drops ($n = 42$, group 1) or a tear substitute ($n = 42$, group 2). Both groups received systemic HRT. A Schirmer test was performed immediately before the start of therapy and after 4 months. In addition, eye symptoms were assessed using a visual analog scale.

All 84 women were given systemic estrogen-gestagen replacement therapy to treat their climacteric symptoms: estradiol valerate 2 mg daily and medrogeston 5 mg for 10 days every month. The women were randomly assigned to one of the following two treatments: group 1, estrogen eye drops (0.005 mg of 17β-estradiol in 20 ml diluent); group 2, a tear substitute. One drop was instilled in each eye every 6 h for 4 months. Simple randomization was performed by the pharmacy using sealed envelopes. Medication was distributed by the pharmacy.

A comparison of visual analog scores at 4 months in the women who received 17β-estradiol eye drops versus those who received a tear substitute demonstrated a statistically significant difference in all observed ocular symptoms ($p < 0.0001$). The Schirmer test revealed a significant difference in results before and after treatment in the estradiol group ($p < 0.001$), while in group 2 no significant difference was found.

This randomized trial demonstrated that topical estrogen therapy is beneficial in the treatment of postmenopausal keratoconjunctivitis sicca. The fact that there is an increasing incidence of keratoconjunctivitis sicca in women during the menopause, compared with a lower incidence in men, suggests an endocrine origin of this complex ocular disease. The normal functioning of the eye is dependent on blinking, on the secretion of lacrimal fluid and on the integrity of the goblet cells of the conjunctiva. A diffuse fibrosis and atrophy of the lacrimal ducts, often found during the menopause, may also contribute to the development of keratoconjunctivitis sicca[10]. The action of estradiol could be explained by a stimulation of nitric oxide synthase and its vasodilatory effect, which may act not only on blood vessels but also on the lacrimal ducts. One interesting finding of the above randomized trial was that little improvement in eye symptoms occurred in the tear substitute group, despite systemic HRT. All the women who received additional topical estrogen reported a subjective improvement or complete remission of symptoms. This suggests the presence of a blood–eye barrier which prevents systemic estrogen from acting on the conjunctivae and lacrimal ducts. The study demonstrates that topical estrogen is successful in treating keratoconjunctivitis sicca.

INTRAOCULAR PRESSURE

Visual acuity usually deteriorates with age. Sometimes this is the result of glaucoma. There are several types of glaucoma, but all involve a build-up of pressure from fluid in the eye; this pressure can damage the optic nerve. The most common form is chronic simple glaucoma, which is responsible for the majority of cases. Early glaucoma is not painful, so it is important for people over the age of 40 to have their eye pressure checked every year.

A number of studies exist that indicate an association between intraocular pressure (IOP) and female sex hormones, or a deficiency of some of these hormones[11]. A gender-based comparison of patients with IOP of more than 22 mmHg found that an increase in pressure is more frequent in women than in men. As an increased IOP is usually first observed when a refraction necessitating a patient's first pair of reading glasses is determined at an age when menopausal symptoms tend to occur, this suggests a connection between a decrease in serum levels of sex steroids and changes in IOP. Investigators have reported changes in IOP during the menstrual cycle, and the successful use of C-18 and C-21 steroids in glaucoma patients, suggesting a possible relationship between IOP and sex steroids[12]. These findings were the rationale for the following study, the purpose of which was to show the impact of natural hormone preparations on IOP in menopausal women.

Little information is available about the effect of HRT on IOP. A prospective clinical study was performed to evaluate the influence of HRT on IOP in menopausal women with a normal ophthalmological history, to obtain a basis for further clinical studies on glaucoma patients[13]. IOP fluctuations were recorded before and 1, 4 and 12 weeks after the start of HRT. These measurements were obtained according to a standardized time schedule. The mean IOP in the left eye decreased from 16.2 ± 2.4 mmHg before therapy to 14.0 ± 2.1 mmHg after 12 weeks of therapy ($p < 0.001$). In the right eye, with a mean IOP of 15.3 ± 2.3 mmHg before therapy, there was a decrease to 14.0 ± 1.9 mmHg after 12 weeks of therapy ($p < 0.001$).

Intraocular pressure is maintained as the result of a balance between the secretion of aqueous humor by the ciliary processes and the reabsorption or outflow of aqueous humor through the trabecular meshwork, into Schlemm's canal, and then through collecting channels to scleral veins. The cells that line the connective tissue trabeculae of the meshwork have long been considered to play a merely passive role in the drainage process and the valve action of the outflow system. Furthermore, it has been shown that meshwork cells have many characteristics in common with smooth muscle cells, and that they contract in the presence of cholinergic agonists but relax with nitric oxide agonists[14]. Nitric oxide is an important intracellular and intercellular regulator in vascular endothelium, smooth muscle cells and certain other cell types. The endothelium in ophthalmological vessels influences local vascular tone by releasing nitric oxide. It is worth noting that Nathanson and McKee have shown that the human outflow system and ciliary muscle are important sites of nitric oxide synthesis[15]. Nitric oxide activity is associated with endothelial nitric oxide synthase located at the meshwork tissue, responsible for regulation of ocular outflow and intraocular pressure. As a consequence of the action of estradiol, there is an increase of the endothelium-based constitutive nitric oxide synthetase. Nitric oxide and estrogen have been shown to play a critical role in the control of intraocular pressure and outflow facility, and results suggest that nitric oxide synthase activity can be positively regulated and influenced by estradiol[16].

As already discussed above, the incidence of increasing intraocular pressure among females rises after the menopause. This rise in incidence is possibly due to a hormonal imbalance brought about by a deficiency of certain hormones such as 17β-estradiol and progesterone. The above results may give a new direction to the treatment of intraocular pressure[13].

AUDITORY BRAINSTEM RESPONSE

A symptom that is given too little attention in menopausal practice is related to changes in the field of auditory perception. A woman's auditory capacity is subject to cyclical fluctuations which can be measured by brainstem audiometry. Since its description by Jewett and Williston in 1971, auditory brainstem response has achieved a prominent role in the fields of audiology and neurology, and has become an important objective measure of hearing[17]. Auditory brainstem response represents the aggregate responses of many neurons from lower portions of the auditory pathway. The physiological process of hearing is based on numerous changes in the bioelectrical potentials in the cochlea, acoustic nerve and central nervous system that can be used objectively to assess auditory function. Clinically, these changes can be registered by electrodes placed on the scalp. The properties and shapes of these waves depend essentially on how long after the instant of stimulation they occur. Brainstem audiometry has been used to measure the cyclical variations in women's auditory capacity. No such fluctuation of auditory capacity was found to occur in men[18]. Menopausal women undergoing cyclical estrogen therapy show changes of the acoustically evoked potentials[19].

Twenty-four postmenopausal women were recruited according to the following criteria: aged between 50 and 65 years; amenorrheic for more than 1 year; not to have received any systemic or local HRT for the past 2 years[13]. Exclusion criteria were hearing loss or any significant medical problem. All subjects had behavior hearing thresholds from 20 dB hearing loss or better at octave interval frequencies from 250 to 8000 Hz. Twelve women each were randomly allocated to receive either oral tibolone therapy or placebo. Otological examinations included otoscopy, pure-tone audiogram and tympanometry. Assessments were performed before and 12 weeks after the start of therapy.

When the auditory brainstem response (ABR) latency data of the women treated with tibolone were compared with those of women taking placebo, there was a significant trend of shortened ABR latencies (waves II, III, V; $p < 0.05$) in the tibolone group. In contrast, the latencies of wave I and wave IV remained unchanged. Moreover, some investigators have reported different degrees of age dependence of ABR latencies in females[20]. As far as the present authors are aware, the above is the first prospective randomized study to investigate the effect of tibolone, an alternative to other standard HRT regimens. The findings in the tibolone group suggest the activation of a brainstem auditory neural pathway through tibolone during replacement therapy.

In conclusion, the above findings suggest that tibolone has a positive effect on ABR latencies in postmenopausal women. The improvement in auditory function after tibolone treatment may be mediated by γ-aminobutyric acid (GABA)-ergic neurons in the auditory pathway[21]. Replacement therapy with tibolone may open up the possibility of new therapeutic strategies for otological disorders.

The University Hospital of Vienna has been one of the forerunners in this area and it is fascinating to see the development of the topics discussed in this paper.

References

1. Leydhecker H. Der intraokuläre Druck menschlicher Augen. *Klin Monatsbl Augenheilkd* 1958;48:4–7
2. Gharagozloo NZ, Brubaker RF. The correlation between serum progesterone and aqueous dynamics during the menstrual cycle. *Acta Ophthalmol* 1991;69:791–5
3. Sano Y. Sexual cycle and intraocular pressure in women. *Acta Soc Ophthalmol Jpn* 1973;57:892–4
4. Metka M, Enzelsberger H, Knogler W, *et al.* Ophthalmic complaints as a climacteric symptom. *Maturitas* 1991;14:3–8
5. Avasthi P, Luthra MC. Effect of sex hormones on intraocular pressure. *Int Surg* 1967;48:4–7
6. Kramer P, Lubkin V, Potter W, *et al.* Cyclic changes in conjunctival smears from menstruating females. *Ophthalmology* 1990;97:303–7
7. Maumenee A, Stark WJ, Maumenee IH, *et al.* Topical retinoid treatment for various dry eye disorders. *Ophthalmology* 1989;96:730–3
8. Liotet S, Van-Bijsterveld OP, Kogbe O, *et al.* A new hypothesis on tear film stability. *Ophthalmologica* 1987;195:119–24
9. Sator M, Joura E, Golaszewski Th, *et al.* Treatment of menopausal keratoconjunctivitis sicca with topical oestradiol. *Br J Obstet Gynaecol* 1998;105:100–2
10. Gilbart JP, Rossi SR, Heyda KG, *et al.* Stimulation of tear secretion by topical agents that increase cyclic nucleotide levels. *Invest Ophthalmol Vis Sci* 1990;3:1381–8
11. Imre J. Die regulatorische Wirkung der endokrinen Drüsen auf den intraokulären Druck. *Arch Augenheilkd* 1921;88:155–7
12. Green K, Cullen PM, Phillips CI. Aqueous humor turnover and intraocular pressure during menstruation. *Br J Ophthalmol* 1984;68:736–40
13. Sator M, Joura E, Frigo P, *et al.* Hormone replacement therapy and intraocular pressure. *Maturitas* 1997;28:55–8
14. Lepple-Weinhues A, Stahl F, Wiederholt M. Differential smooth muscle-like contractile properties of trabecular meshwork and ciliary muscle. *Exp Eye Res* 1991;53:33–8
15. Nathanson JA, McKee M. Alterations of ocular nitric oxide synthase in human glaucoma. *Invest Ophthalmol Vis Sci* 1995;36:1774–84
16. Nathanson JA, McKee M. Identification of an extensive system of nitric oxide-producing cells in the ciliary muscle and outflow pathway of the human eye. *Invest Ophthalmol Vis Sci* 1995;36:1765–72
17. Jewett DL, Williston JS. Auditory-evoked far fields averaged from the scalp of humans. *Brain* 1971; 94:681–96
18. Fagan PL, Church GT. Effect of the menstrual cycle on auditory brainstem response. *Audiology* 1986;25: 321–8
19. Strachan D. Sudden sensorineural deafness and hormone replacement therapy. *J Laryngol Otol* 1996;110:1148–50
20. Elkind-Hirsch KE, Stoner WR, Stach BA, *et al.* Estrogen influences auditory brainstem responses during the normal menstrual cycle. *Hear Res* 1992;60:143–8
21. Perez J, Zucchi I, Maggi A. Sexual dimorphism in the response of the GABAergic system to estrogen administration. *J Neurochem* 1986;47:1798–803

The management of menopausal symptoms after breast cancer

27

J. A. Eden

Breast cancer is the most common malignancy affecting non-smoking women and, with the advent of screening mammography, the disease is frequently detected at a very early stage where the likelihood of cure is extremely high. Thus, many women will survive breast cancer, and so face some of the problems that the menopause presents such as symptoms including hot flushes, aches and pains, irritability and vaginal dryness, as well as the long-term consequences of estrogen deficiency, in particular osteoporosis. However, an added problem is that some breast cancer treatments such as tamoxifen can greatly aggravate menopausal symptoms. Chemotherapy is increasingly being used to treat premenopausal women with breast cancer, and this may induce the menopause and its associated unpleasant symptoms. Women who have had breast cancer are usually told to avoid estrogen for fear of stimulating the growth of their tumor. Also, these women often try unproven herbal therapies, assuming that they are safe and effective.

Table 1 The case against estrogen replacement in women with a history of breast cancer

Breast cancer is much more common among women than among men
Estrogen stimulates the growth of some breast cancer cell lines in culture
Estrogen stimulates proliferation of breast ductal tissue
Breast cancer risk relates to reproductive markers, i.e. age at menarche, first pregnancy and menopause
Premature menopause reduces the risk of breast cancer development and bilateral oophorectomy is an effective palliative therapy for advanced breast cancer

BIOLOGY OF ESTROGEN AND BREAST CANCER

The case against estrogen is summarized in Table 1[1]. Briefly, there is strong evidence that estrogen is a promoter of breast cancer and little evidence to support the contention that estrogen is a carcinogen. Estrogen increases the rate of mitotic division in breast cancer, and it is during cell division that cells are most vulnerable to carcinogens. Breast tissue levels of estradiol are about 20 times higher than serum levels, and this gradient is maintained both before and after the menopause[2]. There is now considerable evidence that the breast is an endocrine organ; in other words, the breast not only reacts to hormones but also synthesizes them. Pasqualini and Nguyen[3] have shown that the sulfatase–sulfakinase enzyme pathway is around 500 times more active in the breast than the aromatase pathway. Estrone sulfate is converted by the breast into estrone, which is further converted by dehydrogenase into estradiol. This local production of estrogens appears to be far more important than the small amount of estradiol taken up from the circulation. Some locally produced estrogens such as the catecholestrogens appear to be particularly harmful, in that some of these compounds can bind irreversibly to the estrogen receptor and permanently activate it[4].

The effect of progesterone and progestogens on the breast appears to be even more complex and seems to depend upon the type, dosage and duration of the progestogen used. Clarke and Sutherland[5] and Musgrove and colleagues[6] have shown that most progestogens do not directly stimulate resting breast cells to proliferate. Rather, cells that are already entering a cell cycle appear to be 'hurried' through that cell cycle and then have their growth arrested early in the next G_1 phase. A modest increase in mitotic activity is seen over the first 24 h in cell culture, followed by profound and continued inhibition of mitotic activity.

HERBALS FOR MENOPAUSAL SYMPTOMS

Many women use herbal supplements in the hope that these will relieve menopausal symptoms. Randomized trials are few, and typically demonstrate a 30% placebo effect over 12 weeks. However, a number of herbals have been put to randomized trial which have given negative results; these include dong quai[7], evening primrose oil[8], wild yam cream[9] and red clover extract[10,11]. There are two dietary studies using soya which show a 50-60% effect over 12 weeks with a placebo effect of 25-30%[12,13]. Certainly, avoiding known aggravators such as overheating, spicy food, alcohol and hot drinks, and stress reduction can be very helpful in reducing the intensity of menopausal flushing.

PROGESTOGENS FOR MENOPAUSAL SYMPTOMS

Moderate doses of progestins (for example medroxyprogesterone acetate in doses of 20-100 mg per day or norethisterone 5-10 mg per day) have been shown to be effective treatments for hot flushes in double-blind controlled trials[14,15]. As high-dose progestins are often used to treat breast cancer, many oncologists try this approach first. Tamoxifen induced flushing can usually be helped by either temporarily stopping the drug or reducing the dose from 20 mg down to 10 mg or even 5 mg daily.

In a small group of patients, all the above measures fail, and consideration should be given to using hormone replacement therapy (HRT).

STUDIES ON HRT AFTER BREAST CANCER

All the published studies to date on this subject are cohort or case-controlled studies, and generally fairly small in numbers. Our group has published regularly in this area, including a recently updated report[16]. The study group comprises 1472 women with invasive breast cancer. A total of 167 had used oral or transdermal estrogen after their treatment for breast cancer. Among these estrogen users, 152 (91%) had also used a moderate dose of progestin. Cox regression analysis was performed, using estrogen as a time-dependent covariate with disease-free interval as the outcome. The hazard ratio for the estrogen-progestin users was 0.67 (95% confidence interval 0.38-1.16). These results are encouraging, but of course this type of study has all the flaws of a non-randomized trial. Several randomized trials of hormone replacement after breast cancer are now under way around the world. Not surprisingly, all of these studies are having difficulty with recruitment.

CONCLUSION

Women who have had breast cancer should avoid estrogen therapy unless their quality of life is so diminished by menopausal symptoms that the only option left is estrogen replacement. This should be a very small group of women, for most menopausal symptoms disappear with time; life-style changes such as the reduction of stress and the avoidance of trigger factors can greatly attenuate the severity of menopausal flushes.

A moderate dose of progestin is probably the least controversial first-line medical therapy if these simple measures fail. Serial bone density measurements would seem prudent, and if a bone therapy is required, then a bisphosphonate or perhaps a selective estrogen receptor modulator (SERM) should be considered.

References

1. Eden JA. Estrogen replacement therapy and survivors of breast cancer. *Drugs Aging* 1996;2:127–33
2. Bulbrook RD, Leake RE, George WD. Oestrogens in initiation and promotion of breast cancer. In Beck JS, ed. *Oestrogen and the Human Breast.* Edinburgh: Royal Society of Edinburgh, 1989: 67–76
3. Pasqualini JR, Nguyen BL. Estrone sulfatase activity and the effect of anti-estrogens on transformation of estrone sulfate in hormone dependent versus independent human breast cancer cell lines. *Breast Cancer Res Treat* 1991;18:93–8
4. Fishman J, Schneider J, Herschopf RJ, *et al.* Increased oestrogen 16α-hydroxylase activity in women with breast and endometrial cancer. *J Steroid Biochem* 1984;20:1077–81
5. Clarke CL, Sutherland RL. Progestin regulation of cellular proliferation. *Endocr Rev* 1990;11:266–301
6. Musgrove BA, Lee CSL, Sutherland RL. Progestins both stimulate and inhibit breast cancer cell cycle progression while increasing expression of transforming growth factor α, epidermal growth factor receptor *c-fos* and *c-myc* genes. *Mol Cell Biol* 1991;11: 5032–43
7. Hirata JD, Swiersz LM, Zell B, *et al.* Does dong quai have estrogenic effects on postmenopausal women? A double-blind placebo controlled trial. *Fertil Steril* 1997;68:981–6
8. Chenoy R, Hussain S, Tayob Y, *et al.* Effects of oral gamolenic acid from evening primrose oil on menopausal flushes. *Br Med J* 1994;308:501–3
9. Komesaroff PA, Black CVS, Cable V. Effects of wild yam extract on menopausal symptoms and hormonal and biochemical parameters. Presented at the *Australasian Menopause Congress*, Auckland, New Zealand, October 1998:abstr
10. Knight DC, Howes JB, Eden JA. The effect of promensil, an isoflavone extract, on menopausal symptoms. *Climacteric* 1999;2:79–84
11. Baber RJ, Templeman C, Moreton T, Kelly GE, West L. Randomised placebo controlled trial of an isoflavone supplement and menopausal symptoms in women. *Climacteric* 1990;2:85–92
12. Brzezianski A, Adlercreutz H, Shaoul R, *et al.* Short-term effects of phytoestrogen-rich diet on postmenopausal women. *Menopause* 1997;4:89–94
13. Albertazzi P, Pansini F, Bonaccorsi G, *et al.* The effects of dietary soy supplementation on hot flushes. *Obstet Gynecol* 1998;1:6–11
14. Schiff I, Tulchinsky D, Kramer D, *et al.* Oral medroxyprogesterone in the treatment of postmenopausal symptoms. *J Am Med Assoc* 1980;244: 1443–5
15. Paterson MEL. A randomised double-blind cross over trial into the effect of norethisterone on climacteric symptoms of biochemical profiles. *Br J Obstet Gynaecol* 1992;70:464–72
16. Dew J, Eden J, Beller E, *et al.* A cohort study of hormone replacement therapy given to women previously treated for breast cancer. *Climacteric* 1998; 1:137–42

Effects of progestogen on the breast 28

B. von Schoultz

INTRODUCTION

The breast is clearly a target organ for both estrogen and progesterone. However, there is still a remarkable lack of basic understanding as to how these sex steroids exert their effects and, in particular, to what extent they influence breast epithelial proliferation and breast cancer risk. Such information is vitally important for the interpretation of epidemiological data and for the evaluation of the potential risk of different hormonal regimens. Estrogen is known to be a growth hormone and to stimulate proliferation in several target tissues, for example the endometrium and vagina. In these biological systems, progestogens tend to counteract the effect of estrogen and cause inhibition of growth. Several *in vitro* studies of both normal and transformed breast cells in culture have shown that estrogen enhances breast cell proliferation and that the addition of progestogen reduces this effect[1]. However, *in vitro* and *in vivo* data are conflicting. The vast majority of *in vivo* studies of the normal breast have shown that the proliferation of breast epithelial cells is increased during the luteal phase of the menstrual cycle when progesterone levels are high[2,3].

ENDOGENOUS PROGESTERONE

The basis of an increased risk associated with hormonal therapies may lie in the regulation of cell proliferation. Within populations of cells *in vitro* and *in vivo*, high rates of cell proliferation increase the risk of transformation to the neoplastic phenotype[4]. Previous *in vivo* studies on the effects of sex steroids on breast tissue have been mainly analyses of mitosis in tissue sections from reduction mammoplasties or from 'normal' breast tissues near benign or malignant lesions[5,6]. Studies that are based on such tissue specimens have their apparent limitations and the proliferation analysis is possible on only one single occasion. The fine-needle aspiration biopsy technique was developed at the Karolinska Hospital and has become an established tool for the pre-operative diagnosis of palpable tumors in the breast. Fine-needle aspiration biopsies imply a minimum of inconvenience for the patient and can be performed repeatedly during the menstrual cycle or before and during different hormonal treatments[7]. The development of monoclonal antibodies has made it possible to assess sex steroid receptor expression and proliferation in cytological breast cell samples. The KI-67/Mib-1 monoclonal antibody reacts with a human nuclear antigen that is present in proliferating, but absent in quiescent, cells. The antigen is expressed during G1, S, G2 and mitosis[8]. The cytospin technique has successfully overcome the problem of low cellularity and yields samples with a higher cellularity than conventional smears and allows evaluation of proliferation in fine-needle aspiration biopsies[9]. Using this method, we found a decline in estrogen receptor expression from the follicular to the luteal phase of the menstrual cycle in healthy women[10]. In contrast, progesterone receptor expression was maintained and even tended to increase during the luteal phase. We also demonstrated an increased proliferative activity in normal breast epithelium during the luteal phase of the menstrual cycle in apparently healthy women[9]. In addition, there was a significant correlation between circulating levels of progesterone and breast epithelial proliferation. Thus, it seems that, in healthy women, the normal breast undergoes cyclic variations during the menstrual cycle, and these variations are characterized by an increased proliferation in the luteal phase. In fact, the same cyclic proliferative pattern has been demonstrated in breast cancer patients of fertile age.

EXOGENOUS PROGESTOGEN

While our understanding of the regulation of proliferation in the normal breast and of the effects of the native hormones estrogen and progesterone is incomplete, we have even less information on the impact of different hormonal treatment regimens. In clinical practice, a variety of estrogen and progestogen combinations are used in many different therapeutic regimens by numerous women receiving hormonal replacement. It is established that the three major therapeutic principles, (i.e. estrogen only, estrogen in cyclic combination with progestogen, and estrogen in continuous combination with progestogen) have quite different effects in the endometrium and other target organs[11,12]. So far there is very little basal knowledge whether, and to what extent, different treatment regimens may also have a different impact on the normal mammary epithelium. The possibility of an increased risk of breast cancer during hormone replacement therapy (HRT) has been discussed extensively. A slight increase in the relative risk of breast cancer during current HRT has been reported in large meta- and reanalyses of epidemiological data[13]. In women on estrogen replacement therapy, the risk is increased during long-term treatment to a relative risk level of approximately 1.3–2. There are few studies on the impact of different treatment regimens and, in particular, on the effects of various types and doses of progestogen. However, it seems clear that the addition of a progestogen during estrogen replacement has no protective effect. In fact, one recent study suggests that progestogen addition and a continuous combined regimen may further increase breast cancer risk[14]. In an animal model for HRT using surgically postmenopausal macaques, we found breast epithelial proliferation to be more pronounced following combined estrogen/progestogen treatment than after treatment with estrogen alone[15,16].

MAMMOGRAPHIC DENSITY – A SURROGATE MARKER?

During recent years, breast parenchymal density as expressed at mammographic examination has emerged as a potential surrogate marker for epithelial proliferation. An increasing number of reports have indicated that HRT is associated with an increased mammographic density in a significant proportion of postmenopausal women[17–19]. The mammographic picture of the breast reflects the relative amount of fat, connective and epithelial tissue. Proliferation and high amounts of connective and epithelial cells yield an increased density on the mammogram. Within the breast, epithelial and stromal cell interaction is critical for both normal and abnormal growth. Data suggest that an increase in mammographic density may be an independent risk factor for breast cancer in women and also in women on HRT[19]. Recently, the ongoing Postmenopausal Estrogen/Progestin Intervention (PEPI) trial reported a more pronounced effect of combined estrogen/progestogen therapy on mammographic density than treatment with estrogen alone[20] (Table 1). Likewise, our group, in a long-term follow-up of a population-based screening study, found that women on continuous estrogen/progestogen HRT were much more likely to respond with increased mammographic density[21] (Table 2). However, at present, there is no consensus about the interpretation of these data and in our understanding of the histological correlates to mammographic density. It

Table 1 The PEPI trial: percentage of women with increase in mammographic density. From reference 20

Treatment	*BI-RADS increase* (%)
Placebo	0
CEE only	3.5
CEE + cyclic MPA	23.5
CEE + continuous MPA	19.4
CEE + cyclic MPA	16.4

CEE, conjugated equine estrogen; MPA, medroxyprogesterone acetate

Table 2 Number of women with increase in mammographic density during hormone replacement therapy. From reference 21

Treatment	*Wolfe increase*	*All increase*
Estrogen + continuous progestogen	15/50 (30%)	26/50 (52%)
Estrogen + cyclic progestogen	0/75 (0%)	10/75 (13%)
Estrogen only	1/50 (2%)	9/50 (18%)

may tentatively be caused by epithelial proliferation, but also by edema, vasodilatation and fibrosis. The significance of different mammographic density patterns on cancer risk in individual women has been unclear. Mammographic screening sensitivity may be reduced by increased breast density, which may hamper the diagnosis of clinically occult cancers.

SUMMARY

It seems reasonable to assume a relationship between the given doses of sex steroid hormones and proliferation of the mammary epithelium. In the endometrium, differences between treatments associated with the progestogen component, its type, dose and duration of administration have been clearly established. The corresponding information about equipotency and specific differences between types of progestogens in respect to their effects on the mammary epithelium is currently lacking. However, according to data available so far, it seems justified to conclude that both native progesterone and exogenous progestogens enhance breast epithelial proliferation and that progestogen addition during estrogen replacement therapy may even increase breast cancer risk. It is also clear that progestogen effects differ according to type, dose, regimen and the estrogen environment, and further research in this field is vitally needed.

ACKNOWLEDGEMENTS

This work was supported by grants from the Swedish Medical Research Council (project no. 5982), the Swedish Cancer Society (Cancerföreningen), the Karolinska Institute Research Funds and the Trygg-Hansa Research Fund and CTRF.

References

1. Gompel A, Malet C, Spritzer P, *et al.* Progestin effect on cell proliferation and 17β-hydroxysteroid dehydrogenase activity in normal human breast cells in culture. *J Clin Endocrinol Metab* 1986;63: 1174–80
2. Vogel PM, Gerogiade NG, Fetter PF, *et al.* The correlation of histologic changes in the human breast with the menstrual cycle. *Am J Pathol* 1981;104: 23–34
3. Longacre TA, Bartow SA. A correlative morphologic study of human breast and endometrium in the menstrual cycle. *Am J Surg Pathol* 1986;10: 382–93
4. Preston-Martin S, Pike MC, Ross RK, Jones PA, Henderson BE. Increased cell division as a cause of human cancer. *Cancer Res* 1990;50:7415–21
5. Willams G, Anderson E, Howell A, *et al.* Oral contraceptive (OCP) use increases proliferation and decreases oestrogen receptor content of epithelial cells in the normal human breast. *Int J Cancer* 1991;48:206–10
6. Anderson TJ, Battersby S, King RJ, *et al.* Oral contraceptive use influences resting breast proliferation. *Hum Pathol* 1989;20:1139–44
7. Franzén S, Zajicek J. Aspiration biopsy in diagnosis of palpable lesions of the breast. Critical review of 3479 consecutive biopsies. *Acta Radiol Ther Phys Biol* 1968;7:241–62
8. Gerdes J, Li L, Schulueter C, *et al.* Immunobiochemical and molecular biologic characterization of the cell proliferation-associated nuclear antigen that is defined by monoclonal antibody Ki-67. *Am J Pathol* 1991;138:867–73
9. Söderqvist G, Isaksson E, von Schoultz B, *et al.* Proliferation of breast epithelial cells in healthy women during the menstrual cycle. *Am J Obstet Gynecol* 1997;176:123–8
10. Söderqvist G, von Schoultz B, Skoog L, *et al.* Estrogen and progesterone receptor content in breast epithelial cells from healthy women during the menstrual cycle. *Am J Obstet Gynecol* 1993;168:874–9
11. Key TJ, Pike MC. The dose-effect relationship between 'unopposed' oestrogens and endometrial mitotic rate: its central role in explaining and predicting endometrial cancer risk. *Br J Cancer* 1988; 57:205–21
12. Vihko R, Isomaa V. Endocrine aspects of endometrial cancer. In Voigt KD, Knabbe C, eds.

Endocrine Dependent Tumors. New York: Raven Press, 1989:197–214

13. Collaborative Group on Hormonal Factors in Breast Cancer. Breast cancer and hormone replacement therapy: collaborative reanalysis of data from 51 epidemiological studies of 52 705 women with breast cancer and 108 411 women without breast cancer. *Lancet* 1997;350:1047–59
14. Magnusson C, Baron JA, Correia N, *et al.* Breast cancer risk following long-term oestrogen- and oestrogen-progestin-replacement therapy. *Int J Cancer* 1999;81:339–44
15. Cline JM, Söderqvist G, von Schoultz E, *et al.* Effects of hormone replacement therapy on the mammary gland of surgically postmenopausal cynomolgus macaques. *Am J Obstet Gynecol* 1996; 174:93–100
16. Isaksson E, Cline JM, Skoog L, *et al.* p53 expression in breast and endometrium during estrogen and tamoxifen treatment of surgically postmenopausal cynomolgus macaques. *Breast Cancer Res Treat* 1999; 53:61–7
17. Kaufman Z, Garstin WIH, Hayes R, *et al.* The mammographic parenchymal patterns of women on hormonal replacement therapy. *Clin Radiol* 1991;43:389–92
18. Persson I, Thurfjell E, Holmberg L. Effect of estrogen and estrogen-progestin replacement regimens on mammographic breast parenchymal density. *J Clin Oncol* 1997;15:3201–7
19. Boyd NF, Lockwood GA, Byng JW, *et al.* Mammographic densities and breast cancer risk. *Cancer Epidemiol Biomarkers Prev* 1999;7:1133–44
20. Greendale GA, Reboussin BA, Sie A, *et al.* Effects of estrogen and estrogen-progestin on mammographic parenchymal density. *Ann Intern Med* 1999; 130:262–9
21. Lundström E, Wilczek B, von Palffy Z, *et al.* Mammographic breast density during hormone replacement therapy: differences according to treatment. *Am J Obstet Gynecol* 1999;181:348-52

Primary care during the menopause in Latin America

29

N. R. Melo, R. M. Neme, A. H. Galvão Giribela and L. Melo Pompei

INTRODUCTION

Data from the World Health Organization show that female life expectancy has increased during recent decades. Nowadays, people over 65 years old represent 15% of the world population[1].

Women's life expectancy in Latin America is around 75 years; the menopause tends to occur around 50 years of age and specialized medical care is recommended at this time.

Therapeutic measures, focusing on the epidemiological and clinical aspects of the menopause, have been proposed to try to improve the medical care of patients in Latin America.

EPIDEMIOLOGICAL CONSIDERATIONS IN THE MENOPAUSE

The Latin American population has been increasing in a constant and accelerated manner since 1700. In 1990, the population in this area was estimated to be 406 million people; 31 million of these were women over 50 years of age. This population is expected to double by the year 2015. The geographic distribution is not homogeneous: more than 70% is concentrated in Brazil, Mexico, Argentina and Colombia.

In Latin America, the distribution of men and women is 49% and 51%, respectively.

Recently, aging of the population has raised new challenges in health care and prevention. Some epidemiological actions have been identified as useful. The aim of these interventions is to provide the aging population with a better lifestyle. The introduction of appropriate diet, obesity control, fitness and estrogen replacement therapy is helping to prevent cardiovascular diseases and systemic hypertension. In addition, good health care, with special attention to diseases such as diabetes mellitus, gynecological cancer and pulmonary infections, should determine better quality of life during old age[2,3].

Life expectancy is increasing in Latin America and is expected to reach 73 years for women and 69 years for men by 2000 (Table 1). Almost 10% of the world population consists of women of postmenopausal age and 25 million women enter this period every year. The menopause is different to other demographic events, occurring in a well-determined part of a woman's life. It is defined as the last menstrual period and is established 12 months after this event[4].

Data estimate that, by the year 2000, 9.23% of the world population will be over 50 years of age (Table 2). At the time of writing, 13.4% of the world population, were over 50 7.0% of whom were women and 6.4% of whom were men. The life expectancy of women is 4.2 years longer than that of men. This is probably due to the higher risk of cardiovascular disease in men. In Argentina, Cuba and Uruguay, more than 20% of the population is over 50 years of age; Chile, Brazil, Panama and Costa Rica have the next highest percentages of people over 50 years old (Table 3).

In 1990, the population of climacteric women (45–65 years) in Latin America was 27.2 million

Table 1 Life expectancy (years) in Latin America

Years	*Women*	*Men*
1920	49	44
1940	54	49
1960	65	58
1980	69	62
1990	72	65
2000	73	69

Table 2 Percentage of women over 50 years of age in different regions

Region	Year 1990	2000	2010	2020	2030
Africa (South Sahara)	5.10	5.00	5.09	5.62	6.62
India	6.78	7.16	8.23	9.96	11.97
China	8.20	8.92	11.28	14.77	17.08
Others in Asia	6.50	7.16	8.96	11.38	13.82
Latin America	7.00	7.97	9.96	12.44	14.99
Middle East	5.87	5.87	6.77	7.86	9.21
Ex-Socialist Europe	16.57	17.37	19.30	19.50	20.41
Market Economies	16.06	17.54	19.72	21.87	22.85
World	8.87	9.23	10.53	12.22	13.73

Table 3 Age distribution in Latin America

	Female population in 1995				*Female population in 2000*				*Percentage change in female population, 1995-2000*			
Country	*45-54 years*	*55-64 years*	*> 65 years*	*> 45 years*	*45-54 years*	*55-64 years*	*> 65 years*	*> 45 years*	*45-54 years*	*55-64 years*	*> 65 years*	*> 45 years*
Argentina	1764	1449	1892	5105	1967	1522	2063	5552	10	5	8	8
Brazil	6852	4630	4291	15 773	8525	5348	4984	18 857	20	13	14	16
Chile	685	478	530	1693	804	552	604	1960	15	13	12	14
Colombia	1396	864	830	3090	1809	1016	945	3770	23	15	12	18
Equador	418	212	240	870	519	320	276	1115	19	34	13	22
Mexico	3307	2207	1980	7494	3989	2533	2454	8976	17	13	19	17
Venezuela	865	523	474	1862	1083	629	574	2286	20	17	17	19
Total	15 287	10 363	10 237	35 887	18 696	11 920	11 900	42 516	18	13	14	16

(6.7%); this will increase to 36.6 million (7.6%) in 2000.

Latin America is the third biggest seller of climacteric or menopause products in the world. This is because the number of people of this age is increasing in the region. The developed countries have a great influence and prescriptions of these products are increasing. The modernization of the pharmaceutical industry allows a great number of women to be treated[4].

The prevalence of hormonal replacement therapy (HRT) in Latin America is growing. In 1990 it was 2.8% and in 2000 it is expected to be 9.6% (Table 4).

Table 4 Prevalence of hormone replacement therapy (HRT) in Latin America

Year	*Percentage of women using HRT*
1990	2.8
1993	4.0
1995	5.2
1996	5.9
2000	9.6

FACTORS THAT INFLUENCE MENOPAUSE AND CONSEQUENCES OF OVARIAN FAILURE

Perimenopause is the period just before the irreversible interruption of menstruation. The progressive ovarian failure causes cyclical disturbance, altered menstrual bleeding, estrogen deficiency symptoms and an increase in gonadotropins[5].

The menopause is influenced by the age at menarche, weight, height, race, and social and economic factors. Compared to multiparity, nulliparity is associated with earlier menopausal age. The most important determinant of menopausal age is smoking, which leads to earlier menopausal age when compared to non-smoking women[6].

Ovarian failure is associated with the exhaustion of the thecal follicular system, the end of menstrual bleeding and the diminution of cyclical production of estrogen and progesterone, thus leading to the disappearance of the negative feedback regulation of follicle stimulating hormone and luteinizing hormone, resulting in an increase in their serum levels.

In the premenopausal period, the ovary is the major source of estrogen production. Estrogen is the sexual steroid with greatest serum levels and it is produced almost exclusively by the mature follicle.

After the menopause, the estradiol and estrone levels are diminished. Alternative sources of estrogen production are required, such as the conversion of androstenedione to estrone in the fat tissue; hence, after the menopause, estrone is the most abundant estrogen in the circulation.

MENOPAUSAL SYMPTOMS AND THEIR SOCIAL IMPACT

Depression, headache, emotional instability, anxiety, irritability and insomnia can be present at the menopause, but these symptoms are not always caused by estrogen deficiency. There is also a reduction in self-respect as an expression of a negative perception of life.

The sexual behavior of women can change after the menopause, because of vaginal relaxation due to cystocele, rectocele and uterine prolapse, mucosal atrophy, dyspareunia, diminution of libido, or presence of chronic disease such as systemic hypertension or coronary disease.

The vasomotor hot flush is viewed as the hallmark of the female climacteric. It is the most common symptom of climacteric women, being experienced by 5–76% of this population, including those in the premenopausal period. In 80% of women, it lasts more than 1 year, and in 25%, more than 5 years[7,8].

Osteoporosis is the major public health problem and is responsible for 1.2 million fractures per year.

Hypertension and atherosclerosis increase in women after the menopause. During the reproductive years, women are protected from coronary heart disease. The reasons for this are related to estrogen action, increasing high-density lipoprotein and decreasing low-density lipoprotein levels and also direct antiatherogenic effects in arteries, leading to vasodilatation and increasing antiplatelet aggregation factors such as nitric acid.

TREATMENT: HORMONAL REPLACEMENT THERAPY

Because of the increases in women over 50 years old and life expectancy, there have been public health efforts to improve life quality, including treatment with HRT. The incidence of HRT in Latin America is low when compared to developed countries. However, the use of HRT shows a continuous increase. In 1990, only 2.8% of postmenopausal women used HRT; in 1996, this number increased to 5.9% and, in the year 2000, this figure is expected to be 9.6%[9].

Usually, women using HRT are from the highest social levels, the prevalence being 18%, because the government does not pay for this kind of treatment.

HRT is the best treatment for the menopause, because it replaces the hormones previously produced by the ovaries. HRT is almost always successful in reversing neurovegetative symptoms and atrophic changes, as well as decreasing the occurrence of cardiovascular disease, bone loss and Alzheimer's disease. With well-established osteoporosis, the results are not good, so prevention is preferred.

Hormonal replacement can be performed with estrogen, progesterone or a combination of the two. The most widely used estrogens are conjugated estrogens, which constitute 70% of the estrogens sold in the USA. The dose is variable, ranging from 0.625 to 1.25 mg daily. Oral administration is more common, but is not always the best route. Parenteral administration bypasses the gastrointestinal route, thus avoiding the passage of estrogens through the liver, which changes the synthesis of liver proteins and alters the estrogen concentration.

Estrogens are highly efficient in preventing female osteoporosis and decreasing bone reabsorption[10]. They should be used as early as possible[11]. Even when started late, HRT guarantees the prevention of bone loss after treatment has begun, but does not restore the bone mass to premenopausal levels[12].

Estrogen replacement therapy decreases serum levels of total cholesterol and high-density lipoprotein, and may increase triglyceride levels.

The use of isolated progestogens is preferred when side-effects or contraindications to estrogen are present. The results are good for the relief of hot flushes and bone loss, but are not as good as with estrogen[9].

The association of estrogen and progestogen is recommended to avoid the hyperplasic effect of estrogen on the endometrium.

In Latin America, the foreseen increase in the use of HRT-related products was 16.1 million units in 1994 and will be 37.5 million units in the year 2000, which is higher than the increase expected in other regions of the world[4].

The most frequently prescribed HRT therapy in Latin American countries is oral HRT (72%). Transdermal and injectable HRT treatments represent 13% of the HRT prescriptions[4]. The main products prescribed in Latin America are conjugated estrogens alone, a combination of estradiol valerate and cyproterone acetate, progestins alone, transdermal estrogens and, finally, a combination of conjugated estrogens and medroxyprogesterone acetate (MPA) or estradiol valerate and MPA (Table 5).

CONCLUSIONS

The menopause and HRT have been more widely studied due to the increase in life expectancy and demographic evolution in the world and Latin America. Unfortunately, at present, HRT is only used by an economically favored population, and there has been no governmental effort to help less well-off women. However, today it is well known that HRT is able to prevent or treat diseases that incur high costs on the governmental budget. It is important that physicians act positively for the whole population, promoting the best treatment for menopausal women, thus contributing to the improvement of life quality and life expectancy.

Table 5 Hormone replacement therapies over the years. All values given are percentages

	Year								
Therapy	*1995*	*1996*	*1997*	*1998*	*1999*	*2000*	*2001*	*2002*	*2003*
Conjugated estrogens	33.2	27.5	25.6	24.9	22.3	21.5	20.6	19.6	18.8
Conjugated estrogens + MPA	0.7	10.4	10.9	12.5	16.3	18.7	21.5	24.8	27.6
Wyeth® patch	0.3	0.7	2.5	2.4	1.7	1.6	1.6	1.6	1.6
Premarin vaginal cream	6.4	4.9	4.3	3.9	3.6	3.4	3.2	2.9	2.8
Wyeth injectable	5.2	4.4	3.7	3.6	3.5	3.3	3.2	3.1	3.0
Premarin family	45.8	47.9	47.0	47.3	47.4	48.5	50.1	52.0	53.8
SERM/raloxifene	0	0	0	0.3	1.1	1.5	2.0	2.1	2.1
Other conjugated estrogens	4.2	4.0	3.9	4.0	3.7	3.3	3.0	2.8	2.7
Other conjugated estrogens + MPA	0.7	4.7	6.8	7.4	7.6	7.6	7.6	7.5	7.5
Other (Estrace® and generics)	26.3	21.8	21.3	20.7	19.9	19.2	18.4	17.3	16.1
Patch	17.0	15.7	15.3	14.6	14.8	14.7	14.1	13.9	13.5
Other cream/gels/spray	4.5	4.5	4.5	4.4	4.1	3.8	3.4	3.1	2.9
Other injectable	1.5	1.4	1.4	1.4	1.4	1.4	1.3	1.3	1.3
Total	100	100	100	100	100	100	100	100	100

MPA, medroxyprogesterone acetate; SERM, selective estrogen receptor modulator

References

1. Lois EM. Epidemiologia del envejecimiento en América Latina. In Campos OG, Urzua EA, Castro PC, eds. *Menopausia y Longevidad.* Santiago, Chile: Sociedad Chilena de Climaterio, 1998:41–8
2. Acevedo PL. Envejecimiento poblacional y menopausia en Latinoamérica. In Campos OG, Urzua EA, Castro PC, eds. *Menopausia y Longevidad.* Santiago, Chile: Sociedad Chilena de Climaterio, 1998:49–72
3. World Health Organization. *Women, Ageing and Health. Achieving Health across the Life Span* WHO/HRP/AHE/HPD/96.1. Geneva: WHO, 1996
4. Armendáriz MP. Realidad demográfica en Latinoamérica y tratamiento hormonal de reemplazo. In Campos OG, Urzua EA, Castro PC, eds. *Menopausia y Longevidad.* Santiago, Chile: Sociedad Chilena de Climaterio, 1998:73–88.
5. Albright F. Studies on ovarian dysfunction. III. The menopause. *Endocrinology* 1936;20:24
6. Jick H, Porter J. Relation between smoking and age of natural menopause. Report from the Boston Collaborative Drug Surveillance Program, Boston University Medical Center. *Lancet* 1977;1:1354–5
7. Neucarten BL, Kriner RG. Menopausal symptoms in women of various ages. *Psychosom Med J* 1966; 27:26
8. Thompson B, Hart AS, Durno D. Menopausal age and symptomatology in general practice. *J Biol Sci* 1973;5:71–82
9. Lindsay R, Hart DM, Purdie D. Comparative effects of oestrogen and a progestogen on bone loss in postmenopausal women. *Clin Sci Mol Med* 1978; 54:193–5
10. Meema S, Bunker ML, Meema HE. Preventive effect of estrogen on postmenopausal bone loss. *Arch Intern Med* 1975;135:1436–40
11. Nachtigall LE, Nachtigall RH, Nachtigall RD, Beckman EM. Estrogen replacement therapy. A 10-year prospective study in the relationship to osteoporosis. *Obstet Gynecol* 1979;53:277–81
12. Recker RR, Saville PD, Heaney RP. Effect of oestrogens and calcium carbonate on bone loss in postmenopausal women. *Ann Intern Med* 1977;87: 649–55

Menopause in the Asia–Pacific region 30

C. J. Haines

INTRODUCTION

In 1999 it was expected that the world's population would reach six billion. Since 1995, the population has been growing at a rate of 1.3% per annum, with the addition of approximately 78 million persons each year[1]. Of the mid-1998 world population, which stood at 5901 million, 4719 million (80%) lived in less developed countries. Asia accounted for 3585 million (61%) of the total. In addition, the top four contributors to world population growth are located within the Asia–Pacific region (Table 1).

The effects of decreased fertility and increased life expectancy also mean that the world's population is growing older. Population estimates for the Asia–Pacific region show that the number of postmenopausal women will increase rapidly in the next 30 years. It is anticipated that, world-wide, twice as many women will reach the menopause by 2030 as in 1990 and that the proportion living in developing countries will have increased from 60% to 76%[2]. China alone, where postmenopausal women will make up 17% of the population, will account for 23% of the total. These figures suggest that into the new millennium, the management of the menopause in the Asia–Pacific region will pose an even greater health-care problem than that which currently exists.

This brief review will concentrate on menopausal symptoms and the menopausal experience in Asian women, as there is currently a great deal of interest in possible differences between Asian women and those from other regions. The problem of coronary heart disease will also be discussed, as the incidence of this disease is increasing throughout the Asia–Pacific region. Osteoporosis will be mentioned briefly, but other conditions associated with the menopause will not be the subject of this discussion.

Table 1 Major contributors to world population growth. From reference 1

No.	*Country*	*Net addition/1000*	*Percentage increase*	*Cumulative percentage increase*
1	India	15 999	20.6	20.6
2	China	11 408	14.7	35.3
3	Pakistan	4 048	5.2	40.5
4	Indonesia	2 929	3.8	44.2

THE EXPERIENCE OF THE MENOPAUSE IN THE ASIA–PACIFIC REGION

Acute menopausal symptoms in Asian women

Whilst there has been little variation in the reported prevalence of acute menopausal symptoms in different groups of Caucasian women, considerable cross-cultural variation has been described in both the frequency and in the severity of symptoms[3,4]. It is a generally held belief that acute symptoms occur less frequently and are less severe in Asian than in Caucasian women, but, although there is considerable evidence to support this view, not all studies have been in agreement. Hot flushes have been described in over 60% of Caucasian women after a natural menopause and in more than 90% after a surgical menopause[5,6]. Comparative figures are generally much lower in Asian women. In 1988, a study of 1141 Japanese women aged 45–55 years found that hot flushes and sweating occurred in 108 (9.5%) and 41 (3.6%) women, respectively[3]. Studies in other parts of Asia, including Indonesia and Pakistan, have also shown that acute symptoms occur relatively infrequently[7,8].

As far as Chinese women in Hong Kong are concerned, we found that hot flushes and sweating following a surgical menopause occurred in 24.2% and 18.2% of cases, respectively[9]. In another study of 1467 Hong Kong Chinese women, hot flushes and night sweats were found in 10–20% of women[10]. In addition, in a subsequent placebo-controlled study on the effect of estrogen on acute symptoms, we found no difference in the frequency of symptoms between those women taking estrogen and those on placebo[11], however, this may have been due to the low background reporting of symptoms in each group.

As previously mentioned, however, not all studies have been in agreement. In a survey of 119 postmenopausal women living in a slum area in Bangkok, 72.3% described vasomotor symptoms, although these were viewed as being a problem in only 29.4% of cases[12]. The differentiation between the presence of symptoms and the extent to which they cause distress is therefore clearly important. In another study also conducted in Bangkok amongst women aged 40 years and above, vasomotor symptoms were reported by 80% of those who were menopausal, but were also noted by 85.8% of menstruating women[13]. The largest multicenter study in the Asian region also demonstrated considerable differences in the reporting of acute symptoms, but, overall, vasomotor symptoms were less common than in Western women[14]. Of particular interest, psychological complaints were more closely related to the menopause than were vasomotor symptoms.

Apart from hot flushes and sweating, it has also been suggested that Asian women may experience some symptoms that differ from those usually described by women in other regions. A recent survey from Taiwan revealed that the most frequent menopausal symptoms were lumbago or low back pain (68%), fatigue (59%) and memory disturbances (55%)[15]. In another study of Taiwanese women, the three most frequently reported symptoms were backache/lumbago, amentia and tiredness[16]. In Korean women, the most serious symptoms were psychosomatic in origin, but vasomotor symptoms were reported in 38.4% of cases[17]. In Thailand, a cross-sectional survey of 268 middle-aged women found that dizziness and tiredness were the most common problems. Night sweats were reported in 32% of these women while hot flushes were found in 33%[18]. In a much larger study of 8300 Thai women, hot flushes ranked 10th (15.8%) and night sweats 15th (9%) in order of symptoms, with backache (26.1%) and headache (25.1%) being the two most frequent complaints[19].

Overall, most studies suggest that the incidence of acute menopausal symptoms is lower in Asian populations. It has been a commonly held belief that Asian women are more stoical and are therefore more tolerant of these symptoms. In addition, it has been suggested that a higher dietary intake of phytoestrogens in Asia may protect women against estrogen deficiency. However, the variation in the reporting of symptoms may also be due in part to methodological differences between the studies. Few of the data originating from the Asian region have been free from methodological problems and, in many cases, the sample sizes have been small and the samples have been taken from women in urban areas, when the majority of the population are rural dwellers.

The perception of the menopause in Asian women

Whilst it is a commonly held belief that the menopause is not a serious life event for most Asian women, there are relatively few scientific data to support this. It is common to group Asian women together, but it should be remembered that they constitute a diverse group both racially and culturally. It is therefore not unexpected that there has also been some inconsistency in the results of studies on the perception of the menopause in different parts of Asia.

Some events which occur around the time of the menopause may be viewed favorably by many women. Not all of these are directly related to the menopause. These include the removal of the need for contraception and the lesser demands of child rearing as children grow older (although in some societies the 'empty nest syndrome' may be regarded as a negative aspect of the menopause). Negative accompaniments include the perception that the menopause is a symbol of aging[20]. However, whilst aging is regarded as being a negative factor in most Western populations, in some parts of Asia, older people are especially respected for their wisdom and experience. In the 1980s, a number of researchers recognized that the menopause in some cultures was associated with the development of increased confidence and a higher achievement of personal goals[21]. More recent studies have supported these views. Kyung identified four interesting changes as part of the menopausal process in middle-aged Korean women[22]. These were described as a change from suffering to comfort, from being a good wife and mother to becoming a woman, from a life of oppression to one of freedom and from the living of a productive life to the living of a transformed life.

George interviewed women from a village on the coast of India and found that, after the menopause, they could devote more time to their businesses; furthermore, none of them sought treatment for the menopause[23]. Other studies have also reported a wide discrepancy between the prevalence of symptoms and the number of women who seek treatment for them[14].

Our experience in Hong Kong is that women lack awareness of the menopause and its potential long-term effects[24]. We found that 73% of mainland Chinese women and 96% of Hong Kong Chinese women could correctly define the menopause, but 73% and 38%, respectively, knew nothing of the effects of the menopause on either the physical or psychological well-being. Their knowledge about the treatment of the menopause was also scant, with 91% of mainland Chinese and 87% of Hong Kong Chinese women not being aware of any treatment for the menopause. In Taiwan, the menopause was perceived as being a natural phenomenon in 91.7% of women, and some of the descriptions of the menopause included 'wisdom and maturation', 'a symbol of achievement' and 'a time to start enjoying life'.

CORONARY HEART DISEASE IN THE ASIA-PACIFIC REGION

Coronary heart disease is an increasing problem in the Asia-Pacific region. Whilst the proportion of deaths due to circulatory disease decreased from 51% to 46% in developed countries between 1985 and 1997, in developing countries the proportion increased from 16% to 24%[25]. Whilst the percentage remains low compared to that in developed countries, considering the size of the population and the rate of increase in the proportion of deaths from circulatory disease, coronary heart disease may become the most important problem to be faced by postmenopausal women in the Asia-Pacific region. Whilst the rates of coronary heart disease in men exceed those for women at any given age, there is little remaining gender difference after the age of 75 years[26].

Coronary heart disease in Hong Kong

An example of the magnitude of the problem can be found in data from the Department of Health in Hong Kong[27], which reported that the average life expectancy had risen steadily over the preceding three decades from 68.5 to 75.2 years in males and from 75.9 to 80.7 years in females. Heart diseases were responsible for 15.6% of all deaths, second only to cancer, which was responsible for 31.1% of all deaths. However, over the preceding 20 years, the crude death rate due to coronary heart disease in Hong Kong had almost doubled, from 28.4/100 000 of the population in 1972 to 54.7/100 000 in 1992[28]. This occurred in association with a longer life expectancy as well as the development of a more atherogenic lipid profile.

The menopause appears to have a similar effect on cardiovascular disease in postmenopausal Asian women as in most other populations. The sex ratio (males : females) of those suffering from coronary heart disease in Hong Kong is 5.1 : 1 in the 30–49-year-old age group, but decreases to 1.2 : 1 in those aged 65 years and over. However, at all ages, the gender difference is not as great as in most Western countries. In the 40–69-year-old age group, for example, the ratio is 2.8 : 1 in the USA and 3.3 : 1 in England and Wales, but in Hong Kong it is only 2.4 : 1[29]. Women in Hong Kong therefore appear to be at relatively greater risk of developing coronary heart disease at a younger age.

OSTEOPOROSIS IN THE ASIA-PACIFIC REGION

In the 1960s, the age-adjusted incidence of hip fracture in Hong Kong was between 13% and 30% of that reported in most studies on Caucasians[30]. Since then, however, the incidence of hip fracture has increased in Chinese and in most other

Table 2 Changes in age-specific fracture rates in women in Hong Kong between 1966 and 1991. From reference 31

Age group (years)	*Fracture rate/100 000*		
	1966	*1985*	*1991*
40–49	7	11	6
50–59	22	32	26
60–69	54	135	112
70–79	173	501	581
≥ 80	716	1521	1916

populations in the Asia–Pacific region. Changes in age-specific fracture rates in women in Hong Kong between 1966 and 1991 are shown in Table 2[31].

This increase has been attributed to greater longevity, reduced exercise and a change towards a diet that is lower in phytoestrogens. The diet in many Asian populations is also relatively low in calcium, and studies of ours and other groups have shown that the dietary calcium intake in postmenopausal Chinese women is less than 500 mg daily[32]. Intervention with dietary calcium supplementation (with or without estrogen) has been shown to increase bone mineral density at the femoral neck[33,34].

The cost and lack of availability of many pharmaceutical preparations used in the prevention and treatment of osteoporosis means that the majority of women in the Asia–Pacific region will not be able to choose whether to use one of these treatments. The available data on the benefits of both calcium supplementation and exercise suggest that, for Asian women, these may be the most appropriate first-line measures until other treatments become available.

SUMMARY

Most studies of postmenopausal women have suggested that the experience of the menopause is less of a problem in Asians than in Caucasians. This conclusion has arisen mainly from the findings that Asian women in general are less troubled by acute menopausal symptoms and that, in some populations, aging is viewed as a positive rather than a negative aspect of life. Whilst symptoms may be less of a problem in Asia, postmenopausal women are still at risk of the long-term complications of the menopause. The incidence of both osteoporosis and coronary heart disease is increasing in most Asia–Pacific countries, but the absence of symptoms removes the opportunity for many women to discuss the consequences of the menopause and its treatment.

References

1. United Nations Population Division. *World Population Prospects, The 1998 Revision*. New York: United Nations, 1998
2. Report of a WHO Scientific Group. *Research on the menopause*. WHO Technical Report Series 670. Geneva: World Health Organization, 1981:8–10
3. Lock M, Kaufert P, Gilbert P. Cultural construction of the menopausal syndrome: the Japanese case. *Maturitas* 1988;10:317–32
4. Beyene Y. Cultural significance and physiological manifestations of menopause. A biocultural analysis. *Cult Med Psychiatry* 1986;10:47–71
5. Hagstad A, Janson PO. The epidemiology of climacteric symptoms. *Acta Obstet Gynecol Scand* 1986;134(Suppl):59–65
6. Chakravarti S, Collins WP, Newton JR, Oram DH, Studd JWW. Endocrine changes and symptomatology after oophorectomy in premenopausal women. *Br J Obstet Gynaecol* 1977;84:769–75
7. Agoestina T, Van Keep P. The climacteric in Bandung, West Java province, Indonesia. *Maturitas* 1984;6:327–33
8. Wasti S, Robinson SC, Akhtar Y, Khan S, Badaruddin N. Characteristics of menopause in three socioeconomic urban groups in Karachi, Pakistan. *Maturitas* 1993;16:61–9
9. Haines CJ, Chung TKH, Leung DHY. A prospective study of the frequency of acute menopausal symptoms in Hong Kong Chinese women. *Maturitas* 1994;18:175–81

10. Tang GWK. Menopausal symptoms. *J Hong Kong Med Assoc* 1993;45:249-54
11. Chung TK, Yip SK, Lam P, Chang AM, Haines CJ. A randomized, double-blind, placebo-controlled, crossover study on the effect of oral oestradiol on acute menopausal symptoms. *Maturitas* 1996;25: 115-23
12. Chaikittisilpa S, Limpaphayom K, Chompootweep S, Taecakraichana N. Symptoms and problems of menopausal women in Klong Toey slum. *J Med Assoc Thailand* 1997;80:257-61
13. Sukwatana P, Meekhangvan J, Tamrongterakul T, Tanapat Y, Asavarait S, Boonjitrpimon P. Menopausal symptoms among Thai women in Bangkok. *Maturitas* 1991;13:217-28
14. Boulet MJ, Oddens BJ, Lehert P, Vemer HM, Visser A. Climacteric and menopause in seven south-east Asian countries. *Maturitas* 1994;19:157-76
15. Chow SN, Huang CC, Lee YT. Demographic characteristics and medical aspects of menopausal women in Taiwan. *J Formosan Med Assoc* 1997;96; 806-11
16. Chang C, Chang CH. Menopause and hormone using experiences of Chinese women in Taiwan. *Health Care Women Int* 1996;17:307-18
17. Chan YN, Kim KJ, Lim HK, Jang HS, Han HS, Chung YH. A study on menopausal symptoms and health needs among middle aged women. *Taehan Kanho [Korean Nurse]* 1995;34:70-82
18. Punyahotra S, Dennerstein L, Lehert P. Menopausal experience of Thai women. Part 1. Symptoms and their correlates. *Maturitas* 1997;26;1-7
19. Punyahotra S, Limpaphayom K. An Asian perspective of the menopause. In Wren B, ed. *Progress in the Management of the Menopause.* New York: Parthenon Publishing, 1996:108-13
20. Datan N. Aging in transitions: cross-cultural perspectives on women at midlife. In Formaner R, ed. *The Meanings of Menopause: Historical, Medical and Clinical Perspectives.* Hilsdale, NJ: Analytic, 1990: 117-32
21. McKinlay JB, McKinlay SM, Brambilla D. The relative contributions of endocrine change and social circumstances to depression in mid-aged women. *J Health Soc Behav* 1987;28:345-63
22. Kyung HL. Korean urban women's experience of menopause: new life. *Health Care Women Int* 1997; 18:139-48
23. George T. Women in a south Indian fishing village: role identity, continuity, and the experience of menopause. *Health Care Women Int* 1996;17:271-9
24. Haines CJ, Li R, Chung TKH, Leung DHY. The perception of the menopause and the climacteric among women in Hong Kong and southern China. *Prev Med* 1995:24:245-8
25. World Health Organization. *The World Health Report 1998.* Geneva: World Health Organization, 1998
26. Stampfer MJ, Colditz GA, Willett WC. Menopause and heart disease: a review. *Ann NY Acad Sci* 1990; 592:193-203
27. Department of Health, Hong Kong. *Annual Report 1993/94.* Hong Kong: Department of Health, 1994
28. Department of Health, Hong Kong. *Public Health Report No. 1. A New Approach to Public Health Report. Coronary Heart Disease and Lung Cancer.* Hong Kong: Department of Health, 1994
29. Beaglehole R. International trends in coronary artery disease mortality, morbidity, and risk factors. *Epidemiol Rev* 1990;12:1-14
30. Chalmers J, Ho KC. Geographical variations in senile osteoporosis. *J Bone Joint Surg* 1970;52B: 667-75
31. Lau EMC. The epidemiology of osteoporosis in Asia. In Lau EMC, ed. *Osteoporosis in Asia.* Singapore: World Scientific, 1997:1-12
32. Haines CJ, Chung TKH, Leung PC, Leung DHY, Wong MY, Lam LL. Dietary calcium intake in postmenopausal Chinese women. *Eur J Clin Nutr* 1994;48:591-4
33. Lau E, Woo J, Leung PC, Swaminathan R, Leung D. The effects of calcium supplementation and exercise on bone density in elderly Chinese women. *Osteoporosis Int* 1992;2:168
34. Haines CJ, Chung TKH, Leung PC, Hsu SYC, Leung DHY. Calcium supplementation and bone mineral density in postmenopausal women using estrogen replacement therapy. *Bone* 1995;16:529-31

Improvement of knowledge and perception of the menopause in the Bulgarian population

31

D. B. Georgiev and E. P. Ratchev

INTRODUCTION

Menopausal knowledge is expanding world-wide among doctors, but also among women and even men. This is mainly due to the education directed at both important groups - medical practitioners and patients. Some countries have organized extensive educational campaigns for a long time, and their success is reflected in the number of women taking hormone replacement therapy (HRT) and visiting menopausal care units there[1]. In a recent survey in France, the UK and Germany, women's magazines were the main source of information on climacteric problems[2]. In other countries, however, there is insufficient knowledge about the dilemmas related to estrogen deficiency, and this is mainly due to a lack of information, among both doctors and patients, about the modern trends in climacteric medicine[1].

Unfortunately, Bulgaria is one of the countries with limited menopause knowledge. For years, the Bulgarian health-care system had a more therapeutic, rather than preventive, approach towards climacteric women. There was insufficient education for medical students, and postgraduate training courses on menopausal medicine were rare. The shift towards a modern health-care system with another type of financing is not finalized yet.

On the other hand, the menopausal population in Bulgaria has increased in absolute and relative terms. At the end of 1997, the Bulgarian Menopause Association estimated that there are approximately 1.2 million women aged above 45, which is 14.6% of the entire population.

The aim of the present paper was to evaluate the level of menopausal knowledge in Bulgaria and to follow the changes in this knowledge over the past few years.

MATERIALS AND METHODS

Three types of survey were used for the description of menopausal knowledge and perceptions in Bulgaria:

(1) One thousand female patients visiting the Perimenopausal Care Unit (MCU) at the Second Obstetrical and Gynecological Hospital in Sofia, Bulgaria for the first time during the period November 1995-January 1998 were interviewed anonymously with a written questionnaire. None of them was taking HRT and almost all of them were visiting a menopausal care unit for the first time. The answers were processed with special software and then analyzed with a statistical package for social surveys (SPSS).

(2) A menopausal hotline was set up at the end of 1997 in order to provide free advice on the menopause. This is a 24-hour telephone line managed by volunteers without medical education, but with adequate experience and understanding of menopausal complaints. The aim of the hotline was to answer queries related to menopause and menopausal care, as well as to collect information about the caller's menopausal perception and problems. The menopause hotline telephone number was advertised in the press and in a television program dedicated to female health. Almost 1900 calls had been answered by August 1999.

(3) In June 1999, a cross-sectional survey of 1640 women aged 45-65 years, drawn from four samples representing the general population of Bulgaria, was performed by Gallup British Balkan Social Surveys. A questionnaire designed by the Bulgarian Menopause Society

and covering some background details, income, general health, menopausal knowledge and HRT use was used. A direct 'face-to-face' interview was performed, but, to avoid eliciting stereotypical views of the menopause, the survey was described as a study of women's health and well-being, and some additional irrelevant questions were attached. The results were analyzed with SPSS.

RESULTS

Menopausal care unit patients

The answers from the questionnaires distributed in the Sheinovo Hospital MCU were divided into the following five groups:

Group 1: Reasons for the visit to the MCU

(1) Are you visiting a menopausal care unit for the first time? Yes, 92%; no, 8%.

(2) Who advised you to visit the MCU? A friend (relative), 62%; a doctor, 28%; no-one, 10%.

(3) What is the reason for your visiting the MCU? Hot flushes and other subjective complaints, 82%; knowledge about the preventive potential of HRT, 11%; menstrual disorders, 4%; a strong wish to do something for my health, 3%.

Group 2: General knowledge about the menopause

(1) How do you estimate your knowledge about the menopause? Insufficient, 95%; sufficient, 5%.

(2) Do you know anything about osteoporosis? Yes, 72%; no, 28%.

(3) Do you know anything about HRT? Yes, 56%; no, 44%.

(4) Have you any concerns about the use of HRT? Yes, 71%; no 29%.

(5) What are your reasons for concern? Getting fat and hairy, 65%; possible breast problems, 27%; don't know, 7%; miscellaneous, 1%.

(6) Do you accept the menopausal status as normal or as morbid? Normal, 61%; morbid, 39%.

(7) Do you miss your regular bleedings (344 postmenopausal women)? Yes, 30%; no, 70%.

(8) Do you think that the menopause should be treated? Yes, 42%; no, 58%.

(9) Do you think that menopausal problems should be treated with hormones? Yes, 25%; no, 75%.

Group 3: Family history

(1) Has your mother had problems with the menopause? Yes, 45%; no, 22%; don't remember 33%.

Group 4: Advanced knowledge

(1) Do you know anything about mammography? Yes, 38%; no, 62%.

(2) Do you know anything about densitometry? Yes, 18%; no, 82%.

(3) Are you aware of the higher risk for cardiovascular diseases after the menopause? Yes, 28%; no, 72%.

(4) Do you know anything about the relation between the menopause and Alzheimer's disease? Yes, 2%; no, 98%.

Group 5: Organization of menopausal care

(1) Who should treat menopausal symptoms and consequences? Obstetrician/gynecologist, 70%; neurologist, 18%; cardiologist, 7%; others, 5%.

(2) Do you consider HRT prices in Bulgaria as reasonable? Yes, 60%; no, 40%.

Menopausal hotline

All conversations were recorded and the important questions asked by calling women were collected in a special file.

The most frequently asked questions were:

(1) Where could I find a doctor who deals with the menopause?

(2) Are hormones dangerous and, if not, are the preparations available in Bulgaria not old-fashioned?

(3) How many women suffer the same symptoms as mine?

(4) When should HRT be stopped and should I consult a doctor for this?

Some women reported their experience with medical practitioners (mainly gynecologists) prescribing HRT. Some statements are intriguing:

(1) HRT was prescribed without any breast examination in at least 30% of the patients contacting the hotline;

(2) Unopposed estrogens were given in women with an intact uterus in 44 cases;

(3) HRT was prescribed only for 6 months with the statement that 'this is enough, longer could be dangerous' in 27 cases;

(4) HRT was taken by the patient after a 'consultation' with non-medical advisors - a neighbour, a relative, etc.;

(5) Approximately 10% of the calling women were hysterectomized, but only 40% of them received HRT.

Questionnaire of the Gallup British Balkan Social Surveys

(1) Do you know what kind of symptoms are typical for the climacteric? Yes, 84.8%; no, 15.2%.

(2) Have you visited a doctor because of climacteric complaints during the past year? Yes, 24.5%; no, 75.5%.

(3) If answer to question (2) is yes, which of the mentioned medical investigations did you have?

   (a) Gynecological check-up, 82.5%;

   (b) Mammography, 15.0%;

   (c) Densitometry, 7.5%;

   (d) Laboratory tests, 35.5%;

   (e) None, 2.4%.

(4) Are you using HRT at the moment? Yes, 2.4%; no, 97.6%.

(5) If no, are you a past user? Yes, 9.3%; no, 90.7%.

(6) If, yes, for how long?

   (a) Up to 6 months, 58%;

   (b) Up to 2 years, 16.7%;

   (c) More than 2 years, 25.3%.

(7) If no, what is the reason?

   (a) Doctor's advice, 8.1%;

   (b) Personal choice, 24%;

   (c) No reason, 25.9%;

   (d) Don't know the problem, 32%;

   (e) Financial reasons, 10%.

(8) Would you accept participation in a medical trial? Yes, 21.5%; no, 78.5%.

(9) Do you think that the price of the HRT preparations is reasonable? Yes, 14%; no, 86%.

(10) Do you think that HRT should be covered by health-care providers? Yes, 94.4%; no, 5.6%.

(11) Do you think that the media provide enough information about climacteric problems? Yes, 17.7%; no, 82.3%.

(12) Which of the following diseases due to estrogen deficiency do you know about?

   (a) Osteoporosis, 41%;

   (b) Atherosclerosis, 39.8%;

   (c) Alzheimer's disease, 7.5%;

   (d) Changes in the urinary tract, 20.9%;

   (e) Skin changes, 33.4%;

   (f) Liver cirrhosis, 0.5%.

DISCUSSION

It is evident that the knowledge of Bulgarian menopausal women concerning climacteric problems and consequences is insufficient. Seventy-two per cent of the patients of the MCU and 41% of those interviewed by Gallup had some idea about osteoporosis, but only 18% were familiar with bone densitometry as a diagnostic tool. Moreover, only 7.5% of the women who visited a doctor for climacteric complaints in the past year had had a bone density evaluation. This chain of 'unrealized knowledge' partly explains the low rate of HRT use in the country - 2.4%. Some findings from the questionnaires require special attention - the worry about the possible connection between HRT and cancer, side-effects and contraindications, and the lack of knowledge about the serious diseases that may be related to estrogen deficiency.

It is also evident that some medical practitioners are reluctant to issue HRT prescriptions in Bulgaria - women who contacted the hotline asked for 'a doctor who deals with menopausal problems'. It could be speculated that they had visited some colleagues who rejected HRT or prescribed it for up to 6 months. This explains the low motivation rate in Bulgarian perimenopausal women towards hormone replacement, which is also probably due to the fact that some women after the menopause are satisfied with their quality of life. Sixty-one per cent of them accept the menopausal status as a normal period of their life, compared to 39% who consider the menopause as a disease. Forty-two per cent of the interviewed patients expect some treatment for menopausal problems, but only 60% of them consider hormones to be the right choice. As in other similar studies worldwide, women visit perimenopausal care units after advice mainly from friends and relatives and because of subjective complaints, and not because of the wish to prevent undesirable effects[3,4]. One positive outcome emerging from the study is that more than 95% of the patients considered their menopausal knowledge to be insufficient in 1997 and 1998, whereas in 1999 85% reported that they were familiar with some symptoms of the climacteric. This awareness indicates the potential of further patient education[5].

The fact that the majority of Bulgarian perimenopausal women still accept the menopause as something natural, rather than as a disease which requires medical assistance and care, is in agreement with unpublished results from other investigations of the Bulgarian Menopause Association which show similar views amongst many physicians. In the end, the cost of replacement therapy seems to be unaffordable for a big percentage of the interviewed women, and only 14% of them considered the price of HRT as 'reasonable'.

The presented surveys have some limitations. A stratification of the participating women according to education level was performed only in the Gallup survey. Furthermore, hysterectomized women, those more health conscious and more physically active, and those with a different lifestyle were not subdivided properly.

However, the analysis of the data shows that a broad educational campaign among both doctors and patients is required to achieve an improvement in perimenopausal care in Bulgaria and a positive shift in consumer and professional attitudes towards the menopause and HRT.

References

1. Rozenbaum H. Menopause in Europe: the state of the art. In Rozenbaum H, Birkhaeuser M, eds. *European Consensus Development Conference on Menopause.* Paris: ESKA Editions, 1996:13–23
2. Rozenberg S, Vandromme J, Kroll M, *et al.* Compliance to HRT. *Int J Fertil* 1996;41(Suppl 1):352–61
3. Itzhak SB, Pines A, Eckstein N, *et al.* Adapting to the menopause: psychological aspects. *Eur Menopause J* 1997;4:91–4

4. Sarrel RS. HRT in the menopause. *Int J Fertil* 1997; 42:78–84
5. Hunter MS. Psychological aspects of the climacteric and postmenopause. In Studd JWW, Whitehead MI, eds. *The Menopause*. Oxford, London, Edinburgh: Blackwell Scientific Publications, 1990:55–62

Women's health care in Sweden: primary care in the menopause, actual versus ideal 32

B.-M. Landgren

Sweden is a country with a population of approximately 8 000 000 inhabitants. Approximately 1.6 million are women at or above the age of 50 years. The use of hormone replacement therapy (HRT) in women aged 50–59 years has increased during recent years, as shown in Figure 1, which shows sale statistics for HRT expressed as daily doses per 1000 individuals from 1980–98. This increase is evenly distributed throughout the country, as shown in Figure 2, which shows the number of prescriptions per county. The use of HRT is thus not concentrated in the large cities, Stockholm, Gothenburg and Malmö, as might be expected. HRT is mainly prescribed by gynecologists and general practitioners. It is approved by the health authorities for the treatment of climacteric symptoms, osteoporosis prophylaxis and the treatment of urogenital symptoms. In Figure 3, the daily doses of HRT, divided into medium-dose oral estrogens, low-dose oral estrogens and low-dose local estrogens, per 1000 women are shown for different age groups. Most HRT, mainly medium-dose oral estrogens, was prescribed to the 50–59-year-old age group. However, there were women as old as 95 years and above using low-dose estrogens. This indicates that the main reason for HRT use is still the treatment of climacteric symptoms, although there are some older women using HRT for osteoporosis prophylaxis and for the treatment of urogenital symptoms. These groups are expected to increase in the future.

Most information about HRT for women is given by the media – mainly women's weekly journals, but also the radio, television and press.

Knowledge and management strategies concerning HRT were investigated among gynecologists and general practitioners in Sweden in 1997[1]. Fifteen per cent of the general practitioners participating in the study often considered it difficult to evaluate the advantages and disadvantages of HRT, compared to 2% of the gynecologists ($p < 0.001$). Almost 100% of the physicians considered hot flushes, night sweats and osteoporosis to be indications for HRT. Significantly more general practitioners than gynecologists (50% versus 24%) stated that estrogen increased the risk of developing a deep venous thrombosis. Significantly more general practitioners than gynecologists performed measurements of blood pressure, weight and lipoprotein levels and palpated the breasts

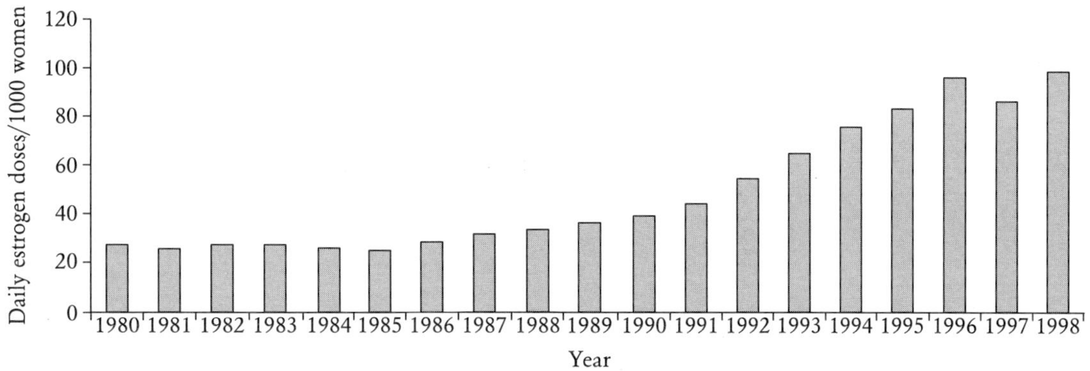

Figure 1 Estrogen use in Sweden from 1980 to 1998, expressed in daily doses sold per 1000 individuals

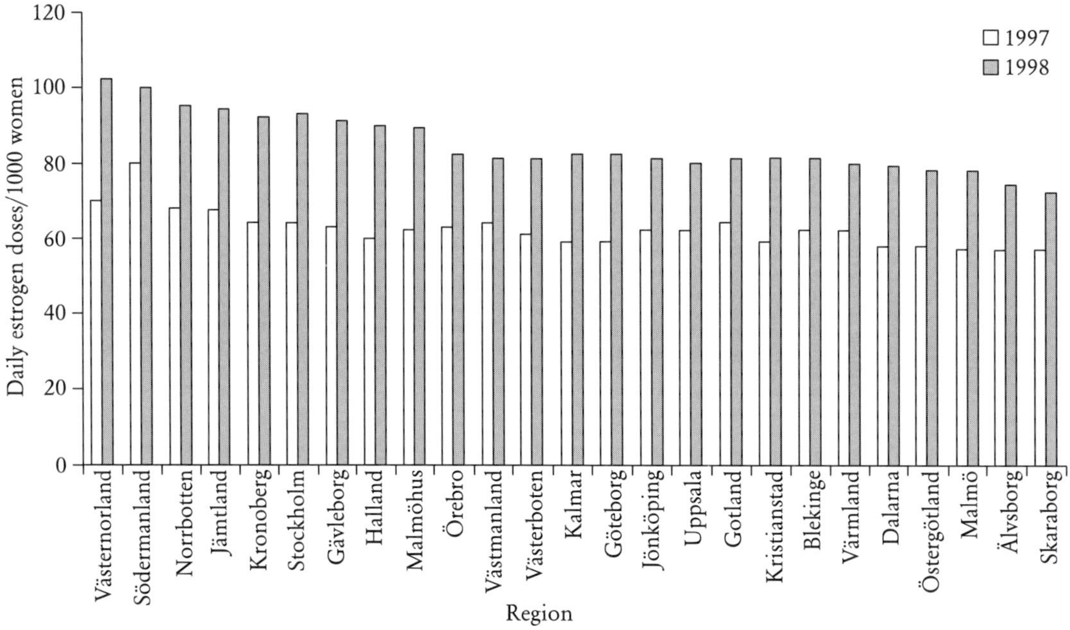

Figure 2 Estrogen use in different regions of Sweden in 1997 and 1998

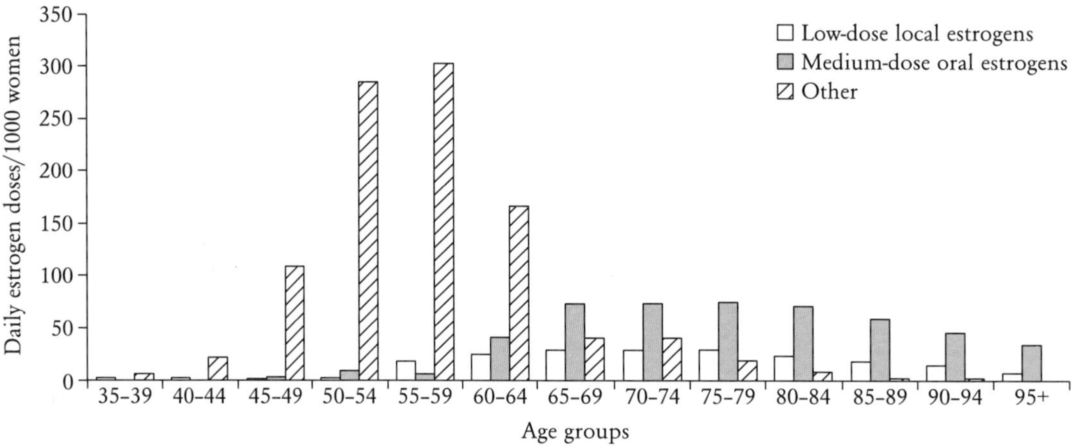

Figure 3 Estrogen use (low-dose local estrogens, medium-dose oral estrogens and other (mainly low-dose oral) estrogens) in different age groups in Sweden, 1998

before starting treatment and at the follow-up visits. Significantly more gynecologists than general practitioners performed pelvic examinations, vaginal sonography, endometrial biopsies and mammography. Among the female doctors who were either postmenopausal or had climacteric symptoms, 72% of the general practitioners and 88% of the gynecologists were current users of HRT ($p < 0.01$). Corresponding figures for the wives were 68% and 86%, respectively ($p < 0.001$). The fact that far more female doctors and doctors' wives use HRT compared to the Swedish female population is important when discussing HRT compliance with patients, and also points to the importance of giving information to women.

In Sweden, we are planning special women's health outpatient clinics, which ideally will meet the special health-care needs of women. These centers will be multidisciplinary and have specialists in the following disciplines: gynecology, oncology, pathology, cardiology, dermatology, urogynecology, internal medicine, physiotherapy, psychiatry and rheumatology. The center will specialize in treating neglected female health problems, such as incontinence, bleeding disturbances, depression, and drug and alcohol addiction. Screening will be performed for human immunodeficiency virus, cervical cancer, breast cancer and osteoporosis. Family planning and sexual advice will be provided by gynecologists and midwives. Women will be offered appointments at short notice (1–2 days) and, as mentioned above, the expertise needed to give them the best health care will be available. The center will give information to women about the menopause, reproductive health and women's health. This information will be given by midwives leading study groups. In addition, lectures will be given by doctors on topics related to women's health. The women will also be advised about literature concerning women's health.

Reference

1. Andersson K, Pedersen AT, Mattsson LÅ, Milson I. Swedish gynecologists' and general practitioners' views on the climacteric period: knowledge, attitudes and management strategies. *Acta Obstet Gynecol Scand* 1998;77:909–16

Diet and exercise: do they influence health outcomes during the menopausal transition? 33

J. R. Guthrie

INTRODUCTION

Diet and exercise are widely recommended to maintain and improve health. Information provided for mid-aged women by menopause clinics and general practitioners includes recommendations on diet and exercise[1]. Books written for the lay public also provide general information on these topics[2]. There is no argument that both these behaviors are important in the maintenance of health and well-being. What is unclear is the best prescription for exercise and dietary intake that will improve health outcomes during the transition from pre- to postmenopause. This menopausal transition phase is associated with the occurrence of a number of bothersome symptoms, in particular vasomotor symptoms[3,4], adverse changes in body composition[5-7] and cardiovascular risk factors[8,9]. These changes have far-reaching consequences on future health status. This article examines evidence of the effect of diet and exercise on vasomotor symptoms, body composition and cardiovascular risk factors during the menopausal transition.

VASOMOTOR SYMPTOMS

Diet

Phytoestrogens are plant compounds which have a close similarity in structure to estrogens, and it is hypothesized that they will have an estrogenic effect in women and relieve vasomotor and other menopausal symptoms. Two review articles[10,11] have reported on the sources, metabolism, intakes and biological effects of these substances in humans. Knight and Eden[10] reviewed 861 articles published between 1980 and 1995, and Murkies and colleagues[11] reviewed over 600 articles between 1975 and 1996. Both reports concluded that phytoestrogens exhibit biological properties in humans, but further work is needed to establish the effect of phytoestrogens on menopausal symptoms.

Evidence for the effects of phytoestrogens on reducing vasomotor symptoms comes from two main sources. The first source is epidemiological data from populations who have high dietary intakes of phytoestrogen compounds, for example Japanese women, who have a very low rate of vasomotor symptoms (5–10% compared with 70–80% in Western women). Japanese women are reported to consume 20–150 mg/day of isoflavones, with levels up to 200 mg/day[11,12], compared to Western women where less than 5 mg/day is consumed[13]. Second, information comes from placebo-controlled trials.

There are problems with both these sources of information. Whether Japanese women do in fact experience a significantly lower frequency of vasomotor symptoms has been challenged[14]. Evidence from controlled trials is limited owing to the difficulty of finding an effective control group, as phytoestrogens are present in so many foods that it is difficult to eliminate them from the diet completely, and the fact that natural improvement of vasomotor symptoms occurs with time. Six studies[15-20] have reported improvement in vasomotor symptoms after dietary supplementation with phytoestrogens. In four of these studies[15-18] there was also an improvement in the placebo groups, and this highlights the limitations of these studies (resolution of vasomotor symptoms over time and placebo effect). In one of these studies[18] there was an increase in urinary isoflavone excretion in the placebo group. Subjects must have obtained isoflavones from their diets. There was a strong correlation between the level of urinary isoflavone excretion and the incidence of vasomotor symptoms in both treatment and placebo groups combined. This further emphasizes the problem with intervention studies using naturally occurring dietary compounds. Larger studies are required in which dietary patterns of both treatment and placebo groups are carefully documented.

Hot beverages can cause flushing through countercurrent heat exchange, mediated via the thermoregulating center of the anterior hypothalamus. Foods containing nitrites and sulfites, and spicy foods such as those containing the active agent in red pepper or capsaicin, may also provoke severe flushing. Avoidance of these foods is recommended in the peri- and postmenopause, to reduce hot flushing due to causes other than declining estrogen levels.

In a cross-sectional population-based study of Australian-born women[21], those who experienced several or more hot flushes a day consumed less caffeine than the women who did not experience hot flushes, although this difference was not statistically significant. The women experiencing these vasomotor symptoms may have reduced their intake of caffeine and/or hot drinks as a coping strategy.

There are no controlled trials looking at the effect of alcohol intake on the severity of menopausal symptoms, in particular vasomotor symptoms. Advice to menopausal women recommends the reduction of alcohol intake[1]. The origin of this advice is probably that alcohol is associated with flushing reactions. The mechanism of alcohol-provoked flushing is complex, but is probably related to the fact that fermented alcoholic beverages contain tyramine or histamine, which induces flushing.

Exercise

It has been suggested that physical activity may have a beneficial effect on reducing vasomotor symptoms in menopausal women. Physical exercise, involving increased energy expenditure, increases hypothalamic β-endorphin production, and β-endorphins are reported to stabilize thermoregulation[22]. However, conflicting evidence exists as to whether exercise does have an effect on menopausal symptoms.

In a cross-sectional study of a population-based sample of 728 Australian-born women[23], physical activity had no significant effect on women's experience of troubling symptoms, including those symptoms associated with their menopausal status such as vasomotor symptoms. Others[24] have reported that women who participated in organized physical exercise on a regular basis had a lower prevalence of moderate to severe vasomotor symptoms compared with women of the same menopausal status from the population. A further study by these researchers[22] reported from a population of 793 women that only 5% of highly physically active women experienced severe vasomotor symptoms, compared with 14–16% of women who had little or no weekly exercise.

The latter study collected data on physical habits and on current and previous experience of vasomotor symptoms. There is the risk of women overestimating the time spent in physical activities as well as the problem of retrospective reporting of vasomotor symptoms. A prospective or intervention study would avoid these problems. However, the fluctuating nature of the experience of vasomotor symptoms and the expectations of participants could affect such studies. A case-control study[25] (82 cases and 89 controls) found that habitual exercise prior to the final menstrual period did not reduce the likelihood of experiencing vasomotor symptoms during the perimenopause.

BONE MINERAL DENSITY

The menopausal transition heralds the start of metabolic changes that, in the postmenopausal years, are associated with an increased incidence of obesity, a change in fat distribution, a decrease in lean body mass, a decrease in bone mineral density (BMD) and an increase in fracture rates[5,26]. The effects of exercise and diet on changes in BMD are dealt with in this section and the other changes are discussed in relation to cardiovascular disease in the following section.

During the transition to postmenopause, i.e. through the perimenopause to 12 months after the final menstrual period, accelerated bone loss from both the lumbar spine and femoral neck has been reported[6,27]. The results, in a population-based cohort of Australian-born women, were a loss of

2.5% per year of BMD from the lumbar spine and 1.7% from the femoral neck over this transition period[6]. These values were similar in other populations, a loss of 2.3% per year for lumbar spine[27] and 1.8% at the femoral neck[28] being reported in European studies.

Diet: calcium

The results of studies concerning the relationship between dietary calcium intake and the effect of calcium supplementation on bone loss during the menopausal transition and in the postmenopause have not been concordant. Heaney[29] reviewed 42 studies published since 1988 that related calcium intake to bone mass, bone loss or bone fragility. Twenty-six reported that calcium intake was associated in some way with bone mass or fracture, and 16 did not. The controlled intervention studies suggest that calcium supplementation (1000 mg or more) can slow down postmenopausal bone loss. This effect can be more easily demonstrated in women who are more than 5 years postmenopausal[29]. The data seem not to support a positive effect of calcium on preventing bone loss in women in the peri- and early-postmenopausal years.

In the Melbourne Women's Mid-life Health Project there was no influence of calcium intake on bone density in both cross-sectional and prospective studies[6,30]. Thirty-three per cent of this cohort did have a calcium intake greater than 1000 mg per day, and in 19% of the women the intake was 400 mg per day with a mean intake of 870 mg per day. During the menopausal transition, bone loss appears to be caused overwhelmingly by estrogen withdrawal, and calcium levels are probably not having a major influence on bone during this period[31].

Other epidemiological studies have variously reported either a weak[32] relationship or no[33,34] relationship at all between diet and bone mass. Earnshaw and colleagues[34] did find a significant positive correlation between dietary calcium and serum osteocalcin, a marker of bone formation, in early-postmenopausal women. The maximal effect of a calcium supplement appears to occur with doses of approximately 1000 mg per day[35], although no published study is able to say how much calcium is actually needed.

Other dietary factors

The evidence relating to the effect of dietary phytoestrogens on bone loss in humans is sparse. Dietary soy supplementation has been reported to increase total bone mineral content in postmenopausal women in one study[36], while another found no preventive effect on postmenopausal cortical bone loss[37]. Vitamin D is necessary for the normal absorption of calcium from the intestine, and a low vitamin D status is attributed to low dietary intake, decreased skin exposure to the sun or impaired synthesis of vitamin D in the skin. Vitamin D deficiency is a problem in institutionalized elderly people, in people not exposed to sufficient sunlight and particularly in countries where fortification of food with this vitamin is not practised. Dietary caffeine induces a negative calcium balance through increased urinary loss, and prospective data show an increase in risk of hip fracture[38]. In cross-sectional studies of perimenopausal women, caffeine intake has been shown to be associated with low bone density of the ultradistal radius[39] but not of the hip and spine[30].

The work of Devine and colleagues, who studied women 10 years past the menopause, found that a high sodium intake, measured as urinary sodium excretion, was associated with increased bone loss at the hip[40]. Data pertaining to effects of moderate amounts of alcohol on bone metabolism, osteoporosis or fracture risk are limited, and evidence from population studies has been conflicting, with most finding no effect of alcohol intake on bone density in pre- and postmenopausal women[41].

Exercise

Cross-sectional studies demonstrate that individuals with a history of exercise in various sports have greater bone mass than their sedentary counterparts[42], as do women who have a history of occupational physical activities[43]. However, these cross-sectional studies on the effect of exercise on bone density are subject to inherent bias, and there is little prospective information on the effects of exercise on bone density during the menopausal transition. A recent study[44] reported that mid-life women who were habitually exercising vigorously more than twice a week had higher total body bone mineral content than those women involved in light to moderate activity no more than once per week. These currently physically active women had also been physically active throughout their lives, so it is difficult to evaluate in this cross-sectional study whether the observed bone mineral content is due to benefits accrued from exercise during growth and development or continued habitual physical activity or, as is most likely, both. There is some evidence that exercise can slow bone loss or add bone mass to the postmenopausal skeleton, although the amounts are site-specific and relatively modest, and the activity needs to be high-load resistance exercises. This evidence comes from prospective intervention studies in which, on the whole, small numbers were involved and studies were short in duration and have the potential for selection and other biases[45–49].

The customary physical activity of an Australian-born population of 224 women has not been shown to have any effect on bone loss at the femoral neck or lumbar spine during the menopausal transition[6]. The effect of hormonal change at this time may over-ride any protective effects of physical activity. However, an 18-month intervention study of a similar menopausal status group[50] reported that an endurance training regime maintained femoral neck BMD, compared with a control group who lost bone at this site. The endurance training was performed four times per week for 18 months, and the 50-min session included intervals of walking, jogging, ergometer cycling, stair-climbing and graded treadmill exercises.

CARDIOVASCULAR RISK FACTORS

Women tend to gain weight and undergo an alteration in their fat distribution in mid-life[51,52]. Whether these changes are related to the menopause, age or life-style remains controversial. The risk of coronary heart disease (CHD) rises with increasing body mass index (BMI)[53]. A major portion of the increase in coronary risk is attributable to the influence of excess weight on blood lipid levels, glucose intolerance and blood pressure, although a moderate residual effect persists which may be due to other mechanisms[53]. In a longitudinal study of risk factors for CHD, only one risk factor, high-density lipoprotein (HDL) cholesterol, showed a statistically significant pattern of change suggesting an association with the menopause itself, although the change in HDL cholesterol across the menopausal transition was small[8]. Observed changes in other blood lipids, diastolic blood pressure and BMI during the menopause were related either to the women's increasing age or to simultaneous changes in other risk factors. The factor that had the most adverse influence on cardiovascular risk was high BMI[8].

Diet

There are two aspects to consider when discussing the effect of diet on cardiovascular risk factors. The first is balancing energy input with energy output, thus preventing weight gain, and this will be considered in the exercise section below. The second is looking at the association of various nutrients and cardiovascular risk factors.

There is little information on dietary and risk-factor data during the actual menopausal transition, but studies on these relationships have been evaluated in pre- and postmenopausal women. A population-based sample of 695 pre- and 727 postmenopausal women reported that plasma triglycerides were inversely related to protein, fiber and polyunsaturated fat and directly related to saturated fat and oleic acid (a monounsaturated fatty acid)[54]. In contrast, other studies have found that oleic acid lowers serum triglyceride levels[55]. This difference can be explained by the source of the oleic acid. If oleic acid in the diet is derived from animal products, which are also high in saturated fat, rather than from vegetable sources of monounsaturated fats, there will be an increase in triglyceride levels. Plasma total and low-density lipoprotein (LDL) cholesterol levels were also directly associated with the intake of total fat, oleic acid and animal fat but not dietary cholesterol, and inversely associated with carbohydrate intake[56]. Millen and colleagues[56] reported that diet explains 2% of the variance in plasma lipid levels in a cross-sectional population-based sample of pre- and postmenopausal women. Alcohol intake has been reported to be significantly directly related to HDL cholesterol levels in pre- and most postmenopausal women[54,57]. However, in certain groups of women categorized by apolipoprotein E phenotype, alcohol consumption may be detrimental to HDL cholesterol levels[54].

While cross-cultural studies have established a cardioprotective effect of phytoestrogens, particularly soy proteins[58], the benefits of these substances in controlled trials have only recently been evaluated and evidence is still accumulating. A meta-analysis of 38 published trials reported prior to 1995 found that soy protein consumption was associated with reductions in total and LDL cholesterol and triglyceride levels. More recently, Washburn and colleagues[59] reported that soy supplementation in the diet of healthy perimenopausal women resulted in significant declines in total and LDL cholesterol and diastolic blood pressure.

Exercise

Cross-sectional studies have found an association between exercise and BMI in mid-life women[23,60]. However, longitudinal studies have not consistently found an association between exercise and weight changes during the mid-life period[7,51]. A mean increase in weight of 2 kg over 5 years was reported in a population-based cohort of mid-life Australian-born women aged 46–57 years at baseline[7]. This weight gain was not related to change in menopausal status or to any life-style factors measured, and women who were older at baseline gained less weight than the younger members. In an American study of mid-life women[51] a weight gain of 2 kg occurred over a 3-year period that was also not related to the menopause *per se*, but women who increased their physical activity over the study period gained significantly less weight.

Weight gain occurs because of a discrepancy between energy intake and energy expenditure. The most variable component of daily energy expenditure is the thermic effect of physical activity, which includes energy expended in addition to that expended due to resting metabolic rate and the thermic effect of a meal. It has been reported that resting metabolic rate declines with age, and that this decline may be accelerated by the normal menopausal transition[5]. This decline in energy expenditure during rest may be related to the increase in body fat and decline in fat-free mass observed in postmenopausal women, and, although there may not be any change in the hours they spend in leisure-time exercise, their energy expenditure may also be reduced. Thus, this general decline in daily energy expenditure without a proportional reduction in food intake would lead to a period of positive energy imbalance and weight gain.

A 6-month randomized clinical trial involving life-style changes in both diet and physical activity in women aged 44–50 years who were pre- or early-perimenopausal resulted in significant weight loss and reductions in serum total cholesterol, LDL cholesterol and triglycerides[61]. Waist/hip ratio and blood pressure also declined, although there was no increase in HDL cholesterol. The life-style intervention included walking 10 miles per week over 3–5 days and reducing the intake of total fat, saturated fat and dietary cholesterol. In another controlled study, postmenopausal women walking for 60 min, 3 or 5 days per week, showed no change in serum lipids after 6 months[62]. However, there was a small (1%) decrease in percentage body fat, significantly different from that in the sedentary control group.

In longitudinal studies[8,51], changes in some cardiovascular risk factors, i.e. HDL cholesterol, LDL cholesterol, triglycerides and blood pressure appear to be more dependent on changes in other risk factors, in particular BMI, rather than changes in menopausal status. Cross-sectional studies of mid-life and older women have found associations between high physical activity levels and low blood pressure, high HDL cholesterol and low BMI[23,63,64]. Several prospective cohort studies found that increases in physical activity were associated with favorable changes in HDL cholesterol[65,66]. In Australian-born women, on average, an increase of 0.04 mmol/l in HDL cholesterol was achieved with an increase of 1000 kcal/week of physical activity[65]. This is approximately equivalent to walking an extra 5 h per week. Smaller decreases in HDL were reported in menopausal American women who exercised at moderate intensity for 20 min three times per week, compared with women who exercised less[66].

CONCLUSIONS

Further large placebo-controlled trials are needed to test the effect of dietary phytoestrogens on vasomotor symptoms before a recommendation about their efficacy can be made. There is little evidence to support an association between exercise and vasomotor symptoms.

More research is needed to find an exercise program that is easy to implement, is inexpensive and could maintain bone density in the perimenopausal and postmenopausal periods. Although calcium may not make a difference to bone loss during the menopausal transition, there is evidence for its benefit in the postmenopause. All women entering the menopausal transition should have their baseline dietary habits assessed, and recommendations should be made to achieve a calcium intake of at least 1000 mg per day.

Evidence for both exercise and dietary interventions in reducing cardiovascular risk is very favorable. Further randomized clinical trials investigating different exercise and dietary regimes to promote weight loss or weight maintenance in menopausal women are needed. An increase in knowledge about the metabolic and body composition changes that are occurring during the normal menopausal transition may help in planning better intervention programs.

References

1. MacLennan A. Running a menopause clinic. *Baillière's Clin Endocrinol Metab* 1993;7:243–53
2. Dennerstein L, Shelley JM, eds. *A Woman's Guide to Menopause and Hormone Replacement Therapy*. Washington, DC: American Psychiatric Press Inc, 1998
3. Dennerstein L, Smith AMA, Morse C, *et al.* Menopausal symptoms in Australian women. *Med J Aust* 1993;159:232–6
4. Avis NE, Kaufert PA, Lock M, *et al.* The evolution of menopausal symptoms. *Baillière's Clin Endocrinol Metab* 1993;7:17–32
5. Poehlman ET, Tchernof A. Traversing the menopause: changes in energy expenditure and body composition. *Coronary Artery Dis* 1998;9:799–803
6. Guthrie JR, Ebeling PR, Hopper JL, *et al.* A prospective study of bone loss in menopausal Australian-born women. *Osteoporosis Int* 1998;8: 282–90
7. Guthrie J, Dennerstein L, Dudley E. Weight gain and the menopause: a 5 year prospective study of a population-based cohort. *Climacteric* 1999;2:205–11
8. Do KA, Green A, Guthrie JR, Dudley EC, Burger HG, Dennerstein L. A longitudinal study of risk factors for coronary heart disease across the menopausal transition. *Am J Epidemiol* 1999; in press
9. Barrett-Connor E. Heart disease in women. *Fertil Steril* 1994;62:127S–32S
10. Knight DC, Eden JA. A review of the clinical effects of phytoestrogens. *Obstet Gynecol* 1996;87:897–904
11. Murkies AJ, Wilcox G, Davis SR. Phytoestrogens. *J Clin Endocrinol Metab* 1998;83:297–303
12. Adlercreutz H, Honjo A, Higashi A, *et al.* Urinary excretion of lignans and isoflavonoid phytoestrogens in Japanese men and women consuming traditional Japanese diet. *Am J Clin Nutr* 1991;54: 1093–100
13. Coward L, Barnes NC, Setchell KDR, Barnes S. The antitumor isoflavones, genistein and daidzein, in soybean foods of American and Asian diets. *J Agric Biol Chem* 1993;41:19961–7
14. Albery N. Plenary lecture. Politics of the menopause. Presented at the *8th International Congress on the Menopause*, Sydney, Australia, November 1996
15. Murkies AL, Lombard C, Strauss BJG. Dietary flour supplementation decreases postmenopausal hot flushes: effect of soy and wheat. *Maturitas* 1995;21:189–95
16. Harding C, Morton M, Gould V. Dietary supplementation is oestrogenic in postmenopausal women. Presented at the *2nd International Symposium on the Role of Soy in Preventing and Treating Chronic Disease*, Brussels, Belgium, September 1996: abstr
17. Knight DC, Howes JB, Eden JA. The effect of Promensil, an isoflavone extract, on menopausal symptoms. *Climacteric* 1999;2:79–84
18. Baber RJ, Templeman T, Morton GE, *et al.* Randomized placebo-controlled trial of an isoflavone supplement and menopausal symptoms in women. *Climacteric* 1999;2:85–92

19. Brzezinski A, Adlercreutz H, Shaoul R. Short-term effects of phytoestrogen-rich diet on postmenopausal women. *Menopause* 1997;4:89–94
20. Albertazzi P, Pansini F, Bonaccorsi G, *et al.* The effect of dietary soy supplementation on hot flushes. *Obstet Gynecol* 1998;1:6–11
21. Guthrie JR, Dennerstein L, Hopper JL, *et al.* Hot flushes, menstrual status, and hormone levels in a population-based sample of midlife women. *Obstet Gynecol* 1996;88:437–42
22. Ivarson T, Spetz A-C, Hammar M. Physical exercise and vasomotor symptoms in postmenopausal women. *Maturitas* 1998;29:139–46
23. Guthrie JR, Smith AMA, Dennerstein L, *et al.* Physical activity and the menopause experience: a cross-sectional study. *Maturitas* 1995;20:71–80
24. Hammar M, Berg G, Lindgren R. Does physical exercise influence the frequency of hot flushes? *Acta Obstet Gynecol Scand* 1990;69:409–12
25. Sternfield B, Quesberry CP, Husson G. Habitual physical activity and menopausal symptoms: a case-control study. *J Women's Health* 1999;8:115–23
26. Greendale GA, Lee NP, Arriola ER. The menopause. *Lancet* 1999;353:571–80
27. Pouilles JM, Tremollieres F, Ribot C. The effects of menopause on longitudinal bone loss from the spine. *Calcif Tissue Int* 1993;52:340–3
28. Pouilles JM, Tremollieres F, Ribot C. Effect of menopause on femoral and vertebral bone loss. *J Bone Miner Res* 1995;10:1531–6
29. Heaney RP. Thinking straight about calcium. *N Engl J Med* 1993;328:503–5
30. Guthrie JR, Ebeling PR, Hopper JL, *et al.* Bone mineral density and hormone levels in menopausal Australian women. *Gynecol Endocrinol* 1996;10: 199–205
31. Nordin BE, Need AG, Steurer T, *et al.* Nutrition, osteoporosis, and aging. *Ann NY Acad Sci* 1998;854: 336–51
32. Elders PJM, Netelenbos JC, Lips P, *et al.* Perimenopausal bone mass and risk factors. *Bone Miner* 1989;7:289–99
33. Stevenson JC, Whitehead MI, Padwick M, *et al.* Dietary intake of calcium and postmenopausal bone loss. *Br Med J* 1988;297:15–17
34. Earnshaw SA, Worley A, Hosking DJ for the Nottingham early postmenopausal intervention cohort study group. Current diet does relate to bone mineral density after the menopause. *Br J Nutr* 1997;78:65–72
35. Dawson-Hughes B. Calcium supplementation and bone loss: a review of controlled clinical trials. *Am J Clin Nutr* 1991;54:274S–80S
36. Dalais FS, Rice GE, Wahlqvist ML, *et al.* Effects of dietary phytoestrogens in postmenopausal women. *Climacteric* 1998;1:124–9
37. Kardinaal AF, Morton MS, Bruggemann-Rotgans IE, *et al.* Phyto-oestrogen excretion and rate of bone loss in postmenopausal women. *Eur J Clin Nutr* 1998;52:850–5
38. Hernandez-Avila M, Colditz GA, Stampfer MJ, *et al.* Caffeine, moderate alcohol intake, and risk of fractures of the hip and forearm in middle-aged women. *Am J Clin Nutr* 1991;54:157–63
39. Hernandez-Avila M, Stampfer MJ, Ravnikar VA, *et al.* Caffeine and other predictors of bone density among pre- and perimenopausal women. *Epidemiology* 1993;4:341–8
40. Devine A, Criddle RA, Dick IM, *et al.* A longitudinal study of the effect of sodium and calcium intakes on regional bone density in postmenopausal women. *Am J Clin Nutr* 1995;62:740–5
41. Faine MP. Dietary factors related to preservation of oral and skeletal bone mass in women. *J Prosthet Dent* 1995;73:65–72
42. Stillman RJ, Lohman TG, Slaughter MH, *et al.* Physical activity and bone mineral content in women aged 30 to 85 years. *Med Sci Sports Exercise* 1986;18:576–80
43. Damalakis J, Perisinakis K, Kontakis G, *et al.* Effect of lifetime occupational physical activity on indices of bone mineral status in healthy postmenopausal women. *Calcif Tissue Int* 1999;64:112–16
44. Uusi-Rasi K, Sievanen H, Vuori I, *et al.* Associations of physical actvity and calcium intake with bone mass and size in healthy women at different ages. *J Bone Miner Res* 1998;13:133–42
45. Pruitt LA, Jackson RD, Bartels RL, Lehnhard HJ. Weight-training effects on bone mineral density in early postmenopausal women. *J Bone Miner Res* 1992;7:179–85
46. Nelson ME, Fiatarone MA, Morganti CM, *et al.* Effects of high-intensity strength training on multiple risk factors for osteoporotic fractures. A randomized controlled trial. *J Am Med Assoc* 1994; 272:1909–14
47. Kerr D, Morton A, Dick IM, *et al.* Exercise effects on bone mass in postmenopausal women are site-specific and load-dependent. *J Bone Miner Res* 1996; 11:218–25
48. Kohrt WM, Ehsani AA, Birge SJ Jr. Effects of exercise involving predominantly either joint-reaction or ground-reaction forces on bone mineral density in older women. *J Bone Miner Res* 1997;12:1253–60
49. Pruitt LA, Taaffe DR, Marcus R. Effects of a one-year high intensity versus low intensity training program on bone mineral density in older women. *J Bone Miner Res* 1995;11:1788–95
50. Heinonen A, Oja P, Sievanen H, *et al.* Effect of two training regimens on bone mineral density in healthy perimenopausal women: a randomized controlled trial. *J Bone Miner Res* 1998;13:483–90

51. Wing RR, Matthews KA, Kuller LH, Meilahn EN, Plantinga PL. Weight gain at the time of the menopause. *Arch Intern Med* 1991;151:97–102
52. Svendsen OL, Hassager C, Christiansen C. Age- and menopause-associated variations in body composition and fat distribution in healthy women as measured by dual-energy X-ray absorptiometry. *Metabolism* 1995;44:369–73
53. Manson JE, Colditz GA, Stampfer MJ, *et al.* A prospective study of obesity and risk of coronary heart disease in women. *N Engl J Med* 1990;322:882–9
54. Sonnenberg LM, Quatromoni PA, Gagnon DR, *et al.* Diet and plasma lipids in women. II. Macronutrients and plasma triglycerides, high-density lipoprotein, and the ratio of total to high-density lipoprotein cholesterol in women: the Framingham nutrition studies. *J Clin Epidemiol* 1996;49:665–72
55. Mensink RP, Katan MB. Effect of monounsaturated fatty acids versus complex carbohydrates on high density lipoproteins in healthy men and women. *Lancet* 1987;1:122–5
56. Millen BE, Franz MM, Quatromoni PA, *et al.* Diet and plasma lipids in women. I. Macronutrients and plasma total and low-density lipoprotein cholesterol in women: the Framingham nutrition studies. *J Clin Epidemiol* 1996;49:657–63
57. Razay G, Heaton KW, Bolton CH, *et al.* Alcohol consumption and its relation to cardiovascular risk factors in British women. *Br Med J* 1992;69:145–53
58. Adlercreutz H. Western diet and western diseases: some hormonal and biochemical mechanisms and associations. *Scand J Clin Lab Suppl* 1990;201:3–23
59. Washburn S, Burke GL, Morgan T, *et al.* Effect of soy protein supplementation on serum lipoproteins, blood pressure, and menopausal symptoms in perimenopausal women. *Menopause* 1999;6:7–13
60. Samaras K, Kelly PJ, Chiano MN, *et al.* Genetic and environmental influences on total-body and central abdominal fat: the effect of physical activity in female twins. *Ann Intern Med* 1999;130:873–82
61. Simkin-Silverman L, Wing RR, Hansen DH, *et al.* Prevention of cardiovascular risk factor elevations in healthy premenopausal women. *Prev Med* 1995; 24:509–17
62. Ready AE, Naimark B, Ducas J, *et al.* Influence of walking volume on health benefits in women postmenopause. *Med Sci Sports Exercise* 1996;28: 1097–105
63. Reaven PD, Barrett-Connor E, Edelstein S. Relation between leisure-time physical activity and blood pressure in older women. *Circulation* 1991; 83:559–65
64. Cauley JA, La Porte RE, Sandler RB, *et al.* The relationship of physical activity to high density lipoprotein cholesterol in postmenopausal women. *J Chronic Dis* 1986;39:687–97
65. Guthrie JR, Dudley EC, Hopper JL, *et al.* Changes in physical activity and health outcomes in a population-based cohort of midlife Australian-born women. *Aust NZ J Public Health* 1997;21:1–6
66. Owens JF, Matthews KA, Wing RR, *et al.* Can physical activity mitigate the effects of aging in middle-aged women? *Circulation* 1992;85:1265–70

Exercise and bone in the postmenopausal years: a reality check

34

B. L. Drinkwater

In 1997, a telephone survey of 751 women was conducted to assess the attitudes of women aged 50 and older towards osteoporosis - what it is, strategies for prevention and treatment options. One of the surprising outcomes of the survey was that only 44% of the women received information about osteoporosis from their primary care physician; most reported getting their knowledge from the news media, books, or community organizations. Perhaps that explains their response to the question, 'What things are most effective in helping to prevent osteoporosis in women past menopause?' The women overwhelmingly identified calcium and exercise as the two most important factors in preventing the disease (Figure 1). Almost three-quarters of the women believed that good posture would prevent bone loss. Hormone replacement therapy (HRT) or other therapies were seldom mentioned. Exercise (87%) and calcium (87%) again ranked high as methods of treating osteoporosis. HRT came in fifth in the voting (57%) following good posture (73%) in popularity.

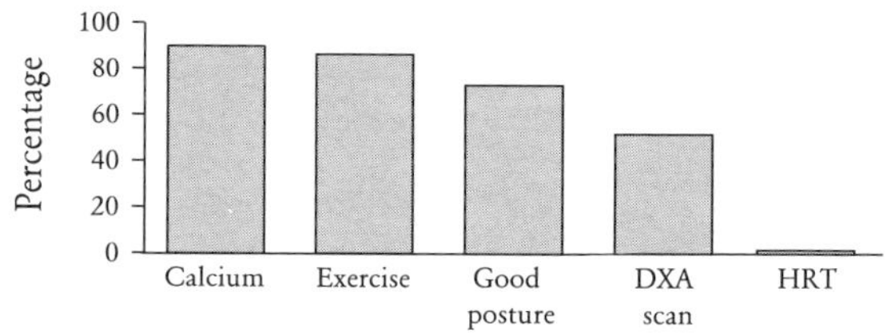

Figure 1 What women 50 years and older believed was most important in preventing osteoporosis. DXA, dual energy X-ray absorptiometry; HRT, hormone replacement therapy

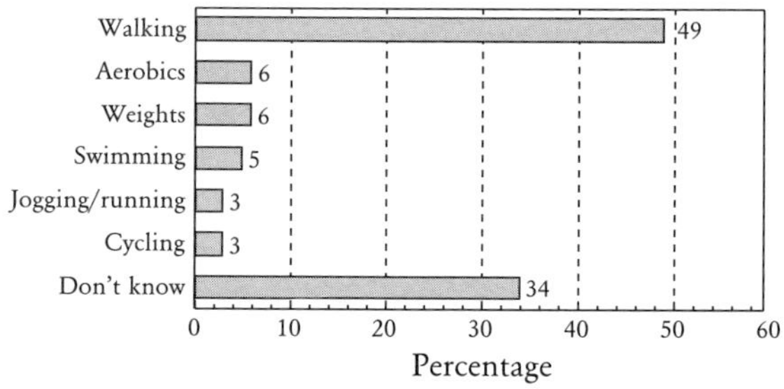

Figure 2 The type of exercise women 50 years and older believed was best for building bone

The exercise most women believed was helpful in building bone was walking (Figure 2). It is not surprising then to find that walking was the most popular form of exercise for these women (75%). We have found a similar reliance on physical activity and calcium as well as 'natural' therapies to prevent bone loss among women who volunteer for our research studies. Are these women correct in their assumptions? What is the role of exercise in the prevention of osteoporosis in the postmenopausal years?

Lanyon[1] theorizes that estrogen and mechanical loading are interrelated in their effect on bone tissue, that a decrease in estrogen diminishes the osteogenic response to mechanical loading. Therefore, to maintain bone mass following the menopause would require an increase in loading beyond that customary in the premenopausal years. If this theory is correct, women choosing exercise in place of HRT would have to increase the intensity of their exercise to prevent bone loss. Whether such an increase in stress on bone is possible or even safe is unknown at this time. On the other hand, the osteogenic effect of physical activity would remain the same in women on HRT and presumably prevent bone loss.

There are other factors to consider as well. The observation that athletes, male and female, have a greater bone mass than sedentary individuals led to the hope that exercise might prevent osteoporosis by enabling young adults to achieve their genetic potential for peak bone mass and then slow or

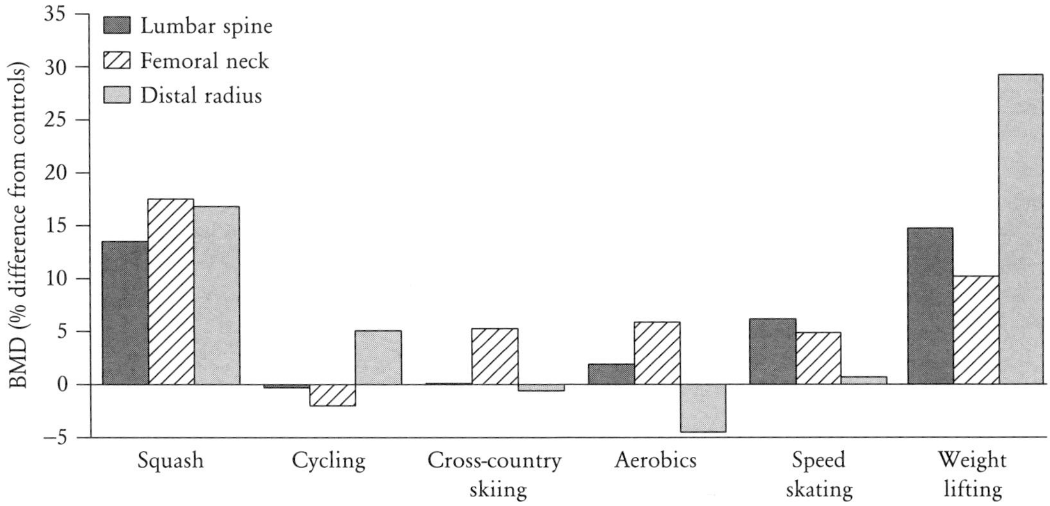

Figure 3 The bone mineral density (BMD) of female athletes at the lumbar spine, the femoral neck and the distal radius

prevent bone loss during the postmenopausal years. Early studies focused on the skeletal effects of a general activity program, with little attention paid to the principles known to be important in training other physiological systems[2]. For example, the effect of mechanical loading on bone mass is specific to the site being loaded (Principle of Specificity) as shown by the bone density data from athletes in different sports (Figure 3)[3]. To prevent osteoporotic fractures, an activity program should be designed to target those skeletal areas where the most serious osteoporotic fractures occur: the hip, spine, wrist and humerus. It is equally important to consider the Principle of Overload: there will be an increase in bone mass *only* if the mechanical stress placed on the bone by the activity exceeds the level to which the bone has adapted[4]. An exercise program, therefore, must be carefully planned to target the areas where fractures occur and continuously increase the load on those sites.

One reason for the lack of a clinically significant increase in bone mineral density (BMD) in the majority of studies[5-8] may be a reluctance to have older women exercise at an intensity that would elicit an osteogenic response. Whether a more demanding protocol would result in a greater gain in bone mass is not known. Obviously the intensity of the activity must be suited not only to a woman's skeletal status but also to her muscular strength, her cardiovascular risk and the condition of other physiological systems. It is understandable why investigators may err on the side of caution in planning their exercise protocols for older women.

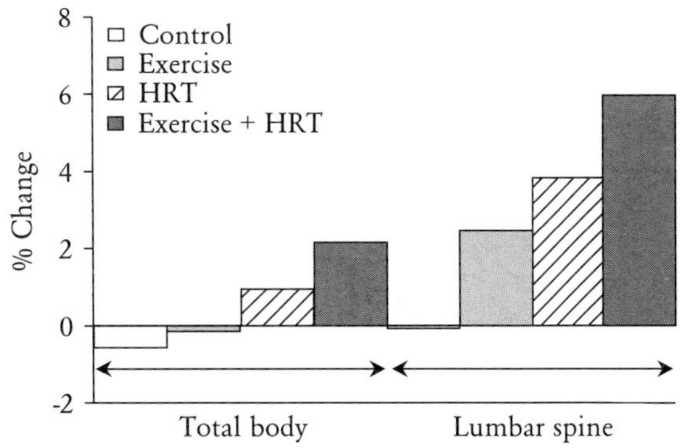

Figure 4 The percentage change in bone mineral density (BMD) of postmenopausal women divided into four groups: controls; those taking exercise only; those on hormone replacement (HRT) only; and those taking exercise plus HRT. Based on data in reference 10

Perhaps a more likely explanation for the seeming lack of effect of the exercise on bone in older women lies in the selection of the study subjects. Invariably the women in these studies are not on hormone therapy. Recent studies by Notelovitz and co-workers[9] and Kohrt and co-workers[10] have demonstrated clearly that women on HRT who exercise gain significantly more bone than women on either HRT or exercise alone (Figure 4). In our laboratory we have looked at the BMD of postmenopausal elite master rowers, women who exercise 5–6 times per week at an intensity far above that possible for the average woman[9]. It is clear from our data that athletes on HRT have significantly higher BMD at both the spine and the proximal femur than those who have chosen not to use HRT (Figure 5).

Although the results of prospective exercise studies in postmenopausal women not on HRT have been rather pessimistic, most do show either a slight increase or no loss in the exercise group. The relatively small increments in BMD are unlikely to show marked effects on the immediate fracture risk for these women. However, if exercise can slow bone loss with increasing age or deter additional decrements in BMD due to inactivity, it may prevent an even greater risk in the future. There are other factors that affect risk as well. While BMD is the best predictor of fracture in the postmenopausal years, the benefit of an active lifestyle may have more to do with these other factors than with changes in bone itself. The active woman is more likely to maintain muscular strength, co-ordination, balance and agility – all factors that decrease the risk of falling and improve her chance of protecting herself from serious injury if she does fall. It is also possible that architectural changes within the bone in response to the mechanical loading may provide protection against fracture but may not be discernable by densitometry measurement.

Clinicians should be assured that they cannot go wrong in prescribing exercise to healthy women of any age. The recent Surgeon General's report in the United States, *Healthy People 2000*[12], listed the following benefits accruing from regular physical activity:

(1) Reduces the risk of:

   (a) Dying from heart disease;
   (b) Developing diabetes;
   (c) Developing hypertension;
   (d) Developing colon cancer;
   (e) Dying prematurely.

(2) Helps:

   (a) Control weight;

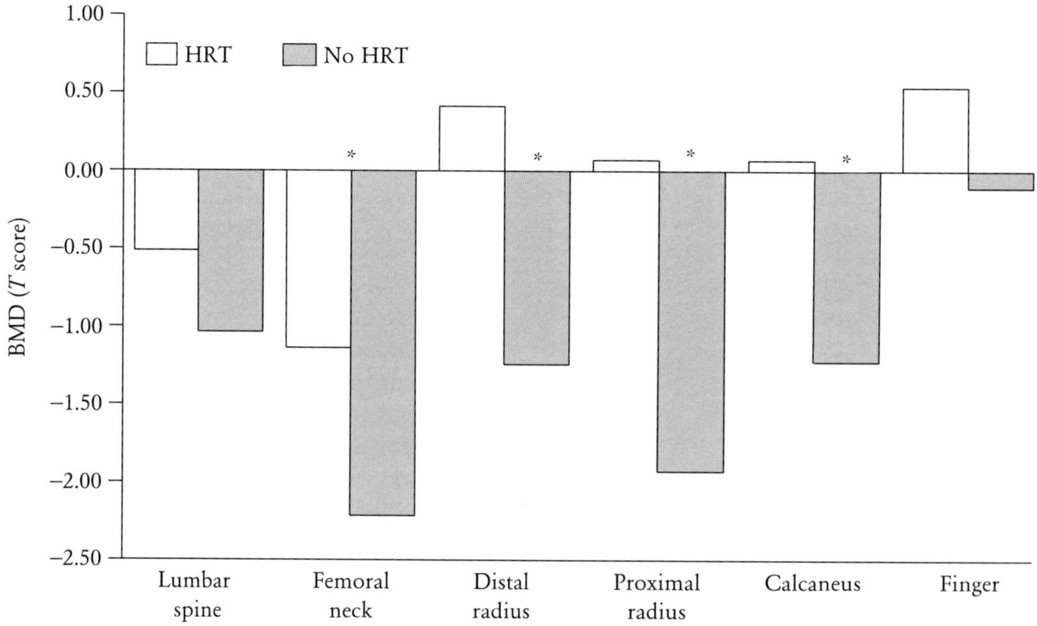

Figure 5 Bone mineral density (BMD) at six skeletal sites for elite master rowers who were more than 4 years postmenopausal. Groups were divided into those women who selected hormone replacement therapy (HRT) and those who did not. Asterisks indicate significant differences ($p < 0.05$)

(b) Build and maintain healthy bones, muscles and joints;
(c) Older adults become stronger and better able to move without falling;
(d) Promote psychological well-being.

As remarkable as these benefits are, postmenopausal women must be cautioned that exercise alone will not prevent bone loss in the postmenopausal years. Further epidemiological research is needed to determine whether a physically active woman, who is stronger and better co-ordinated, and has better balance, has fewer osteoporotic fractures than a sedentary woman with the same BMD.

CONCLUSIONS

On the basis of current research, the best advice for the woman concerned with protecting her bone health is to discuss available therapies with her physician - therapies that have been shown to be effective in preventing both bone loss and osteoporotic fractures. To avoid the bone loss that occurs from inactivity, she should look for opportunities to be physically active. It is important to remember that the skeleton, like all other physiological systems, will retain the beneficial effects of exercise only as long as the activity is continued. If the woman decreases her exercise, bone density will return to its pretraining levels very quickly. It is important to emphasize that exercise is not an alternative to hormone replacement therapy at menopause but an adjunct therapy. At this time there is no evidence that exercise alone can prevent significant bone loss during the postmenopausal years.

References

1. Lanyon LE. Using functional loading to influence bone mass and architecture: objectives, mechanisms, and relationship with estrogen of the mechanically adaptive process in bone. *Bone* 1996; 18:37–43S
2. Drinkwater BL. Does physical activity play a role in preventing osteoporosis? *Res Q Exerc Sport* 1994;65: 197–206
3. Heinonen A, Oja P, Kannus P, *et al.* Bone mineral density in female athletes representing sports with different loading characteristics of the skeleton. *Bone* 1995;17:197–203
4. Frost HM. Skeletal structural adaptations to mechanical usage (SATMU): 2. Redefining Wolff's law: the remodeling problem. *Anat Rec* 1990;226: 414–22
5. Martin D, Notelovitz M. Effects of aerobic training on bone mineral density of postmenopausal women. *J Bone Miner Res* 1993;8:931–6
6. Nelson ME, Fisher EC, Dilmanian FA, Dallal GE, Evans WJ. A 1-y walking program and increased calcium in postmenopausal women: effects on bone. *Am J Clin Nutr* 1991;53:1304–11
7. Nichols JF, Nelson KP, Peterson KK. Bone mineral density responses to high-intensity strength training in active older women. *J Age Phys Act* 1995;3: 26–38
8. Pruitt LA, Jackson RD, Bartels RL, *et al.* Weight-training effects on bone mineral density in early postmenopausal women. *J Bone Miner Res* 1992;7: 179–85
9. Notelovitz M, Martin D, Tesar R, *et al.* Estrogen therapy and variable resistance weight training increases bone mineral in surgically menopausal women. *J Bone Miner Res* 1991;6:583–90
10. Kohrt WM, Snead DB, Slatopolsky E, Birge SJ. Additive effects of weight-bearing exercise and estrogen on bone mineral density in older women. *J Bone Miner Res* 1995;10:1303–11
11. Nattrass SM, Drinkwater BL. Effect of hormone replacement therapy on bone density of postmenopausal master rowers. *Med Sci Sport Exerc* 1999;31: S287
12. DHHS. *Healthy People 2000.* Publication No.(PHS) 91-50212. Washington, DC: US Government Printing Office, 1990:55

Physical activity, obesity and menopause 35

K. Kawakubo and J. S. Lee

INTRODUCTION

Obesity is a major health problem for women, especially during the climacteric. The Japanese National Nutrition Survey in 1997[1] has shown that, in males, the body mass index (BMI) increases during their 30s and reaches a peak in their 40s. On the contrary, in females, the BMI is low in their 20s and increases during their 40s and 50s to reach a peak in their 60s. Furthermore, the incidence of obesity in the middle-age group has increased recently in Japan. Obesity is associated with many metabolic abnormalities, which lead to premature morbidity from cardiovascular disease. Lipoprotein and glucose metabolic abnormalities are the major problems of obese women[2,3]. Metabolic abnormalities of obese women are also influenced by their menopausal state, age and physical activity level. The Japanese National Nutrition Survey[1] found that cholesterol levels in women increase after the age of 50 years and overtake the levels in males. This rise in cholesterol after the age of 50 years is related to the menopause[4]. However, the effects of lifestyle factors, such as physical inactivity and increased energy intake, are more important than the unchangeable menopausal state. The aim of this study was to investigate whether the effects of lifestyle modification on metabolic abnormalities in middle-aged obese women differ depending on their menopausal state. We therefore investigated the effects of a 12-week weight-reduction program on lipoprotein and glucose metabolism in middle-aged obese women. The differences in the effects between premenopausal and postmenopausal women were compared.

METHODS

The 12-week weight-reduction program was performed from 1991 to 1998 at a community-based health promotion center in the metropolitan area of Tokyo. Subjects were 265 women aged 35–65 years, recruited by community-based newsletter during the 8 years of the study. Their mean age was 48.5 years. Among the study subjects were 251 obese women with a clear menstrual history, who had BMI of more than 24. They were divided into premenopausal and postmenopausal groups, according to their menstrual history.

The duration of the weight-reduction program was 12 weeks. The program had a 2-day food intake survey, and energy intake was restricted to 1600 kcal/day. A dietitian was consulted with regard to individual food intake habits. Energy intake was calculated using a semi-quantitative food frequency questionnaire[5]. Subjects had a pedometer and were instructed to increase their daily walking steps to 10 000 per day. They participated in a group lecture concerning obesity, lifestyle factors and nutrition, and attended an aerobics class once a week. The intensity of aerobic exercise was low in order to avoid orthopedic injury.

Medical examinations were performed before and after the program. They consisted of body composition, physical fitness test, blood pressure determination and blood chemistry measurements in the morning fasting state. The percentage of body fat mass was estimated by two-site skinfold measurements (subscapular and mid-triceps), using calipers. Waist and hip circumferences were measured and the waist to hip ratio was calculated. Endurance capacity as a measure of physical fitness was determined using a cycle ergometer, and physical working capacity at 75% of the age-predicted maximum heart rate was calculated. Blood pressure was measured in the sitting position using a sphygmomanometer. Blood chemistry measurements consisted of total cholesterol, high-density lipoprotein (HDL) cholesterol, triglyceride, plasma glucose and fasting insulin. The low-density lipoprotein (LDL) cholesterol value was calculated using the Freidewald equation.

The differences in the measurements between the premenopausal and postmenopausal groups were compared before the program using Student's *t* test. After the program, Welch's test was used to compare the effects of the program on the two groups.

RESULTS

The anthropometric data before the program were compared between the 149 premenopausal women and the 102 postmenopausal women (Table 1). The mean ages of the pre- and postmenopausal women were 43.9 and 55.4 years, respectively. Body weight, BMI and the percentage of body fat mass did not differ between the two groups. Their mean body weights at 20 years old were within the normal range, but the value was lower in postmenopausal women. The waist to hip ratio was significantly higher in the postmenopausal women. Walking steps were higher and energy intake was lower in the postmenopausal group; furthermore, the physical working capacity at 75% of the age-predicted maximum heart rate was lower in the postmenopausal group.

Arterial blood pressure and blood chemistry data before the program are shown in Table 2. Postmenopausal women had higher values of systolic blood pressure, diastolic blood pressure,

Table 1 Anthropometric and lifestyle data before the weight-reduction program. Comparison between the pre- and postmenopausal women. Values are mean ± SD where appropriate

	Premenopausal women (n = 149)	*Postmenopausal women* (n = 102)	*p Value**
Age	43.9 ± 4.9	55.4 ± 5.0	
Body weight (kg)	64.5 ± 8.3	63.0 ± 6.7	NS
Body weight at 20 years (kg)	51.5 ± 7.0	48.8 ± 5.5	0.001
BMI	26.8 ± 3.0	26.8 ± 2.5	NS
Body fat mass (%)	36.5 ± 7.8	36.7 ± 6.8	NS
Waist to hip ratio	0.91 ± 0.07	0.94 ± 0.08	0.006
Walking steps/day	5930 ± 2179	6940 ± 2731	0.003
Energy intake (kcal)	1940 ± 407	1831 ± 372	0.037
PWC at 75% of the age-predicted max. HR	82.4 ± 23.3	74.5 ± 25.6	0.014

*From Student's *t* test; BMI, body mass index; PWC, physical working capacity; max. HR, maximum heart rate; NS, not significant

Table 2 Medical examination data before the weight-reduction program. Comparison between the pre- and postmenopausal women. Values are mean ± SD where appropriate

	Premenopausal women (n = 149)	*Postmenopausal women* (n = 102)	*p Value**
SBP (mmHg)	117.9 ± 15.1	127.4 ± 18.5	0
DBP (mmHg)	76.0 ± 10.4	80.8 ± 11.7	0.001
Total cholesterol (mg/dl)	212.4 ± 41.3	232.3 ± 36.8	0
HDL cholesterol (mg/dl)	56.4 ± 13.2	58.8 ± 15.0	NS
LDL cholesterol (mg/dl)	135.1 ± 38.6	149.4 ± 35.0	0.003
Triglyceride (mg/dl)	106.3 ± 65.7	120.1 ± 65.9	NS
FPG (mg/dl)	97.6 ± 30.3	99.2 ± 17.9	NS
Insulin (μU/ml)	8.7 ± 4.2	8.0 ± 3.4	NS

*From Student's *t* test; SBP, systolic blood pressure; DBP, diastolic blood pressure; HDL, high-density lipoprotein; LDL, low-density lipoprotein; FPG, fasting plasma glucose; NS, not significant total cholesterol and LDL cholesterol than premenopausal women. HDL cholesterol, triglyceride, fasting plasma glucose and fasting insulin did not differ between the two groups.

Among the 251 women who participated in the weight-reduction program, 206 women completed the program (82.1% adherence rate). Anthropometric data before and after the program were compared between the 118 premenopausal women and 88 postmenopausal women (Table 3). The mean body weight decreased by 2.8 kg in both groups and the difference was not significant. The decreases in the percentage of body fat mass and the waist to hip ratio also did not differ significantly between the two groups. The walking steps increased by 3750 steps in the premenopausal group and 3658 steps in the postmenopausal group. These increments were not significantly different between the two groups. The energy intake decreased by 300 kcal in the premenopausal group and 154 kcal in the postmenopausal group. The reduction in energy intake was significantly smaller in the postmenopausal women.

The differences in the medical examination data are shown in Table 4; these results were compared between the premenopausal and postmenopausal women (Table 4). Systolic blood pressure, diastolic blood pressure, total cholesterol, LDL cholesterol, triglyceride, fasting plasma glucose and insulin all significantly decreased after the program. HDL cholesterol did not change significantly. The differences between the premenopausal women and the postmenopausal women were not significant.

Table 3 Anthropometric and lifestyle data before and after the weight-reduction program. Comparison between the pre- and postmenopausal women. Values are mean ± SD where appropriate

	Premenopausal women (n = 118)		*Postmenopausal women* (n = 88)		
	Before	*After*	*Before*	*After*	*Welch's test*†
Body weight (kg)	64.2 ± 7.7	61.4 ± 7.2***	62.6 ± 6.8	59.8 ± 6.6***	NS
Body fat mass (%)	36.3 ± 7.1	33.0 ± 6.4***	36.7 ± 7.0	33.7 ± 6.3***	NS
Waist to hip ratio	0.92 ± 0.07	0.90 ± 0.07***	0.94 ± 0.07	0.92 ± 0.07**	NS
Walking steps/day	5995 ± 2210	9745 ± 2789***	7046 ± 2779	10 704 ± 3566***	NS
Energy intake (kcal)	1919 ± 427	1619 ± 288***	1825 ± 368	1671 ± 300***	**

†Difference between the pre- and postmenopausal women; Student's t test (difference before and after program): *$p < 0.05$, **$p < 0.01$, ***$p < 0.001$; NS, not significant

Table 4 Medical examination data before and after the weight-reduction program. Comparison between the pre- and postmenopausal women. Values are mean ± SD where appropriate

	Premenopausal women (n = 118)		*Postmenopausal women* (n = 88)		
	Before	*After*	*Before*	*After*	*Welch's test*†
SBP (mmHg)	118.6 ± 15.1	109.6 ± 9.0***	127.2 ± 16.7	119.0 ± 16.0***	NS
DBP (mmHg)	76.5 ± 10.1	71.5 ± 8.8***	80.9 ± 11.1	75.8 ± 9.6***	NS
Total cholesterol (mg/dl)	212.9 ± 42.3	200.9 ± 34.5***	233.6 ± 35.9	220.3 ± 32.5***	NS
HDL cholesterol (mg/dl)	56.9 ± 13.5	57.8 ± 12.5	59.7 ± 15.2	60.9 ± 14.9	NS
LDL cholesterol (mg/dl)	136.6 ± 38.6	127.8 ± 33.0***	149.8 ± 34.2	140.6 ± 32.5**	NS
Triglyceride (mg/dl)	101.2 ± 60.7	77.4 ± 40.4***	118.6 ± 66.2	92.7 ± 52.2***	NS
FPG (mg/dl)	99.2 ± 33.7	94.3 ± 18.6*	99.8 ± 18.8	96.1 ± 17.4**	NS
Insulin (μU/ml)	8.7 ± 4.4	7.1 ± 3.1***	8.2 ± 3.5	6.5 ± 2.2***	NS

†Difference between the pre- and postmenopausal women; Student's t test (difference before and after program): *$p < 0.05$, **$p < 0.01$, ***$p < 0.001$; SBP, systolic blood pressure; DBP, diastolic blood pressure; FPG, fasting plasma glucose; NS, not significant

DISCUSSION

In this study, we investigated the differential effects of a weight-reduction program on lipoprotein and glucose metabolism in premenopausal and postmenopausal obese women. Before the program, postmenopausal women had higher values of waist to hip ratio, systolic blood pressure, diastolic blood pressure and LDL cholesterol than premenopausal women, although both groups had the same BMI and percentage body fat mass. The 12-week weight-reduction program was equally effective in reducing LDL cholesterol, triglyceride and fasting plasma glucose in pre- and postmenopausal women.

Postmenopausal women had higher LDL cholesterol levels than premenopausal women, although both groups had the same BMI and percentage body fat mass. The metabolic abnormalities of obese women are influenced by the menopause. After the menopause, estrogen decreases, resulting in increases in LDL cholesterol and triglyceride and a decrease in HDL cholesterol[6]. However, in our study, triglyceride and HDL cholesterol did not differ between pre- and postmenopausal women. Our study subjects were all obese women. The effects of the menopause on HDL cholesterol and triglyceride might be small in obese women.

Postmenopausal women had a higher waist to hip ratio than premenopausal women. The distribution of body fat changes after the menopause and central obesity predominates[7]. Central obesity is more associated with metabolic abnormalities than peripheral obesity[8]. When we perform a body composition study of obese women, we should focus on body fat distributions, such as the waist, waist to hip ratio and waist to stature ratio[9]. Postmenopausal women had a higher blood pressure than the premenopausal group. This may be more related to aging and physical inactivity than the menopause.

Physical activity and fitness also influence metabolic abnormalities of obese women, by increasing blood pressure and glucose and decreasing HDL cholesterol[10,11]. The mean walking steps per day of the study population were approximately 6000–7000. Walking steps per day is a surrogate measure of physical activity. According to the Japanese National Nutrition Survey, the mean walking steps of women in their 40s and 50s were 8200 and 8100, respectively, in 1997[1].

The 12-week weight-reduction program was equally effective in pre- and postmenopausal women. After 12 weeks, mean body weight decreased by 2.8 kg and the waist to hip ratio also decreased. This was achieved by an increase in the number of walking steps and a decrease in energy intake. This indicates that a modification in lifestyle can change the degree of central obesity, irrespective of the menopausal state.

The effects of weight reduction on metabolic abnormalities were the same between pre- and postmenopausal women. All metabolic data except HDL cholesterol improved, irrespective of the menopausal state. Total cholesterol and LDL cholesterol decreased by approximately 10 mg/dl in both groups. According to the National Nutrition Survey in 1997, the mean total cholesterol level of women in their 40s and 50s was 201 mg/dl and 209 mg/dl, respectively. The total cholesterol levels of our study subjects after the program were near these values. In Japan, the cholesterol level has increased by 10 mg/dl over the past 10 years. A modification in lifestyle could reverse this increase in cholesterol levels in obese women. HDL cholesterol did not change significantly, while triglyceride decreased significantly. One study has shown that women only have a small increase in HDL cholesterol after exercise training because of the high value before training[12]. Energy intake restriction might also influence the HDL change after the weight-reduction program.

Fasting plasma glucose and insulin decreased after the program. This indicates that the insulin sensitivity increased after the program, irrespective of the menopausal state. The prevalence of non-insulin-dependent diabetes mellitus has recently increased rapidly in Japan. A national survey on diabetes in 1997 revealed that about one-tenth of people over 40 years of age are diabetic. This rise in diabetes prevalence after the age of 40 years is not related to the menopause. The rapid rise of diabetic prevalence in Japan might be related to the very rapid transition of lifestyle after the war, that is, from poor diets and high physical activity to Western diets and low physical activity.

In conclusion, many factors, such as menopause, aging and physical inactivity, bring about the metabolic abnormalities of obese women. However, by changing the modifiable factors, many of the abnormalities could be changed.

ACKNOWLEDGEMENT

We greatly thank the staff members of the weight-reduction program at the health promotion center.

References

1. Ministry of Health and Welfare. *National Nutrition Survey*, 1997
2. Baumgartner RN, Roche AF, Chumlea WC, *et al.* Fatness and fat patterns: associations with plasma lipids and blood pressures in adults, 18 to 57 years of age. *Am J Epidemiol* 1987;126:614–48
3. Hartz AJ, Rupley DC, Kalkohoff RD, *et al.* Relationship of obesity to diabetes; influence of obesity level and body fat distribution. *Prev Med* 1983;12:351–7
4. Mathews KA, Meilahn E, Kuller LH, *et al.* Menopause and risk factors for coronary heart disease. *N Engl J Med* 1989;321:641–6
5. Katagiri A, Hashimoto S, Ohashi Y, *et al.* Reproducibility and validity of a semi-quantitative food frequency questionnaire. *Jpn J Public Health* 1998; 45:1127–36
6. Bengtsson C, Lindquist O. Menopausal effects on risk factors for ischemic heart disease. *Maturitas* 1979;1:165–70
7. Shimokata H, Tobin JD, Muller DC, *et al.* Studies in the distribution of body fat. 1. Effects of age, sex and obesity. *J Gerontol* 1989;44:M66
8. Sjostrom L, Kvist H. Regional body fat measurements with CT-scan and evaluation of anthropometric predictions. *Acta Med Scand Suppl* 1988;723: 169–77
9. Lee JS, Kawakubo K. A useful index highly correlated with coronary risk factors for community based obesity screening. *Jpn J Public Health* 1999;46: 89–102
10. Owens JW, Matthews KA, Wing RR, *et al.* Physical activity and cardiovascular risk: a cross-sectional study of middle-aged premenopausal women. *Prev Med* 1990;19:147–50
11. Kawakubo K, Yanagibori R, Gunji A. Physical fitness, coronary risk factors and menopause. *J Jpn Menopause Soc* 1994;2:178–84
12. Lokey EA, Tran ZV. Effects of exercise training on serum lipid and lipoprotein in women: a meta-analysis. *Int J Sports Med* 1989;10:424–9

Obesity, stress and menopause

36

T. Moskovic and N. Antic

INTRODUCTION

Obesity is generated by an imbalance between energy (food) intake and energy expenditure (mainly resting metabolism and physical activity) followed by excess storage of triacylglycerides in the adipocytes, resulting in enhancement of total body mass. What causes this imbalance between consuming and burning calories is unclear. Evidence suggests that obesity often has more than one cause. Genetic, ethnic, sex-related, cultural, social, endocrine, metabolic, thermogenetic, psychological, exercise-related, life-style-dependent, and nutrient- as well as drug-induced factors all may play a part.

Obesity in adults is defined in terms of body mass index (BMI), which is weight divided by the square of the height in kg/m^2. A BMI of 25 is ordinarily taken as the upper limit of normal, with the span 25–29.9 considered to be overweight and 30 or greater to be obesity. At the upper cut-off level of 28 kg/m^2 the prevalence of co-morbidity with aging becomes definitively higher than in lean populations[1].

PREVALENCE

In Western culture, women tend to consume high-fat diets, often putting taste and convenience ahead of nutritional content when choosing meals. Most women also do not undertake enough exercise. The prevalence of obesity varies depending on the definition used. In the UK, 39% of men and 32% of women were considered overweight on the basis of a BMI of 25 or greater, but only 6% of men and 8% of women were defined as obese[2]. According to the Nurses' Health Study cohort[3], it has been found that about 25% of American women from 35 to 64 years of age have a BMI of 29 kg/m^2 or higher, leading to the phenomenon that, at any time, 25–50% of adult Americans are attempting to reduce their weight by dieting[4]. Sixteen per cent and 40% of the German population are obese or overweight, respectively[5].

ANATOMICAL OBESITY

Although BMI or measures of total adiposity show important relationships with measures of risk, there are much stronger relationships with the abdominal or visceral partitioning of adipose tissue[6].

Gynoid obesity (pear shape) refers to fat distribution in the lower body, while android obesity (apple shape) refers to central body distribution. Gynoid obesity is more resistant to catecholamines and more sensitive to insulin than abdominal fat. This is associated with minimal fatty acid flux and, therefore, the negative consequences of fatty acid metabolism are less. Android obesity refers to fat located in the abdominal wall and visceral-mesenteric locations. This fat is more sensitive to catecholamines and less sensitive to insulin and, thus, more active metabolically[7].

RELATIONSHIP OF STRESS TO VISCERAL OBESITY

It seems possible that psychological factors might provide a background for visceral obesity. Reactions to stress may be followed by either a fight-or-flight reaction, stimulating mainly the catecholaminergic system, or a depressive, defeatist, helplessness type of response. The latter is characterized endocrinologically by a hyperactivity of the hypothalamic–pituitary–adrenal (HPA) axis. Therefore, a depressive reaction to stress would be an interesting background candidate for pathogenesis of the syndrome of visceral obesity. Various socioeconomic and psychosocial factors (low education, physical type of work, low social class, problems at work, prolonged stress in war condition), amplified by associated alcohol and smoking habits, may be of importance for the induction of a stress reaction of the depressive, helplessness type with activation of the HPA axis and visceral obesity as its somatic consequences[8].

Corticotropin-releasing hormone (CRH) or arginine vasopressin induces the secretion of higher than normal levels of adrenocorticotropic hormone (ACTH) and cortisol[9]. There is considerable evidence that this type of reaction is followed by inhibition of other peripheral endocrine axes by CRH and/or cortisol[10]. An elevated response to challenge of the HPA axis would then be followed not only by increased secretions of adrenal hormones (cortisol and androgens), but also by an inhibition of secretion of growth hormone[11] and sex steroid hormone. Cortisol in the presence of insulin seems to stimulate lipid-accumulating metabolic pathways[12]. These effects are more pronounced in adipose tissue regions that have a high density of steroid hormone receptors, where visceral adipocytes seem to occupy a leading position. Because visceral adipose tissue seems to have a rich blood flow and a dense innervation, endocrine changes resulting in effects on adipose tissue metabolism would be more pronounced in visceral depots than in other depots[13].

PATHOGENIC ROLE OF VISCERAL ADIPOSE TISSUE

Visceral fat has a rapid turnover and high sensitivity for lipolytic stimuli. With excess visceral fat, portal free fatty acids (FFAs) would then be expected to be elevated, particularly in situations such as starvation and stress. Increased FFA levels may indicate signs of insulin resistance. Elevation of insulin secretion may result in fewer inhibitory effects on lipolysis from visceral depots, leaving higher concentrations of uninhibited FFAs in the portal vein. FFAs seem to be the driving mechanism for hepatic synthesis and secretion of very high-density lipoproteins. In addition, FFAs inhibit insulin uptake in hepatocytes and decrease hepatic clearance of insulin in the liver and visceral obesity. This can then contribute to hyperinsulinemia[14]. Both hyperinsulinemia and insulin resistance in obese subjects are seen to be independent risk factors for coronary heart disease (CHD). Visceral obesity is associated with an increase in androgen production rate, decreased levels of sex hormone binding globulin and increases of free testosterone and estradiol.

Obesity and hypertestosteronemia are both independently and synergistically associated with hyperinsulinemia and dyslipidemia[15].

Angiotensinogen is secreted by adipose tissue in quantities second only to those secreted by the liver[16]. Furthermore, tumor necrosis factor-α (TNF-α), which reduces tyrosine kinase activity of the insulin receptor in obese animals, is also secreted, leading to the hypothesis that adipocyte-derived TNF-α might be involved in the development of insulin resistance in obese patients.

WHAT ARE THE CONSEQUENCES OF OBESITY?

Obesity is not just a cosmetic problem but a health hazard. It has been linked to several serious medical conditions.

Diabetes

Hyperinsulinemia in patients with visceral obesity is associated with normal plasma glucose levels, indicating that an excess of insulin is required for glucose homeostasis in such patients (glucose tolerance, euglucemia). If circulating glucose levels exceed the cut-off value in an oral glucose tolerance test, an impaired glucose tolerance (hyper-, normoinsulinemia, glucose intolerance, euglucemia) is diagnosed, which finally results in the non-insulin-dependent diabetes mellitus (NIDDM) (normo-hypoinsulinemia, hyperglycemia).

Hypertension

One of the most common complications of obesity is hypertension, which improves or reverses with weight reduction[2]. The cause of hypertension is uncertain. Peripheral resistance appears to be increased, coupled with a higher cardiac output[17]. Obese subjects have increased basal and stimulated levels of norepinephrine as well as plasma renin and aldosterone[18].

Stroke

Most studies of the association between obesity and stroke have found little if any adverse effect. The search for causality is confounded by the close association between obesity and other risk factors for stroke, although the Framingham Study has suggested that obesity is an independent risk factor if it is given a long enough period of exposure[19]. Because the effects of obesity may be gradual in development, a lifelong history of obesity may be more important in assessment of stroke risk than current weight in middle age.

Cardiovascular disease

In most Western societies, obesity carries a two-fold risk of CHD in both men and women.

It is now well established that those with visceral obesity are at highest risk of cardiovascular disease, so estimates of risk based on BMI or other crude measures alone will underestimate the risk associated with specific types of obesity. Upper-body obesity appears to be associated with a higher risk in older women, probably via its concomitant diabetes, hypertriglyceridemia, hyperinsulinemia and hypertension. A waist/hip ratio greater than 0.8 is associated with substantially greater coronary risk for women[20].

In the Framingham Study[19], obesity was identified as a significant independent predictor of cardiovascular disease, especially among women, although obesity as a CHD risk factor is obviously also mediated by the metabolic consequences of, or factors associated, with obesity: elevated total cholesterol, triglyceride and low-density lipoprotein (LDL) cholesterol levels; lower high-density lipoprotein (HDL) cholesterol levels; glucose intolerance, insulin resistance, hyperuricemia and hypertension. The 16-year follow-up data from the Nurses' Health Study identified a doubled coronary risk in mild to moderate obesity[21]. However, to adjust for factors that are among the mechanisms by which obesity brings about vascular disease seems illogical in trying to establish etiology.

Reproductive system

Obese women have a decreased concentration of sex hormone binding globulin (SHBG). It has been assumed that the percentage of free estradiol is increased. Conversion of androstenedione to estrone is increased in both pre- and postmenopausal women. Premenopausally at least, it has been postulated that the ovarian production of estrogen is so large that the increase from peripheral overproduction of estrone does not contribute to menstrual disorders. Continued overproduction of estrogens peripherally may be important in menopausal obese women, in whom it could play a role in both dysfunctional bleedings and development of uterine cancer. Secondary amenorrhea and hirsutism are not uncommon, nevertheless. The cause appears to be increased androgen production and increased free testosterone fraction. A significant proportion of the androgen excess appears to derive from the adrenal gland.

Cancer

Obesity is also associated with higher rates of certain types of cancer. Obese women are more likely than non-obese women to die from cancer of the gall bladder. In females, there is up to a three-fold increase in the incidence of breast, cervical and ovarian cancer. The risk of endometrial cancer is up to seven times higher for obese women. Obese individuals with increased insulin levels have lower levels of insulin-like growth factor binding protein-1 (IGFBP-1)[22]. This lower level of IGFBP-1 would allow greater local activity of insulin-like growth factor-I (IGF-I) in the ovary and increased androgen production. Greater IGF-I activity in the endometrium due to reduced levels of IGFBP-1, and direct insulin activation of IGF-I receptors, are possible mechanisms of endometrial growth and the increased risk for endometrial cancer in these patients[23].

Osteoporosis

Chronically elevated C-18 steroid levels in obese patients are thought to be responsible for less osteoporosis.

Gall bladder disease

Obesity is also complicated by gallstones. Approximately 25% of obese individuals have gallstones, frequently resulting in surgery. The supersaturated bile, because of enhanced biliary secretion of cholesterols, is one of the major reasons for increased incidence of gallstones.

Degenerative arthritis

Obesity is frequently complicated by osteoarthritis. Increased weight causes more wear and tear on the joints. Adipose tissue produces cytokines that destroy normal cartilage in joints.

Sleep disorders

As people gain weight they tend to feel tired all the time, and may have sleeping problems. Problems with sleep may be indicative of a severe condition called Pickwickian syndrome or sleep apnea.

Psychological-social consequences

One of the most painful aspects of obesity may be the emotional suffering it causes. Modern Western societies place great emphasis on physical appearance, often equating attractiveness with slimness, especially in women. These messages, intended or not, make overweight women unattractive. Many people assume that obese people are gluttonous, lazy or both. Obese people often face prejudice or discrimination at work, at school, while looking for a job and in social situations. Feelings of rejection, shame, guilt, anxiety or depression are common.

EFFECT OF ESTROGEN ON APPETITE

Animal studies

Animal research in rats has clearly linked estradiol to food intake. Female rats' food intake varies dramatically during the ovarian cycle[24,25]. During estrus, food intake and weight decline, attributable to a decrease in the size of meals consumed. Oophorectomy leads to the absence of physiological and behavioral estrus, loss of the ovarian rhythm of eating and an increase in the basal level of food intake[24,25] that leads to an increase in body weight mainly because of an increase in adiposity. Cyclical replacement of estradiol is sufficient to reinstate the normal level and rhythmic pattern of food intake[26]. Progesterone replacement does not result in a return to normal eating, but large doses may antagonize the effects of estradiol.

Relationship of estradiol to food intake in women

Menses-related changes
Human research suggests that women also experience a variation in food intake during the menstrual cycle[27]. Total daily food intake is significantly reduced during the periovulatory period[28]. Some studies also suggest that women eat more during the luteal phase than during the follicular phase. The incidence of food craving also increases during the premenstrual phase.

Menopause
Data from the National Health Nutrition Examination Surveys[29] have led to a provocative suggestion that the end of a woman's reproductive life is associated with significant body weight gain. However, only slight increases in weight and no changes in food intake have been detected in perimenopausal and postmenopausal women[30,31]. A randomized clinical trial indicated that oral conjugated equine estrogen therapy reduced postmenopausal weight gain[32].

Physiological mechanisms of estradiol's effect on eating

Brain
The action of estradiol in the brain involves possibly more than one forebrain site. It was originally hypothesized that estradiol acts in the ventromedial hypothalamic area to inhibit feeding. A more promising site of action appears to be the hypothalamic paraventricular nucleus[33].

Increasing evidence has implicated corticotropin-releasing factor in the inhibitory control of estrogen with regard to eating[34].

Neuropeptide Y delivered into the paraventricular nucleus and the adjacent perifornical hypothalamus potently stimulates eating in animals. Anorectic effects of estrogen may be mediated by decreased neuropeptide Y release in the hypothalamic paraventricular nucleus[35].

The brain serotonin 5-hydroxytryptamine is another neurochemical that should be considered in the investigation of estradiol's effects on eating.

Metabolism

A plausible hypothesis that estradiol affects the availability of circulating metabolic substrate by directing long-chain fatty acids into and out of storage in adipose tissue was not supported in extensive tests[36].

Adipose tissue

Both plasma insulin and Ob protein (leptin) are thought to be endocrine feedback signals that relate level of food intake to adipose tissue mass. Another possible explanation for estradiol's effect on eating is that it influences the secretion of, or sensitivity to, these hormones. In both rats and humans, the ovary expresses functional leptin receptors[37], and estradiol apparently upregulates adipocyte Ob protein production[38]. Basal plasma Ob concentration is greatest in premenopausal women, less in postmenopausal women and lowest in men[39].

Gut peptides

Peptides released from the gut during meals are a crucial part of the mechanism by which preabsorptive food stimuli control satiety. Cholecystokinin (CCK), bombesin-like peptides, glucagon, insulin and amylin are released by preabsorptive food stimuli during the meal and have been implicated as feedback signals for the direct control of meal size.

Estradiol increased the satiating potency of exogenous CCK-8 in oophorectomized rats[40]. The satiating potency of endogenous CCK in non-oophorectomized rats increased during estrus[41]. The potency of glucagon and bombesin-like peptides may also be increased by estradiol in rats. Several lines of investigation have begun to reveal mechanisms by which estradiol exerts its opponent inhibitory effects on eating in rats. If similar mechanisms are presented in women, this may throw more light on not only eating disorders in women but also obesity in the menopause and the relationship between obesity, the menopause and hormone replacement therapy (HRT).

MANAGEMENT OF OBESE MENOPAUSAL WOMEN

Concern about the safety of HRT is frequently cited by doctors and patients alike as the reason for not prescribing or taking it. Much of this concern is misplaced. A recent epidemiological study[42] conducted in northern Italy showed that HRT use was inversely related to BMI. Obesity with its consequences (hypertension, diabetes mellitus, dyslipidemia and hyperandrogenemia) may still be considered as a relative contraindication for HRT.

Several questions must be answered in the treatment approach to obese postmenopausal women.

Is weight gain in menopause myth or reality?

Women tend to gain weight with age, starting around the time of their menopause. Metabolism slows down with advancing age. Additionally, when women become postmenopausal, their metabolic rate decreases significantly. A series of metabolic changes related to hypoestrogenism can cause an increase in body weight, with an android body fat distribution that provokes profound changes in body image. In a prospective 3-year study in 485 middle-aged women[43], it was found that females gained an average of 2.25 kg; 20% of subjects gained 4.5 kg or more, and only 3% lost 4.5 kg or more.

Do estrogens cause weight gain?

The currently available literature clearly indicates that HRT does not cause weight gain in the majority of women, but the effect of progestogen must be considered. Nevertheless, a small subgroup of women experience dramatic weight gain. Various explanations are available: fluid retention is one, progestogen addition is a second, and the third is that estrogens in some women stimulate appetite mediated through changes in mood. Poor appetite can be associated with depressed mood, which may be improved by HRT. Conversely, mood elevation with HRT in some women results in weight loss, because they stop 'comfort eating'.

Are obese women candidates for HRT?

HRT represents the main menopause treatment: a large body of data have demonstrated HRT benefits on menopausal symptoms and on long-term menopausal risks (cardiovascular disease and osteoporosis), showing a reduction of morbidity and mortality in HRT users. Chronically elevated estrone levels in obese patients are thought to be responsible for less osteoporosis and fewer vasomotor symptoms. Obese postmenopausal women are said to suffer less than thin women from estrogen-deficiency symptoms such as hot flushes and night sweats, but data to support this statement are difficult to find. There is some evidence that psychological symptoms are more prevalent in menopausal women with neurotic personality traits, current difficulties in coping with stress and low self-esteem, which can be expected to be found in obese postmenopausal women.

As already mentioned above, obesity is an additional amplificating factor in the network of metabolic dysfunctions and risk factors for CHD in menopause. Obesity, hypertestosteronemia and hypoestronemia are all independently and synergistically associated with hyperinsulinemia and dyslipidemia, which can be decreased by HRT use. The physiological protection afforded by estrogens against CHD in postmenopausal women may be diminished by diabetes mellitus.

How may route of administration be important?

Estradiol decreases tissue resistance to the action of insulin. Transdermal treatment has no effect on glucose tolerance or insulin concentrations[44] but decreases serum triglycerides[45]. As the liver is the principal site of synthesis of various plasma proteins and globulins including clotting factors, SHBG and renin substrate, production of these substances may be influenced more by oral than by non-oral estrogens. A non-oral route of estrogen administration would seem preferable in obese patients, especially when associated with hypertriglyceridemia, diabetes and hypertension.

What is the best progestogen?

Unwanted effects of progestogens include somatic symptoms and psychological symptoms as well as androgenic action (raised insulin level and unfavorable lipid profile). Protection of the endometrium is even more important in obese menopausal women because of the very well known high risk for endometrial carcinoma. However, it is reasonable to prescribe the progestogen with the lowest androgenic activity and minimal effect on insulin activity. Levonorgestrel and medroxyprogesterone induce insulin resistance; natural progesterone and possibly dydrogesterone appear to have minute effects; and norethisterone seems to be relatively inert[46]. Norpregnan derivatives possess a strong progestogenic effect and they have no androgenic activity. Progesterone and dydrogesterone are devoid of any androgenic effect but have a weak antiestrogenic effect. One possible method is the use of a progestogen intrauterine device (IUD) with minimal systemic effects and maximal protection of the endometrium.

With the correct approach to the obese menopausal woman, in the overwhelming majority of patients it will be possible to find a treatment regimen which maximizes benefits yet causes minimal side-effects.

References

1. Hirsch J, Leibel R. Clinical review 28: a biological basis for human obesity. *J Clin Endocrinol Metab* 1991;73:1153–7
2. Black D, James WPT, Besser GM, *et al.* Obesity. A report of the Royal College of Physicians. *J R Coll Physicians London* 1983;17:5–56
3. National Center for Health Statistics. *Anthropometric reference data and relevance of overweight: United States, 1976–80. Vital and health statistics.* Series 11, No. 238. DHHS publication no. (PHS) 87-1688. Washington DC: Government Printing Office, 1989
4. Bouchard C. Is weight a risk factor? *N Engl J Med* 1991;324:1887–9
5. Wechsler JG. Diatetische Therapie der Adipositas. *Dtsches Arzteblatt* 1997;94:2250–6
6. Lean MEJ, Han TS, Morrison CE. Waist circumference as a measure for indicating need for weight management. *Br Med J* 1995;311:158–61
7. Kissebah AH, Krakower GR. Regional adiposity and morbidity. *Physiol Rev* 1994;74:761–811
8. Moyer AE, Rodin J, Grilo CH, *et al.* Stress induced cortisol response and fat distribution in women. *Obesity Res* 1994;17:83–9
9. Pasquali R, Anconetani B, Chattat R, *et al.* The hypothalamic–pituitary–adrenal axis activity and its relationship to the autonomic nervous system in women with visceral and subcutaneous obesity. Effects of the corticotropin-releasing factor arginine vasopressin test and stress. *Metabolism* 1996;45:351–6
10. Chrousos G, Gold P. The concept of stress and stress system disorders. *J Am Med Assoc* 1992;267: 1244–52
11. Iranmanesh A, Lizzarralde G, Veldhuis JD. Age and relative adiposity are specific negative determinants of the frequency and amplitude of growth hormone secretory burst and half life of endogenous GH in healthy men. *J Clin Endocrinol Metab* 1991; 73:1081–8
12. Bjorntrop P. Diabetes. In *The Origins and Consequences of Obesity*. Ciba Foundation Symposium 201. Chichester: John Wiley, 1996:68–89
13. Bjorntrop P. Visceral obesity: a 'civilization syndrome'. *Obesity Res* 1993;1:206–22
14. Bjorntrop P. 'Portal' adipose tissue as a generator of risk factors for cardiovascular disease and diabetes. *Arteriosclerosis* 1990;10:493–6
15. Geisthovel F, Olbrich M, Frorath B, *et al.* Obesity and hypertestosteronaemia are independently and synergistically associated with elevated insulin concentrations and dyslipidaemia in premenopausal women. *Hum Reprod* 1994;9:610–16
16. Loffler G. Pathophysiologie des Fettgewebes. *Dtsches Artzeblatt* 1997;94:2003–6
17. Messerli FH, Ventura HO, Reisin E, *et al.* Borderline hypertension and obesity: two prehypertensive states with elevated cardiac output. *Circulation* 1982;66:55–60
18. Tuck ML, Sowers J, Dornfeld L, *et al.* The effect of weight reduction on blood pressure, plasma renin activity, and plasma aldosterone levels in obese patients. *N Engl J Med* 1981;304:930–3
19. Hubert HB, Feinleib M, McNamara PM, *et al.* Obesity as an independent risk for cardiovascular disease: a 26-year follow up of participants in the Framingham Health Study. *Circulation* 1983;67: 968–77
20. Kissebah A, Peiris A. A biology of regional body fat distribution: relationship to non-insulin-dependent diabetes mellitus. *Diabetes Metab Rev* 1989;5:83–109
21. Manson JE, Willett WC, Stampfer MJ, *et al.* Body weight and mortality among women. *N Engl J Med* 1995;333:677–85
22. Conover CA, Lee PDK, Kanaley JA, *et al.* Insulin regulation of insulin-like growth factor binding protein-1 in obese and nonobese humans. *J Clin Endocrinol Metab* 1992;74:1355
23. Speroff L, Glass RH, Kase NG. Anovulation and the polycystic ovary. In *Clinical Gynecologic Endocrinology and Infertility*. Baltimore, MD: Williams & Wilkins, 1994:457–82
24. Wade GN, Gray JM. Gonadal effects on food intake and adiposity: a metabolic hypothesis. *Physiol Behav* 1979;22:583–93
25. Wade GN, Schneider JE. Metabolic fuels and reproduction in female mammals. *Neurosci Biobehav Rev* 1992;16:235–72
26. Wade GN. Some effects of ovarian hormones on food intake and body weight in female rats. *J Comp Physiol Psychol* 1975;88:183–93
27. Dye L, Blundell JE. Menstrual cycle and appetite control: implications for weight regulation. *Hum Reprod* 1997;12:1142–51
28. Lyons PM, Truswell AS, Mira M, *et al.* Reduction of food intake in the ovulatory phase of the menstrual cycle. *Am J Clin Nutr* 1989;49:1164–8
29. Kuczmarski RJ, Flegal KM, Campbell SM, *et al.* Increasing prevalence of overweight among US adults: the National Health and Nutrition Examination Surveys, 1960 to 1991 [Comments]. *J Am Med Assoc* 1994;272:205–11
30. Pasquali R, Casimirri F, Labate AM, *et al.* Body weight, fat distribution and the menopausal status in women. *Int J Obesity* 1994;18:614–21
31. Poehlman ET, Toth MJ, Gardner AW. Changes in energy balance and body composition at menopause: a controlled longitudinal study. *Ann Intern Med* 1995;123:673–5

32. Espeland MA, Stefanick ML, Kritz-Silverstein D, *et al.* Effect of postmenopausal hormone therapy on body weight and waist and hip girths. *J Clin Endocrinol Metab* 1997;82:1549–56
33. Butera PC. CNS steroids and the control of feeding. In Stone TW, ed. *CNS Neurotransmitters and Neuromodulators: Neuroactive Steroids*. New York: CRC Press, 1996:211–35
34. Dagnault A, Ouerghi D, Richard D. Treatment with α-helical-CRF_{9-41} prevents the anorectic effect of 17β-estradiol. *Brain Res Bull* 1993;32:689–92
35. Bonavera JJ, Dube MG, Kalra PS, *et al.* Anorectic effects of estrogen may be mediated by decreased neuropeptide-Y release in the hypothalamic paraventricular nucleus. *Endocrinology* 1994;134: 2367–70
36. Ramirez I. Estradiol-induced changes in lipoprotein lipase, eating, and body weight in rats. *Am J Physiol* 1981;240:E533–8
37. Karlsson C, Lindell K, Svensson E, *et al.* Expression of functional leptin receptors in the human ovary. *J Clin Endocrinol Metab* 1997;82:4144–8
38. Shimuzu H, Shimomuura Y, Nakanishi Y, *et al.* Estrogen increases in *in vivo* leptin production in rats and human subjects. *J Endocrinol* 1997;154:285–92
39. Rosenbaum M, Nicolson M, Hirsch J, *et al.* Effects of gender, body composition, and menopause on plasma concentrations of leptin. *J Clin Endocrinol Metab* 1996;81:3424–7
40. Linden A, Uvnas-Moberg K, Forsberg G, *et al.* Involvement of cholecystokinin in food intake. III. Oestradiol potentiates the inhibitory effect of cholecystokinin octapeptide on food intake in ovariectomized rats. *J Neuroendocrinol* 1990;2: 797–801
41. Asarian L, Geary N. Cyclic estradiol replacement in ovariectomized rats elicits cyclic changes in food intake without increasing the satiating potency of CCK-8. *Soc Neurosci Abstr* 1997;23:256
42. Parazzini F, La Vecchia C, Negri E, *et al.* Determinants of estrogen replacement use in northern Italy. *Rev Epidem Sante Bubl* 1993;41:53–8
43. Wing RR, Matthews KA, Kuller RH, *et al.* Weight gain at the time of menopause. *Arch Intern Med* 1991;151:97–102
44. Godsland IF, Gangar GF, Walton C, *et al.* Insulin resistance, secretion, and elimination in postmenopausal women receiving oral or transdermal hormone replacement therapy. *Metabolism* 1993;42: 846–53
45. Crook D, Cust MP, Gangar KF, *et al.* Comparison of transdermal and oral estrogen–progestin hormone replacement therapy: effect on serum lipids and lipoproteins. *Am J Obstet Gynecol* 1992;166: 950–5
46. Stevenson JC, Proudler AJ, Walton C, *et al.* HRT mechanism of action. Carbohydrates. *Int J Fertil* 1994;39:50–5

Culture and medical consultation

37

C. A. Gurucharri

INTRODUCTION

In our profession, there are two basic approaches to the subject of the climacteric: to consider it either as an endocrinopathy or a vital crisis, a disease or a moment in life. We support the latter approach. These two different approaches are derived not from medicine but from the perception of what a woman is and who she is. Our domain, gynecology, might find it difficult to explain the perception and idiosyncrasies of a woman.

I believe it would help to remember the words of the Spanish philosopher, Julián Marías[1], in his book *Women in the Twentieth Century*: 'A woman is one of the two components of sexual life but, is she only that? Is it enough to simply say one of the two components? I don't think so. Hasn't she an original and irrefutable space? It is necessary to resort to a concept that I explored many years ago in many books until achieving its complete mastery in the metaphysical anthropology. We must search for the anthropological essence of a woman and not just her anatomical or physiological or psychological characteristics. We should identify all that is involved in being a woman or we may ask ourselves, what does it mean to be a woman?' All of us who develop our daily activities with women patients might benefit from sharing the concerns of the Spanish philosopher Julián Marías.

THE EVOLUTION: FROM GYNECOLOGY TO THE HEALTH CARE OF WOMEN

Gynecologists face an important handicap when understanding the climacteric. Part of the reason for this concerns the history of medicine and part concerns gynecology itself. Medicine as a science began with the structuring of anatomy. The body was thoroughly studied, but it was divided into areas or sections. The concept of function arose centuries after anatomical knowledge, first through the circulation (Harvey, 1628) and then through the physiology (Claude Bernard, 1813–78). This latter investigator emphasized 'how' and not 'the reason why'.

Medical knowledge in the past emphasized the parts and not the whole, the biological issue over the psychosocial aspect and sickness over health. In so far as gynecology is concerned, we must recall that, in the same way that obstetrics preceded medicine itself, in the last century gynecology separated from general surgery. For this reason, gynecology was originally considered as a genital, organic and surgical discipline.

If we analyze our curriculum, we will find subjects such as tumors, dystopias, infections and cycle disorders. But where is the woman? This genital vision of the woman prevailed for the first 50 years of this century until genetics, immunology, infectology and neurobiology, among others, made a breakthrough in science.

It has been said that medicine did not become concerned with women for a considerable time. This changed in 1924 when Halban and Seitz started publishing *Biologie und Pathologie des Weibes*, which is a real masterpiece on women. Facts concerning women as human beings were further explained through techniques developed in the medical field. In fact, psychology, anthropology and sociology developed theories, proposed systems and analyzed roles. Our health-care system, governed by the medical authorities, resisted exploring these areas of knowledge. However, little by little, and through interdisciplinary work, some groups of physicians started to develop an overall vision of the patient.

To go on to the subject of this paper, culture[2] can be defined in the following ways:

(1) The total pattern of human behavior and its products embodied in thought, speech, action and artefacts, which are dependent upon man's capacity for learning and transmitting knowledge to succeeding generations through the use of tools, language and systems of abstract thought.

(2) The body of customary beliefs, social forms and material traits constituting a distinct complex of tradition of a racial, religious or social group.

(3) A complex of typical behaviors of standardized social characteristics peculiar to a specific group, occupation or profession, sex, age, grade or social class.

Analyzing the definition, it is obvious that there are no clear limits separating cultural, anthropological and educational factors. We could add the following: do psychology and religion constitute factors separate from culture?

Culture influences any personal activity, but it is very important when it is associated with our medical actions. There are many factors involved, from the wording of the reason for the consultation (educational background) up to the meaning assigned to those words (anthropological and family traditions). Culture modulates the interpretation and the meaning of the menopause (both in patients and in physicians) and the consultation itself (where, why, when and how).

A DIFFERENT CONSULTATION

Traditional medicine is not sufficient or totally competent to be of help in vital crises: adolescence and the climacteric. The cultural factor will bear a higher importance in the final stage of fertility than in the case of an ovarian cyst. The consultation involves medical and non-medical factors. According to the teachings of Ortega y Gasset, we believe that a man is the man himself together with his own circumstances. Consequently, we will review some aspects that are involved in the medical consultation between the patient and the physician and their relationship with culture.

As regards the patient, her own interpretation of what is happening to her depends on her knowledge about health, her biography, her personality, her culture and her family tradition.

When a patient comes to our office, we must realize that she is a woman with her own experience of life. In most cases, her biographical, affective and social experiences are much more important than her high follicle stimulating hormone or low estradiol levels. This does not imply that the physician must disregard his obligation to carry out a primary examination, detect risk factors, prevent pathologies and relieve symptoms. Nevertheless, the consultation should not be limited to analyzing a lipid test or a bone densitometry, thus minimizing the woman to some biological apparatus that must be repaired.

The medical consultation makes us face the difficulty in discerning between being sick and feeling sick. This circumstance, analyzed by von Weiszaecker from a medical point of view, may be linked to the antinomy of nature and culture. Claude Levi-Strauss[3], in the first chapter of *The Elemental Structures of Kinship* (1949), develops the imprecise limits distinguishing between a condition of nature and a society status (culture). 'Everything that is universal in men corresponds to nature and its main feature is the spontaneity, while all that is subject to rules belongs to culture and bears relative and particular attributes'.

The difference between a symptomatic and an asymptomatic woman is not clear. In 1997, Avis and colleagues[4] analyzed the variables that are involved in this binomial. Some of the factors involved are education, utilization of health services, lifestyle and attitude towards the menopause. Culture indirectly influences signs and symptoms, but it is directly related to the meaning attributed to a certain clinical condition; with regard to this, beliefs regarding health based on experience, culture, personality, family traditions and the collective unconscious bear importance.

Cobb[5] concludes, on the basis of a survey performed by means of 7000 letters, that the basic needs of a woman going through the climacteric are reassurance and reliable information. During the premenopause stage, women want to know what is ahead, during the menopause they want to know if their experiences are normal and during the postmenopause period they need help to decide on whether or not to take hormone replacement therapy (HRT).

PATIENT-DOCTOR RELATIONSHIP

When we speak about the risk-benefit of hormonal therapy for endometriosis, a question needs to be answered: what does the patient know and think about it? When we speak about the risk-benefit of HRT for the menopause, does the patient listen in the same manner as in the case of endometriosis? Or are there many other factors involved? Are these health factors only or are they mainly factors other than those relating to health?

Is the very important subject of compliance a medical circumstance or is it also a cultural circumstance? Do we evaluate all the factors that influence treatment compliance or non-compliance? What words do we use? And what about our non-verbal speech?

Cultural factors demand that we should be humbler in our conclusions and opinions.

When we say that postmenopause is an estrogen failure, then isn't childhood a size failure? When we say that a woman over 50 years of age, being 60, 70 or 80 years old, is in the 'postmenopause stage', isn't this just as true or false as saying that a 2-year-old girl is in the 'pre-menarche phase'? Usually, a medical issue is linked to a cultural issue. For example, Leo Speroff claims that 75% of women in the USA and Europe had hot flushes compared to 25% of Japanese women. He also states that 15–20% of American women had daily hot flushes versus 3% of Japanese women. Today, we know that soybean and tofu contain phytoestrogens. Cooking, food and estrogens are medical and cultural concepts. Where does the limit lie?

It is important for a medical team to have a positive attitude toward the menopause. The mature woman is labelled as less productive and healthy on the basis that she has reached the end of her fertile life and may request hormone therapy. Wright's[6] challenge is to be more realistic when he affirms that the menopause is more the beginning than the end of a cycle.

One of the risks of a poor understanding of the menopause is to consider this stage as a period in which health is at risk and requires pharmacological treatment. According to Palmlund[7], the social consideration of the menopause as a health risk is becoming more prominent in popular culture and in the medical field and it involves the medicalization of women's live. Generally, this medicalization refers to the process by which the normal situations of pregnancy, lactation, menstruation and menopause have been claimed and redefined by medicine.

Kaufert[8] has analyzed how the menopausal woman is represented in pharmaceutical product information and in the media. In the same manner as a woman was presented as depressed or sick in the 1970s, in the 1990s she is shown as the example of fitness and in the height of her physical splendor, with no mention of possible future risks. This is the changing expression of society's vision of the menopause: 'It will all depend on what I do when I reach menopause'. The final image should be real: neither so sick nor so healthy.

Sociocultural aspects of sexuality can be hindering factors in the secondary prevention of cervicouterine cancer. Silvia Lamadrid Alvarez[9] analyzed this and proposed exploring some characteristics of the vision that women have regarding their sexuality, as there is information that relates a population's sexual culture to the incidence of cervicouterine cancer. She also explored the recognition of sexual pleasure, engaging in sex after menopause and the ways to prevent cervical cancer, through the results of a survey. The survey was carried out with a group of women who visited the Primary Assistance Health Services in Santiago, Chile, and who had not had a Papanicolaou (Pap) smear in the past year. This survey indicates that, compared to prior studies carried out in Chile, women show a more positive attitude toward their sexuality and that they are willing to learn more about their body, even though there is a minority group that continues to have negative visions about their sexuality. This opens up new perspectives for an educational program on the part of the health services, not only to enhance the benefits of the Pap test, but also to improve women's quality of life.

OTHER LITERATURE

Many times we are not sure what basic literature on the menopause should be recommended to a young colleague. Our doubts grow by the day, but we always insist on giving this reply: 'It is not only a question of medicine'. Two years ago, the Argentine Association for the Study of Menopause reached a consensus on different aspects of the menopause. The following films, among others, were recommended to enlighten women's knowledge on this stage of life: *Same Time, Next Year*, *Madison Bridges*, *I love Shirley Vallantine* and *Secrets and Lies*.

A Spanish doctor, Gregorio Marañón[10], put forward some basic knowledge to understand menopause and contribute to women's welfare. He pointed out that the following factors were important: internal medicine, pathology, physiopathology, etiology and life experience. However, the latter involves not only being somewhat mature, but also resorting to the literature. In his book *The Critical Age*, together with Cannon, Houssay, Brown Sequard, Levy and Culberton, he mentions authors such as Feuillet (*La Crise*), Michaelis (*L'Age Dangereux*), Estene (*L'Heredite Romantique*), Saint Augustine, Ovid, Michelet, Perez de Ayala and D'Ors. Marañón claims: 'Today we are better off studying human feelings in Shakespeare books than in *A Masterpiece on Passions* by Descartes'.

Albarracin Teulón[11] published an article on the menopause found in the Spanish literature of the 20th century. He also quotes Marañón who, in 1919, stated that an artist obtains his impressions directly from reality, without the scientific prejudices that do not consider the human being. 'Physicians cannot penetrate in the spiritual privacy of suffering people because their excessive contact with the physical matter blunts their psychological penetration.' 'This phenomenon is especially true with gynecologists, who are never capable of surmounting the barrier of the genital organs, which is the least intimate part of a woman.'

If we put together all aspects, i.e. cultural, anthropological, psychological and social, we will achieve a more comprehensive and, thus, a more real 'construction' of the menopause. Culture assigns meanings to signs and symptoms not only for the patient, but also for the physician.

As long as the acting physician takes into account non-medical aspects of the consultation, the physician in question will be able to overcome two prejudicial situations: medicalization and psychiatrization of the menopause. As we believe that 'Truth is found in science and reality in art', I would like to finish by quoting the Spanish author, Jacinto Benavente[12], who states in his book *Autumn Roses*: 'Autumns and sunsets, not to mention a sunset in autumn, is nature at its full height'. Why can't this also be true for a woman? Autumn is still very beautiful.

ACKNOWLEDGEMENT

The author is grateful to Miriam Golia for her translation and assistance in the English version of this paper.

References

1. Marias J. *La Mujer en en Siglo XX.* Madrid: Alianza, 1980
2. *Webster's Third New International Dictionary*. USA: Merriam Webster Inc., 1986
3. Levi Strauss C. *Las Estructuras Elementales del Parentezco.* Paidós, 1949
4. Avis NE, Crawford SL, McKinlay SM. *Women's Health* 1997;3:103
5. Cobb JO. *Patient Educ Couns* 1998;33:281
6. Wright J. *Nurs Stand* 1998;12:46
7. Palmlund L. *J Psychosom Obstet Gynaecol* 1997;18: 87–94
8. Kaufert BA, Lock M. *J Psychosom Obstet Gynaecol* 1997;18:81–6
9. Lamadrid Alvarez S. *Cad Saude Publica* 1998;14 (Suppl 1):33–40
10. Marañón G. *Soc Esp De Pub Med* Madrid, 1919
11. Albarracín Teulon A. *Acta Ginecológica* 1991;48:327
12. Benavente J. *Rosas de Otoño.* Madrid: Nelson, 1924

Attitudes to and practice of hormone replacement therapy in Central and Eastern Europe

38

L. Kovács

INTRODUCTION

For most women, the natural menopause takes place at around the age of 50 years. As life expectancy increases, more women spend a larger proportion of their lives in the postmenopausal state. In 1990, somewhat less than 500 million women were aged 50 years or over around the world, but this level is expected to rise to 1200 million by the year 2030.

As people live longer, the years after the menopause represent a significant proportion (usually more than one-third) of a woman's life, and she has every right to want to enjoy this time to the full. Women's health, the condition of their lives in the postmenopause and their life expectancy are linked strongly with their lifestyle in these years and are highly dependent on their health care, including hormone replacement therapy (HRT) provided by the health system.

Most women require some medical assistance to alleviate their more or less pronounced discomforts due to the symptoms that occur around and after the menopause, such as hot flushes, night sweats, insomnia, vaginal dryness, discomfort during sexual intercourse, decreasing libido and urinary problems. There is no doubt that these symptoms need to be alleviated in order to provide these women with a better quality of life. The real health hazards, however, remain unrevealed by symptoms in the early postmenopausal years: the progressive decrease in bone mineral density and its consequence, osteoporosis; atherosclerosis in the arteries, with serious circulatory consequences; and the progressive loss in cognitive function of the brain and Alzheimer's disease.

This list is far from complete, but it can serve to underline the need for the prevention that has now been properly developed: estrogen replacement therapy. We can correctly refer to this therapeutic activity as HRT, because all those who have their endometrium (e.g. those who have not undergone hysterectomy) will also need progestogen supplementation to prevent endometrial hyperplasia and cancer.

I do not wish to deal with questions of progestogen supplementation such as the timing of administration, the selection of the progestogen and its influence on the cardioprotective action of the estrogen.

The first investigations relating to the benefits of estrogen replacement, both in experimental studies and clinically as HRT in postmenopausal women, date back to the 1940s in the USA[1]. The number of estrogen prescriptions reached a peak of 28 million by 1975[2].

However, the number then fell significantly following reports of the association of estrogens and adenocarcinoma of the endometrium. With the recommendation of the addition of progestogens to the estrogen to prevent the development of endometrial cancer, the frequency of use of HRT by postmenopausal women in the USA is currently about 35%[1].

In Europe, HRT was introduced somewhat later than in the USA, about 25-30 years ago, and its use varies widely from country to country and even from one region to another within the same country[3]. The different reports indicate that its use is about 15-20% in Scandinavia[4], 12% in the Netherlands[5], about 10% in the UK, 25% in France[4], and only 2% in women aged 50-59 years in Italy, where it is used much more in the north than in the south of the country[6].

In Central and Eastern Europe, HRT has been used only during the past 7–10 years, because HRT preparations have only been available in the area during this time. Both oral tablets and transdermal patches are marketed. All of them are imported products of western pharmaceutical companies, because for historical reasons the local pharmaceutical industry in Eastern Europe did not establish research and development in this field.

The number of postmenopausal women in the area is quite high, but unfortunately only a rather small proportion of them use HRT, largely because most remain poorly informed about the therapy. Fewer than 5% of the postmenopausal population is making use of HRT. There are few published reports on HRT use; most of our information is based on data from industry, on personal experience from our own Department, on a few presentations at local congresses and on personal communications from colleagues in neighboring countries.

The region of Central and Eastern Europe has a female population of about 190 million and the number of postmenopausal women is estimated to be 38–40 million. The number of those who receive HRT is very low. According to the available data, mainly based on market penetration reports from the pharmaceutical industry, the number of those who have ever used HRT is below 5%. The number of actual users has been assessed as being between 1 and 4%. The highest numbers of users are probably observed in Hungary, Poland and Slovenia, at about 5%. A recent report from the Czech Republic suggested that the number of users was 12%, but this appears most likely to be an unrealistic overestimation.

Most women begin treatment for the unpleasant symptoms of the climacteric, but compliance is poor and consequently the number of discontinuations is high: about half of the starters discontinue within the first year of use.

The reasons for discontinuation are the same as in the developed countries: primarily bleeding and several fears, mainly concerning malignancies (cancer of the breast and cancer of the uterus), but the fear of weight gain and the unpleasant feeling of interference with the normal process of life are also common. Unfortunately, publications in the mass media referring to HRT and carcinogenesis, which are mainly unrealistic non-professional reports, can have an adverse effect. The attitude of some doctors and the cost of the treatment also tend to promote discontinuation. I will deal with these points later.

The supply of preparations for HRT in Central and Eastern Europe is generally sufficient. Different estrogens and progestogens are available, as are several sequential and continuous combined preparations for oral or transdermal application. Oral medication is preferred to transdermal, the ratio being approximately 75 : 25.

The primary prescribers are almost exclusively gynecologists, while repeat prescriptions can also be provided by general practitioners.

HRT is relatively expensive in many countries in Central and Eastern Europe and this is one reason for the poor continuation rates. In several of these countries, imported pharmaceutical products (and all HRT preparations are imported ones) have to be paid for by the patients at full price, without any reimbursement from health insurance schemes. In other countries, including Hungary, 50% of the price of most preparations is reimbursed. In cases of proven osteoporosis, 90% reimbursement is provided for the treatment in most countries; this also relates to the costs of HRT preparations.

The negative attitude of some doctors, mainly general practitioners, originates from the confusion caused by not differentiating properly between estradiol and ethinylestradiol. It is therefore important for us to make it clear that, while it may be correct to withdraw ethinylestradiol (the basic component of most combined oral contraceptive pills) from women at cardiovascular or thromboembolic risk with increasing age, and not to use this estrogen for the treatment of postmenopausal women, 17β-estradiol is harmless for these patients. Doctors should be aware, however, of the risks of unopposed estrogen therapy in non-hysterectomized women.

Most general practitioners working today did not encounter postmenopausal hormone replacement during their university education and they are therefore not familiar with this topic. As a consequence, they never recommend this therapy to their patients or, even worse, they discourage those who have already been correctly counselled by an up-to-date gynecologist. We therefore need to organize postgraduate courses for general practitioners on this topic and also to provide them with sufficient information in their continuous medical education.

To improve the poor use of HRT, we must make more information available to women. In doctor-patient communications, more intensive counselling is needed to convince patients of the benefits of HRT. More broadly, the media, predominantly magazines targeted at women, should be used to distribute realistic information on the postmenopausal period of women's lives, emphasizing the need for HRT to provide the best possible quality of life. In several countries, e.g. in Hungary, non-profit-making civil organizations support clubs for climacteric women, where, within the scope of social programs, education and also some psychological support can be provided.

Innovations in the health services can also improve the situation. In our experience, the organization of menopause clinics providing a gynecological examination with oncological screening, including mammography and easy access to bone mineral density measurements, proved very effective in the introduction and good continuation of HRT.

From a scientific point of view, any new treatment modality that could reduce bleeding in the course of HRT would be very beneficial, and research in this direction should be encouraged and supported. From recent reports, the lower-dose continuous combined regimens (with a daily estradiol dose of 1 mg) seem to be favorable.

It is clear from the data presented that a difference exists in HRT practice between Western Europe and Eastern and Central Europe. We must endeavor to achieve the same standard for the Central and Eastern European population as that found in Western Europe. This requires much education, with emphasis on the fact that the menopausal transition is not an end to life or normalcy, but is a normal biological event caused by changes in hormone secretion. It will undoubtedly create a period of increasing health and situational concerns, but all these can be overcome with assistance from health-care systems and in part by a change in lifestyle.

Education of the population and also of health professionals is the primary demand, and much of our time should be spent on this. As women live longer, it is essential for us to do our part to ensure that they have better lives.

References

1. Carr BC. HRT management: the American experience. *Eur J Obstet Gynecol Reprod Biol* 1996;64 (Suppl 1):17–20
2. Kennedy DL, Baum C, Forbes MB. Noncontraceptive estrogens and progestins: use patterns over time. *Obstet Gynecol* 1985;65:441–6
3. Schneider HPG. Cross-national study of women's use of hormone replacement therapy (HRT) in Europe. *Int J Fertil* 1997:42(Suppl 2):365–75
4. Mattson LA, Stadberg E, Milsom J. Management of hormone replacement therapy: the Swedish experience. *Eur J Obstet Gynecol Reprod Biol* 1996;64(Suppl 1):3–5
5. Barentsen R. The climacteric in the Netherlands: a review of Dutch studies on epidemiology, attitudes and use of hormone replacement therapy. *Eur J Obstet Gynecol Reprod Biol* 1996;64(Suppl 1): 7–11
6. Crosignani PG. Management of hormone replacement therapy: the Italian experience. *Eur J Obstet Gynecol Reprod Biol* 1996;64(Suppl 1):13–15

Culture and aging of the female: a case of Japanese society 39

E. Namihira

MENSTRUATION AND MENOPAUSE IN PUBLIC CONTEXT

Menarche, menstruation and menopause are very private physical phenomena that occur within the female body. They may be referred to in the context of biomedicine, medical care or sanitation, but in daily life they are rarely referred to or discussed in public. These topics are reserved only for intimate female interlocutors.

However, in many societies, including Japanese society, menarche, menstruation and menopause are publicly acknowledged[1]. In such societies, a menstruating woman is thought to be polluted and polluting, and is prohibited from approaching sacred matters because it is believed that her pollution angers the gods and deities. Their anger, in turn, brings misfortune upon the woman's family and the entire community. Since a menstruating woman cannot enter sacred places or make offerings to the gods and deities during her period, other female members or her children sometimes do so on her behalf. As a result, her family and community members recognize that she is menstruating without even having been told. In those societies where people believe that menstrual blood and a menstruating woman are polluting, women are forced to stay in secluded huts during menstruation so as not to contaminate other members of the communal living space and everyday utensils[2-4].

One of the reasons postulated for why such private, physical phenomena are acknowledged socially is that society needs to know the exact number of women with reproductive potential and to identify each female member with such potential.

In the 1960s and 1970s, feminist anthropologists argued that pollution beliefs reveal social prejudice and discrimination towards women, not only in the religious, but also in the social and political realms. That is, by expelling female members from those sacred matters that often represent the core of a society's value system, society can confine female members to inferior positions vis-à-vis men. Furthermore, some anthropologists have attributed women's universal subordination to their biological and reproductive features[5-7].

In the societies referred to above, a girl's menarche is celebrated by her family and sometimes by her community members. This celebration informs other members of society that the girl has entered the reproductive stage. Even nowadays in Japan, a girl's menarche is celebrated by her family. The girl's mother cooks red-colored rice and serves it for the celebration dinner. The rice is sometimes shared by the girl's grandparents if they live nearby. At the dinner, neither the girl nor her mother refers to the girl's menarche, but family members recognize that the girl's menstruation has begun. The girl will be given her own bedroom soon afterwards in those cases where she has been sharing a bedroom with her male siblings.

Acknowledging menarche and menstruation in public results in dividing all of the female members of society into two groups: namely, women with reproductive potential and women without reproductive potential.

In contrast to menarch, menopause is not celebrated by a woman's family, but is acknowledged publicly as menopausal and postmenopausal women become free of the prohibition against participating in sacred matters. By means of the beliefs concerning the pollution of menstruation, a woman's private and physical affairs are translated into public and social events.

POSTMENOPAUSE AND 'REPRODUCTIVE POWER' OF POSTMENOPAUSAL WOMEN

Each society constructs human life socially and culturally and gives cultural meaning to the aging process[8,9]. The life process is divided into several stages: for example, childhood, adolescence, adulthood and old age. An individual moves from one stage to the next in the process of aging. When an individual moves from one stage to the next, the transition is celebrated by members of his/her society. In cultural anthropology, these celebrations are called 'rites of passage'[10]. Celebrations for girls at menarche are rites of passage in which they make the transition from sexual immaturity to sexual maturity or from the pre-reproductive period to the reproductive period.

The social functions and purposes of rites of passage are to let other members of society recognize the person's new status and to encourage the person concerned to confirm his/her new status and status obligations. After the celebration of menarche, girls are made to be more sensitive to their reproductive potential. They are taught with whom they can have sexual relations and with whom sexual relations are strictly prohibited.

In societies where women's reproductive phenomena are publicly recognized, women's social activities are determined by their reproductive abilities and women's reproduction always attracts social concern. However, it never means that menopausal and postmenopausal women are inferior to women in their reproductive period. In the Japanese case, menopausal and postmenopausal women are thought to have other kinds of power and abilities relating to human reproduction. At this stage, they are believed to gain guardian powers over newborn babies, young children and pregnant women. Additionally, they are more active in the public sphere because they are free from the many taboos that regulate women in the reproductive period.

Although Japan is now a highly industrialized society, it still maintains its traditional culture because of the rapidity with which industrialization and urbanization occurred. Among my first-hand data, collected since 1964, and literary data, we can find religious folk groups called 'kan-non-koh' or 'koyasu-koh' all over Japan. The members of each group are menopausal and post-menopausal women from the community. They gather together in a communal Buddhist hall once a month and chant a Buddhist folk Sutra. They pray for the good health of newborn babies, young children and pregnant women in their community. In the last month of pregnancy, the pregnant woman asks the group to offer an extra prayer for her and her unborn baby[11]. In the case of a certain mountain village in Niigata Prefecture, where I conducted field surveys from 1980–93, the male members of the community never referred to the group or to the group's meetings, even though they knew about them. It seems to be taboo for male members to approach the small Buddhist hall during the prayer. Incidentally, many men could not take meals in their own houses for 2 weeks after a female member of the family bore a child, until 1960, when the site of childbearing moved to hospitals. This was because childbearing was believed to be so polluting as to contaminate everything in the house and the pollution was believed to bring danger to the male members of the household.

The idea that menopausal and postmenopausal women have other kinds of reproductive power can also be found in traditional Japanese attitudes toward the midwife. A midwife is 'san-ba' in the Japanese language. The literal meaning of the word is 'an old woman who helps with child delivery'. More traditionally, a midwife is called 'toriage-bah-san' or 'hikiage-bah-san'. The terms mean 'an old woman who draws up or draws out a pre-human baby into the human world'[12]. In previous times, toriage-bah-san practiced infanticide when the baby's mother asked her to. Therefore, a midwife used to be the person who determined a baby's future life. In many cases, quasi-grandmother–grandchild relationships were formed between midwives and these babies.

When we discuss Japanese postmenopausal women's reproductive power, it is noteworthy that they are of the grandmother's generation. A traditional Japanese family consists of grandparents, children and grandchildren. Sometimes great-grandparents are also members. Women of the grandmother's generation are key persons in the family, because they are in a mediatory position between three generations and between those persons who were born into the family and those who were married into it. They take the initiative in most domestic affairs.

A young bride usually marries a man and begins her marital life in her husband's house with his parents, his unmarried brothers and sisters, and sometimes with his grandparents. In the beginning, her status is the lowest in the family because she is the newest member. However, within a few decades, she gains strong influences over her husband, children, her first son's wife and her grandchildren. That is, menopausal and postmenopausal women's 'reproductive power' coincides with their social and domestic power, because they are prized for overseeing the family's continuity and succession.

THE JAPANESE LIFE CYCLE AND RITES OF PASSAGE FOR THE LIVING AND THE DEAD

Like many other traditional societies, Japanese people celebrate rites of passage for dead persons. For 49 years, each dead person is celebrated by his/her children and grandchildren. After 49 years, each dead person loses his/her individuality and is unified with former generations of ancestors. In traditional thought, ancestors will be born into the family. This means that newborn babies, living family members, and ancestors are positioned in a cyclic form. This calls to mind the belief that old and postmenopausal women gain a new kind of reproductive power. Such thinking is also cyclic. For most Japanese aged women, aging and postmenopause are not devaluating features, as they have fulfilled their reproductive roles and have confirmed the succession of their families. Even the women who could not bear their own children are evaluated as having 'reproductive power' if they have managed their households well and have brought up adopted children. Furthermore, the children of the adopted child are categorized as the women's grandchildren in the Japanese family system.

It is predicted that the traditional Japanese idea of human reproduction and a woman's life cycle will be changed. The causes bringing the change are the weakened ideology of family succession and the concept of the cyclic process of living, 'afterlife' and pre-living. Statistical data from 1997 show that, in 1996, a Japanese woman bore only 1.43 children during her lifetime. On the other hand, data from 1925 show that, on average, a woman bore more than four children. Furthermore, data from 1947–49 show that a woman bore more than five children[13]. Such changes force us to change our ideas about women and reproduction. Women are no longer defined as the childbearing sex. Menstruation is not only associated with reproduction. Therefore, menopause and the menopausal period have gained new social and cultural meanings.

As mentioned above, each society constructs human life socially and culturally and each society gives cultural meaning to the aging process. In cultural anthropology, the construction of the lifespan, its meaning and ideas about aging are all considered part of a society's culture. Culture gives people a way of life, but people can also act to change culture. In the newly given circumstances, where women have a long lifespan and short reproductive period, we are trying to establish a new culture of aging and reproduction. The medicalization of the menopausal period is part, but not all, of the newly formed culture of aging. Even if medicine relieves the problem caused by the menopause, women still feel anxiety or fear of aging because it reminds them of death. As mentioned above, Japanese women have been evaluated for their 'reproductive power' even after the postmenopause. However, the situation has changed because of the change of the family system. Our task now is to establish a new culture of death in which people can give a positive value to death, as traditional societies (and cultures) have done.

The traditional Japanese cyclic cosmology, in which, for example, dead persons and ancestors are unified with newborn babies, and menopausal women with women in the reproductive stage, is one of the cultures of aging and death. If we cannot any longer expect Japanese people to reconstruct the traditional ideology of family succession or attribute women as the childbearing sex, we may be able to construct cyclic cosmology in the global context, i.e. sustainable relations between human life and ecological situations. Since the 1970s, active movements for preventing ecological pollution have been increasing. Most members of groups who undertake the activities are elderly women, both in urban and rural areas. It is presumed that such phenomena are signs of the construction of a new cyclic cosmology.

References

1. Buckley T, Gottlieb A. *Black Magic: The Anthropology of Menstruation*. Berkeley: University of California Press, 1988
2. Douglas M. *Purity and Danger*. Baltimore: Penguin Books, 1966:166–87
3. Namihira E. Tsukagirei niokeru 'hare' to 'kegare' no kan-nen no bunseki. [Analysis of 'hare' and 'kegare' in Japanese rites of passage.] *Minzougaku kenkyu [Jpn J Ethnol]* 1976;40:350–68
4. Namihira E. Pollution in the folk belief system. *Curr Anthropol* 1987;28:567–9
5. Rosald MZ, Lamphere L, eds. *Woman, Culture, and Society*. Stanford: Stanford University Press, 1974
6. MacCormack C, Strathern M, eds. *Nature, Culture and Gender*. Cambridge: Cambridge University Press, 1980
7. Moore HL. *Feminism and Anthropology*. Cambridge: Polity Press, 1988
8. Sokolovsky J, ed. *The Cultural Context of Aging: Worldwide Perspectives*. New York: Bergin & Garvey Publishers, 1990
9. Lock M. *Encounters with Aging*. Berkeley: University of California Press, 1993
10. Van Gennep A. *The Rites of Passage*. Chicago: University of Chicago Press, 1960
11. Onshizaidan-boshi-aiikukai. *Nihon Sanniku Shuzoku Shiryou Shusei*. [*Compiled Data on Japanese Custom of Childbearing and Child Caring.*] Tokyo: Daiichi-hoki Shuppan, 1975
12. Iijima Y. Kodomo no hakken to jidouyuugi no sekai. [Discovery of child and the children's world.] In Tsuboi Y, Amino Y, Tanigaura K, *et al.*, eds. *Ie to Josei*. [*Japanese Family and the Female.*] Tokyo: Shohgaku-kan, 1985:250–1
13. Jyosei-joho. Jinko-doutai tokei geppo nenkei no gaikyo. [Monthly report of demographic data by the Ministry of Health and Welfare.] In *Monthly Journal of Josei Joho*. Tokyo: Pado Women's Office, 1996:13–15

The current status of Chinese traditional medicine treatment of postmenopausal women in Taiwan

40

K.-E. Huang

INTRODUCTION

One of the oldest textbooks of Chinese medicine, *Huang-di Nei-jing Su-wen* (Yellow Emperor's Inner Classic of Medicine), which first appeared c. 100 BC, described the menopause, stating that cessation of menstruation may occur at age 7 × 7 (49) years; women lose their ability to reproduce and their body configurations change and deteriorate. In spite of this long-standing insight about the menopause, the treatment of postmenopausal women started in Taiwan only a few decades ago. The main reason for the late commencement of postmenopausal treatment was the fact that people thought the menopause was a natural phenomenon that did not need to be treated. Only in recent years, with the establishment of the Taiwanese Menopause Society, which provided intensive education programs, did the terms climacteric and menopause, and the associated problems, become familiar to the public and hormone replacement therapy (HRT) become acceptable to women in Taiwan.

Nevertheless, the concerns about the side-effects of HRT have never been eradicated. Some people believe that Chinese medicines, which mainly consist of herbs, are 'natural' and are safer than hormones. Moreover, Chinese traditional medicines, which have been used for symptom relief, have long existed in Taiwan and have been used for the treatment of climacteric symptoms for many generations. Many postmenopausal women in Taiwan, who have easy access to doctors providing Chinese medicine, prefer to take herbs as an alternative to HRT treatment for climacteric symptoms.

However, the use of Chinese medicine among postmenopausal women in Taiwan has never been studied. The purpose of this study was to evaluate the current status of the use of Chinese traditional medicine, including the rates of use, kinds of herb used, length of use, continuation rates and results of treatment, among Taiwanese postmenopausal women.

MATERIALS AND METHODS

This study was carried out by questionnaires filled in by postmenopausal women who were visiting the menopause clinic at university-affiliated teaching hospitals or were attending menopause seminars provided in large cities over the island of Taiwan. Those women who had had spontaneous amenorrhea for more than 1 year; who were healthy and self-content; and who had experienced at least one symptom that was considered menopause-related were included in this study. Those women who were known to be physically ill, who had undergone hysterectomy; or were asymptomatic were excluded from this study. A total of 1045 women were studied. The effects of medications on the climacteric symptoms were evaluated by questionnaires and/or interviews. The bone mineral density (BMD) of the lumbar spine was measured with dual energy X-ray absorptiometry (DXA) in 50 volunteers who were taking Chinese medicine at the time of enrolment, and again in 32 of them after 6 months and 23 after 12 months of treatment. The significance of changes was evaluated using Student's *t* test.

RESULTS

The ages of the 1045 women included in this study ranged from 44 to 72 years with a mean of 54.5 years. Their educational levels were 258 (25%) college and above, 585 (56%) middle/high school and 202 (19%) primary school or under. Among these 1045 women, 212 (20.3%) indicated that they had used Chinese medicine in order to relieve climacteric symptom(s). Of these 212 women, 100 (9.6% of total women) had, at some point in time, used some kind of Western medicines, mainly HRT, concomitantly and 112 (10.7% of total women) had used Chinese medicine only. Fifty-nine women (5.6%) indicated that they were using Chinese traditional medicine alone at the time the questionnaire was completed. Among those women who had used Chinese medicine, 97 indicated that they knew at least one herb in the medicine they were taking. The three most frequently used herbs were *Dong-gui* (radix *Angelicae sinensis*), *Chuan-xiong* (rhizoma *Ligustici wallichii szechuanensis*) and *Bai-shao* (radix *Paeoniae albae*), and were used in 78%, 64% and 54% of women, respectively. The average length of use of Chinese medicine was 6 months among all women and was 3 months in those under 55 years of age and 8 months in those over 56 years of age. They indicated that symptoms were improved during the use of Chinese medicine, significantly in 14%, moderately in 40% and slightly in 22%. In 24%, it was indicated that symptoms had not improved.

The average BMD of the lumbar spine of 50 volunteers showed osteopenia compared to that of a normal young adult with a *T* score of −1.12. The BMD decreased in 1.1% after 6 months of treatment and in 1.6% after 12 months of treatment. The latter was statistically significant when compared with the initial measurement.

DISCUSSION

This study was done to evaluate the current status of the use of Chinese herbal medicine among postmenopausal women in Taiwan. The survey was based on the questionnaires filled in by women who were attending the menopause clinic or menopause educational seminars. The study therefore provides epidemiological data on selected groups of women. These women who attended the clinic or the seminars might have been more symptomatic or more aware of postmenopausal problems than the general population and, therefore, more prone to seek treatment than the general population. The prevalence of the use of Chinese herbal medicine among Taiwanese postmenopausal women in general might be lower than that shown in this study. However, on the other hand, the incidence might be higher, because the menopause clinics that those women attended provided only conventional HRT and all the speakers at the seminars were physicians who provide only Western medicine.

People in Taiwan have gradually come to acknowledge postmenopausal problems, such as vasomotor symptoms, osteoporosis and cardiovascular diseases, and the beneficial effects of HRT. However, fear of breast cancer and other side-effects has limited the long-term use of conventional HRT. The use of an alternative to such preparations would therefore have a considerable potential. Perimenopausal women appear to be among the greatest users of unconventional medicine[1]. An Australian survey of some 3000 individuals showed that alternative medicine was used in 48.5% of those interviewed and was more frequently used by better-educated women and the perimenopausal[1]. In our study, Chinese herbal medicines were used more often by women of low education than by women of high education. A Swedish study indicated that 21% of postmenopausal women were on HRT, whereas 45% took non-hormonal preparations[2].

While most (76%) of the women in this study indicated that there was at least a slight improvement in their symptoms with the use of Chinese herbal medicine, the results were based on their subjective feelings. The BMD of the lumbar spine of those women showed continuous decay during the time they were taking Chinese medicine and to a significant degree after 12 months of medication. Thus, the results of this study showed that the Chinese medicines used by these women did not improve or maintain the lumbar spine BMD which was measured with the use of DXA. However, the number of women studied was too small to reach an appropriate conclusion. A placebo-controlled randomized trial to evaluate the efficacy, safety and side-effects of Chinese herbal medicines is desperately needed in Taiwan, particularly when there has been an indication that some Chinese medicine may contain potent contaminants, such as steroids[3]. The other obstacle in this study was that those women surveyed did not take the same kind of herbal medicine. Chinese medicines almost always consist of several herbal ingredients, with each doctor using different ingredients in their prescription. These facts may make the evaluation of treatment results of Chinese medicine very difficult.

It would be interesting to evaluate whether there are estrogenic components or estrogenic effects in the traditional Chinese medicines that are used for treatment of postmenopausal women. Hirata and colleagues reported that there was no estrogen component in *Dong-gui*[4], one of the most commonly used herbs in Chinese medicine. Moreover, it would also be interesting to evaluate whether there is any interaction between Chinese medicines and estrogen receptors.

CONCLUSION

The rate of use of Chinese traditional medicine was 20.3% in this study. The herbs used had improved postmenopausal symptoms at least slightly in most (76%) of the women. There was a tendency of sporadic rather than continuous use of Chinese medicine among postmenopausal women in Taiwan. In this study, the BMD of the lumbar spine showed a decrease during Chinese medicine treatment. We conclude that Chinese traditional medicine could be used effectively for relief of postmenopausal symptoms, but not for loss of bone mass.

References

1. MacLennan AH, Wilson DH, Taylor AW. Prevalence and cost of alternative medicine in Australia. *Lancet* 1996;347:569–73
2. Stadberg E, Mattsson L, Milson I, *et al.* The prevalence and severity of climacteric symptoms and the use of different treatment regimens in a Swedish population. *Acta Obstet Gynecol Scand* 1997;76:442–8
3. Ernst E. Harmless herbs? A review of the recent literature. *Am J Med* 1998;104:170–8
4. Hirata JD, Swierz LM, Zell B, *et al.* Does dong guai have estrogenic effects in postmenopausal women? A double-blind, placebo-controlled trial. *Fertil Steril* 1997;68:981–6

Dietary strategy for postmenopausal women 41

H. M. Park

INTRODUCTION

After the menopause, estrogen deficiency due to loss of ovarian function results in various metabolic changes. Weight gain occurs in the majority of women, even without estrogen/hormone replacement therapy (ERT/HRT), with changes to the lipid profile, body composition and insulin sensitivity, leading to increased risk of chronic metabolic diseases.

Troublesome menopausal symptoms, vasomotor and/or psychological, are the first to develop, followed by various kinds of disorder related to estrogen deficiency such as genitourinary atrophy, involutional osteoporosis, cardiovascular disease and Alzheimer's disease. Of these, two major long-term consequences of ovarian failure are osteoporosis and cardiovascular disease, which are the major causes of morbidity, mortality and financial costs.

ERT/HRT has been recommended as the first-line measure to prevent and treat estrogen deficiencies. However, it is clear that ERT/HRT is not suitable for all postmenopausal women and long-term compliance is low because of side-effects, concerns about the associated risk of cancer, absolute contraindications and reluctance to use it. For these postmenopausal women, in whom HRT is not acceptable or contraindicated, alternative non-estrogen-based therapies are needed.

Good nutrition is fundamental to good health. There is good evidence that diet and nutritional status are factors in the development of cardiovascular disease, certain cancers and other chronic conditions that are leading causes of death and disability. Therefore, dietary modification can improve health and reduce the disease incidence in women.

The Third Gallop Survey commissioned by the North American Menopause Society in 1998 reported that approximately 75% of postmenopausal women changed their lifestyles and 50% made dietary changes to enhance their health at mid-life or the menopause[1].

Appropriate evidence-based dietary and natural nutraceutical therapies are viewed as alternatives to traditional HRT/ERT. In this paper, various dietary strategies for the prevention of cardiovascular disease and osteoporosis are discussed with regard to their efficacy.

DIETARY STRATEGY FOR THE PREVENTION OF CARDIOVASCULAR DISEASE

Coronary heart disease is the leading cause of mortality and a significant cause of morbidity among women in developed countries. It is increasingly recognized as an important cause of mortality and morbidity in developing countries as well.

The level of risk for coronary heart disease is determined by a combination of risk factors, modifiable and non-modifiable. The risk factors can be attenuated through HRT, physical exercise with other lifestyle changes and appropriate diet in postmenopausal women. Dietary modification is the first step for the prevention and treatment of coronary heart disease. Diet can alter the risk of coronary heart disease through the alteration of several modifiable risk factors such as the serum lipid and lipoprotein profile, lipid peroxidation, blood pressure and coagulation.

Dietary fat

A low-fat diet may reduce the risk of a wide variety of chronic diseases such as cardiovascular disease, hypertension and some cancers. Dietary guidelines recommend consumption of no more than 30% of total daily calories from fat[2]. However, a recent study[3] suggested that total fat intake is not significantly related to the risk of coronary heart disease, because of the opposing effects of different fats. The type of fats consumed may be more important than total fat intake in determining the risk of coronary heart disease in women.

Triglycerides make up 95% of the fats we eat, which consist of three fatty acids attached to glycerol. There are three major classes of fatty acid: saturated, monounsaturated and polyunsaturated fatty acids (Table 1).

Saturated fatty acids

The sources of saturated fatty acids include most animal fats and a few tropical vegetable oils such as palm, palm kernel and coconut. Four saturated fatty acids - lauric, myristic, palmitic and stearic acid - account for most of the saturated fatty acids in the diet and, except stearic acid, raise serum cholesterol levels[4].

From metabolic ward studies, a change in saturated fatty acid intake explains 60–80% of the change observed in total cholesterol levels[5,6]. Other dietary factors make up the remainder of the cholesterol-lowering response. For this reason, reduced intake of dietary saturated fatty acids is the most important focus of a cholesterol-lowering diet. Reduced intake to less than 10% of calories as saturated fat is recommended[2].

Increased saturated fatty acid intake was associated with an increase in total cholesterol, low-density lipoprotein (LDL) cholesterol and a smaller increase in high-density lipoprotein (HDL) cholesterol[7]. In general, ingestion of 10 g of saturated fatty acids daily for several weeks raises total and LDL cholesterol levels 8–10 mg/dl[5,6].

According to the Nurses' Health Study[3], each 5% increase of energy intake from saturated fat was associated with a 17% increase in risk of coronary heart disease as compared with equivalent energy intake from carbohydrate.

Monounsaturated fatty acids

The most common monounsaturated fatty acid is oleic acid, which can be synthesized in the human body and is found in small amounts in butter and animal fat. Oleic acid is the predominant fatty acid found in olive and canola oils. It comprises up to 70% of the fat in a Mediterranean diet.

Monounsaturated fatty acids have no significant effect on total cholesterol and LDL cholesterol, but increase HDL cholesterol and decrease triglycerides[7]. Monounsaturated fatty acids may have additional benefits over polyunsaturated fatty acids by improving insulin sensitivity[8] and resistance to oxidative modification[9].

Increased intake of monounsaturated fatty acid is associated with a reduced risk of coronary heart disease and mortality due to cardiovascular disease[10,11]. The relative risk of coronary heart disease for a 5% increase in energy intake from monounsaturated fatty acid was 0.81 as compared with equivalent energy intake from carbohydrate according to the Nurses' Health Study[3].

Polyunsaturated fatty acids

There are two types of polyunsaturated fatty acids: omega-6 polyunsaturated fatty acids and omega-3 polyunsaturated fatty acids.

Omega-6 polyunsaturated fatty acids The most common ω-6 polyunsaturated fatty acid in the diet is linoleic acid. Omega-6 polyunsaturated fatty acids are primarily found in vegetable oils. Vegetable oils that are low in saturated fatty acids and high in polyunsaturated fatty acids as more than

Table 1 Classification of commonly used oils and fats

		Polyunsaturated		
Saturated	*Monounsaturated*	*Omega-3*	*Omega-6*	*Trans-unsaturated*
Animal fat	olive oil	fish oil	corn oil	margarine
Cotton oil	canola oil	flaxseed oil	peanut oil	shortening
Palm oil		canola oil	sesame oil	
Palm kernel oil			soybean oil	
			safflower oil	

50% of their fatty acids are corn oil, safflower oil and soybean oil.

Polyunsaturated fatty acid intake decreases serum total cholesterol and LDL cholesterol and increases HDL cholesterol[7].

The relative risk for coronary heart disease for a 5% increase in energy intake from polyunsaturated fat was 0.62 as compared with equivalent energy intake from carbohydrate[3]. Replacement of 5% energy from saturated fats with energy from unsaturated fats (monounsaturated fatty acids and polyunsaturated fatty acids) reduced the risk of coronary heart disease by 42%[3].

Omega-3 polyunsaturated fatty acids The most common long-chain ω-3 polyunsaturated fatty acids are eicosapentaenoic acid and docosahexaenoic acid, which are primarily found in fish oils. Some vegetable oils such as canola oil and flaxseed oil contain a shorter-chain ω-3 polyunsaturated fatty acid, α-linolenic acid. In the body, α-linolenic acid is elongated and desaturated to form eicosapentaenoic acid and docosahexaenoic acid.

Omega-3 polyunsaturated fatty acids are neutral in their effects on total cholesterol, LDL cholesterol and HDL cholesterol levels, but long-chain ω-3 polyunsaturated fatty acids have the most potent effect on serum triglyceride levels among all dietary constituents.

The eicosanoids derived from eicosapentaenoic acid and docosahexaenoic acid are capable of inhibiting thromboxane A_2 production while stimulating prostacyclin I_3 production, leading to vasodilatation and reduced thrombosis[12,13].

The consumption of fish and fish oils containing ω-3 polyunsaturated fatty acids including eicosapentaenoic acid and docosahexaenoic acid reduces the risk of coronary heart disease and associated mortality through numerous mechanisms such as decreased platelet aggregation, reduced blood pressure and blood viscosity and prevention of cardiac arrhythmia[14-16]. Therefore, consumption of fresh fish two to three times a week is a reasonable recommendation based on current scientific knowledge.

Trans-unsaturated fatty acids

Trans-unsaturated fatty acids occur when unsaturated fatty acids such as vegetable oils are partially or completely hydrogenated by having hydrogen atoms added to double bonds. Hydrogenation changes the configuration of carbon moieties around a double bond from the natural bent *cis*-configuration to an artificial straight *trans*-configuration. This process hardens the oil to a solid state. It allows greater product stability and thus extends the shelf-life of processed foods.

These are usually found in almost all processed snack foods. They are used for the production of butter substitutes (margarine) and in fast-food chains for deep fat frying of their foods.

Trans-unsaturated fatty acids increase the total cholesterol, LDL cholesterol, triglyceride and lipoprotein(a) levels and decrease HDL cholesterol levels. The adverse effects of *trans*-unsaturated fatty acids are stronger than those of saturated fatty acids[17].

Trans-unsaturated fatty acid intake is directly related to the risk of coronary heart disease. The relative risk of coronary heart disease for each 2% increment in energy intake from *trans*-unsaturated fat was 1.93, as compared with equivalent energy intake from carbohydrate. Replacement of 2% energy from *trans* fats with energy from non-hydrogenated unsaturated fats reduced coronary heart disease risk by 53%[3].

Dietary cholesterol

Most cholesterol is formed in the liver and some cholesterol is absorbed from dietary intake of cholesterol. Dietary cholesterol is present in all animal products, dairy products and egg yolks. More than 95% of fatty acids is absorbed while only 40–60% of dietary cholesterol is absorbed[18].

Dietary cholesterol influences total cholesterol and LDL cholesterol levels within the usual range of dietary intake. The predicted plasma cholesterol response to a 25 mg/day increase in dietary cholesterol intake is 1 mg/dl.

Consumption of 300 mg or less of dietary cholesterol per day is recommended for healthy adults, with more stringent reductions recommended for those with coronary heart disease or risk factors[2].

Dietary fiber

Dietary fiber includes substances such as cellulose, pectins and brans. Dietary fiber provides cardioprotection. The daily recommended amount is 20–30 g. The best way to get enough dietary fiber is to consume a wide variety of unrefined versions of foods, such as brown rice over white rice, whenever possible.

Dietary fiber is divided into two types: soluble and insoluble. Each type of fiber has different physiological effects. Soluble fibers, rich in fruits, vegetables, seeds and oats, modestly reduce total cholesterol and LDL cholesterol levels through increased bile acid excretion and decreased hepatic synthesis of cholesterol and have little or no effect on HDL cholesterol, while insoluble fibers increase the stool bulk, help to relieve constipation and prevent colon cancer.

Daily intake of 3 g of soluble fiber, equivalent to one large bowl of oat bran cereal or three packets of instant oatmeal, can lower the total cholesterol level by 5–6 mg/dl. The reduction is greater in those with initially higher blood cholesterol levels[19].

Diets high in fiber also have other beneficial effects such as increased insulin sensitivity[20], lower triglyceride levels[21] and favorable effects on plasminogen activator inhibitor (PAI) type I[22] and factor VII activity[23].

According to the Nurses' Health Study[24], higher fiber intake, particularly from cereal products, reduces the risk of coronary heart disease: a 19% risk reduction per 10 g/day increase of total dietary fiber and a 23% risk reduction of major coronary heart disease events for the highest compared with the lowest quintile.

Vitamins

Antioxidant vitamins

Three major nutrient antioxidants – tocopherol, ascorbic acid and β-carotene – can be obtained from the diet. Vitamin C and β-carotene are primarily obtained by intake of fruits and vegetables. Vitamin E is obtained through ingestion of vegetable oils (Table 2).

Vitamin C is the major water-soluble antioxidant and vitamin E is the major lipid-soluble antioxidant. Preformed vitamin A is referred to as vitamin A, which is known collectively as retinoids. This is not an antioxidant, but provitamin A (carotenoids) is an antioxidant. Of these carotenoids, 17% can be metabolized to vitamin A (retinol)[25]. Beta-carotene, one of the carotenoids, is the most widely distributed carotenoid in nature and the most thoroughly investigated. As an antioxidant, β-carotene is relatively weak, and functions primarily after other antioxidants have been used up.

Table 2 Recommended* daily allowance (RDA) and food sources of vitamins for women over 50 years

Nutrient	*RDA*	*Food sources*
Vitamin C	60 mg	green leafy vegetables, cauliflower, citrus fruits
Vitamin D		fish, fish oils
age 50+	400 IU (10 mg)	
age 70+	600 IU (15 mg)	
Vitamin E	30 IU	vegetable oils
Folic acid	400 mg	fresh vegetables, wheatgerm, brewer's yeast
Vitamin B_6	1.5 mg	whole grains, fish, nuts animal products
Vitamin B_{12}	2.4 μg	

*Recommended by the National Academy of Sciences, USA

The basic physiological function of antioxidants is to neutralize highly reactive free radical oxygen intermediates.

Epidemiological studies have shown that intake of these antioxidant vitamins was associated with a decreased risk of cardiovascular disease and associated mortality. Their major effect on protection from cardiovascular disease is protection from LDL cholesterol oxidation.

Beta-carotene

Consumption of increased dietary β-carotene or fruits and vegetables rich in β-carotene was found to be inversely related to the risk of cardiovascular disease[26,27]. However, large trials[28,29] with β-carotene supplementation did not show a protective effect on cardiovascular disease and was even associated with an increased risk of cancer.

Vitamin C

Many studies[30,31] have shown that increased intake of fruits and vegetables rich in vitamin C or increased serum ascorbic acid level was associated with a decreased risk of coronary heart disease and stroke.

Vitamin E

The main source of vitamin E is vegetable oils, and of those wheat germ oil has the highest concentration. Animal products are not a good source.

Vitamin E prevents oxidation of LDL cholesterol and also reduces platelet aggregation. Many studies have shown an inverse association between vitamin E intake and coronary heart disease risk. The strongest association was shown in the Nurses' Health Study[32]. The relative risk of major coronary disease for women in the highest fifth of vitamin E intake was 0.66 as compared with women in the lowest fifth. The cardioprotective benefit from vitamin E was due to supplements and was not related to dietary consumption. To obtain this vitamin E level by diet alone, three tablespoons of wheat germ oil or 0.75–1 cup of other vegetable oils daily would have to be consumed. This would significantly increase calories (1600 kcal/one cup of oil) and free radical production from the metabolism of unsaturated fatty acids in the oil. For cardioprotection, supplementation is the logical method.

However, recent studies - the Iowa Women's Health Study[33] and a Finnish study[34] - have provided evidence of an inverse association between mortality from coronary heart disease and intake of vitamin E from food. These findings suggest that modification of dietary habit to increase vitamin E intake may be worthwhile in preventing coronary heart disease.

Homocysteine-related vitamins

Homocysteine is a sulfur-containing amino acid and an intermediate metabolite formed during methionine metabolism. Homocysteine concentration is an independent risk factor for cardiovascular disease. Like cholesterol, the effects of homocysteine on cardiovascular disease are linearly related. Higher concentrations of plasma homocysteine are associated with a higher risk of cardiovascular disease such as coronary heart disease, stroke and peripheral vascular disease[35].

Plasma homocysteine concentrations are significantly increased after the menopause[36]. Plasma homocysteine levels are inversely related to plasma levels of folic acid, vitamin B_6 and vitamin B_{12}[37]. Intake of vitamin B_6 and folic acid are related to the plasma concentration of these vitamins except vitamin B_{12}. Gastric acid is necessary for the absorption of food-derived vitamin B_{12}. Malabsorption of vitamin B_{12} due to an increased prevalence of atrophic gastritis in aging people prevents adequate plasma levels being reached, even with the intake of an adequate amount of vitamin B_{12}. However, vitamin B_{12} is absorbed from supplements even in the presence of gastric atrophy.

One cup of cooked spinach and one cup of orange juice per day easily provide 400 mg of folic acid. Vitamin-fortified cereals and milk are the main sources of folic acid, vitamin B_6 and vitamin B_{12} in the diets of many elderly people.

The Hordaland Homocysteine Study[38] showed a relationship between higher intake of fruits and vegetables and decreased levels of homocysteine. There has been no definitive trial demonstrating that a reduction in homocysteine through supplementation with vitamin B_6, vitamin B_{12} and folic acid will reduce the incidence of cadiovascular disease, but recent data from the Nurses' Health Study[39] showed that a higher intake of vitamin B_6 and folate from food and/or supplement reduced the risk of coronary heart disease.

Minerals

Micronutrients, such as the minerals sodium, potassium, calcium and magnesium, can affect the cardiovascular system mainly through the effect on blood pressure.

Sodium

Sodium is ubiquitous in the diet. Controversy exists as to whether sodium intake contributes to elevations in blood pressure. Dietary sodium plays a relatively minor role in determining blood pressure[40], but some people are 'sodium sensitive' and high sodium intake in these women contributes to an elevation of blood pressure.

Increased sensitization to high sodium intake appears as people age[41]. High sodium intake becomes clinically important as a risk factor for postmenopausal hypertension. Persons with hypertension and/or obesity are more likely to be sodium sensitive[42,43]. Therefore, it seems prudent to restrict dietary sodium in individuals who are older, overweight or hypertensive.

Potassium/calcium

Increased dietary intake of potassium or calcium decreases blood pressure[44].

Magnesium

The recommended daily allowance (RDA) for magnesium in women is 280 mg/day. A significant inverse relationship was found between magnesium intake or intracellular magnesium and hypertension[45,46].

The cardiovascular effects of magnesium extend beyond its effect on blood pressure. Low serum and intracellular magnesium levels contribute to an increase in vascular thrombosis and cardiac dysrhythmia. Magnesium supplementation also benefits serum levels of lipids, decreasing triglycerides and very-low-density lipoprotein (VLDL) cholesterol with a trend toward increasing HDL cholesterol.

Phytochemicals

Carotenoids

Carotenoids are fat-soluble plant pigments providing the bright color of various fruits and vegetables. There are over 600 naturally occurring carotenoids. They can prevent lipid peroxidation. The major precursor of vitamin A, β-carotene, is found in many yellow, orange and dark-green leafy vegetables and in some yellow fruits. As an antioxidant, β-carotene is relatively weak as compared with other antioxidant vitamins.

Lycopene gives tomatoes their red color. Lycopene appears to be a more potent antioxidant than β-carotene. The EURAMIC study[47] showed that high tissue levels of lycopene were associated with a decreased risk of myocardial infarction.

Flavonoids

There are over 4000 naturally occurring flavonoids identified in fruits and vegetables, providing color, texture and taste.

Flavonoids prevent lipid peroxidation, promote vascular relaxation and have antihypertensive and antiarrhythmic properties.

Several studies[48–50] have found an inverse association between flavonoid intake and coronary heart disease and associated mortality. Flavonoid-rich food products such as soybean products, red wine and blueberries may provide cardioprotective benefits.

Isoflavones, one class of phytoestrogens, are found almost exclusively in soybeans. Three primary soy isoflavones are genistein, daidzein and glycitein. Soybeans are rich sources of phytoestrogens, containing 1–2 mg of phytoestrogen per gram of soy protein.

The intake of soy protein was shown to reduce total cholesterol and LDL cholesterol, suggesting beneficial effects of isoflavones on plasma lipid levels[51]. In addition to reducing the blood cholesterol level, isoflavones, especially genistein, alter the specific cellular atherosclerotic process through antioxidation, reduced platelet activity and accumulation, reduced platelet-derived growth factor (PDGF) production and thrombin action in *in vitro* studies[52,53]. Soy isoflavones also enhance coronary vascular reactivity[54].

The incorporation of food containing as little as 20–25 g of soy protein with isoflavones per day into the diet may provide a safe, inexpensive method to reduce an elevated cholesterol level and to decrease coronary heart disease. It can be recommended as a basic part of a healthy diet to benefit the heart in postmenopausal women.

Red wine contains quercetin in abundance, which is responsible for a cardioprotective effect[55]. The aqueous extract of blueberries is rich in antioxidants and appears to be more potent than vitamin C[56].

Alcohol

Consumption of alcoholic beverages in moderation, that is one or two alcoholic drinks daily, especially red wine, is associated with a decrease of cardiovascular disease and total mortality[57,58].

Moderate alcohol intake increases serum HDL cholesterol and decreases LDL cholesterol, which accounts for half of the beneficial effects[59]. A moderate intake of alcohol is also associated with an increase in endogenous tissue-type plasminogen activator, promoting fibrinolysis[60].

Red wine contains abundant quercetin and resveratrol. This flavonoid inhibits platelet aggregation and/or LDL cholesterol oxidation; this is responsible for additional cardioprotective effects[61]. Red grape juice has the same antioxidant and may give the same cardiovascular benefits. Therefore, consumption of red grape juice on a daily basis can be an alternative to red wine if alcohol is a problem.

DIETARY STRATEGY FOR THE PREVENTION OF OSTEOPOROSIS

Bone is a living structure. Hence, a wide range of adequate nutrition is needed for good bone health throughout life. Calcium is clearly the most important component of bone and essential for the formation of bone. However, for adequate bone health, more than just adequate amounts of calcium are required. The nutrients considered necessary for a healthy skeleton include macronutrients, bone mineral nutrients and bone matrix nutrients.

Calcium

Calcium is the most abundant mineral in the body and the dominant mineral of bone. Ninty-nine per cent of calcium is present in the bone, existing as hydroxyapatite. Low dietary intake and/or great loss of calcium leads to the demineralization of bone, to maintain the normal plasma calcium level.

The menopause is associated with an increase in bone resorption, a decrease in calcium absorption in the intestine and an increase in calcium excretion in the urine.

The RDA for calcium varies over the woman's lifespan. The RDA is 800 mg/day for women over 25 years of age. The National Institutes of Health (NIH) Consensus issues on the optimal calcium requirement were significantly different from the current RDA. Postmenopausal women on ERT/HRT are recommended to have a calcium intake of 1000 mg/day and postmenopausal women who are not receiving ERT/HRT or who are over the age of 65 are recommended to take 1500 mg/day. Regardless of these recommendations, postmenopausal women usually take less calcium than even the RDA of 800 mg calcium/day.

Dietary calcium intake and postmenopausal bone loss

It is not yet clear whether a high postmenopausal intake of calcium, either from the diet or from supplement, can prevent bone loss and subsequent fractures.

Bone turnover is very rapid and bone loss is accelerated during the immediate postmenopausal period. Estrogen deprivation plays the most significant role in this accelerated bone loss.

High calcium intake does not appear to protect against bone loss in the early postmenopausal period[62–64]. Even calcium supplementation of 1500–2000 mg/day has no effect on trabecular bone loss from the spine, but reduces cortical bone loss in the radius[60].

This finding suggests that calcium does not prevent the rapid decrease of bone density soon after the menopause. Estrogen therapy should be used. Calcium should not be considered as a substitute for estrogen in preventing osteoporosis.

Once the estrogen deprivation effect on bone has passed its maximum effect 5–6 years after the menopause, high calcium intake with supplementation may be beneficial, especially in women with inadequate calcium intake[64].

There is also some evidence that high calcium intake may have a synergistic bone-protective effect with antiresorptive agents such as estrogen or calcitonin[65].

Dietary calcium sources

Dairy products such as milk, hard cheese and yogurt are the best and major sources of calcium. They account for 60–75% of calcium intake. Three servings of dairy products meet the RDA of 800 mg/day. For postmenopausal women who do not like or cannot ingest dairy products, other good food sources of calcium – green vegetables such as kale and broccoli, turnips, fish containing bones, legumes including tofu, nuts and fruits - can be substitutes for dairy products (Table 3).

A concern with increased dairy consumption for dietary calcium sources is the possible adverse effects of excessive caloric intake from increased fat intake; therefore the use of low-fat or non-fat dairy products is recommended.

Dietary factors related to calcium absorption

Approximately one-fifth of oral calcium is absorbed. The degree of calcium absorption depends on various factors: calcium intake, the level of 1,25-$(OH)_2$ vitamin D, the pH in the gut lumen and dietary factors such as fiber or certain anions.

The adaptation phenomenon is well known in which calcium absorption is increased when calcium intake is low, and decreased when intake is high. The process is regulated by 1,25-$(OH)_2$ vitamin D.

Lactose and other sugars such as xylose and sorbitol increase calcium absorption, but it is not clear whether lactase deficiency decreases calcium absorption[66,67]. For lactose-intolerant individuals who have very low calcium intake because of avoidance of milk products, such dairy products with reduced lactose content as cheese and yogurt and the addition of lactase to milk are recommended[68,69].

High-fiber diets may reduce calcium absorption. It has been estimated that an increase in fiber intake of 26 g/day could increase the calcium requirement by 150 mg/day. Foods high in phytates such as wheat bran and beans decrease calcium absorption across the gut[70], and so do high-oxalate foods such as spinach and rhubarb[71].

Table 3 Food sources of calcium. Adapted from reference 91

Food	*Amount*	*Calcium* (mg)
Dairy products		
milk	1 cup	300
yogurt	1 cup	400
hard cheese	1 oz	200
Green vegetables	½ cup	175
Canned fish*	3 oz	200
Legumes		
all	½ cup	100
Others		
almonds	¼ cup	80
oranges	1 medium	30
oatmeal	1 cup	20

*Salmon/sardines with bones

Dietary factors related to calcium excretion

Sodium across the full range of its intake increases urinary calcium loss owing to the decrease in renal tubular reabsorption of calcium[72]. Therefore, urinary calcium is usually proportional to urinary sodium. A diet low in sodium, causing reduction in urinary calcium excretion and conservation of calcium, eventually reduces the bone resorption.

Adequate protein intake is necessary for bone health. However, excessive protein intake negatively affects calcium balance[73]. The effect of animal protein with sulfur-containing amino acids on the kidney is to increase the clearance and also to decrease the tubular reabsorption of calcium, thus increasing the urinary excretion of calcium[74]. In practical terms, with any given dietary protein intake, a doubling of protein intake results in an approximately 50% increase in urine calcium excretion[75].

Not all proteins have the same effect in increasing calcium excretion. Compared with animal protein, soy protein does not result in an increased loss of calcium in the urine. Additionally, isoflavones in soy may inhibit the resorption of bone.

The role of phosphorus in calcium metabolism is controversial. Phosphorus reduces urinary calcium excretion but it enhances endogenous fecal loss of calcium. The net result is no real change in calcium balance[76]. However, high-phosphate diets may induce secondary hyperparathyroidism and hypercalciuria. Excessive phosphorus intake in animal studies has also increased urinary calcium loss causing osteoporosis. High-phosphorus drinks such as colas which also contain high sugar and caffeine levels are of recent concern[77].

Caffeine increases urinary calcium excretion in a dose-dependent fashion[78]. A cup of coffee reduces the calcium balance by 2-3 mg/day[79]. There have been cohort studies[80,81] that have observed a positive association between high caffeine consumption and risk of hip fracture.

Tea also contains caffeine, but appears to be associated with a decrease in hip fracture risk, perhaps due to estrogenic flavonoids.

Magnesium

Sixty per cent of the body magnesium is found in the bone. Magnesium is required for the bone matrix and mineral metabolism. It may also increase bone quality by decreasing the size of hydroxyapatite crystals.

Dairy products are good sources of dietary magnesium. Other sources include whole grains, green leafy vegetables and nuts.

Calcium and magnesium compete for absorption across the gut[82]; magnesium absorption becomes positive when the ratio of calcium to magnesium intake is approximately 2 : 1. High doses of calcium for osteoporosis, as recently recommended, will deleteriously affect magnesium homeostasis. Therefore, if postmenopausal women have a high calcium intake, supplemental magnesium in doses of 250–500 mg/day should be advised.

Copper, manganese and zinc

Copper, manganese and zinc are classified as bone matrix nutrients. Copper is a cofactor for lysyl oxidase, an enzyme required for the formation of collagen cross-links[83]. Manganese is required as a coenzyme in the production of mucopolysaccharides, upon which mineralization occurs[84]. Zinc is required for cellular proliferation and protein synthesis. It enhances the effect of vitamin D[85]. Therefore, dietary deficiencies of these trace minerals are associated with osteoporosis.

Copper and manganese are present abundantly in unrefined whole grains, leafy vegetables and nuts. Zinc is abundant in oysters, unrefined sugar and flour.

Vitamins

The vitamins to consider in terms of bone health are folic acid, vitamin B, vitamin C, vitamin D and vitamin K.

Vitamin D is needed to maintain skeletal integrity and calcium homeostasis through the intestinal and renal absorption of calcium. Women over age 50 and 70 years are recommended to take daily 400 IU and 600 IU of vitamin D, respectively. Vitamin D is formed in the skin with exposure to sunlight but synthesis may be compromised as people age, because of less exposure to sunlight and less production of 7-dehydrocholesterol in the skin[86].

Vitamin D is also obtained from the diet. The main food sources of vitamin D are oily fish, fish liver oil, egg yolk and vitamin-fortified dairy products, but it is difficult to obtain enough vitamin D from food alone.

Homocysteine, increasing after the menopause, interferes with collagen cross-linking in the bone matrix. Vitamin B_6 and folic acid may be used for elimination from the metabolism of the harmful metabolite. Vitamin C is necessary for hydroxylation of protein. Vitamin K is a cofactor of γ-carboxylase, being required to synthesize osteocalcin[87]. The sources and the recommended daily allowances of these vitamins are seen in Table 2.

Isoflavones

Isoflavones, one of three main classes of phytoestrogens, are found richly in soybean and soy products. Limited short-term human studies[88,89] revealed that isoflavones or soy protein reduced bone turnover and increased bone mineral density in postmenopausal women. However, there are no long-term study data evaluating the effect of isoflavones on bone mineral density or fracture rates in postmenopausal women.

Alcohol

High alcohol consumption appears to be a significant risk factor for osteoporosis. Alcohol reduces bone formation[90] and this may be due to a primary effect of ethanol toxicity on bone. High intake of alcohol is associated with marked dietary disturbances such as protein malnutrition.

CONCLUSION

Decreasing serum levels of atherogenic lipoproteins reduces the incidence of atherosclerosis and thus the risk of coronary heart disease. This can be accomplished by a reduction of total dietary fat. The type of fat in the diet is more important. Therefore, after reducing the total fat intake, the substitution of ω-3 polyunsaturated and monounsaturated fats for other fats may be healthful. The intake of any foods containing hydrogenated oil should be avoided or limited.

The increased consumption of vegetables, fruits and unrefined whole grains is recommended, because these plant foods provide cardioprotective soluble fibers, antioxidant vitamins, ample cardioprotective minerals and various non-nutritive phytochemicals in addition to a reduction in serum cholesterol levels.

A moderate consumption of alcohol, not more than one glass of red wine per day, may provide cardiovascular benefits.

The intake of calcium as well as other bone minerals and matrix nutrients such as magnesium, copper, zinc and some vitamins is important for the prevention of osteoporosis.

References

1. Utian WH, Boggs PP. The North American Menopause Society 1998 menopause survey. Part I: Postmenopausal women's perceptions about menopause and midlife. *Menopause* 1998;6:122–8
2. American Heart Association. Dietary guidelines for healthy American adults. *Circulation* 1996;94: 1795–800
3. Hu FB, Stampfer MJ, Manson JE, *et al.* Dietary fat intake and the risk of coronary heart disease in women. *N Engl J Med* 1997;337:1491–9
4. Grundy SM, Denke MA. Dietary influences on serum lipids and lipoproteins. *J Lipid Res* 1990; 31:1149–72
5. Hegsted DM, McGandy RB, Myers ML, *et al.* Quantitative effects of dietary fat on serum cholesterol in man. *Am J Clin Nutr* 1965;7:281–95
6. Keys A, Anderson JT, Grande F. Prediction of serum cholesterol responses of man to changes in fats in the diet. *Lancet* 1957;1:966–8
7. Clarke R, Frost C, Collins R, *et al.* Dietary lipids and blood cholesterol: quantitative meta-analysis of metabolic ward studies. *Br Med J* 1997;314: 112–17
8. Garg A, Grundy SM, Koffler M. Effect of high carbohydrate intake on hyperglycemia, islet function, and plasma lipoproteins in NIDDM. *Diabetes Care* 1992;15:1572–80
9. Parthasarathy S, Khoo JC, Miller E, *et al.* Low density lipoprotein rich in oleic acid is protected against oxidative modification: implications for dietary prevention of atherosclerosis. *Proc Natl Acad Sci USA* 1990;87:3894–8
10. de Lorgeril M, Renaud S, Mamelle N, *et al.* Mediterranean alpha-linolenic acid-rich diet in secondary prevention of coronary heart disease. *Lancet* 1994; 343:1454–9
11. Jacobs D, Blackburn H, Higgins M, *et al.* Report of the conference on low blood cholesterol: mortality associations. *Circulation* 1992;86:1046–60
12. Zollner N, Tato F. Fatty acid composition of the diet: impact on serum lipids and atherosclerosis. *Clin Invest* 1992;70:968–1009
13. Knapp HR, Reilly IAG, Alessandrini P, *et al. In vivo* indexes of platelet and vascular function during fish-oil administration in patients with atherosclerosis. *N Engl J Med* 1986;314:937–42
14. Herold PM, Kinsella JE. Fish oil consumption and decreased risk of cardiovascular disease: a comparison of findings from animal and human feeding trials. *Am J Clin Nutr* 1986;43:566–98
15. Rogers S, James KS, Butland BK, *et al.* Effects of a fish oil supplement on serum lipids, blood pressure, bleeding time, haemostatic and rheological variables. *Atherosclerosis* 1987;53:137–43
16. Woodcock BE, Smith E, Lambert WH, *et al.* Beneficial effect of fish oil on blood viscosity in peripheral vascular disease. *Br Med J* 1984;288:592–4
17. Ascherio A, Willett WC. Health effects of *trans* fatty acids. *Am J Clin Nutr* 1997;66(Suppl): 1006S–10S
18. Conner WE, Lin DS. The intestinal absorption of dietary cholesterol by hypercholesterolemic (type II) and normocholesterolemic humans. *J Clin Invest* 1974;553:1062–71
19. Ripsin CM, Keenan JM, Jacobs DR Jr, *et al.* Oat products and lipid lowering: a meta-analysis. *J Am Med Assoc* 1992;267:3317–25
20. Hallfrisch J, Scholfield DH, Behall KM. Diets containing soluble oat extracts improve glucose and insulin responses of moderately hypercholesterolemic men and women. *Am J Clin Nutr* 1995;61: 379–84

21. Anderson JW, Chen WL, Sieling B. Hypolipidemic effects of high-carbohydrate, high-fiber diets. *Metabolism* 1980;29:551–8
22. Sundell IB, Ranby M. Oat husk fiber decreases plasminogen activator inhibitor type 1 activity. *Haemostasis* 1993;23:45–50
23. Marckmann P, Sandstrom B, Jespersen J. Favorable long-term effect of a low-fat/high-fiber diet on human blood coagulation and fibrinolysis. *Arterioscler Thromb* 1993;13:505–11
24. Wolk A, Manson JE, Stampfer MJ, *et al.* Long-term intake of dietary fiber and decreased risk of coronary heart disease among women. *J Am Med Assoc* 1999;281:1998–2004
25. Bendich A. Biological functions of dietary carotenoids. *Ann NY Acad Sci* 1993;691:61–7
26. Gaziano JM, Manson JE, Buring JE, *et al.* Dietary antioxidants and cardiovascular disease. *Ann NY Acad Sci* 1992;669:249–59
27. Gaziano JM, Manson JE, Branch LG, *et al.* Dietary beta carotene and decreased cardiovascular mortality in an elderly cohort [abstract]. *J Am Coll Cardiol* 1992;19(Suppl A):377A
28. The Alpha-Tocopherol, Beta Carotene Cancer Prevention Study Group. The effect of vitamin E and beta carotene on the incidence of lung cancer and other cancers in male smokers. *N Engl J Med* 1994;330:1029–35
29. Omenn GS, Goodman GE, Thornquist MD, *et al.* Risk factors for lung cancer and for intervention effects in CARET, the beta-carotene, and retinol efficacy trial. *J Natl Cancer Inst* 1996;88:1550–9
30. Ginter E. Decline of coronary mortality in the United States and vitamin C. *Am J Clin Nutr* 1979;32:511–12
31. Simon JA, Hudes ES, Browner WS. Serum ascorbic acid and cardiovascular disease prevalence in US adults. *Epidemiology* 1998;9:316–21
32. Stampfer MJ, Hennekens CH, Manson JE, *et al.* Vitamin E consumption and the risk of coronary disease in women. *N Engl J Med* 1993;328:1444–9
33. Kushi LH, Folson AR, Prineas RJ, *et al.* Dietary antioxidant vitamins and death from coronary heart disease in postmenopausal women. *N Engl J Med* 1996;334:1156–62
34. Knekt P, Reunanen A, Jarvinen R, *et al.* Antioxidant vitamin intake and coronary mortality in a longitudinal population study. *Am J Epidemiol* 1994;139:1180–9
35. Stein JH, McBride PE. Hyperhomocysteinemia and atherosclerotic vascular disease. *Arch Int Med* 1998;158:1301–6
36. Wouters MG, Moorrees MT, van der Mooren MJ, *et al.* Plasma homocysteine and menopausal status. *Eur J Clin Invest* 1995;25:80–5
37. Selhub J, Jacques PF, Wilson PWF, *et al.* Vitamin status and intake as primary determinants of homocysteinemia in an elderly population. *J Am Med Assoc* 1993;270:2693–8
38. Nygard O, Vollset SE, Refsum H, *et al.* Total plasma homocysteine and cardiovascular risk profile; the Hordaland Homocysteine Study. *J Am Med Assoc* 1995;274:1526–33
39. Rimm EB, Willett WC, Hu FB, *et al.* Folate and vitamin B6 from diet and supplements in relation to risk of coronary heart disease among women. *J Am Med Assoc* 1998;279:359–64
40. The Intersalt Cooperative Research Group. Intersalt: an international study of electrolyte excretion and blood pressure. Results for a 24-hour urinary sodium and potassium excretion. *Br Med J* 1998;297:319–28
41. Rosenfield J. Hypertension in the elderly. *Kidney Int* 1983;23:540–7
42. Law MR, Frost CD, Wald NJ. By how much does dietary salt reduction lower blood pressure? III. Analysis of data from trials of salt reduction. *Br Med J* 1991;302:819–24
43. Rocchini AP, Key J, Bondie D, *et al.* The effect of weight loss on the sensitivity of blood pressure to sodium in obese adolescents. *N Engl J Med* 1989;321:580–5
44. Langford HG. Dietary potassium and hypertension: epidemiological data. *Ann Intern Med* 1983;98:770–2
45. Witteman JC, Willett WC, Stampfer M, *et al.* A prospective study of nutritional factors and hypertension among U.S. women. *Circulation* 1989;80:1320–7
46. Resnick LM, Gupta RK, Lavagh JH. Intracellular free magnesium in erythrocytes of essential hypertension: relation to blood pressure and serum divalent cations. *Proc Natl Acad Sci USA* 1984;81:6511–15
47. Kohlmeier L, Kark JD, Gomez-Garcia E, *et al.* Lycopene and myocardial infarction risk in the EURAMIC Study. *Am J Epidemiol* 1997;146:618–26
48. Hertog MG, Feskens EJ, Hollman PC, *et al.* Dietary antioxidant flavonoids and risk of coronary heart disease: the Zutphen elderly study. *Lancet* 1993;342:1007–11
49. Hertog MG, Kromhout D, Aravanis C, *et al.* Flavonoid intake and long-term risk of coronary heart disease and cancer in the seven countries study. *Arch Intern Med* 1995;155:381–6
50. Knekt P, Jarvinen R, Reunanen A, *et al.* Flavonoid intake and coronary mortality in Finland: a cohort study. *Br Med J* 1996;312:478–81
51. Anderson JW, Johnstone BM, Cook-Newwell ME. Meta-analysis of the effects of soy protein intake on serum lipids. *N Engl J Med* 1995;333:276–82
52. Tikkanen MH, Walhala K, Ojala S, *et al.* Effect of soybean phytoestrogen intake on low density lipoprotein oxidation resistance. *Proc Natl Acad Sci USA* 1998;95:3106–10
53. Potter SM. Soy protein and serum lipids. *Curr Opin Lipidol* 1996;7:260–4

54. Honore EK, Williams JK, Anthony MS, *et al.* Soy isoflavones enhance coronary vascular reactivity in atherosclerotic female macaques. *Fertil Steril* 1997; 67:148–54
55. Formica JV, Regelson W. Review of the biology of quercetin and related bioflavonoids. *Food Chem Toxicol* 1995;33:1061–80
56. Laplaud PM, Lelubre A, Chapman MJ. Antioxidant action of *Vaccinium myrtillus* extract on human low density lipoproteins *in vitro*: initial observations. *Fundam Clin Pharmacol* 1997;11:35–40
57. Moore RD, Pearson TA. Moderate alcohol consumption and coronary artery disease: a review. *Medicine (Baltimore)* 1986;65:242–67
58. Jackson R, Scragg R, Beagle Hole R. Does recent alcohol consumption reduce the risk of acute myocardial infarction and coronary death in regular drinkers? *Am J Epidemiol* 1992;136:819–24
59. Thorton J, Symes C, Heaton K. Moderate alcohol intake reduces bile cholesterol saturation and raises HDL cholesterol. *Lancet* 1983;2:819–22
60. Ridker PM, Vaughan DE, Stampfer MJ, *et al.* Association of moderate alcohol consumption and plasma concentration of endogenous tissue-type plasminogen activator. *J Am Med Assoc* 1994;272: 929–33
61. Sharp D. When wine is red. *Lancet* 1993;341:27–8
62. Riis B, Thomson K, Christiansen C. Does calcium supplementation prevent postmenopausal bone loss? A double-blind, controlled clinical study. *N Engl J Med* 1987;316:173–7
63. Riggs BL, Wahner HW, Melton LJ III, *et al.* Dietary calcium intake and rates of bone loss in women. *J Clin Invest* 1987;80:979–82
64. Dawson-Hughes B, Dallal GE, Krall EA, *et al.* A controlled trial of the effect of calcium supplementation on bone density in postmenopausal women. *N Engl J Med* 1990;323:878–83
65. Genant HK, Baylink DJ, Gallagher JC, *et al.* Effect of estrone sulfate on postmenopausal bone loss. *Obstet Gynecol* 1990;76:579–84
66. Cochet B, Jung A, Griessen M, *et al.* Effects of lactose on intestinal calcium absorption in normal and lactase-deficient subjects. *Gastroenterology* 1983; 84:935–40
67. Griessen M, Cochet B, Infante F, *et al.* Calcium absorption from milk in lactase-deficient subjects. *Am J Clin Nutr* 1989;49:377–84
68. Gallagher JC, Fillion A. Calcium and vitamin B. In Lorrain J, Plouffe L Jr, Ravnikar V, eds. *Comprehensive Management of Menopause.* New York: Springer-Verlag, 1993:137–58
69. Kelsay J, Behall KM, Prather ES. Effect of fiber from fruits and vegetables on metabolic responses of human subjects. II. Calcium, magnesium, iron and silicon balances. *Am J Clin Nutr* 1979;32: 1876–80
70. Weaver CM, Heaney RP, Martin BR, *et al.* Human calcium absorption from whole wheat products. *J Nutr* 1991;121:1769–75
71. Heaney RP, Weaver CM. Oxalate in vegetables: effect on calcium absorbability. *J Bone Miner Res* 1993;8:S333–7
72. McParland BE, Goulding A, Campbell AH. Dietary salt affects biochemical markers of resorption and formation of bone in elderly women. *Br Med J* 1989;299:834–5
73. Johnson NE, Alcantara EN, Linkswiler HM. Effect of protein intake on urinary and fecal calcium and calcium retention of young adult males. *J Nutr* 1970;100:1425–8
74. Schuette SA, Zemel MB, Linkswiler HM. Studies on the mechanisms of protein induced hypercalciuria in older men and women. *J Nutr* 1980;110:305–15
75. Kontessis P, Hones R, Dodd R, *et al.* Renal, metabolic and hormonal responses to ingestion of animal and vegetable proteins. *Kidney Int* 1990;38: 136–44
76. Heaney RP, Recker RR. Effects of nitrogen, phosphorus, and caffeine on calcium balance in women. *J Lab Clin Med* 1982;99:46–55
77. Carey A, Carey B. Nutritional support for osteoporosis. In Studd J, ed. *The Management of the Menopause: Annual Review 1998.* Carnforth, UK: Parthenon Publishing, 1998:159–68
78. Hollingbery PW, Bergman EA, Massey LK. Effect of dietary caffeine and aspirin on urinary calcium and hydroxyproline excretion in pre- and postmenopausal women. *Fed Proc* 1985;44: 1149
79. Heaney RP, Recker RR. Effects of nitrogen, phosphorus, and caffeine on calcium balance in women. *J Lab Clin Med* 1982;99:46–55
80. Kiel DP, Felson DT, Hannan MT, *et al.* Caffeine and the risk of hip fracture: the Framingham study. *Am J Epidemiol* 1990;132:675–84
81. Hernandez-Avila M, Colditz GA, Stampfer MJ, *et al.* Caffeine, moderate alcohol intake, and risk of fractures of the hip and forearm in middle-aged women. *Am J Clin Nutr* 1991;54:157–63
82. Seelig MS. The requirement of magnesium by the normal adult. *Am J Clin Nutr* 1964;14:342–90
83. Weaver CM, Peacock M, Johnston CC. Adolescent nutrition in the prevention of postmenopausal osteoporosis. *J Clin Endocrinol Metab* 1999;84: 1839–43
84. Leach RM, Muenster AM, Wein EM. Studies on the role of manganese in bone formation. II. Effect upon chondroitin sulfate synthesis in chick epiphyseal cartilage. *Arch Biochem Biophys* 1969;133: 22–8
85. Yamaguchi M, Sakashita T. Enhancement of vitamin D3 effect on bone metabolism in weanling rats

orally administered zinc sulphate. *Acta Endocrinol* 1986;11:285–8

86. Riggs B, Melton LJ. Involutional osteoporosis. In Evans JG, Williams TF, eds. *Oxford Textbook of Geriatric Medicine.* Oxford: Oxford University Press, 1992:405–11
87. Dodds RA, Catterall A, Bitensky L, *et al.* Effects on fracture healing of an antagonist of the vitamin K cycle. *Calcif Tissue Int* 1984;36:233–8
88. Potter SM, Baum JA, Teng H, *et al.* Soy protein and isoflavones: their effects on blood lipids and bone density in postmenopausal women. *Am J Clin Nutr* 1998;6(Suppl 6):1375S–9S
89. Bonaccorsi G, Albertazzi P, Constantino D, *et al.* Soy phytoestrogens and bone. Presented at the *Meeting of the North American Menopause Society*, 1997: abstr 44
90. Dimond T, Stiel D, Lunzer M, *et al.* Ethanol reduces bone formation and may cause osteoporosis. *Am J Med* 1989;86:282–8
91. Pennington JA, Churchill HN. *Food Values of Portions Commonly Used*, 13th edn. New York: Harper & Row, 1980

Optimal treatment of menopausal disorder based on differential diagnosis of mental disorders

42

T. Ushiroyama

The menopausal transition is frequently associated with an increase in psychological as well as physical symptoms. Vasomotor and atrophic symptoms are recognized as being associated with estrogen deficiency, and widely accepted as common symptoms of the menopause or undefined syndromes in the perimenopause. There is much debate about the etiology of menopausal disorder, because of the many complex related factors. Furthermore, psychological complaints are frequently observed, such as depressive mood, irritability and difficulty in concentrating, and it is still not fully understood whether these can be attributed to endocrine changes or whether they are mainly brought about by other factors such as stressful life events, cultural and socioeconomic factors, or patient characteristics.

Several mental disorders are observed during the perimenopausal period. One of the more intriguing dilemmas in menopause research is that different people, from different disciplines, at different points in time have asked the same question about the relationship between menopause and depression, or anxiety disorder, (for example 'panic disorder'), and have returned with quite different answers.

It has been established that hormone replacement therapy (HRT) improves menopausal symptoms, particularly vasomotor disturbance, such as hot flushes or sweating. However, HRT is not always effective in menopausal disorder, because several complaints occurring in the perimenopause remain undefined. Although apparently these complaints are seen as menopausal disorder, they may actually be related to depression or anxiety disorder. For this reason, it is difficult to find the most suitable HRT. Ideally, we should choose the optimum treatment for each disease. In most of these cases, women come to out-patient clinics with undefined complaints, and are diagnosed with menopausal disorder through wide interpretation. Therefore, accurate differential diagnosis is necessary.

INCIDENCE OF UNDEFINED SYNDROMES IN PERIMENOPAUSE

We investigated psychological and physical problems occurring around the time of the menopause in healthy Japanese women during 10 years after the onset of the menopausal transition (Figure 1). About one in ten women consulted a doctor because of physical or psychological complaints during the perimenopause. Some 12.8% of women experienced several symptoms for more than 1 year, but they were patient and did not receive any medication. However, the proportion of women who never experienced unfavorable psychosomatic symptoms and never had undefined complaints during the perimenopausal period was 51.2%. These data show that acute endocrine changes do not always cause undefined symptoms, and that cultural and socioeconomic factors or patient characteristics are clearly involved in the problem of menopausal disorder and related diseases.

CAUSES OF AND FACTORS IN MENOPAUSAL DISORDER

A large number of epidemiological studies have reported that HRT is optimal or recommended for the relief of undefined complaints during the menopausal period. However, in clinical practice,

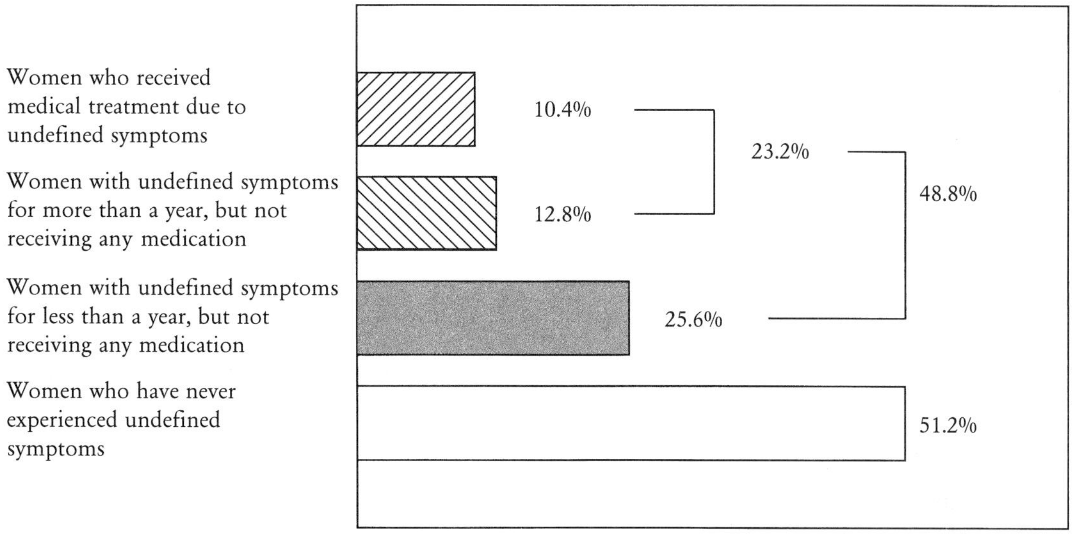

Figure 1 Incidence of undefined symptoms in perimenopausal period

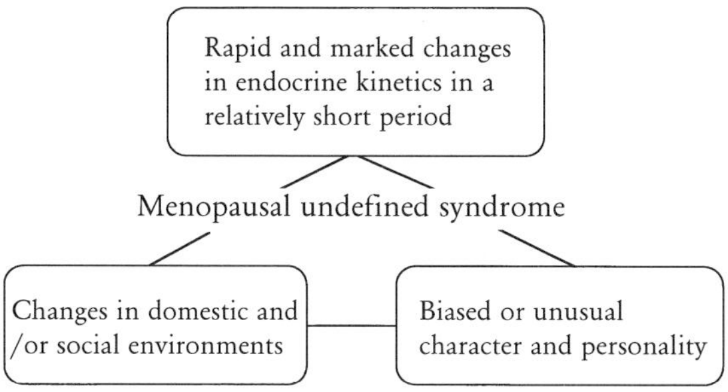

Figure 2 Factor triangle for menopausal undefined syndrome

Table 1 Factors affecting undefined symptoms in perimenopausal women

Rapid and marked changes in endocrine kinetics in a relatively short period
elevation of plasma gonadotropin levels
reduction of plasma estradiol level
Changes in domestic and/or social environments
empty-nest syndrome
loneliness in the home
separation experience
relationship with spouse
mid-life crisis
economic problems
Biased or unusual character and personality
seriousness
punctiliousness
strong sense of responsibility
melancholic
self-sacrificing

unfavorable psychological and physical conditions, mainly involving vegetative nerve disturbance in patients with acute menopausal disorder, do not always respond to hormone treatment. This is because marked changes in endocrine kinetics[1,2], as well as domestic and social environments during the perimenopausal period, are involved in the etiology, and because the patient's condition is modified by deviations in character or personality. These three factors are considered to be the main causes of menopausal disorder (Figure 2). For instance, specific situations such as the terminated role of mother, the 'empty-nest' syndrome, a separation experience or an unhappy spousal relationship may be observed as changes in circumstances in perimenopausal women (Table 1). These are conditions that easily result in emotional disturbances. In addition to these factors, some physical problems also cause vegetative nerve disturbances in menopausal women ('Mid-life crisis'). In sensitive women, symptoms may be triggered by some very small endocrinological change, if great mental stress already exists. Therefore, attention should be paid to background factors, such as circumstances, socioeconomic factors and cultural factors, of menopausal women who come to out-patient clinics with symptoms. The menopausal woman is surrounded by many stress-related factors, resulting in psychological conflict.

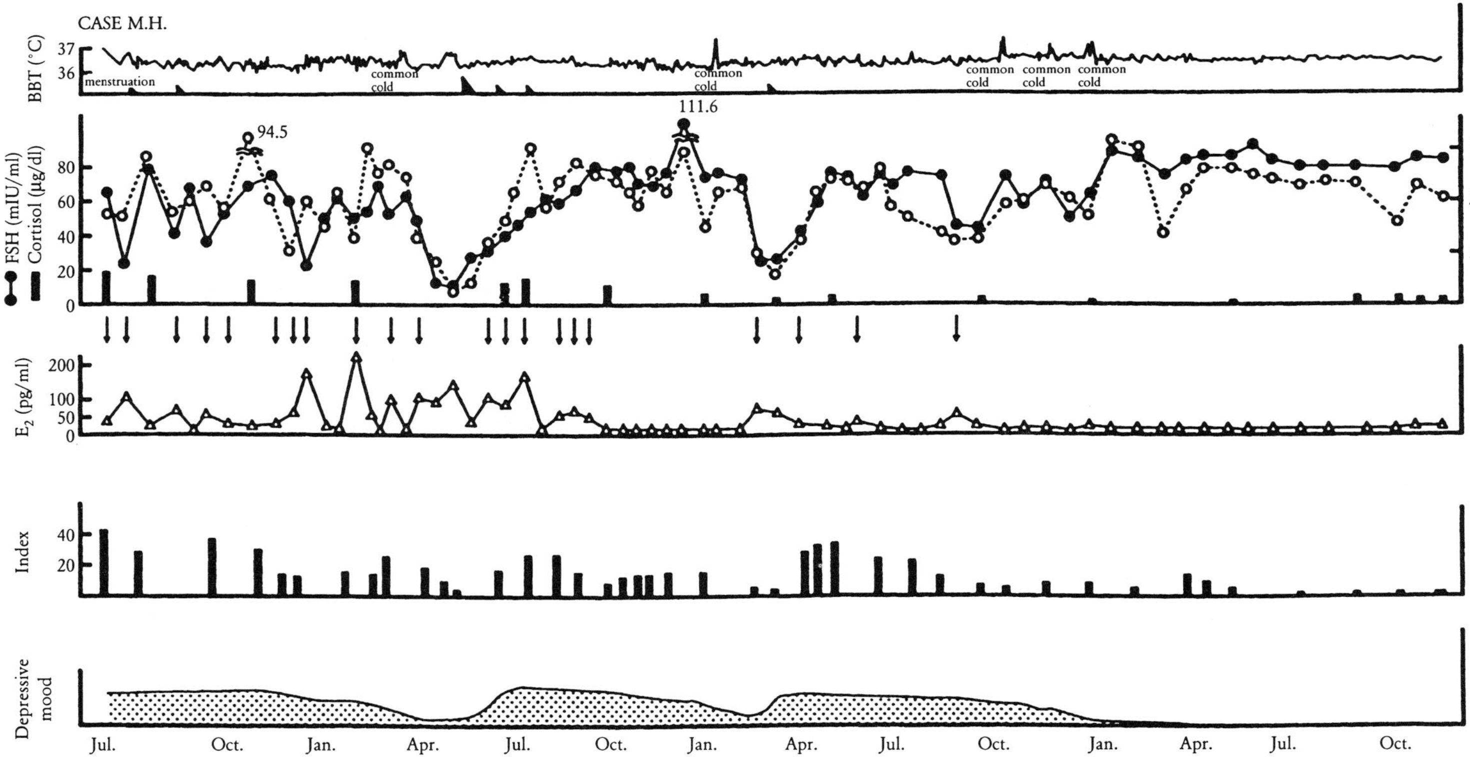

Figure 3 Daily concentrations of plasma luteinizing hormone (LH), follicle stimulating hormone (FSH), cortisol and estradiol (E_2) in one 48-year-old mood disorder patient during menopausal transition. Arrows indicate hypergonadotropinemia with estradiol secretion. BBT, basal body temperature

Figure 3 illustrates the endocrine profiles associated with changes in symptoms or depressive mood during multiple cycles in a woman studied 3.5 years into the menopausal trasition. In the first year, gonadotropin levels were clearly in the menopausal range, with sporadic rises in estradiol. The mean estradiol concentration during this period was 66 ± 60 pg/ml with maximum levels of 250 pg/ml. In the second year, mean estradiol levels decreased to 36 ± 38 pg/ml. The increase in physical symptoms and depressive mood distinctly synchronized with the rise in plasma gonadotropin concentrations. In the final 1.5 years, gonadotropin levels remained high, while estradiol concentrations fell to 20 pg/ml. Depressive mood and other physical symptoms disappeared in correlation with the development of sustained hypergonadotropinemia and hypogonadism. The possible explanation of this clinical course is related to endocrine changes; rapid elevation of gonadotropins probably promotes a sympathoadrenal response to a variety of simple physiological stimuli[3]. On the other hand, we found that the plasma estradiol levels of depressive perimenopausal women (56 ± 6.8 pg/ml) whose menstrual periods had recently become irregular were significantly higher than in those with menopausal disorder without mental symptoms (30 ± 4.4 pg/ml; $p < 0.05$) or in healthy women (37 ± 2.0 pg/ml; $p < 0.05$). We observed the same significant differences in postmenopausal women (Figure 4). These findings suggest that endocrine changes are one of the causes of undefined symptoms during the menopausal period.

It has also been suggested that undefined complaints are associated with personal characteristics, as well as rapid endocrine changes and socioeconomic environments in the perimenopause. Table 2 gives the results of character or psychological tests considering various diseases that were accompanied by undefined complaints. In the Minnesota Multiphasic Personality Inventory - alexithymia scale (MMPI-AS) test, which is used for screening alexithymia, the mean scores of patients with mental disorders were higher than those of patients with menopausal disorder or ovarian deficiency syndrome. Similarly, the mean scores of patients with menopausal disorder were higher than those of healthy middle-aged women[4,5].

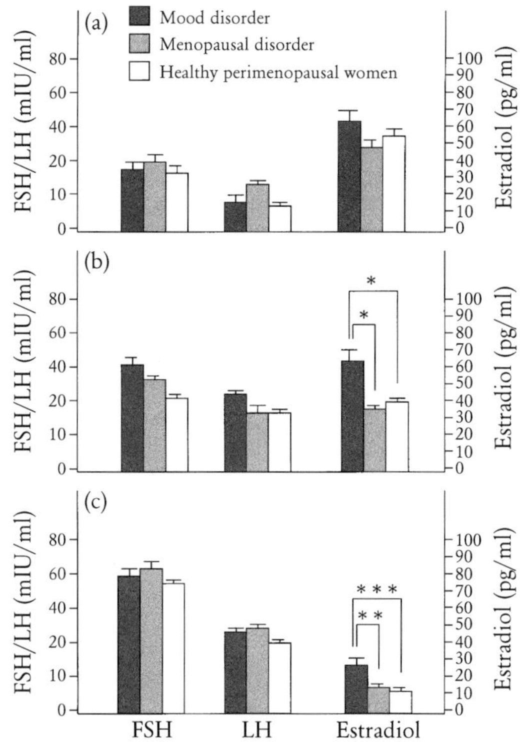

Figure 4 Serum follicle stimulating hormone (FSH), luteinizing hormone (LH) and estradiol levels in mood disorder, menopausal disorder and healthy women with different menstrual patterns: (a) perimenopausal women with regular menstrual periods; (b) perimenopausal women whose menstrual periods have recently become irregular; (c) postmenopausal women. Results are given as mean ± SE. *, **, ***, statistically significant difference at $p < 0.05$, < 0.01, < 0.001, respectively

PREVALENCE OF MENOPAUSAL DISORDER AND MENTAL DISORDERS IN WOMEN WITH UNDEFINED COMPLAINTS IN THE PERIMENOPAUSAL PERIOD

In patients with undefined symptoms during the perimenopausal period, mental and psychosomatic disorders develop concurrently for the reasons described above. Figure 5 shows the final diagnoses of 1000 patients with undefined complaints during the menopausal period. We diagnosed mental disorders using the specified diagnostic criteria for each mental disorder, the Diagnostic and Statistical Manual of Mental Disorders, 3rd edn (DSM-III) revised[6] of the American Psychiatric Association. Overall, 33.3%

(333/1000) of the women with undefined symptoms were diagnosed with menopausal disorder, showing hypergonadotropinemia and estradiol deficiency, but neither a psychosomatic relationship nor psychological abnormalities. Women who were diagnosed with a psychosomatic disorder made up 12.3% (123/1000) and those with vegetative disorder 5.0% (50/1000) of the total population. It is worthy of note that half of the total population of 1000 women with undefined complaints (49.4%) were reported as having mental disorders. In the population with mental

Table 2 Personality inventory in perimenopausal women with undefined complaints. Values are expressed as mean (SD)

		Personality test							
				Egogram comparison					
Disease type	*Age* (years)	*SRQ-D*	*MMPI-AS*	*CP*	*NP*	*A*	*FC*	*AC*
Mood disorder ($n = 226$)	48.1 (3.6)	23.1 (3.9)	15.2 (2.6)	3.4 (1.5)	4.8 (1.8)	4.5 (1.3)	4.4 (1.9)	5.3 (1.1)
Anxiety disorder ($n = 118$)	49.5 (6.1)	22.2 (5.3)	13.5 (4.3)	3.3 (1.3)	5.5 (2.0)	3.9 (1.4)	4.5 (1.4)	5.5 (2.2)
Somatoform disorder ($n = 44$)	50.0 (4.6)	18.3 (5.7)	14.7 (3.6)	3.2 (1.0)	4.8 (1.4)	4.2 (1.2)	4.5 (1.5)	4.6 (1.5)
Menopausal disorder ($n = 209$)	49.5 (4.3)	10.9 (3.0)	11.9 (1.8)	4.0 (1.4)	5.0 (1.4)	4.2 (1.5)	5.0 (1.3)	4.6 (1.4)
Ovarian deficiency syndrome ($n = 245$)	45.4 (5.1)	11.1 (3.2)	11.9 (2.0)	4.1 (1.5)	6.4 (0.9)	5.6 (0.2)	5.1 (0.2)	4.0 (0.3)
Healthy middle-aged women ($n = 287$)	47.9 (4.7)	9.9 (1.9)	9.6 (2.1)	3.8 (1.3)	5.5 (1.7)	4.3 (1.3)	4.9 (1.3)	3.9 (1.4)

SRQ-D, Self Rating Questionnaire for Depression; MMPI-AS, Minnesota Multiphasic Personality Inventory-alexithymia scale; CP, Critical Parents; NP, Nursing Parents; A, Adult; FC, Free Child; AC, Adapted Child

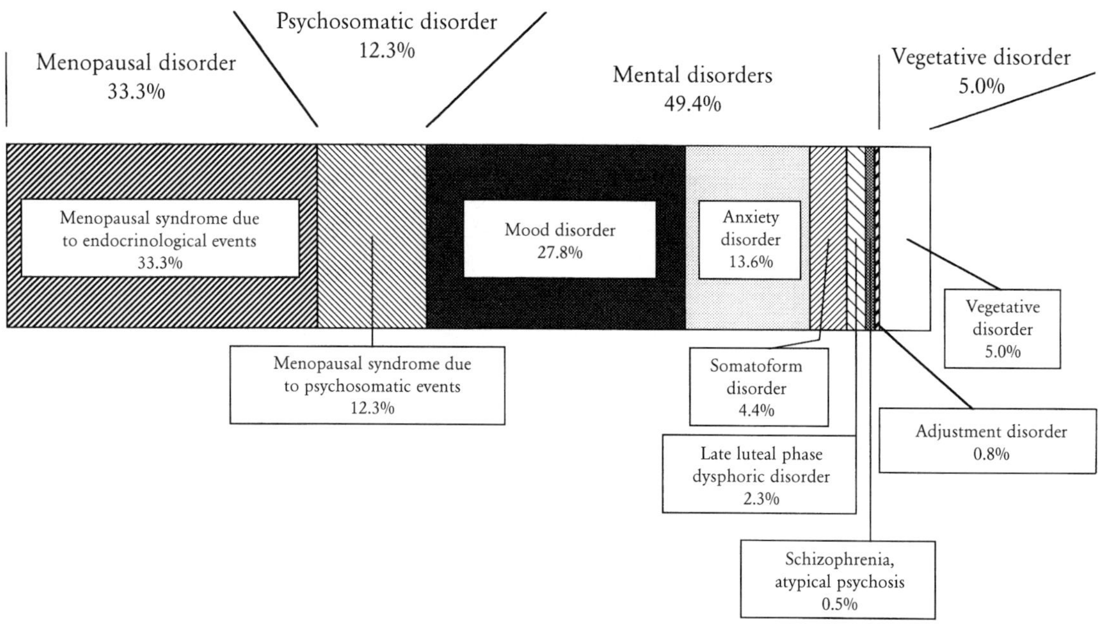

Figure 5 Distribution of final diagnoses of perimenopausal women with undefined symptoms

disorders, the rates of mood disorder and anxiety disorder, which includes generalized anxiety disorder and panic disorder, were 56.3% and 27.5%, respectively. It is a feature of perimenopausal patients with undefined complaints that the incidence of mood disorder is high for those with menopausal disorder.

DIFFERENTIAL DIAGNOSIS OF MENTAL DISORDERS

Complaints observed in the patients with undefined symptoms were very similar in each disease described above. Table 3 compares the top five symptoms for menopausal disorder, mood disorder, anxiety disorder and somatoform disorder in perimenopausal women. We observed that the symptoms of hot sensations and hot flushes, and general fatigue or malaise, were placed within the top five in each case. Furthermore, these symptoms are multiple, undefined and non-specific. Accurate diagnosis for undefined symptoms is therefore not always easy from clinical manifestations. Therefore, in the case of differential diagnosis, a past medical record, life events, psychological features and personal characteristics as well as changes in situation and crisis management should be considered. Moreover, a well-informed, total image of patients is necessary for differential diagnosis. In climacteric medicine, an accurate diagnosis should guarantee good efficacy in the treatment of women with undefined symptoms.

The psychological complaints presented by women of menopausal age may be severe and persistent enough to meet the diagnosis of mental disorders. In most cases, menopausal complaints which occur mainly as a result of estrogen deficiency are less severe, and are not continuous, but fluctuating. As mood and anxiety disorders are especially important for differential diagnoses in patients with undefined symptoms, a short description of each follows.

Mood disorder is a disorder in which there is a persistent lowering of mood as the primary feature. Almost all patients with mood disorder report complaints suggesting physical illness, such as menopausal disorder. Other features of mood disorder include general fatigue, decreased energy, hot sensation, shoulder and neck stiffness, appetite disturbance, weight loss, bodily aches and pains, difficulty in breathing, dry mouth, and an unusual sensation in the abdomen, chest or head. In addition to a feeling of sadness and depressive mood, patients often suffer anxiety, loss of interest, difficulty in concentration, painful thoughts and suicidal feelings. It is important to note that mental and physical symptoms often change, improving from morning to evening. The diagnosis of depression is made on the basis of persistent and prominent lowering of mood, combined with the presence of at least five of the accompanying symptoms in which at least one of the symptoms is either depressive mood, or loss of interest or feeling of pleasure, every day for at least 2 weeks (DSM-IV).

Anxiety disorder is a disorder in which anxiety is the primary and dominant feature of the clinical picture. The severity, frequency or duration of the anxiety interferes with the individual's well-being, occupation or interpersonal relationships. Anxiety is a complex emotion which comes from an underlying feeling of fear or apprehension. The woman

Table 3 Common complaints in perimenopausal women with undefined symptoms

Ranking	*Menopausal disorder*	*Mood disorder*	*Anxiety disorder*	*Somatoform disorder*
1	hot sensations, hot flushes	general fatigue, malaise	anxiety, jitters	physical pain
2	shoulder stiffness, muscle pain	shoulder stiffness	insomnia	anxiety
3	numbness	hot sensations, hot flushes	hot sensations, hot flushes	insomnia
4	general fatigue, malaise	headaches	general fatigue, malaise	hot sensations, hot flushes
5	loss of energy, unsteady sensation	depressive mood	palpitations	general fatigue, malaise

in an anxious state looks tense, and may be restless during the interview or show other signs of motor tension. She may complain of autonomic concomitants of anxiety such as a dry mouth, sweating, hot flushes, palpitations and tachycardia, headaches, nausea, difficulty in breathing, and aches and pains. The clinician needs to distinguish such symptoms from other mental disorders in which anxiety is frequently present, such as depression, and from physical disorders that may present in this way, such as menopausal disorder or hyperthyroidism. Generalized anxiety disorder and panic disorder are commonly observed in perimenopausal patients with undefined symptoms. The criteria for diagnosis of generalized anxiety disorder in DSM-IV are at least three of six symptoms from the categories of motor tension, autonomic hyperactivity, vigilance and scanning. These must be present continuously for at least 6 months. In contrast, the severity of the psychological complaints of the menopausal years is lower, and the symptomatology is not continuous. Additionally, panic disorder usually occurs with panic attacks, i.e. discrete periods of intense fear or discomfort, with at least four characteristic associated symptoms. The panic attacks usually last for minutes, and are at least initially unexpected, and not triggered by any particular situation. In contrast, menopausal disorder never occurs initially accompanied by a panic attack.

TREATMENT OF MENOPAUSAL DISORDER

In treating patients with undefined complaints, differential diagnosis may be extremely important for the above reasons. Concerning treatment, HRT was administered in 351 of the 1000 patients (35.1%). Traditional Japanese herbal medicines were concurrently administered to 418 patients. To treat mental disorders, psychosomatic disorders and partial menopausal disorder, minor tranquillizers and antidepressant agents were administered to 50.2% and 44.5% of patients, respectively. It is important to note that psychotherapy was given to 927 patients. In other words, perimenopausal women with undefined complaints should be treated with both pharmacotherapy and psychotherapy (Figure 6).

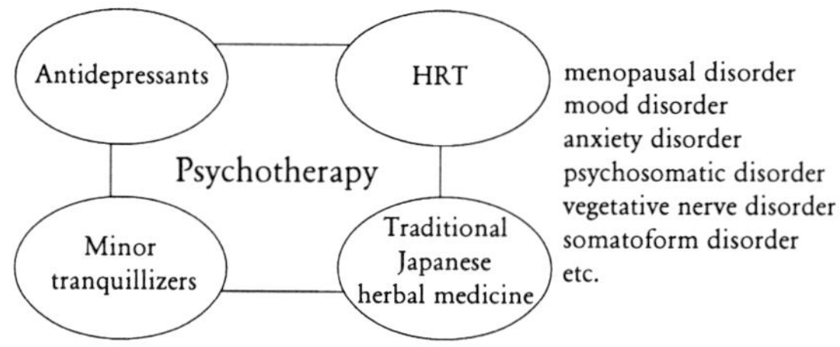

Figure 6 Optimal and desirable treatment for women with undefined symptoms. HRT, hormone replacement therapy

The main points of the psychotherapy are as follows. Acceptance, support and reassurance are three important elements of psychotherapy. Listening is the main therapeutic method in acceptance and support for the patient. The reassurance involves promising that the patient's poor psychological and physical conditions will return to their original healthy condition. By repeating psychotherapy as above, it is important to establish a fiduciary relationship between patient and doctor. This is indispensable when treating patients with undefined symptoms. There are many cases in which patients with depression and anxiety disorders are not thought by their families to have serious illness. That the family does not understand the distress of the patients will mentally trouble them. Furthermore, the patients often believe that the distress or suffering in the present will continue for life. Thus, it is necessary to tell patients that the optimum treatment will immediately relieve their distress.

Pharmacotherapy appropriately combines drugs such as antidepressants, minor tranquillizers, estrogen and autonomic nerve-stabilizing drugs. In the present study, patients received HRT with conjugated estrogen and medroxyprogesterone, and for overall symptoms improvement was observed in 28.5% and 39.2% within 2 and 4 weeks, respectively. Estriol therapy also brought about marked improvement in symptoms. The efficacy of administration of Japanese herbal medicine, which has traditionally been widely used in Japan, particularly in the treatment of patients with undefined complaints, was improvement within 2 weeks in 34.7%, i.e. markedly effective. In other words, traditional Japanese herbal medicine has a good efficacy compared with HRT in Japanese women (Figure 7).

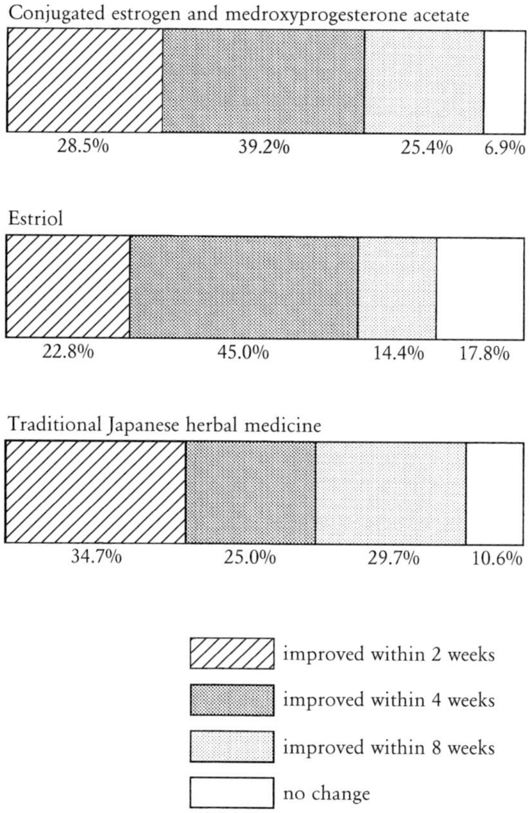

Figure 7 Assessment of efficacies of hormone replacement therapy and traditional Japanese herbal medicine in treatment of menopausal disorder

Figure 8 shows the improvement in symptoms of mood and anxiety disorders with optimal treatment, which involved combined therapy with antidepressants, minor tranquillizers, traditional Japanese herbal medicine and vegetative nerve-stabilizing drugs. Overall improvement was observed in more than 40% of patients within 2 weeks of administration. For mood disorder, improvement was observed in 83.4% of patients within 2–4 weeks. Not only pharmacotherapy, but also behavior therapy such as exposure, systematic desensitization or operant techniques is useful in mental and psychosomatic disorders.

MANAGEMENT OF PERIMENOPAUSAL PATIENTS WITH UNDEFINED COMPLAINTS

When perimenopausal women with undefined complaints come to hospital, it is important that

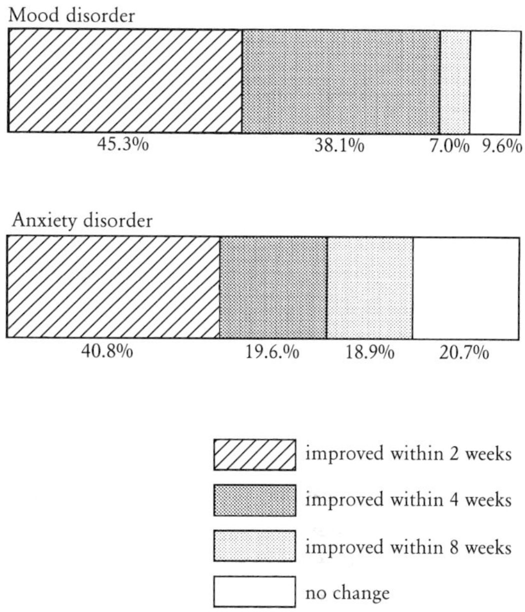

Figure 8 Improvement in symptoms of mood and anxiety disorders with optimal treatment

the physician distinguishes whether or not the patient suffers from some mental disorder. The following items should be added in the diagnosis of some diseases of perimenopausal women with undefined symptoms. What kind of symptoms appear as undefined, and how do they appear? How does the patient's character contribute to the occurrence of symptoms? In addition, it may also help the diagnosis to check whether or not the patient is experiencing changes in circumstances or major life events. When the patient is diagnosed with a mental disorder, psychosomatic disorder or menopausal disorder with psychological factors, it is very important to have sufficient conversation with the patient and establish good communication. As part of treatment, psychotherapy should be carried out for all patients. Depending on the case, we should also try to guide the adjustment of the circumstances in which the patient works and lives.

CONCLUSIONS

In summary, it would appear that many psychosocial and characteristic variables may be important in determining women's experience of the menopause. These factors include the meaning of changes produced by climacteric processes within the setting of a particular culture, the woman's social class, her work status (whether or not she works outside the home), the adequacy of her social network, the degree of her involvement with her children, and the occurrence of undesirable life events. In other words, biological, psychological and sociological factors are probably all important in the development of these complaints. Underlying endocrinological changes may in themselves be sufficient to trigger emotional changes leading to distress. In other women, these changes may lead only to physical or psychological complaints when other factors are present. Personality factors including anxiety, or melancholic or alexithymic proneness, have also been found to be associated with more psychological complaints. These findings support an interactive biopsychological model of the psychological complaints experienced in the climacteric years. In conclusion, to achieve potent curative effects on menopausal disorder, careful, rapid and accurate diagnosis, especially differential diagnosis from mental disorders, and detection of sociocultural and characteristic factors involved in the onset of undefined symptoms are important. Furthermore, it is important for the physician to have a heartfelt and psychosomatic attitude in the examination of perimenopausal patients with undefined symptoms.

ACKNOWLEDGEMENTS

We would like to thank Ms Akiko Yoshida and Ms Kyoko Shiraishi for their helpful assistance, and gratefully acknowledge President Professor Takeshi Aso for the opportunity to conduct this study.

References

1. Ushiroyama T, Sugimoto O. Endocrine function of the peri- and postmenopausal ovary. *Horm Res* 1995; 44:64–8
2. Ushiroyama T, Ikeda A, Ueki M. Evidence for attenuation of gonadotropin pulse frequency in hypergonadotropic women with estradiol secretion in the menopausal transition. *Psychoneuroendocrinology* 1999;24:85–97
3. Ushiroyama T, Toyoda K, Okamoto Y. Contribution of endocrine changes to depressive mood in peri- and postmenopausal women. *Bull Osaka Med Coll* 1991;37:81–6
4. Ushiroyama T, Sugimoto O. Clinical observation of personality characteristics of perimenopausal women with undefined complaints. *Asia-Oceania J Obstet Gynecol* 1993;19:67–70
5. Ushiroyama T, Ueki M, Orino I, *et al.* Alexithymia and undefined complaints in climacteric women: prevalence, correlates and personality traits. *Res Commun Psychol Psychiatr Behav* 1994;19:49–58
6. American Psychiatric Association. *Diagnostic and Statistical Manual of Mental Disorders*, 3rd edn revised. Washington, DC: American Psychiatry Press, 1987: 213–68

A patient-centered approach to managing the menopause

43

J. Rymer

INTRODUCTION

Hormone replacement therapy (HRT) is prescribed for the relief of the acute symptoms of estrogen deficiency as well as the long-term sequelae, namely osteoporosis, prevention of cardiovascular disease risk, prevention of Alzheimer's disease and protection against colorectal cancer (Table 1). Despite these benefits, adherence rates with HRT remain low. On examining the literature, one finds that few women seek advice regarding HRT and, of those women who do, few take it and, of those who commence it, few continue it. It appears that doctors like HRT but patients do not. Therefore it is time that we adopted a patient-centered approach to the management of the menopause and give women a choice.

Table 1 Reasons why women take hormone replacement therapy (HRT)

Acute symptoms of estrogen deficiency
Vasomotor symptoms
Mood disturbances
Urogenital symptoms
Memory changes
Long-term benefits of HRT
Protects the female skeleton
Decreases cardiovascular risk
Prevents Alzheimer's disease
Protects against colorectal cancer

Table 2 Factors determining adherence to hormone replacement therapy

Patient
Doctor
Medication
Other factors

Adherence is influenced by patient factors, doctor factors, the medication itself and other factors (Table 2). The patient factors involve the decision to seek health care, the expectation of the consultation and the expectations of the prescription. The decision to seek health care is influenced by a woman's previous experiences and her pre-existing attitudes. Whether or not she takes the medication depends upon her understanding of the need for the therapy, but this is influenced by the experiences of her friends and relatives and what she has read in the media. Interestingly, Graziottin[1], on questioning women about whether or not they would take HRT, found that the women were concerned much more with self-image and sexual identity rather than medical consequences. Eisenberg and colleagues[2] found that 72% of patients using alternative therapies did not tell their physician. When talking about ovarian failure, the experience of symptoms will change a woman's attitude as to whether or not she will take hormone replacement therapy (or any other therapy). Therefore, surveying premenopausal women about whether or not they would take HRT postmenopausally is not a true reflection of what will happen, as they are not motivated by experiencing negative symptoms[3].

The 'doctor' factors involve the doctor's knowledge of the condition and his confidence and competence in managing the postmenopausal woman. They also include the doctor's ability to negotiate and agree the management strategy with the patient. Ghali and colleagues[4] surveyed primary-care physicians' awareness of patients in the menopausal consultation. The surveys contained questions from four established (five-point) attitudinal scales. They found that doctors were aware of the patients' desire for autonomy, but underestimated the patients' desire for information and patients' perceptions of barriers to using HRT. They also underestimated the extent to which the patient viewed menopause as a medical problem. Interestingly, the patients overestimated concern regarding heart disease and breast cancer. The conclusion of Ghali and colleagues[4] was that, to optimize HRT counselling, physicians may need to increase their awareness of patients' attitudes.

The 'medication' factor involves the convenience of taking the drug, the evidence of benefit, the side-effects one may experience and the cost.

In the doctor/menopausal relationship, there must be negotiation at the outset so that both parties have realistic expectations. There must be scope for asking and answering difficult questions and the woman must feel that she has an escape route if there are irreconcilable problems with the doctor.

Topo and co-workers[5] described this interaction as the physician's willingness to prescribe (the push effect) versus the woman's desire to use medication (the pull effect). Therefore, at the initial consultation, one needs to ascertain women's health beliefs, discuss the benefits of HRT and quality-of-life issues, discuss risks, suggest the most appropriate therapy and arrange follow-up.

WHY DO WOMEN TAKE HRT?

Women take HRT for preventative reasons, therapeutic reasons, or because their doctor has recommended it. Why don't women take HRT over a long period of time? Because they do not want to make this commitment and because there is unsatisfactory communication with the physician.

The Adelphi Women's Health Programme focused on pre- and postmenopausal women between 45 and 65 years of age, with a special emphasis on management of the menopause, use of HRT, and prevention and treatment of osteoporosis. Both doctors and women were studied and the investigation included face-to-face interviews with doctors, patient recording by doctors and confidential questions by patients. When patients were asked why they discontinued therapy, they said that the doctor recommended them to stop, there was lack of efficacy of the drug, breast tenderness, weight gain, inconvenient breakthrough bleeding and they claimed that the drug made them more moody and depressed. In contrast, the six main reasons that doctors identified for discontinuation of therapy were side-effects/tolerability, bleeding, weight gain, lack of efficacy, long-term safety concern and difficulties with compliance. Weight gain is quoted by patients and doctors as a significant side-effect. Unfortunately, women do gain weight at this time of life (irrespective of whether or not they take HRT), but women perceive that they gain weight on HRT. Whether or not this is true is irrelevant if it actually affects their adherence. We therefore have to acknowledge that a significant proportion of women do not want to take HRT. This is because they are afraid of or dislike possible side-effects, they are concerned about the long-term risks of HRT, they are disenchanted with conventional medicine or they have an inherent belief in the safety of 'natural' products. Therefore, we must be able to offer alternatives to HRT.

WHAT ARE THE ALTERNATIVES?

They can be broadly divided into four categories, namely diet, exercise, relaxation and alternative therapies (Table 3).

Diet

There are essential elements in the diet and we must check that women have an adequate diet. Their diet should include dairy products, meat and fish, fruit and vegetables, grain products, and fats and oils, as they provide vitamins, minerals, proteins, carbohydrates, fats and water.

Exercise

With regard to exercise, women must understand that weight is dependent upon diet and exercise. The exercise should be regular, of an appropriate

Table 3 Alternatives to hormone replacement therapy

Diet
Exercise
Relaxation
Alternative therapies

intensity and without a break. This should occur three times a week, each session lasting for 30 min, and a significant rise in pulse rate should be observed.

Relaxation

At this time of life, women may be experiencing significant stress and we need to identify the stressor, eliminate the stressor and recommend relaxation and recreation. Freedman and Woodward[6] performed a prospective randomized controlled trial on 33 postmenopausal women experiencing hot flushes and showed that paced respiration training reduced their frequency by 30% during the 4 weeks of the trial. Another group carrying out a randomized controlled trial used relaxation response training and over 10 weeks showed a reduction in hot flush intensity (but not frequency), anxiety and depressed mood[7].

Alternative therapies

These appeal to women as they are less invasive and are considered more natural. These may include Western herbal medicines, ginseng, homeopathy, aromatherapy and traditional Chinese medicines. In the UK lay press, there was an article that identified the top ten natural alternatives. These were plant hormones (phytoestrogens), natural progesterone, altering diet, herbal remedies, vitamins, ginkgo biloba, vitamin E for vaginal dryness, calcium, all-in-one remedies and exercise. Unfortunately, there are very few randomized controlled trials assessing efficacy.

A QUALITY-OF-LIFE PARAMETER: SEXUALITY

As mentioned above[1], women are very concerned about their self-image and sexuality, so it is also important to consider sexual function in our postmenopausal patient. In the elderly, sexual expression is a predictor of general health, and the consideration of aging patients' sexual function can affect medical care and improve quality of life.

Why do we not discuss sexuality in old age?

Mainly because we are embarrassed and we do not want to talk about it or offend our patients. Therefore, the problems go unreported and unaddressed. Sexual function involves both motivational behavior (testosterone-related) and biological response. With ovarian failure, serum testosterone becomes decreased and there are significant resultant biological changes in the female. Women of this age may also be experiencing chronic disease and be on medication that may affect sexual function. They may have undergone surgical procedures which make sexual activity difficult or make them feel that they are unattractive because of physical deformity. We therefore need to take a proactive role to assist them in improving their quality of life. We need to ask the questions, take an appropriate history, be open to discussion, perform an adequate examination, advise simple techniques to improve sexual activity, exclude depression, check medications, give medications if appropriate and facilitate sexual counselling if needed. Many women seek HRT purely with the aim of improving sexual function.

CONCORDANCE

The clinical encounter is concerned with two sets of contrasted, but equally cogent, health beliefs – those of the patient and those of the doctor. This means there is a process of negotiation between the lay and the professional perspectives. However, the most important determinations are those made by the patient, as it is the patient who decides, on a daily basis, whether to take the medication or not.

CONCLUSION

In managing the menopause, we must remember that the patient is the focus; therefore, we need to discuss the problems and offer appropriate solutions. We must offer HRT, but also be able to discuss alternatives. We need to identify their current lifestyle patterns and offer changes regarding diet, exercise, sexual function, stress relief and emotional support. The menopause can be a difficult time for many women and HRT is not always the answer. Let us focus on the woman.

ACKNOWLEDGEMENTS

I would like to thank Professor Roger Jones and Dr Nicky Britten from the Department of General Practice Primary Care (Guy's, King's and St Thomas' Medical School) for their help in preparing this manuscript, and Ms Tracy Alderton for typing the manuscript.

References

1. Graziottin A. HRT: the woman's perspective. *Int J Gynaecol Obstet* 1996;52(Suppl 1):S11–16
2. Eisenberg DM, Kessler RC, Foster C, Norlock FE, Calkins DR, Delbanco TL. Unconventional medicine in the United States. Prevalence, costs, and patterns of use. *N Engl J Med* 1993;328:246–52
3. Hunter MS, Liao KL. Determinants of treatment choice for menopausal hot flushes: hormonal versus psychological versus no treatment. *J Psychosom Obstet Gynaecol* 1995;16:101–8
4. Ghali WA, Freund KM, Boss RD, Ryan CA, Moskowitz MA. Menopausal hormone therapy: physician awareness of patient attitudes. *Am J Med* 1997;103:3–10
5. Topo P, Hemminki E, Uutela A. Women's choice and physicians' advice on use of menopausal and postmenopausal hormone therapy. *Int J Health Sci* 1993;4:101–9
6. Freedman RR, Woodward S. Behavioral treatment of menopausal hot flushes: evaluation by ambulatory monitoring. *Am J Obstet Gynecol* 1992;167:436–9
7. Irvin JH, Domar AD, Clark C, Zuttermeister PC, Friedman R. The effects of relaxation response training on menopausal symptoms. *J Psychosom Obstet Gynaecol* 1996;17:202–7

When hormone replacement therapy is not possible

44

M. Neves-e-Castro

INTRODUCTION

Hormone replacement therapy (HRT) has been one of the more convincing approaches to add quality and years to the life of postmenopausal women. The concept of HRT is open to discussion[1].

After the onset of menopause many women complain of disturbing symptoms that may adversely affect their quality of life. Vasomotor symptoms (hot flushes), irritability, depressive mood, insomnia, sexual dysfunction, bone and joint pains, weight gain, etc., are among those that more often cause discomfort and determine that a woman seeks medical support.

Alternatively, it is well established that after the menopause there is a clear increase in the risk for cardiovascular diseases and osteoporosis.

Both the often incapacitating symptoms and the risk for diseases later in life are accepted to be mainly due to the pronounced fall in circulating estrogens that is a characteristic of the primary ovarian failure, a landmark of the physiological menopause, in middle-aged women. Treatment with estrogens is effective in the relief of most symptoms and in the favorable modification of the above-mentioned risk factors.

Hormones have long been considered by many women either as wonder drugs or as very dangerous medications that may be related to cancer, hirsutism, weight gain, etc. Conversely, there are a few absolute and relative medical contraindications that may prevent the use of HRT by some women. However, in the majority of cases, HRT may be not possible because it is not wanted by the women, who are negatively affected by the 'bad news' that is often inaccurately transmitted by the media. Unfortunately, in many cases, 'bad news is good news' and that is what sells best.

The symptomatology of menopausal women is not universal. In a number of studies, among several ethnic and cultural groups in the world, it was found that there are 'important differences in women's experiences of symptoms and their responses to them, reflecting cultural influences on explanatory models of menopause, lifeways, and in turn, biology' . . . 'Their lifeways, including exercise and nutritional intake, affect symptom experiences and symptom distress'[2]. Filipino American midlife women consider the perimenopausal transition in a positive light, as part of normal life that does not warrant concern[3].

The 1998 North American Menopause Society Survey concluded that the majority of women viewed the menopause and midlife as the beginning of many positive changes in their lives and health[4]. Thus, some women may not feel the need for HRT, whereas others may not want to take it.

In a recent study involving 3000 women > 50 years old, 1350 were not on HRT. Of those, 82% were menopausal out of which only 21% had been treated with HRT in the past. The reasons for not taking HRT included the following: 49% no longer had menopausal symptoms, 45% did not want to take HRT, 33% were not offered it by their doctors, 28% were afraid to use it[5].

Therefore, HRT is sometimes not possible, either because women do not feel the need, or

This chapter has been reproduced with permission from Neves-e-Castro M. When hormone replacement therapy is not possible. In Studd J, ed. *The Management of the Menopause: the Millennium Review*. Carnforth, UK: Parthenon Publishing, 1999:91–102 because they are afraid. Often this is due to lack of information for which health providers are responsible.

OBJECTIVES

Assuming that, no matter why, HRT is either not possible or not wanted, which are the goals of the attending physician and what can be offered to a menopausal woman who seeks support?

Basically, with or without HRT, there are always three fundamental objectives:

(1) Relief of symptoms,

(2) Maintenance and improvement of health,

(3) Prevention (primary or secondary) of diseases.

The assessment of health is far more difficult than the diagnosis of disease. However, the World Health Organization (WHO) has given a definition of health that can be very useful as a guide line: 'Health is a condition of physical, mental and social well-being and not only the absence of disease'.

Thus, the attending physician must adopt a holistic vision of the middle-age woman who comes to him for support. He must be concerned and involved in all the aspects that define health. If he is a gynecologist he should be aware of the etymology of this word, of Greek origin (*gyneka* = woman/*logos* = science). Gynecology in its broader dimension means the science or the knowledge of women, and not only the treatment of the diseases of the reproductive tract. Perhaps one should invent another designation (hybrid from Latin and Greek) like *feminology* or *holistic feminology* to better define the role of a modern gynecologist. As a matter of fact, if he is only a good specialist, with an average knowledge of internal medicine and little time or talent to establish a good empathic relationship with a human being, he is certainly not a good gynecologist.

Middle-aged women do not routinely visit a cardiologist or a rheumatologist, but they go regularly to their gynecologists for a routine pelvic examination, a Papanicolaou smear, mammography, etc.

It is the responsibility of the modern gynecologist to take advantage of this opportunity to perform the necessary screenings to identify risks (cardiovascular, osteoporosis, cancer, etc.) and to attempt to modify them to the extent of his capacities and possibilities.

THE WOMAN

She may be defined as:

(1) A menopausal woman - if one considers that the shut down of ovarian function and the consequent hypoestrogenism is the key problem; or as

(2) A middle-aged woman - in whom natural aging is already playing a role, both from a biological and a psychological perspective.

In both cases she may suffer from a lack of estrogens and from aging. Biological age and chronological age run in parallel. She may complain of somatic and of psychic symptoms. For practical purposes one must accept that there is a biological syndrome and a psychological syndrome that affect these women. The purpose of the anti-aging interventions is to dissociate the biological age from the chronological age[6] and thus to compress morbidity as late as possible in the life time[7]. Adding life to the years and years to life is the target to hit. That is to say longer life but with greater quality.

The biological syndrome

Estrogens have profound effects in almost every organ and tissue of the body. Be it through genomic (α and β receptors) or non-genomic mechanisms the fact is that estrogen deprivation may cause dysfunctions and that treatment with estrogens may have corrective effects.

With aging and lack of estrogens the development of insulin resistance, increase in blood pressure, changes in lipid metabolism, a decrease in immune function, and increase in stored fat are almost universal phenomena.

These are the major factors for the high cardiovascular morbidity from which women were protected until the onset of menopause.

Insulin resistance (with hyperinsulinemia) seems to be one of the major factors of aging. It has profound impact on other hormonal systems, in particular eicosanoids, considered to be the molecular foundation of aging[6]. Insulin causes the production of more 'bad' (vasoconstrictor) than 'good' (vasodilator) eicosanoids. Insulin also increases the fat stores in the body.

Besides hyperinsulinemia there is also an excess in free radicals and cortisol, both with dangerous effects in the aging process. According to Sears[6], excessive insulin, excess in glucose, excess in free radicals and excess in cortisol, cause increased caloric consumption, increased DNA turnover, increased formation of advanced glycosylated end products (AGEs), neural death in some areas of the brain and an imbalance in eicosanoid synthesis, considered to be the molecular nature of chronic diseases.

From the above it can already be inferred that nutrition, exercise and life-style are closely related to these problems, as will be discussed later.

The lack of estrogens, lower amounts of vitamin D, lack of exercise and poor calcium intake are some of the factors that contribute to osteopenia and osteoporosis. Therefore, osteoclasts become more active (due to increased parathyroid hormone secretion resulting from a lesser negative feedback of calcium) and osteoblasts are not stimulated by the low levels of estrogens and androgens.

These woman seek help mostly because of the following:

(1) Weight gain,

(2) Different body fat distribution,

(3) Increased appetite,

(4) Asthenia, tiredness,

(5) Pain in the bones and joints,

(6) Precordial pressure,

(7) Hypertension,

(8) Dyspareunia (dry vagina),

(9) Stress incontinence,

(10) Breast tenderness (in early menopause).

The following are markers of good health[6,8,9]:

(1) Fasting insulin levels less than 10 μU/ml,

(2) Fasting glucose/insulin ratio (mg/dl : μU/ml) greater than 4.5,

(3) Glycosylated hemoglobin less than 5%,

(4) Fasting triglycerides less than 140 mg/dl,

(5) Low total cholesterol (less than 200 mg/dl),

(6) Low-density lipoprotein less than 130 mg/dl and high-density lipoprotein greater than 50 mg/dl,

(7) Triglycerides/HDL ratio less than 2,

(8) Total cholesterol/HDL less than 4.5,

(9) BMI (body mass index) 20–25 kg/m^2,

(10) Body fat less than 22%,

(11) Blood pressure: diastolic less than 90 mmHg and systolic less than 140 mmHg,

(12) Bone mineral density: T above –1.0 SD.

The psychic and neurovegetative syndromes

Vasomotor symptoms (hot flushes),
Insomnia,
Irritability,
Depressive mood,
Frigidity,
Headaches and migraine,
Poor memory.

These symptoms are not necessarily estrogen related, other than the hot flushes. However, since the brain is a target for estrogens that act via several neurotransmitters, it is likely that its lower levels after the menopause may have an impact on mood, sleep and memory.

Since in industrialized countries the menopause has for many women (and men, too) a negative connotation, being considered the beginning of the end, the lack of femininity, etc., it is conceivable that menopausal women consider themselves very insecure (feelings of jealousy, need of reaffirmation, etc.). The unhappiness they may feel needs compensatory gratification (food, sweets, etc.). The 'empty nest' syndrome does not help them to reformulate their lifestyles; they do not feel any interest in life, they become inactive and do not want to exercise, and they may often feel miserable.

Estrogens also act on the arterial wall and stimulate the synthesis of nitric oxide (NO) by the endothelium. NO is a potent vasodilator. The lack of nitric oxide may cause vasospasm and cause headaches and migraine.

STRATEGIES

It is obvious that despite the fact that HRT is very important to help in the maintenance of health, the prevention of diseases and the relief of symptoms, there are many other possibilities, other than the use of hormones, to help those women who cannot or do not want to take HRT.

It is beyond the scope of this chapter to go through all the steps that are applicable to all women who are in this phase of their lives. Instead, reference will be made to a number of interventions that are usually omitted despite their proven efficacy as anti-aging, anti-cardiovascular disease, anti-osteoporosis and even anti-cancer. The following topics deserve far greater attention than they have had so far. As a matter of fact it is easier and less time consuming to prescribe pills than to persuade a woman to change her lifestyle, nutrition, etc.

Time to listen

The most important single measure is to have time to listen and to talk. Many of the problems faced by these women can be solved or greatly alleviated if the attending physician believes that he is capable of understanding and supporting and giving, sometimes for the first time, the information those women are lacking. If a woman is properly informed about the physiology of this change in her life, and that most other women do have similar complaints, then the mystery starts fading and doors can be opened to establish a positive dialog. Sometimes if one explains to them the meaning of some clinical trials they may understand what is a benefit–risk analysis, or a relative risk, and eventually change their minds. But, assuming that HRT is out of the question what should be the next step?

Physical activity

It is well established that well-planned physical exercise has very positive effects on mood and on the sense of well being (due to the release of beta-endorphins by the brain). It helps to develop motivation. It contributes to weight loss, to muscle strength, to a better cardiovascular function, and it helps the bone and joint function. It also decreases stress.

Women who took part in moderate exercise, as little as once a week, were 24% less likely to die prematurely than women who did not exercise. Women who took part in vigorous exercise (jogging, swimming, etc) more than four times a week had 43% lower risk of premature death[10].

Anti-stress

The attending physician, with time (!) is often in a better position than a psychotherapist to give the support and advice that may help to decrease psychological stress and distress. Explaining how the central and autonomic nervous systems and the adrenal glands may cause vasospasm (headaches, migraine, hypertension), increase cortisol secretion (with all the metabolic consequences) and make one feel unhappy, is one of the first steps to help that woman look into herself, in the mirror, to start equating her problems and maybe solving some of them. Stress is a major risk for coronary heart disease. If needed, the attending physician should not refrain from complementing his mild psychotherapy with mild tranquillizers or antidepressants. It is expected that he knows how to manipulate these psychopharmacological medicines and that he is also capable of identifying mental disorders that should be treated by another specialist.

Vasomotor symptoms

Sometimes these are intense and require treatment. Antidopaminergics (veralipride) and $\alpha 2$ blockers (clonidine) have been used with some success. However, even when HRT is not possible, an injection of 150 mg medroxyprogesterone acetate is more effective. The side-effect to be considered is on mood.

Insomnia

There is no problem in prescribing mild sedatives and hypnogens.

Headaches and migraine

If acetylsalicylic acid is well tolerated, for short periods, it is acceptable since it also has anti-aggregating effects, preventing atheromatous plaque formation. Otherwise, other mild analgesics are to be recommended. Ergot derivatives should be used with caution. A balanced diet may help. Smoking should be proscribed, since it causes vasoconstriction.

Dyspareunia and frigidity

Only later in the menopause is the vaginal epithelium atrophic enough to cause dyspareunia. In the majority of cases, in the early menopause, dyspareunia is psychogenic and due to perineal muscle spasm. The same is true with frigidity and anorgasmia, which are seldom hormone-related. Lubricant jellies are effective. Even when HRT is not possible there is no reason to avoid estrogen vaginal suppositories or creams. When possible it is advisable to have a joint conversation with the partner to demystify the problem and to propose some techniques that may be less traumatic and more gratifying.

Nutrition and weight control

There is a significant association between younger age at menopause and higher risk of coronary heart disease among women who experienced natural menopause and never used hormone therapy[11]. Therefore, particular attention must be paid to this group of women, particularly if they are obese. Obesity is a significant independent predictor of cardiovascular disease[12].

Aerobic exercise plays an important role in preventing obesity in most persons. Genetic factors do not predispose to obesity as has sometimes been accepted. In a study conducted in 970 healthy female twins (mean age 55.5 years) it was concluded that physical activity is the strongest independent predictor of total body fat and central abdominal fat, far greater than other environmental factors[13].

Higher levels of physical activity lessen total body and abdominal fat, and prevent insulin resistance, hypertension and cardiovascular diseases. This can be achieved with 2 h of sport or 15 km of walking per week. Weight-bearing sport of any intensity was related to lower fat deposits and greater muscle strength. Therefore, physical activity seems to be, according to this study, the strongest determinant of body fat, more than diet. It should be, together with physical activity, another leg of the tripod that supports good health and longevity. (The third leg, pharmacological intervention, will be discussed later.)

This does not mean, of course, that the food intake is not extremely important both quantitatively and qualitatively.

One should never talk about a diet. The woman has already followed many of them and is frustrated by not achieving what she expected.

What is important is to explain how the body functions. How much protein, fat and carbohydrate are needed for that particular person, with that type of energy consumption. It is mandatory to take measures to determine the body mass index, the percentage of body fat and to set the objectives.

One must take the time to explain the nutritional value of food and its content of substances that are health-protective. This may be reinforced by the information of the high or low prevalence of several diseases in different areas of the world as a function of their nutrition.

Many women ignore that excessive weight and a high consumption of animal fat raises the risk for breast cancer more than does HRT. A high consumption of vegetables, fruit and fiber is linked with a lesser prevalence of cardiovascular events, and cancer of the colon and breast.

It can be stated that modern nutritional advice is very effective for the prevention of cancer and cardiovascular diseases. It is this type of information that motivates a woman to change her dietary habits. The objective is not to start on a diet but to change and incorporate the change. This is fundamental for behavior support.

Antioxidants

It was previously mentioned that a typical marker of aging is an increase in oxygen free radicals that damage cells. Antioxidants prevent free radicals from damaging the cells. Aging appears to be due, in good part, to the oxidants produced by mitochondria as by-products of normal metabolism. Vitamins C, E and betacarotene are good antioxidants which are contained in certain foods (fruit, vegetables). Olive oil is a powerful antioxidant, too. Oxygen free radicals oxidize low-density lipoprotein cholesterol particles, which are atherogenic. Antioxidants may prevent heart disease, and also cancer[14].

Tomatoes are rich in antioxidants (lycopene and carotenoids) and do protect from coronary heart disease and cancer[15].

In a recent study involving 2400 Greek women it was shown that the incidence of breast cancer dropped with a higher intake of olive oil, certain vegetables and fruits[16].

Similar conclusions were reported in other studies[17,18].

Frequent nut consumption is associated with a reduced risk of both fatal coronary heart disease and non-fatal myocardial infarction (relative risk 0.65, 95% confidence interval 0.47–0.89, p for trend = 0.0009). Adjustment for intakes of dietary fats, fiber, vegetables and fruit did not alter these results derived from the Nurses' Health Study[19].

Phytoestrogens

Red clover and soy are particularly rich in phytoestrogens[20]. Green split peas, chick peas and broad beans are also rich in some isoflavones (genistein, daidzein, biochamin, formononetin) that have special estrogenic effects. Perhaps this is why traditional legume-based diets used by Asiatic populations are associated with reduced heart disease and also breast cancer.

Some commercial preparations containing these isoflavones are available and have been tested in clinical trials[21,22]. Isoflavones are also strong antioxidants.

Dietary fiber

Wolk and colleagues[23] examined the association between long-term intake of total dietary fibre and the risk of coronary heart disease in women aged 37–64 years, followed for 10 years, without evidence of heart disease, hypercholesterolemia or diabetes at baseline. The age-adjusted relative risk (RR) for major coronary heart disease was 0.53 for the highest quintile of total dietary fibre intake (median, 22.9 g/day) compared with women in the lowest quintile (median, 11.5 g/day). After controlling for age, cardiovascular risk factors and multivitamin supplement use, the RR was 0.77. Only cereal fiber was strongly associated with a reduced risk of coronary heart disease. These fiber-rich diets may also increase insulin sensitivity (reduce insulin resistance) and lower triglyceride levels. The recommended daily intake of fiber is 20–35 g. Rich in fiber are: wholegrain bread, oatmeal, brown rice, apple (with skin), avocado, oranges, prunes, raspberries, kidney beans, etc.

Vitamins (C, A and β-carotene)

Vegetables and fruit are very good vitamin sources, namely, broccoli, Brussels sprouts, chicory, tomatoes, carrots, kiwi fruit, citrus fruits, raspberries and strawberries, watermelons and many others.

The natural micronutrients contained in food seem to be more protective than in their pure form. Deficiency of vitamins B12, folic acid, B6, niacin, C or E, or iron or zinc, appears to mimic radiation in damaging DNA by causing single and double strand breaks, oxidative lesions, or both.

Micronutrient deficiency may explain, in good part, why the quarter of the North American population that eats the fewest fruits and vegetables (five portions a day is advised) has approximately double the cancer rate for most types of cancer when compared to the quarter with the highest intake[24].

Whole foods and fibers

Even if one takes tablets, daily, with vitamins and minerals, a balanced diet with whole foods must be a centerpiece. An orange or a glass of milk supply much more than vitamin C or protein.

Dietary fibers are important for digestion. Soluble fiber (in most fruits, certain beans and grains, some vegetables) may help prevent heart diseases and diabetes. Insoluble fibers, found in most vegetables, some fruits and breakfast cereals, can prevent constipation and colon cancer.

A diet high in fruits and vegetables reduces the risk of cancer, heart diseases and stroke.

High intake of whole-grain products is linked to reduced mortality among older women by 15% compared to non-users[25].

Fish

The more fish one eats the less coronary artery disease one has. Salmon, tuna fish and sardines are particularly rich in omega-3 polyunsaturated fatty acids. Eating these fish can reduce triglycerides and cholesterol because of their content of omega-3 fatty acids. The American Heart Association recommends eating fish two or three times a week.

It is of interest to note that a reduction in total or saturated fat intake, or cholesterol intake, is significantly associated with a reduction in area of breast density on mammography. A dense breast tissue is a risk for breast cancer, i.e. because it may disguise occult minor atypical lesions[26].

MORE SPECIFIC INTERVENTIONS

Again the targets for primary and secondary prevention will be the cardiovascular system and the bones. Cancer is not the women's big killer. They live and suffer with their heart, and it is ultimately the heart that will kill most of them!

(1) What to do to prevent coronary heart disease?

(2) What to do to decrease insulin resistance?

(3) What to do in cases of resistant obesity?

(4) What to do to prevent osteoporosis?

Coronary heart disease

Reducing cholesterol and blood pressure, as well as stopping smoking, are effective strategies to prevent cardiovascular disease. There are many convincing coronary primary prevention trials, all showing that either with diet or with lipid-lowering agents (cholestyramine, gemfibrozil, nicotinic acid, simvastatin, pravastatin, pravachol) there was a decrease in mortality due to coronary heart disease. Unfortunately, these trials were conducted only in men. It is hoped that the same conclusions may apply to women; this seems to be the case at least with the statins[27,28].

There are some new preventive strategies that include the liberal use of antioxidants, the use of angiotensin-converting enzyme inhibitors and homocystein lowering[29].

Cholesterol lowering by pharmacological means prevents atherosclerotic plaque progression and it has been shown to reduce both fatal and non-fatal coronary events in patients with or without coronary heart disease. Simvastatin for secondary prevention and lovastatin for primary prevention have a very favorable cost-effect profile[30].

Vitamin E seems to be a good choice in doses of 200 mg/day although the final proof in terms of death reduction is not yet known since the ongoing trials have not yet been reported[31].

Vitamin E, besides being a powerful antioxidant (inhibiting the oxidation of low-density lipoprotein cholesterol), also has a biological anti-inflammatory effect that contributes to the prevention of fatty plaque formation on the arterial walls. Recent studies suggest that plaque formation is an inflammatory process.

Of greater interest seem to be the angiotensin-converting enzyme inhibitors that are antiproliferative, improve endothelial function, may act as antioxidants, decrease platelet aggregation and enhance fibrinolysis.

Homocysteine, an amino acid, can experimentally induce vascular damage. It was demonstrated that there is a non-linear relation between homocysteine concentration and cardiovascular risk[32].

Low circulating concentrations of folic acid and vitamins B6 and B12 increase the risk of cardiovascular disease and cause a rise in homocysteinemia. Administration of folic acid and those vitamins rapidly decreases the levels of homocysteine. Clinical trials are underway to determine if these strategies are cardioprotective. It has been suggested that even people with normal levels of homocysteine might benefit from its reduction. Elderly patients taking vitamin B6 supplements of 100–200 mg/day showed a 73%

reduction in the risk of angina and myocardial infarction with an average increase in lifespan of 8 years[33]. In the Nurses' Health Study it was found that the intake of folate and vitamin B6 above the current recommended dietary allowance may be important in the primary prevention of coronary heart disease among women[34].

The understanding of coronary artery disease risk and atherogenesis has changed very much in recent years. It is the unstable soft plaque, that cannot be seen in angiography, that is prone to rupture and results in infarction. There are also important changes in vascular reactivity that result from diet. Most infarctions occur in patients who have normal total cholesterol levels. At-risk patients can be identified using the ratios of total cholesterol to high-density lipoprotein, and triglycerides to high-density lipoprotein. Primary prevention trials demonstrate that coronary artery disease risk can be lowered dramatically with diet and drug therapy[35].

Insulin resistance

A fasting glucose/insulin (G : I) ratio (md/dl : µU/ml) less than 4.5 is the single best screening measure for detecting insulin resistance[36].

Strong physical activity and a properly balanced diet are the best initial approaches. The so-called insulin sensitizers can be used, with caution, as if these women had type 2 diabetes. For this purpose, biguanides (like metformin) have been widely used. A new class of compounds, the glitazones[37], was recently introduced in the market; but they may have some liver toxicity.

Obesity

In most cases, obesity is psychogenic in its origin. If general measures[38] (physical exercise, balanced nutrition) do not work it is essential to refer the woman to a behavioral psychotherapist. Two new compounds have been introduced in the market. Orlistat[39] decreases the intestinal absorption of dietary fat. Sibutramine[40] inhibits the reuptake of both serotonin and norepinephrine; it reduces food intake and increases thermogenesis, thus contributing to weight loss.

Obesity, *per se*, is a cause of insulin resistance which, in turn, can also cause obesity. In such cases, when hyperinsulinemia is present, these cases should be managed as in insulin resistance.

Osteopenia and osteoporosis

In a recent study[41] it was concluded that subclinical vitamin D deficiency may contribute to increased fractures. Low levels of vitamin D are associated with high levels of parathyroid hormone, and may cause parathyroid hormone-mediated bone loss. Vitamin D and calcium therapy reduce parathyroid hormone and decrease bone resorption, with a consequent decrease in fractures. It is estimated that 800 IU of vitamin D and 1 g elemental calcium per day are needed to reduce fractures. This is a recommendation for the primary prevention of bone loss.

Fatty fish is a good source of vitamin D. Too much protein in the diet can result in increased loss of calcium in the urine; the same is true of too much sodium, caffeine and alcohol. Smoking increases the risk for osteoporosis.

If one has to complement these measures with drugs, specific estrogen receptor modulators like raloxifene cannot be considered as being hormones and may safely be used. Besides increasing bone mineral density and preventing osteoporosis, they also have a positive effect in lipid metabolism, they do not stimulate the endometrium and may even protect against breast cancer[42,43]. Bisphosphonates[44] have a very positive effect on the bone and are used with success for the treatment of osteoporosis.

Breast cancer

Other important information from the Nurses' Health Study suggests that folates, which are involved in DNA synthesis, may reduce breast cancer risk, particularly among women with greater alcohol consumption (at least 15 g/day of alcohol)[45]. (The relative risk of breast cancer for current users of folate supplements versus never users was RR 0.74; 95% CI, 0.59–0.93). It is also known that alcohol increases breast cancer risk.

This study did not show any association between total folate intake and breast cancer risk among women who consumed less than 15 g/day of alcohol. Thus, a decrease in alcohol, and also in animal fat consumption, seems a wise measure to decrease the risk of breast cancer, even more so if one also eats more fruits and vegetables containing isoflavones.

CONCLUDING REMARKS AND PRACTICAL GUIDELINES

There seems to be little doubt that Hippocrates was right when he said 2500 years ago 'Let food be your Medicine, and let Medicine be your food'. Barry Sears[7] has made a monumental contribution to the science of nutrition with a very comprehensive and highly scientific logical approach to anti-aging. Public health authorities are concerned with the little attention that is paid to the urgent need to change alimentary habits and lifestyles, as a cheap and very effective strategy to prevent many diseases. Health-care providers are also not motivated to implement and reinforce such life-saving strategies.

There is nowadays an abuse of drug consumption. Most people do not know, or do not believe, that many a time proper nutrition, good physical exercise and changes in lifestyle can achieve more, in terms of disease prevention and health maintenance, than some tablets taken by mouth.

When HRT is not possible, what can be done for menopausal women? It is unquestionable that estrogens can be of great help during the early and late postmenopausal phases of a woman's life. Nevertheless one can often achieve as much with non-hormonal medication or even without drugs. It may take longer but, in the long run, it pays.

The following suggestions and recommendations should be made to *all* middle-aged women whether or not they are on HRT.

(1) Start a Mediterranean diet[46] or a 'zone' diet[6], eating:
   (a) More whole breads and cereals,
   (b) More root vegetables, green vegetables and legumes (beans, peas, carrots, broccoli, tomatoes, etc.),
   (c) More fish (salmon, tuna, etc.),
   (d) More fresh fruit (apples, citrus, etc.),
   (e) Replace beef with poultry,
   (f) No butter,
   (g) Plenty of olive oil,
   (h) Some red wine,
   (i) Plenty of black or green tea,
   (j) Nuts;

(2) Start a program of physical fitness, and exercise as much as possible;

(3) Keep mentally active;

(4) Reformulate the life-style;

(5) Take the following nutrients (essential):
   (a) Vitamin A 4.000 IU/day,
   (b) Vitamin B6 5–10 mg/day,
   (c) Vitamin C 500–1000 mg/day,
   (d) Vitamin D 400–800 IU/day,
   (e) Vitamin E 200–400 IU/day,
   (f) Folic acid 0.5–1.0 mg/day,
   (g) Calcium 500–1000 mg/day,
   (h) Magnesium 250–400 mg/day,
   (i) β-carotene 5000 IU/day;

(6) For the prevention of atherosclerosis (advisable):
   (a) Lovastatin or simvastatin (for primary and secondary prevention, respectively),
   (b) Aspirin (50–100 mg/day),
   (c) Angiotensin-converting enzyme inhibitors.

References

1. Speroff L. It's time to stop using the word 'replacement'. *Maturitas* 1999;in press
2. Woods NF. Symptoms among midlife women: cultural lenses, research, and health care. Editorial. *Menopause* 1999;6:90–1
3. Berg DA, Taylor DL. Symptom experience of Filipino American midlife women. *Menopause* 1999;6:105–14
4. Utian WH, Boggs PP. The North American Menopause Society 1998 Menopause Survey. Part I: Postmenopausal women's perception about menopause and midlife. *Menopause* 1999;6:122–8
5. Rabin DS, Cipparrone N, Linn ES, *et al.* Why menopausal women do not want to take hormone replacement therapy. *Menopause* 1999;6:61–7
6. Sears B. *The Anti-aging Zone.* New York, NY: Harper Collins Publisher Inc., 1999
7. Speroff L. Women's health care in the 21st century. *Maturitas* 1999;in press
8. Notelovitz M, Tonnessen D. *The Essential Heart Book for Women.* New York: St. Martin's Griffin, 1997.
9. Byyny RL, Speroff L. *A Clinical Guide for the Care of Older Women.* Baltimore: Williams and Wilkins, 1990
10. Kushi LH, Fee RM, Fulson AR, *et al.* Physical activity and mortality in postmenopausal women. *J Am Med Assoc* 1997;227:1287–92
11. Hu FB, Grodstein F, Hennekens CH, *et al.* Age at natural menopause and risk of cardiovascular disease. *Arch Intern Med* 1999;159:1061–6
12. Tamaka K, Nakamishi T. Obesity as a risk factor for various diseases: necessity for lifestyle changes for healthy aging. *Appl Human Sci* 1996;15:139–48
13. Samaras K, Kelly PJ, Chiano MN, *et al.* Genetic and environmental influences on total-body and central abdominal fat: the effect of physical activity in female twins. *Ann Intern Med* 1999;13:873–82
14. Stampfer MJ, Hennekens CH, Manson JE, *et al.* Vitamin E consumption and the risk of coronary disease in women. *N Engl J Med* 1993;328:1444–9
15. Giovannuci E. Tomatoes, tomato-based products, lycopene and cancer: review of the epidemiological literature. *J Natl Cancer Inst* 1999;91:317–31
16. Trichopoulou A, Katsouyanni K, Stuver S, *et al.* Consumption of olive oil and specific food groups in relation to cancer in Greece. *J Natl Cancer Inst* 1995;87:110–16
17. Block G, Patterson B, Subar A. Fruit, vegetables and cancer prevention: a review of epidemiological evidence. *Nutr Cancer* 1992;18:1–29
18. Tavani A, La Vechia C. Fruit and vegetable consumption and cancer risk in a Mediterranean population. *Am J Clin Nutr* 1995;61(Suppl):1374S–7S
19. Hu FB, Stampfer MJ, Manson JE, *et al.* Frequent nut consumption and risk of coronary heart disease in women: prospective cohort study. *Br Med J* 1998;317:1341–5
20. Reinil K, Block G. Phytoestrogen content of food – a compendium of literature values. *Nutr Cancer* 1996;26:123–48
21. Nachtigall L, Fenichel R, Lagregal L, *et al.* The effects of isoflavone derived from red clover on vasomotor symptoms, endometrial thickness and reproductive hormone concentrations in menopausal women. Poster 2-59, The 81st Hormonal Meeting of the Endocrine Society, USA, 1999
22. Washbuen S, Burke GL, Morgan T, *et al.* Effect of soy protein supplement on serum lipoproteins, blood pressure, and menopausal symptoms in perimenopausal women. *Menopause* 1999;6:7–13
23. Wolk A, Manson JE, Stampfer MS, *et al.* Long-term intake of dietary fiber and decreased risk of coronary heart disease among women. *J Am Med Assoc* 1999;281:1998–2004
24. Ames BN. Micronutrients prevent cancer and delay aging. *Toxicol Lett* 1998;102–3:5–18
25. Jacobs DR Jr, Meyer KA, Kushi LH, *et al.* Is whole grain intake associated with reduced total and cause-specific death rates in older women? The Iowa Women's Health Study. *Am J Public Health* 1999;89: 322–9
26. Knight JA, Martin LJ, Greenberg CV, *et al.* Macronutrient intake and change in mammography density at menopause: results from a randomised trial. *Cancer Epidemiol Biomarkers Prev* 1999;8:123–8
27. Williamson DR, Pharand C. Statins in the prevention of coronary heart disease. *Pharmacotherapy* 1998;18:242–54
28. Downs JR, Clerfield M, Weis S, *et al.* Primary prevention of acute coronary events with lovastatin in men and women with average cholesterol levels. *J Am Med Assoc* 1998;279:1615–22
29. Lonn EM, Yusuf S. Emerging approaches in preventing cardiovascular disease. *Br Med J* 1999;318: 1337–41
30. Hay JN, Yu WM, Ashraf T. Pharmacoeconomics of lipid-lowering agents for primary and secondary prevention of coronary artery disease. *Pharmacoeconomics* 1999;15:47–74
31. Devaraj S, Jialal I. Alpha-tocopherol-2 decreases interleukin-1-beta release from activated human monocytes by inhibition of 5-lipoxygenase. *Atheroscler Thromb Vasc Biol* (United States) 1999;19: 1125–33
32. Boushey CJ, Beresford SAA, Omenn GS, *et al.* A quantitative assessment of plasma homocysteine as a risk factor for vascular disease. Probable benefits

of increasing folic acid intakes. *J Am Med Assoc* 1995;274:1049–57
33. Ellis JM, Mckully KS. Prevention of myocardial infarction by vitamin B6. *Res Comm Mol Pathol Pharmacol* 1995;89:208–20
34. Rimm EB, Willett WC, Hu FB, *et al.* Folate and vitamin B6 from diet and supplements in relation to risk of coronary heart diseases among women. *J Am Med Assoc* 1998;279:359–64
35. Castelli WP. The new pathophysiology of coronary artery disease. *Am J Cardiol* 1998;82:60T–65T
36. Legro RS, Finegood D, Dunaif A. A fasting glucose to insulin ratio is a useful measure of insulin sensitivity in women with polycystic ovary syndrome. *J Clin Endocrinol Metab* 1998;83:2694–8
37. Nolan JJ, Ludvik B, Beerdsen P, *et al.* Improvement in glucose tolerance and insulin resistance in obese subjects treated with troglitazone. *N Engl J Med* 1994;331:1188–93
38. Anderson DA, Wadden TA. Treating the obese patient. Suggestions for primary care practice. *Arch Fam Med* 1999;8:156–67
39. Sjöström L, Rissanen A, Andersen T, *et al.* Controlled trial of Orlistat for weight loss and prevention of weight regain in obese patients. *Lancet* 1998;352:167–72
40. Bray GA, Blackburn GL, Fergunson JM, *et al.* Sibutramine produces dose-related weight loss. *Obesity Res* 1999;7:189–98
41. LeBoff MS, Kohlmeier L, Hurwitz S, *et al.* Occult vitamin D deficiency in postmenopausal US women with acute hip fracture. *J Am Med Assoc* 1999;281:1505–11
42. Delmas P, Bjarnason NH, Mitlak BH, *et al.* Effects of raloxifene on bone mineral density, serum cholesterol concentrations, and uterine endometrium in postmenopausal women. *N Engl J Med* 1997;337:1641–7
43. Walsh BW, Kuller LH, Wild RA, *et al.* Effects of raloxifene on serum lipids and coagulation in healthy post-menopausal women. *J Am Med Assoc* 1998;279:1445–50
44. Ensrud K, Black DM, Palermo L, *et al.* Treatment with alendronate prevents fractures in women at highest risk: results from the Fracture Intervention Trial. *Arch Intern Med* 1997;157:2617–24
45. Zhang S, Hunter DJ, Hankinson SE, *et al.* A prospective study of folate intake and the risk of breast cancer. *J Am Med Assoc* 1999;281:1632–7
46. Greenwood S. The Mediterranean diet: acceptable and effective for Americans? *Menopause Management* (NAMS) 1999;8:16–19

Suggested reading

Notelovitz M, Tonnessen D. *Menopause and Midlife Health.* New York: St. Martin's Press, 1993

Neves-e-Castro M, Birkhäuser M, Clarkson TB, Collins P, eds. *Menopause and the Heart.* Carnforth, UK: Parthenon Publishing, 1999

Web sites

Mayo Clinic – http://*www.mayo.health.org/* (women's health and diets)

Tufts University – http://*www.navigator.tufts.edu/* (excellent for nutrition)

Biological actions of progesterone and progestins on breast epithelial cell cycle progression

45

E. A. Musgrove and R. L. Sutherland

INTRODUCTION

Combinations of steroid and polypeptide hormones, growth factors and cytokines provide the signals necessary to orchestrate the development and differentiated function of the breast and reproductive organs by eliciting a suite of cell type-specific responses. Progesterone can be viewed as balancing the proliferative effects of estrogen by directing the tissue toward its normal differentiated function. In the mammary gland, estrogen appears to be the main drive to proliferation, particularly in the formation of the mammary ducts, while progesterone acts in concert with other hormones, particularly prolactin, to induce the alveolar development necessary for subsequent milk production. Increasing evidence from studies of the murine mammary gland suggests that this lobuloalveolar development results from progesterone stimulation of epithelial cell proliferation. However, the role of progesterone in mediating breast epithelial cell proliferation in humans remains a controversial area.

Despite the physiological importance of progesterone and the widespread pharmacological use of synthetic progestins, progesterone and synthetic progestin effects on cell proliferation have not been widely studied from a mechanistic viewpoint. Nevertheless, significant recent advances have been made towards understanding this aspect of progestin action at both the whole cell and the molecular level.

EFFECTS ON NORMAL BREAST EPITHELIAL CELL PROLIFERATION

The hormonal control of mammary gland development and function has been the subject of extensive investigation, with immature or ovariectomized mice being the most extensively utilized experimental model. These studies demonstrate that a minimal hormonal requirement for ductal development is estrogen and either prolactin or growth hormone; lobuloalveolar development requires progesterone in addition[1]. Progesterone stimulates the proliferation of the mammary epithelium in mature animals and is, indeed, more effective than estrogen[2]. The impaired mammary development in mice lacking progesterone receptor ($PR^{-/-}$)[3-5], indicating a requirement for progestin action for the formation of the lobular alveoli during pregnancy, adds further support to these observations. It should be noted, however, that progesterone is not the sole factor required for lobuloalveolar proliferation and differentiation, as illustrated by the similar phenotype of the mammary gland in $PR^{-/-}$ mice and mice lacking either prolactin or its receptor[3,4,6-8], and that the response to progesterone alone and the effect of combined estrogen and progesterone treatment vary with the maturity of the animal[2]. Experiments in which $PR^{-/-}$ epithelium is transplanted onto wild-type stroma and vice versa indicate that, at least in the mouse, the effect of progesterone on lobuloalveolar development is mediated via the epithelium, although ductal development appears to depend on a progesterone-dependent signal from the stroma[4,5,9]. In contrast, the effect of estrogen appears to be mediated indirectly, via stromal rather than epithelial receptors[10].

In comparison with the situation in mice, our understanding of the control of normal human breast proliferation and differentiation is rudimentary. In part, this is due to difficulties in obtaining tissue, particularly after hormonal manipulation. Studies in which mitoses or DNA synthesis were evaluated histologically in breast biopsies showed that both varied in a cyclical manner during the menstrual cycle, reaching maxima during the luteal phase[11,12] (Figure 1). While the stimulus for the wave of proliferation is unknown, it coincides with, or immediately follows, a rise in the serum concentrations of both estrogen and progesterone[11]. Interestingly, the increased proliferation in the breast epithelium is followed by increased cell death via apoptosis in the late luteal phase, when hormone levels are decreasing, suggesting that the apoptosis may be a response to hormone withdrawal[13]. In distinct contrast with the timing of proliferation in breast epithelium, the peak of response in the endometrium occurs early in the cycle and proliferation is low or absent after ovulation[11]; this is thought to be an estrogen-mediated effect, which is opposed by the additional presence of progesterone in the luteal phase.

Various approaches have been used to examine the effects of steroid manipulation on breast epithelial cell proliferation. However, no clear consensus on a stimulatory role for progesterone or an ability to inhibit estrogen-mediated proliferation has yet emerged. In one study, topical application of a gel containing estradiol, progesterone or both for 10–13 days preceding breast surgery was used to increase the steroid accumulation within the breast tissue. The growth fraction of breast epithelial cells, as measured by proliferating cell nuclear antigen (PCNA) immunoreactivity, was reduced following progestin exposure[14]. Similarly, progestin treatment inhibited the proliferation of steroid-responsive breast epithelial cells in short-term culture[15]. A more recent study addressed the issue by implanting normal breast tissue into nude mice, which was followed by treatment with estradiol and progesterone. Estradiol stimulated the thymidine labelling index, while progesterone had no effect, either when administered alone or in combination with estradiol, despite the presence of estrogen-inducible progesterone receptors in this tissue[16]. These results argue for a predominantly antiproliferative role for progestins in human breast epithelial cells, consistent with the use of progestins as therapy for breast cancer, but the possibility that a short-term increase in proliferation precedes progestin-mediated inhibition, as observed in breast cancer cells (see below) cannot

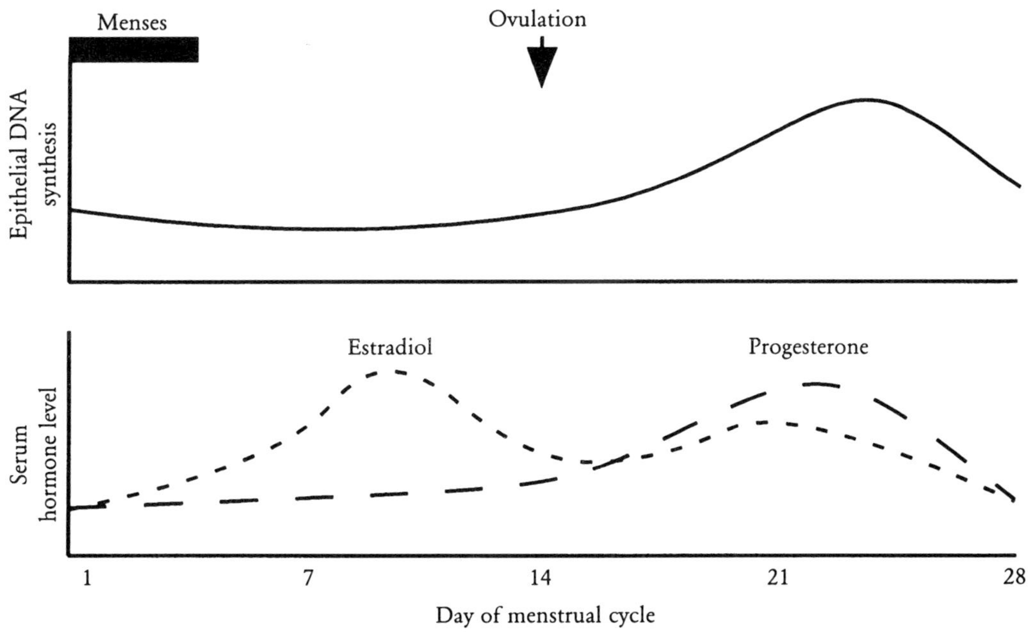

Figure 1 Changes in breast epithelial DNA synthesis and serum hormone levels during the human menstrual cycle. Based on data published in references 40 and 41

yet be excluded. Further experimentation in this area is critical to understanding the role of progesterone in the control of cell proliferation in the human breast.

EFFECTS ON BREAST CANCER CELL PROLIFERATION

Early studies demonstrated direct growth-inhibitory effects of synthetic progestins on proliferation in progesterone receptor-positive human breast cancer cell lines[17,18], consistent with the efficacy of progestins as therapy for breast cancer. This is the result of a cell cycle stage-specific action in the early G_1 phase[19]. Cells that have passed the arrest point begin DNA synthesis in the presence of progestin, subsequently completing a round of replication and undergoing cell division, but are arrested upon re-entry into the G_1 phase. Cells initially in the G_1 phase fail to initiate DNA synthesis and remain in the G_1 phase.

Experiments using breast cancer cells proliferating under conditions where either stimulation or inhibition could be detected have indicated that both responses to progestin treatment could occur in the one cell type[20]. During initial exposure, the proportion of cells initiating DNA synthesis increased as a result of progestin-induced acceleration through the G_1 phase, partially synchronizing a cohort of cells which then completed a round of replication. Consistent with the earlier experiments, cells that were originally later in the cell cycle continued through the cell cycle, but were arrested in the G_1 phase at the beginning of the next cell cycle. Thus, the initial stimulation was transient, with the later inhibition predominating, and together these responses resulted in a biphasic change in the proportion of cells undergoing DNA synthesis (Figure 2).

Despite the presence of functional receptors and the rapid metabolism of progesterone, progesterone-inhibited breast cancer cells are resistant to further stimulation by progestin for approximately 72 h[21], a time similar to that taken for the spontaneous resumption of cell cycle progression[19,21]. However, progesterone-inhibited cells become sensitive to the mitogenic effects of epidermal growth factor much earlier, within 46 h[21], suggesting that this is a specific resistance to progestins. These data suggest that cyclic exposure to progesterone *in vivo* may lead to successive single rounds of proliferation.

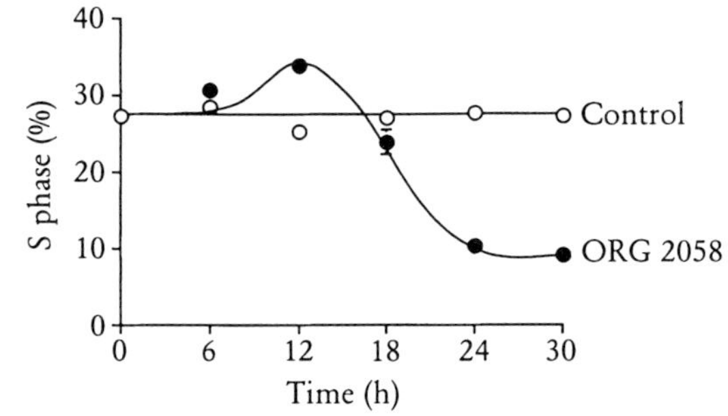

Figure 2 Effect of progestin treatment on T-47D breast cancer cell proliferation. Exponentially proliferating T-47D cells were treated with progestin and the proportion of cells undergoing DNA synthesis (S-phase fraction) was determined by flow cytometry

EFFECTS ON BREAST CANCER CELL CYCLE CONTROL MECHANISMS

The direct action of progestins on epithelial cell proliferation implies that progestin-regulated genes will include genes that either have a role in cell cycle control or are regulators of such genes. Recent experiments in this laboratory have thus concentrated on investigating the effects of progestins on cyclins and their associated cyclin-dependent kinases (CDKs), proteins that are regulators of key transitions during the cell cycle. An evolutionarily conserved class of serine/threonine protein kinases, the CDKs, are regulated by their association with cyclins, members of another well-conserved class of proteins. Additional controls include the phosphorylation of activating or inhibitory residues on the CDK and the abundance of CDK inhibitor proteins. Together, these regulate the sequential activation of a series of CDKs to ensure passage through a series of checkpoints and hence orderly progression through the cell cycle (Figure 3).

The major CDKs active in the G_1 phase in breast cancer cells are cyclin D-Cdk4 and cyclin E-Cdk2[22], as illustrated in Figure 3. Opposing CDK activation by cyclins are the CDK inhibitors p21 (Waf1, Cip1, Sdi1) and p27 (Kip1), although not all cyclin-CDK complexes containing these 'inhibitor' proteins are inactive[23]. Rather, p21 and

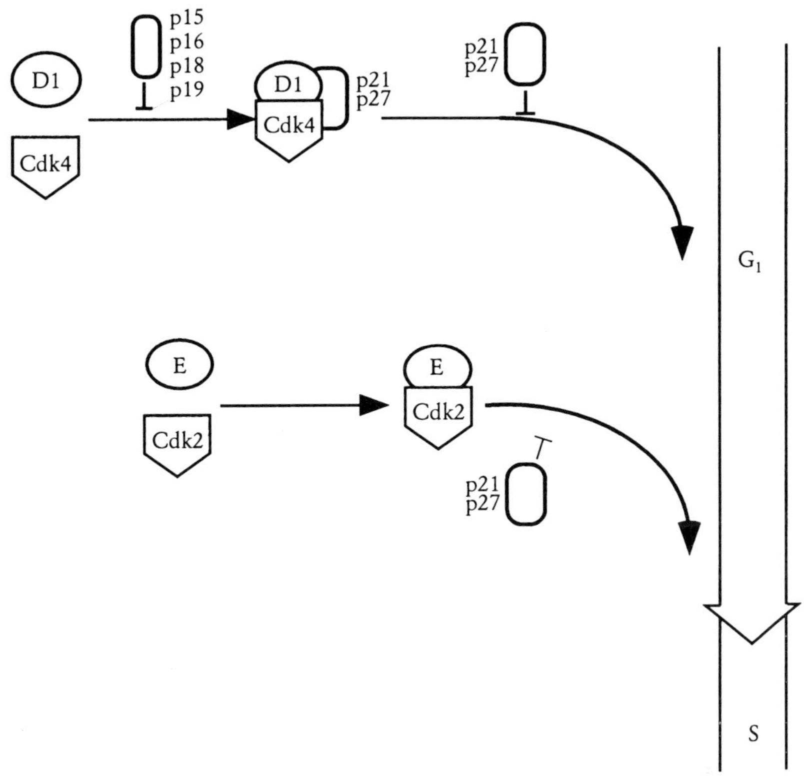

Figure 3 Cell cycle regulation during the G_1 phase. Progress from the G_1 to the S phase depends on the actions of the molecular pathways illustrated schematically. The major G_1 cyclin complexes in breast cancer cells, cyclin D1-Cdk4 and cyclin E-Cdk2, are illustrated. These cyclin-dependent kinases (CDKs) phosphorylate key substrates, thus allowing entry into the S phase. Their activity is regulated at several levels, including assembly and activation. The CDK inhibitors p21 and p27 inhibit active CDK complexes, but also act as assembly factors for cyclin D1-Cdk4. A major function of the INK4 CDK inhibitors p15, p16, p18 and p19 is to inhibit the assembly of cyclin D1-Cdk4 complexes

p27 appear also to function as adaptors that promote the assembly of cyclin D-CDK complexes and perhaps target these complexes to specific intracellular compartments or substrates[24]. An unrelated family of CDK inhibitors, characterized by an ankyrin repeat structure (including $p16^{INK4a}$ and $p18^{INK4c}$), more specifically target cyclin D-associated kinases[23]. Their inhibitory action appears to be largely due to competition with the cyclin for CDK binding.

Progestin stimulation of cyclin-CDK activity

Initial investigations of the possible effects of progestins on CDK function showed that the entry of progestin-stimulated T-47D human breast cancer cells into the S phase was preceded by an increase in cyclin D1 mRNA and protein abundance[25]. Cyclin D1 mRNA levels increased only transiently, however, returning to control levels as progestin-stimulated cells entered the S phase[25]. Cyclin D1 expression is high in murine mammary epithelium during pregnancy, when serum steroid levels are high, but largely undetectable in mammary epithelium from virgin or lactating animals[26]. In ovariectomized mice, estrogen increases cyclin D1 mRNA and protein expression in the mammary epithelium, and the addition of progesterone as well as estrogen further increases cyclin D1 levels[27]. The correspondence between the induction of cyclin D1 and subsequent proliferation suggests cyclin D1 induction as one of the elements coupling steroid hormone action with cell cycle control mechanisms. This conclusion is strongly supported by data from several experimental models. For example, experiments using T-47D breast cancer cells expressing cyclin D1 under the control of an inducible promoter indicated that cyclin D1 induction led to an increase in the rate of G_1 transit[28]. Thus, a progestin-induced increase in cyclin D1 abundance could account for the acceleration in G_1 phase progression. Furthermore, overexpression of cyclin D1 in the mammary gland of transgenic mice led to increased lobuloalveolar development, reminiscent of the changes associated with pregnancy, while, conversely, development of the lobular alveoli did not occur in pregnant cyclin D1-null mice[29-31], indicating a very specific requirement for cyclin D1 in alveolar proliferation. In cyclin D1-null mice, ductal proliferation apparently occurs normally, allowing both pubertal development of the gland and some side-branching during pregnancy[30,31]. Since progesterone is also necessary for alveolar, but not ductal, proliferation, cyclin D1 action may be essential for progesterone-driven mammary epithelial proliferation.

Progestin inhibition of cyclin-CDK activity

Progestin inhibition of T-47D breast cancer cell entry into the S phase is associated with decreased phosphorylation of the CDK substrates pRB and p107[21,32] and decreases in both cyclin D-Cdk4[32] and cyclin E-Cdk2 activity[21,32], accompanying or slightly preceding the decrease in the fraction of S-phase cells. Downregulation of kinase activity was accompanied by decreases in the expression of cyclin D1 and cyclin E, followed later by a decrease in cyclin D3 expression[21,32]. However, the decreases in cyclin abundance were generally more modest than the decreases in kinase activity, suggesting that other mechanisms are also involved. More detailed studies showed that, following progestin treatment, almost all of the cyclin E was in a low specific activity, p21- and p27-bound, form[32]. These data suggest preferential formation of a CDK inhibitor-bound species as a further mechanism for the decreased cyclin E-associated kinase activity following progestin treatment. An additional factor in the decrease in cyclin D-Cdk4 activity is likely to be an increase in the abundance of the INK4 family inhibitor $p18^{INK4c}$, since progestin induction of $p18^{INK4c}$ mRNA and protein is apparent before the decrease in Cdk4 activity[32,33]. Together, these data suggest a model for progestin inhibition of proliferation in which $p27^{Kip1}$ inhibition of cyclin E-Cdk2 and $p18^{INK4c}$ inhibition of Cdk4/6 co-operate with reduced cyclin D and E abundance to bring about growth inhibition (Figure 4). In progestin-treated breast cancer cells, increased $p18^{INK4c}$ and decreased cyclin D1 may together increase the availability of $p27^{Kip1}$ for binding to cyclin E-Cdk2, accounting for increased $p27^{Kip1}$ binding to this complex before substantial changes in $p27^{Kip1}$ abundance are observed[32,33]. While this model provides an explanation of the effects on CDK activity associated with progestin inhibition of proliferation, it is important to note that extended progestin treatment (> 12 h) is required before these responses are manifest[19,21,32], and the basis of this delay remains to be defined.

CONCLUSIONS

While it is apparent that substantial recent progress has been made towards understanding the potential molecular interactions leading to progestin regulation of cell proliferation in breast epithelium, much remains to be learnt. Potential models for progestin effects have largely been based on data obtained using breast cancer cells in tissue culture. A critical issue is the degree to which the general features of these models can be applied to other progestin-responsive model systems, particularly human breast epithelium, although it will be necessary first to define more clearly the effects of progestins on cell cycle progression in this tissue. A further challenge arises from the interactions between progesterone and other hormones. For example, both progesterone and prolactin are required for the control of proliferation and differentiation in the lobular alveoli. While progress towards answering these questions remains a goal of ongoing research, the evidence that cell cycle regulatory molecules, in particular cyclin D1, play a critical role in progestin action suggests that their aberrant expression may contribute to alterations in steroid sensitivity in breast cancer.

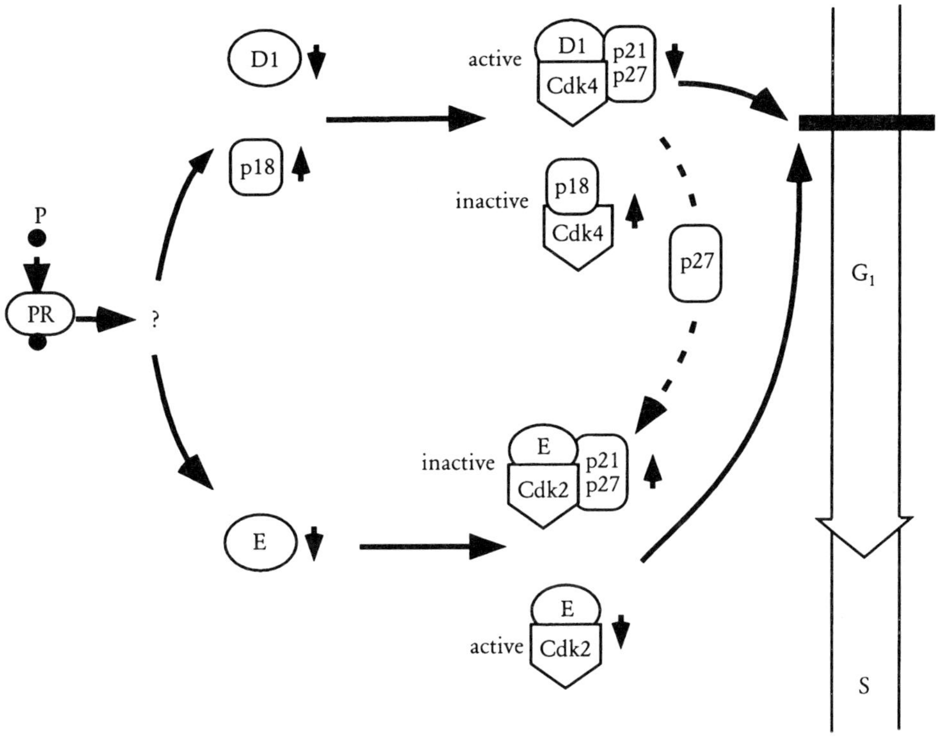

Figure 4 Progestin inhibition of cell cycle progression. Potential models of progestin inhibition of cyclin-dependent kinase (CDK) activity, and hence cell cycle progression, are illustrated. Progestin (P) inhibition of entry into the S phase is preceded by decreased activity of cyclin D1-Cdk4, cyclin D3-Cdk4 and cyclin E-Cdk2. This is accompanied by decreases in the expression of cyclins D1 and E, and the induction of p18. Decreased cyclin D1 and increased p18 together make p27 increasingly available to bind to, and inhibit the activity of, cyclin E-Cdk2. PR, progestin receptor

Additional impetus towards the further definition of progestin effects on normal and neoplastic breast epithelium is provided by the possibility that exposure to exogenous steroid hormones through the use of oral contraceptives and hormone replacement therapies might influence the risk of developing hormone-responsive cancer, including breast cancer. Indeed, there appears to be a slight increase in breast cancer risk in recent or current users[34,35], and the risk associated with estrogen use does not appear to be reduced by the addition of progestin[36], in marked contrast to the protective effects of progestins against the risk of endometrial cancer. However, synthetic progestins have an established role in the therapy of breast cancers[37-39]. Whether the apparent conflict between these findings relates simply to differences in the type or dose of progestins used, or reflects the complexity of progestin action, remains to be determined.

ACKNOWLEDGEMENTS

Research in this laboratory has been supported by the National Health and Medical Research Council of Australia and the New South Wales State Cancer Council. We thank Christine Lee, Alex Swarbrick and Ann Cornish for their invaluable assistance with our studies of progestin action on cell progression.

References

1. Imagawa W, Bandyopadhyay GK, Nandi S. Regulation of mammary epithelial cell growth in mice and rats. *Endocr Rev* 1990;11:494-523
2. Haslam SZ. Progesterone effects on deoxyribonucleic acid synthesis in normal mouse mammary glands. *Endocrinology* 1988;122:464-70
3. Lyndon JP, DeMayo FJ, Funk CR, *et al.* Mice lacking progesterone receptor exhibit pleiotrophic reproductive abnormalities. *Genes Dev* 1995;9: 2266-78
4. Humphreys RC, Lyndon JP, O'Malley BW, *et al.* Use of PRKO mice to study the role of progesterone in mammary gland development. *J Mamm Gland Biol Neoplasia* 1997;2:343-54
5. Brisken C, Park S, Vass T, *et al.* A paracrine role for the epithelial progesterone receptor in mammary gland development. *Proc Natl Acad Sci USA* 1998;95:5076-81
6. Horseman N, Zhao W, Montecino-Rodriguez E, *et al.* Defective mammopoiesis, but normal hematopoiesis, in mice with a targeted disruption of the prolactin gene. *EMBO J* 1997;16:6926-35
7. Ormandy CJ, Camus A, Barra J, *et al.* Null mutation of the prolactin receptor gene produces multiple reproductive defects in the mouse. *Genes Dev* 1997;11:167-78
8. Ormandy CJ, Binart N, Kelly PA. Mammary gland development in prolactin receptor knockout mice. *J Mamm Gland Biol Neoplasia* 1997;2:355-64
9. Humphreys RC, Lyndon J, O'Malley BW, *et al.* Mammary gland development is mediated by both stromal and epithelial progesterone receptors. *Mol Endocrinol* 1997;11:801-11
10. Cunha GR, Young P, Hom YK, *et al.* Elucidation of a role for stromal steroid hormone receptors in mammary gland growth and development using tissue recombinants. *J Mamm Gland Biol Neoplasia* 1997;2:393-402
11. Clarke CL, Sutherland RL. Progestin regulation of cellular proliferation. *Endocr Rev* 1990;11:266-302
12. Anderson E, Clarke RB, Howell A. Estrogen responsiveness and control of normal human breast proliferation. *J Mamm Gland Biol Neoplasia* 1998;3:23-35
13. Ferguson DJP, Anderson PJ. Morphological evaluation of cell turnover in relation to the menstrual cycle in the 'resting' human breast. *Br J Cancer* 1981;44:177-81
14. Chang K-J, Lee TTY, Linares-Cruz G, *et al.* Influences of percutaneous administration of estradiol and progesterone on human breast epithelial cell cycle *in vivo*. *Fertil Steril* 1995;63:785-91
15. Gompel A, Malet C, Spritzer P, *et al.* Progestin effect on cell proliferation and 17β-hydroxysteroid dehydrogenase activity in normal human breast cells in culture. *J Clin Endocrinol Metab* 1986;63: 1174-80
16. Laidlaw IJ, Clarke RB, Howell A, *et al.* The proliferation of normal human breast tissue implanted into athymic nude mice is stimulated by oestrogen but not progesterone. *Endocrinology* 1995;136:164-71
17. Vignon F, Bardon S, Chalbos D, *et al.* Antiestrogenic effect of R5020, a synthetic progestin in human breast cancer cells in culture. *J Clin Endocrinol Metab* 1983;56:1124-30
18. Horwitz KB, Freidenberg GR. Growth inhibition and increase of insulin receptors in antiestrogen-resistant $T47D_{co}$ human breast cancer cells by progestins: implications for endocrine therapies. *Cancer Res* 1985;45:167-73
19. Sutherland RL, Hall RE, Pang GYN, *et al.* Effect of medroxyprogesterone acetate on proliferation and cell cycle kinetics of human mammary carcinoma cells. *Cancer Res* 1988;48:5084-91
20. Musgrove EA, Lee CSL, Sutherland RL. Progestins both stimulate and inhibit breast cancer cell cycle progression while increasing expression of transforming growth factor α, epidermal growth factor receptor, *c-fos* and *c-myc* genes. *Mol Cell Biol* 1991; 11:5032-43
21. Groshong SD, Owen GI, Grimison B, *et al.* Biphasic regulation of breast cancer cell growth by progesterone: role of the cyclin-dependent kinase inhibitors, p21 and $p27^{Kip1}$. *Mol Endocrinol* 1997;11:1593-607
22. Sherr CJ. Cancer cell cycles. *Science* 1996;274: 1672-7
23. Sherr CJ, Roberts JM. CDK inhibitors: positive and negative regulators of G_1 phase progression. *Genes Dev* 1999;13:1501-12
24. LaBaer J, Garrett MD, Stevenson LF, *et al.* New functional activities for the p21 family of CDK inhibitors. *Genes Dev* 1997;11:847-62
25. Musgrove EA, Hamilton JA, Lee CSL, *et al.* Growth factor, steroid and steroid antagonist regulation of cyclin gene expression associated with changes in T-47D human breast cancer cell cycle progression. *Mol Cell Biol* 1993;13:3577-87
26. Stepanova L, Leng X, Parker SB, *et al.* Mammalian $p50^{Cdc37}$ is a protein kinase-targeting subunit of Hsp90 that binds and stabilises Cdk4. *Genes Dev* 1996;10:1491-502
27. Said TK, Conneely OM, Medina D, *et al.* Progesterone, in addition to estrogen, induces cyclin D1 expression in the murine mammary epithelial cell, *in vivo*. *Endocrinology* 1997;138:3933-9
28. Musgrove EA, Lee CSL, Buckley MF, *et al.* Cyclin D1 induction in breast cancer cells shortens G_1 and is sufficient for cells arrested in G_1 to complete the cell cycle. *Proc Natl Acad Sci USA* 1994;91: 8022-6

29. Wang TC, Cardiff RD, Zukerberg L, *et al.* Mammary hyperplasia and carcinoma in MMTV-cyclin D1 transgenic mice. *Nature (London)* 1994; 369:669-71
30. Sicinski P, Liu Donaher J, Parker SB, *et al.* Cyclin D1 provides a link between development and oncogenesis in the retina and breast. *Cell* 1995;82:621-30
31. Fantl V, Stamp G, Andrews A, *et al.* Mice lacking cyclin D1 are small and show defects in eye and mammary gland development. *Genes Dev* 1995;9: 2364-72
32. Musgrove EA, Swarbrick A, Lee CSL, *et al.* Mechanisms of CDK inactivation by progestins. *Mol Cell Biol* 1998;18:1812-25
33. Swarbrick A, Lee CSL, Sutherland RL, *et al.* Cooperation of $p27^{Kip1}$ and $p18^{INK4c}$ in progestin-mediated cell cycle arrest in T-47D breast cancer cells. *Mol Cell Biol* 2000; in press
34. Collaborative Group on Hormonal Factors in Breast Cancer. Breast cancer and hormonal contraceptives: collaborative reanalysis of individual data on 53 297 women with breast cancer and 100 239 women without breast cancer from 54 epidemiological studies. *Lancet* 1996;347:1713-27
35. Collaborative Group on Hormonal Factors in Breast Cancer. Breast cancer and hormone replacement therapy: collaborative reanalysis of data from 51 epidemiological studies of 52 705 women with breast cancer and 108 411 women without breast cancer. *Lancet* 1997;350:1047-59
36. Colditz GA, Hankinson SE, Hunter DJ, *et al.* The use of estrogens and progestins and the risk of breast cancer in postmenopausal women. *N Engl J Med* 1995;332:1589-93
37. Veronesi U, Goldhirsch A, Yarnold J. Breast cancer. In Peckham M, Pinedo HM, Veronesi U, eds. *Oxford Textbook of Oncology*. Oxford: Oxford University Press, 1995:1243-89
38. Santen RJ, Manni A, Harvey H, *et al.* Endocrine treatment of breast cancer in women. *Endocr Rev* 1990;11:221-65
39. Rose PG. Endometrial cancer. *N Engl J Med* 1996; 335:640-9
40. Longacre TA, Bartow SA. A correlative morphologic study of human breast and endometrium in the menstrual cycle. *Am J Surg Pathol* 1986;10: 382-93
41. Going JJ, Anderson TJ, Battersby S, *et al.* Proliferative and secretory activity in human breast during natural and artificial menstrual cycles. *Am J Pathol* 1988;130:193-204

Endometrial effects of progesterone versus progestins

46

B. de Lignieres

INTRODUCTION

Since the mid 1970s, unopposed estrogen use has been clearly established as resulting in a high risk of endometrial cancer[1]. The addition of a progestin for at least 10 days per month was soon afterwards shown to reduce this endometrial risk, a fact that has been consistently confirmed by subsequent studies. Then, in the 1980s, the almost universal recommendation was to prescribe progestins for 12–14 days each calendar month. Medroxyprogesterone acetate ≤ 10 mg/day and norethisterone ≥ 2.5 mg/day were the most prescribed treatments in North America[2]. However, large discrepancies between theory and practice remain despite almost 30 years of consistent warnings. In two recent US case-control studies conducted in non-hysterectomized women, the use of estrogen, either unopposed or opposed by fewer than 10 days of progestin treatment each month, has been identified in 42–59% of all cases of endometrial cancer and in 71–74% of the cases discovered in hormone replacement therapy (HRT) users. This unsafe use of estrogens was also found in 47–65% of HRT users among controls[3,4]. Similarly, in the Nurses' Health Study, no more than 25% of current estrogen users were also progestin users, whatever the dose and schedule, while 45% of them were not hysterectomized[5].

It was found that, even among US users of opposed estrogens, the overall relative risk of endometrial cancer remained around 1.6-2.0, mainly due to the 25% of women using less than 10 days of progestins[3,4]. This situation was probably related to the low acceptability of the recommended progestin regimens.

The progestogens can be classified according to their chemical structure. Progesterone (4-pregnene-3,20-dione) is the only progestogen naturally secreted by the ovaries of mammals. Progestins are derivatives that are modified mainly to increase the oral bioavailability of progesterone by decreasing its clearance rate by gut and liver enzymes, while retaining its effects on the endometrium. The pregnane derivatives (such as medroxyprogesterone acetate) are synthesized from 17-hydroxyprogesterone or 19-norprogesterone. The androstane or estrane derivatives (such as norethisterone) are synthesized from 19-nortestosterone. All these compounds achieve their main goal by reducing at least ten-fold the oral dose to be administered in comparison with oral progesterone. However, whether these progestins retain the favorable safety/efficacy ratio of progesterone is far from being established. For example, the use of classical synthetic progestins is thought to produce a drop in high-density lipoprotein (HDL) cholesterol levels[6-8], to impair glucose metabolism[8,9], to limit vasodilatation[10-12] and to alter the histological appearance of the artery walls[13-15], showing that a reduction in the daily dose (in comparison with progesterone) does not necessarily mean an improvement in safety.

The need for new compounds with safer profiles was understood in the early 1980s in Europe, where new progestogens, including an oral progesterone formulation, have been studied. These progestogens were expected to be more appropriate to the specific situation of postmenopausal women, who have more estrone than estradiol, increased cardiovascular risks and no need for an antigonadotropic activity[16]. Since 1980, with time and experience, the relevant criteria to evaluate not only the safety of these steroids, but also their efficacy on the endometrium, have dramatically changed.

EFFECTS ON ENDOMETRIAL GLANDS

In the early 1980s, the major concerns were focused on epithelial cells, which are the potential providers of adenocarcinoma. Stroma and blood vessels were thought to follow the same 'stop and go' schedule under the same hormonal control. A nuclear estradiol receptor was known to control the cell cycle of glandular epithelial cells; this receptor is activated by estrogens and down-regulated by endogenous progesterone or exogenous synthetic progestogens in the same manner, but at different doses[17].

The optimal dose of any progestogenic compound was first determined on its ability to reproduce within 6 to 10 days in estrogen-treated postmenopausal women, all the morphological and biochemical changes being observed in the normal endometrium of premenopausal women during a physiological luteal phase. The effects of progestins were measured by the suppression of DNA synthesis and the nuclear estradiol receptor (antiestrogenic effect) and by the increase in the activities of progestin-sensitive enzymes such as estradiol and isocitric dehydrogenases (secretory effect). The morphological changes were assessed by light and transmission electron microscopy. It was believed that the safe control of epithelial proliferation could not be obtained without inducing full secretory transformation followed by endometrial sloughing.

The induction of bleeding on or after the 11th day of the cyclic progestogen treatment was recognized as reassurance of effective endometrial protection[18]. However, the need for a precisely scheduled vaginal bleeding, proposed as the most simple clinical evidence of an individually adapted combination of estrogen and progestogen[18], soon created serious problems, not only to women willing to remain amenorrheic, but also to numerous women bleeding before the 11th day of the progestogen sequence.

In the early 1990s, several studies demonstrated that the induction of cyclic bleeding and endometrial secretory transformation, requiring on average a larger daily dose of progestogens, was not providing any measurable benefit for the prevention of estrogen-induced hyperplasia[19,20]. Since it is clear that withdrawal bleeding, secretory changes and arrest in proliferation can be dissociated, the optimal daily dose of a progestogen is the dose that is able to slow down mitotic activity in glands and prevent hyperplasia[19,21]. The main end-points for an effective progestogen then became a low mitotic activity in glands in the short term (≤ 2 mitoses per 1000 gland cells at the end of one cycle of treatment) and no hyperplasia in the long term (≤ 2 cases of hyperplasia per 100 treated women at 12 months). All other descriptive characteristics of the endometrium (e.g. atrophy, blocked proliferation, mild or full secretory changes, focal hyperplasia) were considered as unpredictive[1].

EFFECTS ON ANGIOGENESIS

The control of bleeding, however, appeared to be more difficult than expected. Because the main mechanism for the induction of cyclic bleeding was thought to be related mostly to the withdrawal of both estrogen and progestogen, a continuous combined regimen was proposed to patients in the hope of suppressing any bleeding. Unfortunately it was soon discovered that this simple recommendation had to be adjusted, since 35–70% of patients using the continuous combined regimens experienced some episodes of irregular bleeding[22,23]. Numerous hysteroscopic studies were conducted in postmenopausal women experiencing unscheduled bleeding during continuous combined HRT. When no polyp or submucosal myoma was visible, the most common finding was a subatrophic endometrium without hyperplasia, but with dilated vessels and superficial spots of bleeding. Thus, the continuous combined regimen does not fail to control endometrial growth in most of these patients, but seems to maintain or even stimulate an inappropriate angiogenesis[24,25].

One of the most attractive explanations for this involves the role of vascular endometrial growth factor in the formation of new vessels and their progression within the endometrial tissue through the synthesis and release of enzymes able to destroy the extracellular matrix[26]. Usually found only in injured tissues or around rapidly growing tumors, vascular endometrial growth factor has been identified in human corpus luteum and endometrium.

That its concentration in the endometrium increases during the follicular phase and even more during the luteal phase suggests that progesterone is an agonist rather than an antagonist with respect to this specific target[27]. Moreover, the effects on the histology of new microvessel walls seem to vary according to the type of progestogen used, which may explain the different bleeding patterns observed with different progestogens used in similar schedules[24,25]. Some progestogens induce defects in vessel walls more frequently than others, specifically dilatation with irregular endothelium, facilitating blood leakage. Endothelial cell proliferation and adherence to artery walls is upregulated by estrogens and downregulated by progestins[28,29], which may induce defects in the endothelium when synthetic hormones bind in an unphysiological manner to this target.

Efforts are in progress to standardize the evaluation of the effects of various progestogens on endometrial angiogenesis, either through hysteroscopic controls[30] or through histological analysis[31].

MAIN EFFECTS OF PROGESTERONE

In HRT regimens for postmenopausal women, progesterone is almost exclusively administered orally as a micronized formulation[32,33]. The vaginal route, frequently recommended for short-term treatment in infertility, results in a high concentration of progesterone in the vaginal mucosa through a first-pass effect. This may modify the microbicide efficacy of vaginal secretions in a manner not suitable for long-term treatment[34,35].

The daily doses effective in preventing estrogen-dependent endometrial hyperplasia have been identified[32,33]. Despite the relatively short half-life of progesterone in serum, the endometrial concentration remains high enough after a once-daily administration to ensure a level of efficacy similar to that of synthetic progestins. The lowest effective doses of progesterone tested are 200 mg per day, 12 days per month, and 100 mg per day, 25 days per month. There is a clear dose-effect relationship of progesterone with both serum levels[36] and endometrial histology[37].

Some preliminary information on endometrial angiogenesis during treatment that combines estrogens and micronized progesterone is available. Endothelial morphological disturbances in endometrial vessels seem quite limited[25] and coincide with a low incidence of bleeding in users of the 100 mg/day regimen[38-40]. Around 90% of women remain amenorrheic, without bleeding or spotting episodes, after 6 months of this treatment regimen.

MAIN EFFECTS OF PROGESTINS

In HRT regimens for postmenopausal women, progestins are administered orally once a day. With medroxyprogesterone acetate, 2.5 or 5 mg per day continuously, and 10 mg per day, 12–14 days per month, combined with an estrogen, the annual incidence of endometrial hyperplasia remains below 2%[2,22]. With the cyclic schedule, most women (80%) experience around 7 days of bleeding per month. With both continuous schedules, only around 50% of women experience stable amenorrhea without bleeding or spotting episodes[22]. This suggests that this progestin is less than optimal for women wanting to avoid bleeding and related gynecological investigations.

With norethisterone acetate, 0.1, 0.25 or 0.5 mg per day continuously, and 2.5 or 5 mg per day, 12–14 days per month, combined with an estrogen, the annual incidence of endometrial hyperplasia remains low[41]. With the cyclic regimens, most women experience scheduled bleeding, while with the continuous regimens, the incidence of bleeding or spotting episodes still remains around 20–25% of cycles after 6 months of treatment[41]. There is a tendency for a slightly lower incidence of bleeding in the 0.5 mg treatment group.

CONCLUSION

Recent information about the poor adherence of postmenopausal women to some combined progestogen and estrogen treatments[3,4], as well as their relatively disappointing results on endometrial[42,43] and cardiovascular protection[44], clearly suggests that not all progestogens are equal and that a more careful selection of the optimal ones is necessary. Simply decreasing the daily doses or selecting steroid structures closer to progesterone than to testosterone may not be translated into an improved efficacy/safety ratio.

Besides the various influences on the cardiovascular system, the current criteria with which to select optimal progestogens for the endometrial target should be the control of the cell cycle in endometrial glands in the short term and the incidence of hyperplasia in the long term (≥ 1 year). Progesterone and progestins seem to be equally effective in this field.

The doses and schedules that induce no alteration in the endothelium or the endometrial microvessels should also be identified in the short term, and the rate of amenorrhea measured in the long term. Most of this pivotal information has only recently become available, and, with regard to the histology of endometrial vessels and bleeding patterns, micronized progesterone seems to be more beneficial than traditional progestins. Progesterone may be a better choice not only for women with cardiovascular risks, but also for postmenopausal women looking for stable amenorrhea.

References

1. De Lignieres B, Moyer DL. Influence of sex hormones on hyperplasia/carcinoma risks. In Lobo RA, ed. *Treatment of the Postmenopausal Woman: Basic and Clinical Aspects*. New York: Raven Press, 1994:373–83
2. Gambrel RD. The prevention of endometrial cancer in postmenopausal women with progestogens. *Maturitas* 1978;1:107–12
3. Pike MC, Peters RK, Cozen W, *et al.* Estrogen-progestin replacement therapy and endometrial cancer. *J Natl Cancer Inst* 1997;89:1110–16
4. Shapiro JA, Weiss NS, Beresford SA, Voigt LR. Menopausal hormone use and endometrial cancer by tumor grade and invasion. *Epidemiology* 1998; 9:99–101
5. Grodstein F, Stampfer MJ, Manson JE, *et al.* Postmenopausal estrogen and progestin use and the risk of cardiovascular disease. *N Engl J Med* 1996;335: 453–61
6. Farheus L, Larsson-Cohn U, Wallentin L. L-norgestrel and progesterone have different influences on plasma lipoproteins. *Eur J Clin Invest* 1983;13:447–53
7. Ottosson UB, Johansson BG, von Schoultz B. Subfractions of high-density lipoprotein cholesterol during estrogen replacement therapy: a comparison between progestogens and natural progesterone. *Am J Obstet Gynecol* 1985;151:746–50
8. Writing Group of the PEPI Trial. Effects of estrogen or estrogen/progestin regimens on heart disease risk factors in postmenopausal women. *J Am Med Assoc* 1995;273:199–208
9. Elkind-Hirsch KE, Sherman LD, Malinak R. Hormone replacement therapy alters insulin sensitivity in young women with premature ovarian failure. *J Clin Endocrinol Metab* 1993;76:472–5
10. Sullivan JM, Shala BA, Miller LA, *et al.* Progestin enhances vasoconstrictor responses in postmenopausal women receiving estrogen replacement therapy. *J North Am Menopause Soc* 1995;2:193–9
11. Miyagawa K, Rosch J, Stanczyk F, Hermsmeyer K. Medroxyprogesterone interferes with ovarian steroid protection against coronary vasospasm. *Nat Med* 1997;3:324–7
12. Sorensen K, Dorup I, Hermann A, Mosekide L. Combined hormone replacement therapy does not protect women against the age-related decline in endothelium dependent vasomotor function. *Circulation* 1998;97:1234–8
13. Adams MR, Golden DL. Atheroprotective effects of estrogen replacement therapy are antagonized by medroxyprogesterone acetate in monkeys. *Circulation* 1995;92:1–627
14. Oparil S, Levine RL, Chen SJ, *et al.* Sexually dimorphic response of the balloon-injured rat carotid artery to hormone treatment. *Circulation* 1997; 95:1301–7
15. Register TC, Adams MR, Golden DL, Clarkson TB. Conjugated equine estrogens alone, but not in combination with medroxyprogesterone acetate, inhibit aortic connective tissue remodeling after plasma lipid lowering in female monkeys. *Arterioscler Thromb Vasc Biol* 1998;18:1164–71
16. Kuhl H. Pharmakologie von sexualsteroiden. *Gynakologe* 1998;31:832–47
17. Whitehead MJ, Townsend PT, Pryse-Davies J, *et al.* Effects of estrogens and progestins on the biochemistry and morphology of the postmenopausal endometrium. *N Engl J Med* 1981;305:1599–605

18. Padwick ML, Pryse-Davies J, Whitehead MI. A simple method for determining the optimal dosage of progestin in postmenopausal women receiving estrogens. *N Engl J Med* 1986;315:930–4
19. Moyer DL, De Lignieres B, Driguez P, Pez JP. Prevention of endometrial hyperplasia by progesterone during long-term estradiol replacement: influence of bleeding pattern and secretory changes. *Fertil Steril* 1993;59:992–7
20. Sturdee DW, Barlow DH, Ulrich LG, *et al.* Is the timing of withdrawal bleeding a guide to endometrial safety during sequential oestrogen-progestagen replacement therapy? *Lancet* 1994;343: 979–82
21. Kim S, Snipes W, Korhonen M, *et al.* Antiproliferative effects of low-dose micronized progesterone. *Fertil Steril* 1996;65:323–31
22. Hillard TC, Siddle NC, Whitehead MI, *et al.* Continuous combined conjugated equine estrogen-progestogen therapy: effects of medroxyprogesterone acetate and norethindrone acetate on bleeding patterns and endometrial histologic diagnosis. *Am J Obstet Gynecol* 1992;167:1–7
23. Archer DF, Pickar JH, Bottiglioni F, *et al.* Bleeding patterns in postmenopausal women taking continuous or sequential regimens of conjugated estrogen with medroxyprogesterone acetate. *Obstet Gynecol* 1994;83:686–92
24. Fraser IS, Hickey M, Song JY. A comparison of mechanisms underlying disturbance of bleeding caused by spontaneous dysfunction, uterine bleeding or hormonal contraception. *Hum Reprod* 1996; 11:165–8
25. De Lignieres B, Driguez PC. Long-term experience with oral micronized progesterone and effects on the endometrium. *Contemp Obstet Gynecol* 1998; Suppl:10–17
26. Torry DS, Harris G, Holt VJ, *et al.* Vascular endothelial growth factor expression in cycling human endometrium. *Fertil Steril* 1996;66:72–80
27. Smith SK. Angiogenesis, vascular endothelial growth factor and the endometrium. *Hum Reprod Update* 1998;4:509–19
28. Alvarez RJ, Gips SJ, Moldovan N, *et al.* 17β-Estradiol inhibits apoptosis of endothelial cells. *Biochem Biophys Res Commun* 1997;237:372–81
29. Vasquez F, Rodriquez-Manzaneque JC, Lydon JP, *et al.* Progesterone regulates proliferation of endothelial cells. *J Biol Chem* 1999;274:2185–92
30. Hickey M, Dwarte D, Fraser IS. Precise measurements of intrauterine vascular structures at hysteroscopy in menorrhagia and during Norplant use. *Hum Reprod* 1998;13:3190–6
31. Hansen S, Grabau DA, Rose C, *et al.* Angiogenesis in breast cancer: a comparative study of the observer variability of methods for determining microvessel density. *Lab Invest* 1998;78:1563–73
32. De Lignieres B. Oral micronized progesterone. *Clin Ther* 1999;1:41–60
33. Fitzpatrick LA, Good A. Micronized progesterone: clinical indications and comparison with current treatments. *Fertil Steril* 1999;72:389–97
34. Marx PA, Spira AI, Gettie A, *et al.* Progesterone implants enhance SIV vaginal transmission and early virus load. *Nat Med* 1996;2:1084–9
35. Kaushic C, Murdin A, Underdown B, *et al.* *Chlamydia trachomatis* infection in the female reproductive tract of the rat: influence of progesterone on infectivity and immune response. *Infect Immun* 1998;66:893–909
36. Simon JA, Rocci ML, Robinson DE, *et al.* The absorption of oral micronized progesterone: the effect of food, dose proportionality and comparison with intramuscular progesterone. *Fertil Steril* 1993;60:26–33
37. Lane G, Siddle NC, Ryder TA, *et al.* Dose dependent effects of oral progesterone on the oestrogenised postmenopausal endometrium. *Br Med J* 1983;287: 1241–5
38. Foidart JM, Dombrowicz D, Roelandt L, *et al.* Impact on the endometrium of hormone replacement with combined progesterone and percutaneous estradiol. In Christiansen C, Riis B, eds. *Proceedings of 4th International Symposium on Osteoporosis.* Aalborg, Denmark: APS, 1993:331–3
39. Gillet JY, Andre G, Faguer B, *et al.* Induction of amenorrhea during hormone replacement therapy: optimal micronized progesterone dose. A multicenter study. *Maturitas* 1994;19:103–15
40. Marengo M, Rodriguez Vidal D, Gil Deza E, *et al.* Evaluation of a novel 25-day regimen with percutaneous estradiol and micronized progesterone. Presented at *8th International Congress on the Menopause*, Sidney, 1996:299
41. Archer DF, Dorin MH, Heine W, *et al.* Uterine bleeding in postmenopausal women on continuous therapy with estradiol and norethindrone acetate. *Obstet Gynecol* 1999;94:323–9
42. Grady D, Ernster VL. Hormone replacement therapy and endometrial cancer: are current regimens safe? *J Natl Cancer Inst* 1997;98:1088–9
43. Weiderpass E, Adami HO, Baron JA, *et al.* Risk of endometrial cancer following estrogen replacement with and without progestins. *J Natl Cancer Inst* 1999;91:1131–7
44. Hulley S, Grady D, Bush T, *et al.* Randomized trial of estrogen plus progestin for secondary prevention of coronary heart disease in postmenopausal women. *J Am Med Assoc* 1998;280:605–13

The vascular effects of progesterone/progestogens

47

S. H. Cho

INTRODUCTION

Cardiovascular disease, including coronary artery disease and stroke, is the leading cause of death not only in most Western societies[1,2] but also in Korea[3]. The most common cause of death in Korean women aged over 65 is also cardiovascular disease (Figure 1). It is well established that coronary heart disease is reduced by 50% in postmenopausal women who take estrogen replacement therapy[4]. However, long-term estrogen use is associated with an increased risk of endometrial cancer. To prevent this risk, progesterone/progestogens are prescribed with estrogen. However, the impact of estrogen in combination with progesterone/progestogens on the cardioprotective effects is unclear.

Approximately one-third of the cardioprotective effect of estrogen is thought to be due to beneficial changes in circulating lipids and lipoproteins[5]. Another important mechanism is its direct effect on blood vessels, and there are considerable data supporting this issue. Estrogen stimulates vascular endothelial cell secretion of nitric oxide[6], affects a number of vascular smooth muscle cell functions, including contractility and growth[7], and promotes neovascularization as well as migration, proliferation and differentiation of endothelial cells both *in vitro* and *in vivo*[8]. On the other hand, the direct effects of progesterone/progestogens remain unclear and the results are inconsistent among the researchers.

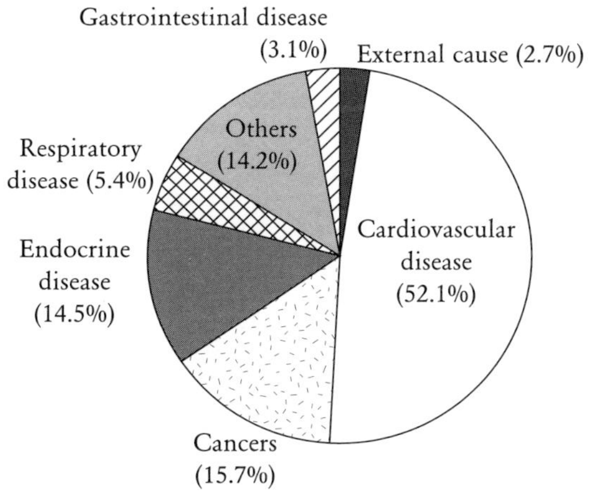

Figure 1 Causes of death in women aged ≥ 65 years in Korea, 1997

Many women who have an intact uterus and take hormone replacement therapy (HRT) are on the regimen of progesterone/progestogens combined with estrogen. Therefore, it is clinically important to evaluate the combined effects of progesterone/progestogens and estrogen on cardiovascular disease. This paper covers some reviews in this field, and describes our *in vitro* experimental results.

OBSERVATIONAL STUDIES OF EFFECTS OF ESTROGEN AND PROGESTERONE/PROGESTOGENS ON CARDIOVASCULAR RISK FACTORS

An observational report from the Nurses' Health Study with up to 16 years of follow-up in 59 337 women found a decrease in the risk of major coronary heart disease among the women who took estrogen with progestogen compared with the women who took estrogen alone or who did not use hormones[9]. In this study, it was suggested that the addition of progestogen did not appear to attenuate the cardioprotective effects of postmenopausal estrogen therapy. Other studies have also found that progesterone in combination with estrogen had no adverse effects, compared with estrogen alone, on the risk of myocardial infarction and stroke[10-12].

EFFECTS OF PROGESTERONE/PROGESTOGEN ON PERIPHERAL ARTERIES

It is not clear whether progesterone/progestogens diminish the favorable endothelial effects of estrogen in postmenopausal women. Several studies have attempted to answer this problem by measuring the changes in blood flow and the artery diameter after combined HRT or progesterone therapy alone. Six months' administration of estradiol and norethisterone was associated with a significant reduction of the pulsatility index in peripheral arteries, and the increase in blood flow was not affected by the addition of progestogen[13]. In another study of combined transdermal estradiol and vaginal micronized progesterone therapy, flow-mediated vasodilatation of the brachial artery was increased and this finding was the same as with estradiol alone[14]. In contrast, a study measuring the flow-mediated vascular dilatation of the brachial artery after estradiol and norethisterone treatment reported that progestogen may attenuate the beneficial effects of unopposed estrogen replacement[15]. It has been reported that vaginal natural progesterone alone sharply decreased forearm blood flow through an increase in local vascular resistance in healthy postmenopausal women[16]. Therefore, the effects of progesterone/progestogens on peripheral arteries are not agreed among different studies, and the reason is not clear. It has been suggested that the effects of progesterone/progestogens on vascular endothelium depend on several factors, including dose, potency and route or pattern of administration[17].

DIRECT VASCULAR EFFECTS OF PROGESTERONE/PROGESTOGEN IN *IN VITRO* ANIMAL STUDIES

Many studies have been performed to observe the direct vascular effects of progesterone/progestogens using animals *in vitro*. Below is a brief summary of our experiment. Eight weeks after bilateral oophorectomy, Sprague-Dawley rats under light ether anesthesia were killed by cervical dislocation and bled. The descending aorta and renal artery were quickly removed and placed in Krebs solution. The aorta, after careful cleaning of adhering connective tissues, was cut into rings of 2–3 mm in length. Each ring was suspended between L-shaped hooks, placed in a 5 ml organ bath containing Krebs solution and bubbled with carbogen (95% O_2 and 5% CO_2). Each vascular ring was connected to an isometric force transducer (FT 03, Grass, USA) and the changes in tension were recorded with an AD converter system (MP100, Biopac Inc, USA) in a personal computer. To test the vasodilatory activity of the hormone, rings were precontracted with norepinephrine (1 μmol/l) or KCl (40 mmol/l). After precontraction, estradiol, progesterone, medroxyprogesterone acetate and norethisterone (10 μmol/l each) were added to each ring and they were incubated for 15 min. The relaxation was expressed as a percentage of the tonic contraction.

In our experiment, not only estrogen but also progesterone, medroxyprogesterone acetate and norethisterone relaxed both the rat aorta and the renal artery. The degree of relaxing effects was the same when estrogen and progesterone/progestogens were compared. Combination of estrogen and progesterone/progestogens did not attenuate the effects of estrogen (Figure 2). Nitro-L-arginine methyl ester (an inhibitor of prostaglandin synthesis), glibenclimide (an inhibitor of ATP-sensitive potassium channels) and methylene blue (an inhibitor of cyclic GMP synthesis) did not affect the relaxation induced by

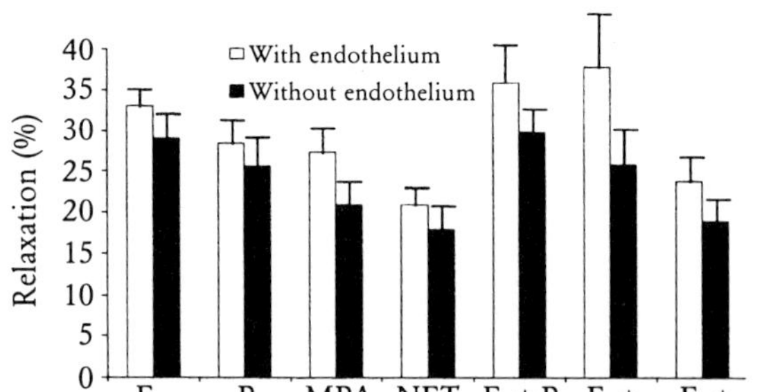

Figure 2 Relaxant effects of steroids (10 μmol/l each) in rat aorta precontracted by norepinephrine. Mean ± SEM; n = 4–6. E_2, 17β-estradiol; P, progesterone; MPA, medroxyprogesterone acetate; NET, norethisterone

progesterone/progestogens. According to our results, shown in Figure 3, it may be suggested that progesterone/progestogens interfere with calcium influx through the voltage-operated and the receptor-operated calcium channels. In agreement with these findings, Glusa and colleagues[18] also suggested that the vasodilatory effects of progesterone/progestogen as well as estrogen seemed to be due to the inhibition of Ca^{2+} uptake.

DIRECT VASCULAR EFFECTS OF PROGESTERONE/PROGESTOGEN ON ARTERIAL SMOOTH MUSCLE CELLS

Estrogen affects a number of vascular smooth muscle cell (VSMC) functions, including contractility and growth[7]. Direct action of estrogen on VSMCs is also an important antiatherogenic effect. Estrogen inhibits VSMC growth and proliferation, and estradiol inhibits neointimal formation (VSMC proliferation and extracellular matrix formation) after balloon injury of the iliac arteries of rabbits[19] and myointimal proliferation after balloon injury of the carotid artery in the rat[20]. Estradiol may also alter VSMC production of matrix elements, attenuate inflammatory responses[21] and regulate VSMC proliferation through an alteration in early response gene expression and the synthesis of proteins involved in the regulation of the VSMC cycle. Inhibition of endothelial cell apoptosis and preservation of endothelial integrity by estrogen represent another

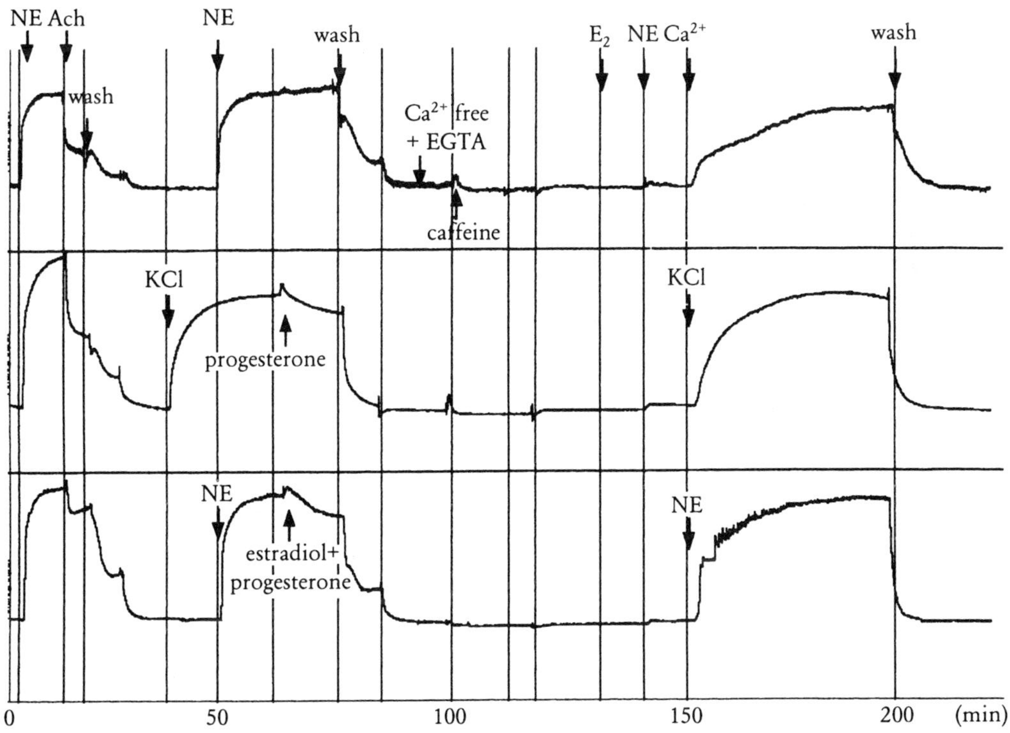

Figure 3 Tension recordings of aortic rings. Contractions were induced by norepinephrine (NE) (1 μmol/l) and relaxed after acetylcholine (Ach) (1 μmol/l) treatment in each channel. In the upper channel, the ring was contracted with norepinephrine followed by washing at the peak of contraction. Calcium-free solution with EGTA (ethylene glycol tetra-acetic acid) was added. Estradiol (E_2) (10 μmol/l) and norepinephrine were added. The tension induced by calcium (2.5 mmol/l) treatment was lower than that from previous norepinephrine treatment. In the middle channel, contraction induced with KCl (40 mmol/l) was relaxed by progesterone (10 μmol/l) treatment. The tension of the final contraction induced by norepinephrine was the same as that of the previous norepinephrine-induced contraction. In the lower channel, the estradiol and progesterone combination treatment induced relaxation. The tension of the final contraction induced by norepinephrine was the same as those of the previous contractions

mechanism that may account for the atheroprotective effects[22].

However, there has been little evidence of the effects of progesterone/progestogens on smooth muscle cells or endothelial cell apoptosis, except for their acute effect on vascular tone. Recently, Lee and co-workers[23] reported that progesterone at physiological levels inhibited DNA synthesis and proliferation in human and rat aorta smooth muscle cells in a dose-dependent manner, and that pretreatment with the progesterone receptor antagonist RU486 blocked inhibition. In another study[24], it has been reported that progesterone as well as estrogen inhibited rat cardiac fibroblast growth.

To evaluate the effects of progesterone/progestogens on endothelial cell apoptosis, we performed a study as described below.

Human umbilical vein endothelial cells (HUVEC) (Clonetics, USA) at a density of 4×10^5 cells per well were cultured for 24 h with tumor necrosis factor (TNF)-α (40 ng/ml) alone or in combination with estradiol, progesterone, medroxyprogesterone acetate or norethisterone (10^{-11} to 10^{-9} mol/l, each). The cell viability was assessed by trypan blue staining and cells were counted in a hemocytometer. Compared to the control group, TNF-α treatment significantly reduced the viable cell counts. Estrogen treatment in all concentrations increased the viable cell counts. All concentrations of progesterone, medroxyprogesterone acetate and norethisterone inhibited the action of TNF-α on induced apoptosis of endothelial cells except for the instance of 10^{-11} mol/l norethisterone. The degrees of inhibition between estradiol and medroxyprogesterone acetate were the same. Those of progesterone and norethisterone, however, were lower than that of estradiol. Norethisterone, if added to estradiol, blocked the effects of estradiol (Table 1).

Table 1 Total count of viable human umbilical vein endothelial cells ($\times 10^4$) after 24 h of exposure to tumor necrosis factor (TNF)-α (40 ng/ml) and TNF-α with estrogen, progesterone, medroxyprogesterone acetate (MPA) and norethisterone (NET) (100 nmol/l each)

	Cell count $\times 10^4$ *(mean* ± *SD)*
Control	20.5 ± 2.8
TNF-α	1.3 ± 0.6
TNF-α + estrogen	$10.5 \pm 1.7^*$
TNF-α + progesterone	$6.5 \pm 1.3^*$
TNF-α + MPA	$4.3 \pm 2.1^*$
TNF-α + NET	$4.0 \pm 1.4^*$
TNF-α + estrogen + MPA	$8.3 \pm 1.7^*$
TNF-α + estrogen + NET	$4.3 \pm 1.6^{*,\dagger}$

$^*p < 0.001$ compared to TNF-α; $^\dagger p < 0.01$ compared to TNF-α + estrogen

CONCLUSION

For postmenopausal HRT, the impact of progesterone/progestogens on cardiovascular disease is important, because most women with an intact uterus are prescribed combination HRT. There is much evidence of the direct vascular effects of progesterone/progestogens. They may relax arteries and inhibit endothelial cell apoptosis, and have not been found to attenuate the action of estrogen in our animal *in vitro* study. The effect of progesterone/progestogens on coronary and cerebral vessels is clinically important but still remains unclear. Further research in this field is necessary.

References

1. Mosca L, Manson JE, Sutherland SE, *et al.* Cardiovascular disease in women: statement for healthcare professionals from American Heart Association. *Circulation* 1997;96:2468–82
2. Gorodeski GI, Utian WH. Epidemiology and risk factors of cardiovascular disease in postmenopausal women. In Lobo RA, ed. *Treatment of the Postmenopausal Woman.* New York: Raven Press, 1994:199–221

3. National Statistical Office, Republic of Korea. *Annual Report on the Cause of Death Statistics*. Seoul, 1998
4. Barrett-Connor E, Bush TL. Estrogen and coronary heart disease in women. *J Am Med Assoc* 1991; 265:1861-7
5. Orimo A, Inoue S, Ikegami A, *et al.* Vascular smooth muscle cells as target for estrogen. *Biochem Biophys Res Commun* 1993;195:730-6
6. Hayashi T, Fukuto JM, Ignarro LJ, *et al.* Basal release of nitric oxide from aorta rings is greater in female rabbits than in male rabbits; implications for atherosclerosis. *Proc Natl Acad Sci USA* 1992;89: 112509-63
7. Oparil S, Levin RL, Chen YF. Sex hormones and the vasculature. In Sowers JR, ed. *Endocrinology of the Vasculature*. Totowa: Humana Press, 1996:225-38
8. Morales DE, McGowan KA, Grant DS, *et al.* Estrogen promotes angiogenesis activity in human umbilical vein endothelial cells *in vitro* and in a murine model. *Circ Res* 1995;91:755-63
9. Grodstein F, Stampfer MJ, Manson JE. Postmenopausal estrogen and progestin use and the risk of cardiovascular disease. *N Engl J Med* 1996;335: 453-6
10. Falkeborn M, Persson I, Terent A, *et al.* Hormone replacement therapy and risk of stroke: follow-up of a population based cohort in Sweden. *Arch Intern Med* 1993;153:1201-9
11. Falkeborn M, Persson I, Adami HO, *et al.* The risk of acute myocardial infarction after oestrogen and oestrogen-progestogen replacement. *Br J Obstet Gynaecol* 1992;99:821-8
12. Psatty BM, Heckbert SR, Atkins D, *et al.* The risk of myocardial infarction associated with the combination use of estrogens and progestins in postmenopausal women. *Arch Intern Med* 1994;154:1333-9
13. Lau TK, Wan D, Yim SF, *et al.* Prospective, randomized, controlled study of the effect of hormone replacement therapy on peripheral blood flow velocity in postmenopausal women. *Fertil Steril* 1998;70:284-8
14. Gerhard M, Walsh BW, Tawakol A, *et al.* Estradiol therapy combined with progesterone and endothelium-dependent vasodilatation in postmenopausal women. *Circulation* 1998;98:1158-63
15. Sorensen KE, Dorup I, Hermann AP, *et al.* Combined hormone replacement therapy does not protect women against the age-related decline in endothelium-dependent vasomotor function. *Circulation* 1998;97:1234-8
16. Mercuro G, Pitzalis L, Podda A, *et al.* Effects of acute administration of natural progesterone on peripheral vascular responsiveness in healthy postmenopausal women. *Am J Cardiol* 1999;84:214-18
17. Williams JK, Adams MR. Estrogen, progestins and coronary artery reactivity. *Nature Med* 1997;3:273-4
18. Glusa E, Graser T, Wagner S, *et al.* Mechanisms of relaxation of rat aorta in response to progesterone and synthetic progestins. *Maturitas* 1997;28:181-91
19. Foegh M, Asotra S, Howell M, *et al.* Estradiol inhibition of arterial neointimal hyperplasia after balloon injury. *J Vasc Surg* 1994;19:722-6
20. Chen SJ, Li H, Durand J, *et al.* βE2 reduces myointimal proliferation after balloon injury of rat carotid artery. *Circulation* 1996;93:577-84
21. Sullivan TR Jr, Karas RH, Aronovitz M, *et al.* Estrogen inhibits the response-to-injury in a mouse carotid artery model. *J Clin Invest* 1995;96:2482-8
22. Spyridopulos I, Sullivan AB, Kearney M, *et al.* Estrogen-receptor-mediated inhibition of human endothelial cell apoptosis; estradiol as a survival factor. *Circulation* 1997;95:1505-14
23. Lee WS, Harder JA, Yoshizumi M, *et al.* Progesterone inhibits arterial smooth muscle cell proliferation. *Nature Med* 1997;3:1005-8
24. Dubey RK, Gillespie DG, Jackson EK, *et al.* 17-β-estradiol, its metabolites, and progesterone inhibit cardiac fibroblast growth. *Hypertension* 1998;31: 522-8

Progestogens, progesterone: their clinical application and problems

48

B. G. Wren

INTRODUCTION

Progesterone has long been regarded as the hormone of pregnancy. It is produced in large amounts in the second half of the menstrual cycle following ovulation. If the ovum is fertilized and implants in a secretory endometrium then the production of progesterone is maintained, initially from the corpus luteum and then from the placenta. During the luteal phase, the main function of progesterone is to convert the proliferating endometrium into secretory phase activity with inhibition of endometrial mitosis, production of nutrients in endometrial glands and decidualization of the stroma. Later, throughout pregnancy, the presence of progesterone maintains the integrity of the decidualized endometrium and also inhibits contraction of the smooth muscle of the uterus.

While these pregnancy-related effects of progesterone are accepted as its main physiological function, progesterone is also known to have many other actions in the human female. Progesterone is responsible for growth and maturation of alveolar cells in the breast as well as influencing other cellular responses including gut motility, brain cell response, electrolyte balance and carbohydrate metabolism.

It is the variation in production and in the circulating level of progesterone occurring in the female body which leads to considerable fluctuations in both physical and emotional responses in women. Progesterone not only inhibits uterine contractions, but also slows all other smooth muscle activity, causing bloating, constipation, and gall bladder and urinary bladder symptoms. Progesterone also induces presecretory changes in the breast including an increase in accumulation of secretions in alveolar cells, thus causing mastalgia. Secretions in the vagina and cervix are also changed, with a thickened plug in the os and less vaginal lubricant. Most of all, progesterone appears to have a depressant effect on certain neurotransmitters in the brain. Women may be calm and placid under the influence of progesterone, but some experience depression, and somnolence. Among the many metabolic actions of progesterone are its salt- and water-losing properties, and its effect on carbohydrate metabolism.

For the above reasons, some women complain of distressing symptoms related to the production of progesterone. This group of women have a heightened sensitivity to their own natural progesterone, and the symptoms induced form part of the complex syndrome now called premenstrual tension (PMT).

While progesterone has an important role to play in reproduction, it also has a significant impact in maintaining normal growth, maturation and shedding of the endometrium and, to an extent, the normal physiological processes in the breast.

Without adequate progesterone, estrogen induces proliferation, hyperplasia, atypical hyperplasia or even cancer of the endometrium[1-3]. These adverse endometrial changes can be inhibited or reversed by the availability of 10 or more days of progesterone[4]. For this reason, the use of progesterone is advocated for women receiving estrogen for postmenopausal hormone deficiency.

PROGESTERONE

Progesterone is carried in the blood by transcortin (corticosteroid-binding globulin) and attaches to progesterone receptors within target cells. There are two progesterone receptors in humans (A and

B) with different molecular weights and inducing different intracellular responses[5]. Human breast tissue contains both progesterone receptors, but the ratio of A to B varies within different cells. Progesterone receptor A has been shown to diminish the response of other hormone receptors including progesterone receptor B, androgen receptor, glucocorticoid receptor, mineralocorticoid receptor and estrogen receptor. These variations in the activity, the amount and the ratio of the progesterone receptors play a significant role in the response of cells to progesterone.

Progesterone receptors have been found in the uterus, endometrium, ovary, testes, vagina, cervix, breast, brain, vascular endothelium and human osteoblast cells. However, estrogen is necessary to stimulate cells to produce progesterone receptors, whereas progesterone down-regulates its own receptor production.

Within the endometrium, progesterone has been shown to suppress the production of a variety of growth factors while at the same time enhancing transforming growth factor-β production. One important extracellular signal in the endometrium is thrombospondin-l, which inhibits angiogenesis and is increased by progesterone[6]. By this complex process, progesterone is capable of inhibiting abnormal growth of estrogen-stimulated endometrium and maintaining control over the function of the uterine tissue.

Unfortunately natural oral progesterone is very unstable, being rapidly broken down by enzymes in the gut and liver. Because of this rapid degradation of natural progesterone, large amounts must be administered to ensure reasonable circulating blood levels, or the progesterone must be administered by a process that bypasses the gut and liver. To achieve this, a variety of techniques have been used including micronizing the progesterone, delivering the small particles through the skin, the vagina or the buccal mucous membrane. Although a variety of claims for all forms of delivery have been made, there is still no clear evidence that the transdermal or buccal system is capable of inhibiting mitosis and growth of endometrial cells or inducing appropriate biological responses.

PROGESTOGENS

Because of the difficulty in achieving appropriate responses with natural progesterone, a variety of steroid compounds have been developed to simulate the action of endogenous progesterone. These steroids all have the capacity to convert proliferative endometrium into a secretory pattern and they are known as the progestogens. Basically they are of two main types, known as pregnanes and androstanes.

Pregnanes have acetylation of the steroid molecule at the carbon-17 site and include megestrol acetate (Megace®), medroxyprogesterone acetate (Provera®), chlormadinone acetate, dydrogesterone (Duphaston®) and cyproterone acetate (Androcur®).

Androstanes were developed by removing the 19-carbon atom from ethisterone, thus creating the compound 19-norethisterone. This molecule was found to be more stable and more potent than the pregnane compounds. Since its development, a number of other androstane compounds have been developed including levonorgestrel, desogestrel, gestodene and norgestimate. Androstanes are between ten and 100 times more potent with regard to the endometrium than pregnanes (Table 1)[7].

The progestogens are degraded at a much slower rate than natural progesterone, and therefore are more amenable for use as an oral compound. Some may be absorbed through the skin or the vaginal epithelium or have a direct effect on the endometrium when used in an intrauterine device.

Because of variations in molecular structure, affinity for the progesterone receptor, possible binding to other steroid receptors, doses required

Table 1 Potency of progestogens: endometrial response. Data from reference 7

Hormone	*Dose* (mg)	*Secretory response* (%)
Medroxyprogesterone	10	72
Norethisterone	1	61
Levonorgestrel	0.15	75
Micronized progesterone	300	75

and other non-genomic effects, different progestogens may produce entirely different responses and side-effects in different women. Over 80% of women have no problems with progestogens, but some find it difficult to use any without inducing an adverse reaction.

To overcome possible side-effects, a variety of delivery techniques and dosage regimens have been employed to achieve protection of the endometrium without inducing a problem with compliance.

SIDE-EFFECTS AND POSSIBLE SOLUTIONS

Bloating

Because all progestogens may affect smooth muscle motility, thus slowing the gut and allowing organisms to produce more gas, it is advisable to either reduce the dose of the oral progestogen tablet or attempt to bypass the gut and the liver. The androstane group of progestins are much more potent than pregnanes, so if bloating is a problem, the use of very small doses of an androstane may achieve endometrial protection without causing bloating and discomfort. Levonorgestrel is about 100 times more potent than medroxyprogesterone acetate, so very small amounts can be used to achieve inhibition of endometrial proliferation without producing an adverse response from the gastrointestinal system.

Another technique to avoid bloating is to use a transdermal or intrauterine progestogen in an attempt to avoid a direct action on the gut. Transdermal norethisterone has been used in commercial preparations, and the results appear to be successful in that the endometrium is protected and gastrointestinal symptoms are reduced. The use of levonorgestrel intrauterine devices, releasing a progestogen locally over a period of 5 years, also appears to be successful.

Transdermal natural progesterone in a micronized form has been used, but the results from sequential transdermal estrogen and transdermal progesterone show that this regimen of therapy is not sufficient to protect the endometrium from proliferative change. In a study conducted at the Sydney Menopause Centre, 27 women were recruited to receive a continuous transdermal estrogen patch (Climara 100®; Schering) for 12 weeks. Subjects were randomly allocated to receive transdermal progesterone cream delivering 16 mg ($n = 9$), 32 mg ($n = 8$) or 64 mg ($n = 10$) of micronized progesterone (Pro-Femme®; Lawley Pharmaceuticals) applied for 14 days each month in three cycles of therapy. Endometrial biopsy was carried out prior to treatment, on day 14 of the first cycle of transdermal estrogen and on day 27 or 28 of the third cycle of micronized transdermal progesterone. Blood was also obtained for hormonal assay. The study demonstrated that transdermal micronized progesterone administered for 14 days over three cycles, even in doses as high as 64 mg daily, failed to increase circulatory blood progesterone levels sufficiently to induce any evidence of a secretory effect on the endometrium (Table 2).

One study from Europe used a progesterone vaginal gel to bypass the gut and the skin. Ross and colleagues[8] found that a 45–90 mg gel, administered per vaginum sequentially to women every second day over 12 days, was sufficient to induce a secretory change in the endometrium in 84% of women. They hypothesized that this effect occurred because vaginal progesterone achieved a first-pass through the uterus rather than being dissipated by general diffusion through the body.

Lee (personal communication) has hypothesized that transdermal progesterone is sufficient to inhibit endometrial proliferation when given in a

Table 2 Results from trial of transdermal estrogen and transdermal micronized progesterone

	Pretreatment	*Cycle 1* (day 14)*	*Cycle 3* (day 27–28)*
Endometrial biopsy			
Proliferative (n)	6	20	19
Secretory (n)	0	0	0
No endometrium obtained (n)	21	2	2
Total (n)	27	22	21
Blood hormone levels			
Estradiol (pmol/l)	80–110	116–603	114–1394
Progesterone (nmol/l)	0.1–1.1	0.1–1.4	0.6–3.2

*On three occasions cervix was found to be stenosed and four women did not complete study

continuous regimen, and he has cited the presence of salivary levels of progesterone in an attempt to explain and support his hypothesis. Unfortunately there is no scientific evidence that salivary progesterone shows any relationship to the biological response of the endometrium. Studies conducted in clinical departments, including our own, fail to support the extravagant claims made by Lee[9].

Breakthrough bleeding

One of the most common side-effects of hormone replacement therapy (HRT) usage is breakthrough and/or withdrawal bleeding, and these are two of the reasons why women often fail to continue to use hormonal therapy. When using sequential HRT, there may be an increase in endometrial proliferation owing to unopposed estrogen activity for 10–20 days in each cycle. This problem is best treated by using a higher dosage of progestogen for a longer period of time. However, continuous combined HRT is becoming more popular as a regimen of therapy. Breakthrough bleeding in these cases is generally found to be associated with an atrophic endometrium. Continuous combined estrogen/progestogen therapy may result in fluctuation of endometrial growth factors, including vascular endothelial growth factor, adrenomedullin or thymidine phosphorylase[6].

Inhibition of endometrial activity occurs in the majority of women using continuous progestogen, but about 10–20% do experience breakthrough bleeding as a result of vascular breakdown. The use of progestogen may lead to continued, recurrent, slight 'spotting', with occasional heavy blood loss. These women are best treated by stopping the progestogen for a period of time, by introducing a higher dosage of estrogen or by changing continuous combined HRT to a sequential regimen.

Breast cancer

One of the great fears of postmenopausal women is that, by using HRT, they will increase their risk of developing breast cancer. However, all biological, epidemiological and clinical evidencesuggests that hormones are not mutagenic for breast cancer. Unopposed estrogens may, however, influence the rate of mitosis of breast cells and thus increase the growth of a pre-existing cancer, or increase the incidence of spontaneous oncogenic mutations[10].

Estrogen appears to increase the rate of cell division of both ductal and alveolar cells, while progestogens have a biphasic action. Short-term or intermittent use of progestogens increases mitosis, whereas continuous progestogen use reduces breast cell division while directing cells to maturation and specialized function. In this manner, continuous combined estrogen and progestogen therapy should reduce the risk of oncogenic mutations in much the same way that pregnancy following breast cancer reduces the risk of new or recurrent cancer[11]. While there are as yet no large prospective studies to confirm this hypothesis, several reports suggest that continuous progestogen therapy is associated with a reduced risk of breast cancer[12–14].

Other reported complications and side-effects of progestogen use include weight gain, depression, headaches and cardiovascular changes. These are being addressed by other contributors so are not mentioned here.

CONCLUSION

Progesterone and progestogens are essential hormones in managing postmenopausal women receiving estrogen replacement therapy to protect the endometrium (and the breast), but care must be exercised to avoid inducing abnormal side-effects. While natural micronized progesterone has been beneficial when administered orally, there is much doubt regarding its effect when given by the transdermal route. Progestogens are very effective but, because of variations in origin, dosage, absorption, degradation and side-effects, they produce vastly differing biological responses at equivalent dosages. Changing the type of progestogen, the dosage and the regimen of postmenopausal therapy may relieve women of unwanted side-effects.

References

1. Smith DC, Prentice R, Thompson DJ, Herman WL. Association of exogenous estrogen and endometrial cancer. *N Engl J Med* 1975;293:1164–8
2. Mack TM, Dike MC, Henderson BE, *et al.* Estrogens and endometrial cancer in a retirement community. *N Engl J Med* 1976;294:1262–7
3. Antunes CMF, Stolley PD, Rosenstein MB, *et al.* Endometrial cancer and estrogen use. *N Engl J Med* 1979;300:9–13
4. Beresford SAA, Weiss NS, Voigt LF, McKnight B. Risk of endometrial cancer in relation to use of oestrogen combined with cyclic progestagen therapy in postmenopausal women. *Lancet* 1997; 349:458–61
5. Groshong SD, Owen GL, Grimison B, *et al.* Biphasic regulation of breast cancer cell growth by progesterone. Role of the cyclin dependent kinase inhibitors, p21, p27. *Mol Endocrinol* 1997;11: 1593–607
6. Rees M, Hague S, Oehler MK, Bicknell R. Regulation of endometrial angiogenesis. *Climacteric* 1999; 2:52–8
7. Hirvonen E. Progestins. *Maturitas.* 1996;23(Suppl): S13–18
8. Ross D, Cooper AJ, Pryse-Davies J, Bergeron C, Collins WP, Whitehead MI. Randomized, double-blind, dose ranging study of the endometrial effects of a vaginal progesterone gel in estrogen treated postmenopausal women. *Am J Obstet Gynecol* 1997; 177:937–41
9. Lee JR. Osteoporosis reversal with transdermal progesterone. *Lancet* 1990;336:1327
10. Wren BG. Hormonal replacement therapy and breast cancer. *Eur Menopause J* 1995;2:13–19
11. Royal College of Obstetricians and Gynaecologists. *Pregnancy after breast cancer*, Guideline 12. London: RCOG, July 1997
12. Plu-Bureau G, Sitruk-Ware R, Thalabard JC, Mauvais-Jarvis P. Progestogen use and the decreased risk of breast cancer in a cohort of premenopausal women with benign breast disease. *Br J Cancer* 1994;70:270–7
13. Dew J, Eden J, Beller E, *et al.* A cohort study of hormone replacement therapy given to women previously treated for breast cancer. *Climacteric* 1998; 1:137–42
14. Eden JA, Bush T, Nand S, Wren BG. A case-controlled study of combined continuous oestrogen–progestin replacement therapy among women with a personal history of breast cancer. *J North Am Menopause Soc* 1995;2:67–72

Potential roles of estrogen receptor-α and -β in the regulation of human osteoblast functions and gene expression 49

K. M. Waters, D. J. Rickard, J. B. Gebhart, M. Subramaniam, S. Khosla, B. L. Riggs, J. Moore and T. C. Spelsberg

INTRODUCTION

In prior decades, estrogen was believed to be primarily a reproductive hormone, with effects limited to the uterus and mammary glands. Evidence now suggests that estrogens exert effects in tissues such as bone, brain, eyes, teeth, vasomotor system, heart, colon and the urogenital tract[1]. The realization that estrogen affected so many functionally distinct tissues stimulated a re-examination of the models involving a single estrogen receptor species. Estrogen is also the most important sex steroid for the maintenance of skeletal homeostasis, as reflected in the widespread and beneficial use of estrogen replacement therapy to combat postmenopausal osteoporosis in women[2]. Clinical studies have highlighted the importance of estrogen deficiency for causing not only the rapid and transient bone loss that accompanies menopause in women, but also in contributing to the slower, sustained age-related bone loss in elderly women and men[2].

Discovery of the estrogen receptor-β species

As outlined in Figure 1, estrogen functions by binding to and activating nuclear receptors, which then act as transcription factors, interacting with other transcription activators and repressors to induce or repress target gene expression[3,4]. The discovery of a second estrogen receptor (ER-β), with tissue distribution, ligand binding and transcriptional regulatory properties distinct from the classical ER-α has widened the potential actions of estrogen and has provided new explanations for the tissue/cell type-specific effects of partial estrogen agonists, i.e. the selective ER modulators (SERMs)[5]. As outlined in Figure 2, ER-α and ER-β share a highly conserved central DNA binding domain, a moderately conserved, C-terminal, ligand binding domain, with a divergent N-terminal A/B domain that contains a transactivation activity (AF-1) responsible for interacting with proteins of the core transcriptional machinery[5]. The two isoforms bind the same consensus estrogen response elements (ERE) in DNA, as either homodimers or as α/β heterodimers, and both can regulate transcription using this element (shown in Figure 1).

Estrogen and the partial estrogen agonist, tamoxifen, differentially regulate the gene transcription, depending on the ER isoform (α or β) expressed, using two types of inducible promoters (containing an ERE or an AP-1 site)[6]. Since ER-α and ER-β adopt distinct conformations upon binding the various ER modulators (SERMs), it is hypothesized that this will determine the repertoire of protein cofactors interacting with each ligand-activated, DNA-bound receptor and thus participating in the transcription initiation complex[7]. The tissue and cell type-specific effects of SERMs on a given promoter may therefore be explained by the ratio of ER-α to ER-β and by the particular cofactors present. This mechanism may in reality be even more complex due to the identification of functional variants of ER-α and ER-β[8].

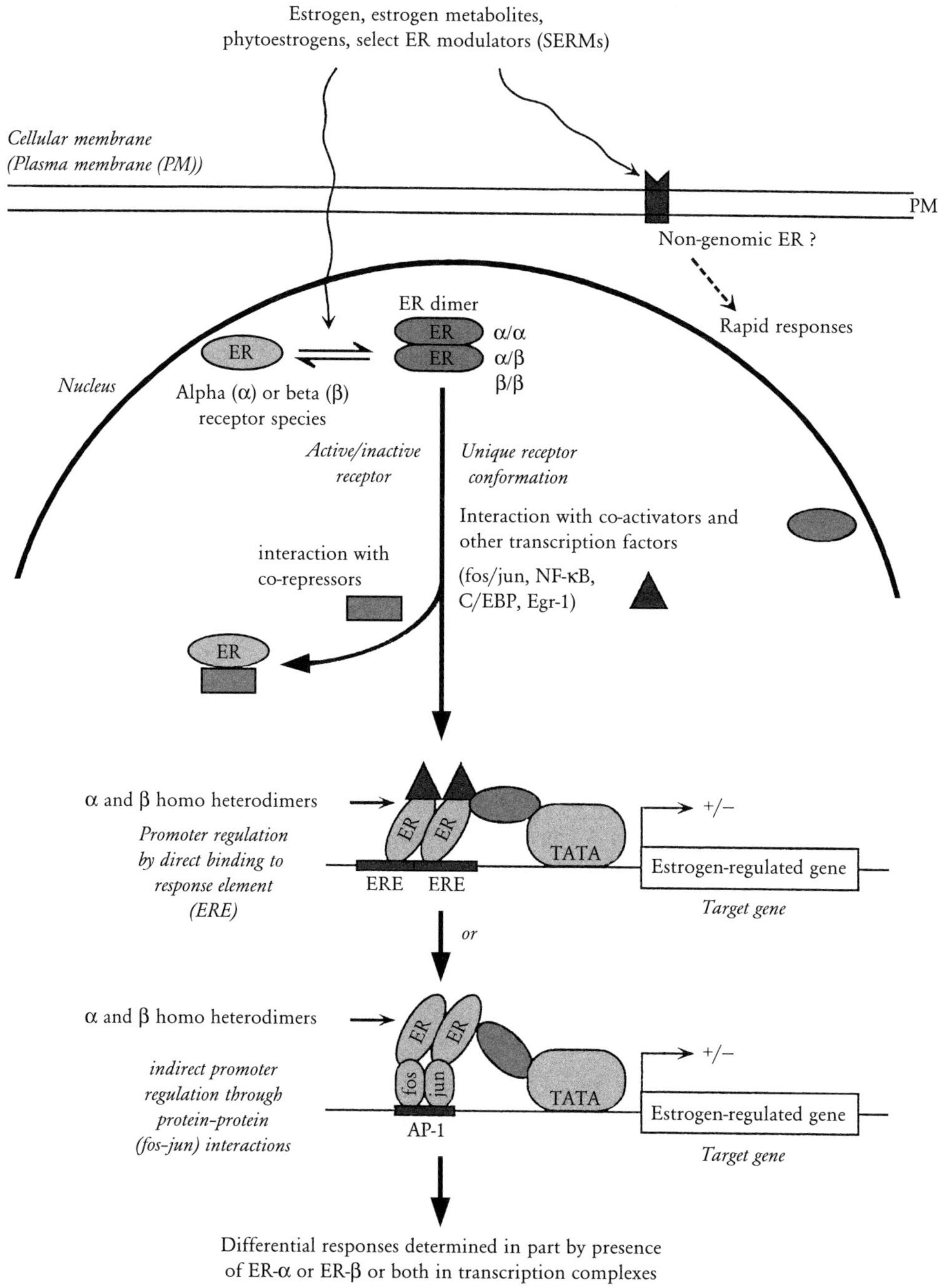

Figure 1 Model of the sequential steps of estrogen action. Ligand binds to ER-α and ER-β isoforms, inducing receptor dimerization and conformational changes, allowing for protein–protein interactions with co-regulators (co-activators and co-repressors) and other families of transcription factors (such as fos/jun, C/EBP, NF-κB). These multiprotein complexes stabilize binding to DNA response elements located within the promoter regions of target genes, either enhancing or inhibiting transcription initiation through the formation of productive or non-productive interactions with the basal transcription machinery. Consequently, estrogen can exert a wide spectrum of effects on promoter activity, depending on a combination of variables, including the ER isoforms present, the nature of the ligand, the balance between co-activators and co-repressors and, finally, the type of DNA response element. Estrogen also induces rapid and transient non-genomic responses in certain types of cell by binding to a putative plasma membrane receptor. Revised from reference 4

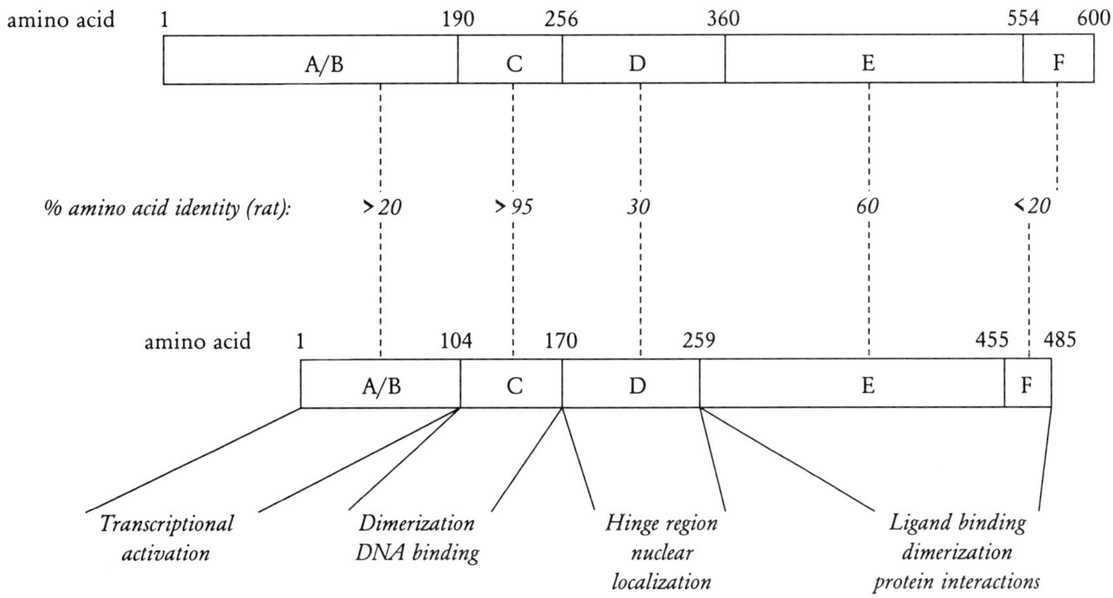

	ER-α	*ER-β*
17β-Estradiol K_d (nM)	0.13	0.4
Protein molecular weight (kDa)	64	55
mRNA (kb)	~ 6.4	10, 8, 1.3
mRNA tissue distribution	uterus, testis, ovary, kidney, epididymis, adrenal, pituitary	uterus, ovary, prostate, lung, testis, bladder, brain, thymus, hypothalamus

Figure 2 Comparisons of the structures of ER-α and ER-β. This information was taken from a variety of sources (references 3–9, 22 and 23)

Expression of ER isoforms in reproductive tissues

Estrogens, acting via ER-α and ER-β, must play important roles in regulating the growth, differentiation and functions of many reproductive tissues, including the uterus, vagina, ovary, oviduct and mammary gland. Estrogen influence on the uterus is manifest through the interaction of the receptor isoforms in the endometrium. The beneficial effects of estrogen replacement therapy in menopausal and postmenopausal women, and thus increased use of estrogens, revealed the potential for carcinomatous change of the endometrium.

Estrogen deprivation during the menopause results in atrophic changes in the vaginal mucosa, characterized by a thinning of the epithelium, a loss of vaginal rugae and a reduction in vaginal lubrication. Loss of vaginal elasticity occurs and the pH rises. Estrogen replacement reduces the vaginal pH, increases the quantity of vaginal fluid and increases vaginal blood flow. The presence of specific estrogen receptors in human vaginal tissue in pre- and postmenopausal women has been described[10]. Histological studies have shown that 17β-estradiol promotes vaginal epithelial proliferation and differentiation[11]. Estrogen receptors are normally present in both vaginal epithelial and stromal cells[12]. These estradiol-induced events require the ER-α isoform, as shown by the lack of vaginal epithelial proliferation, stratification and cornification in estradiol-treated ER-α knockout mice[13]. Both epithelial and stromal ER-α were required for estradiol-induced cornification and normal epithelial stratification[14]. Recent studies have shown the presence of ER-α and ER-β mRNA in human vaginal tissue[15]; ER-α and ER-β have also been localized immunohistochemically to the vagina[16]. Our laboratory has identified ER-α and -β in human vaginal tissues via Northern blot analyses (J. B. Gebhart and colleagues, in preparation).

Expression of the ER isoforms in skeletal cells *in vivo* and *in vitro*

The earliest discovery of estrogen receptors in the skeleton involved human osteoblasts *in vitro*[17,18]. In bone, ER-α transcripts were localized by *in situ* polymerase chain reaction predominantly to trabecular osteoblasts and lining cells with lower levels in osteocytes, osteoclasts and bone marrow[19]. In primary cultures, the expression levels represent the average for all the cells present and it is possible that only a subset of cells actually express estrogen receptors, but at a higher level. Confirmation that ER-α is expressed and functional in at least some osteoblasts has been demonstrated by the isolation of ER-α-positive and estrogen-responsive cell lines from primary cultures, as well as immortalized human bone-derived cultures[17,20]. The cellular distribution of ER-β in bone is unknown at present, but higher ER-β mRNA levels have been reported in trabecular compared to cortical bone. More recent *in vitro* studies of differentiating osteoblasts showed a progressive increase in the expression of both ER isoforms during differentiation[21,22]. In a comparison of the relative mRNA levels for the two ER isoforms in rat skeleton, ER-α was the predominant form expressed in both osteoblast precursors (bone marrow stromal cells) and trabecular bone[23]. Ovariectomy resulted in decreases in the mRNA levels of both ER-α and ER-β in the skeleton. Taken together, these findings suggest that the concentrations of ER-α are higher than ER-β in bone and in osteoblasts at most stages of differentiation, at least in animal skeletal tissue. Interestingly, recent studies suggest that, in the human skeletal tissues, ER-β levels predominate over ER-α levels.

Effects of estrogen on skeletal growth and bone remodelling

The rapid and transient postmenopausal bone loss (type I osteoporosis) and the slower, age-related bone loss occurring in the elderly (type II osteoporosis) may both be caused by reduced estrogen[2]. Early postmenopausal bone loss affects mostly trabecular bone and is the result of increased bone remodelling, where the rate of bone resorption outpaces the rate of bone formation. Figure 3 identifies the locales of estrogen actions in bone, with reported direct actions on the bone forming osteoblasts and bone-resorbing osteoclasts. The osteoblasts appear to be the major target cell, releasing important growth factors and cytokines which extend the actions of estrogen well beyond the mature osteoblast cells to many other cell types in bone.

In the ovariectomized rodent model of osteopenia, most studies have shown reduced bone turnover (i.e. a reduction in both formation and resorption) after estrogen treatment, but some evidence suggests that resorption is inhibited to a greater extent than formation at both pharmacological and physiological estrogen concentrations[24]. By analyzing markers of bone formation within hours of estrogen treatment of ovariectomized rats, possible inhibitory effects on osteoblast metabolism have been measured that cannot be explained as occurring secondarily to decreased bone resorption[25]. The results of estrogen withdrawal and replenishment on bone at the cellular level are outlined in Figure 4.

In vitro effects of estrogen on osteoblasts

Despite exhaustive attempts, it has proved difficult to demonstrate consistent effects of estrogen on

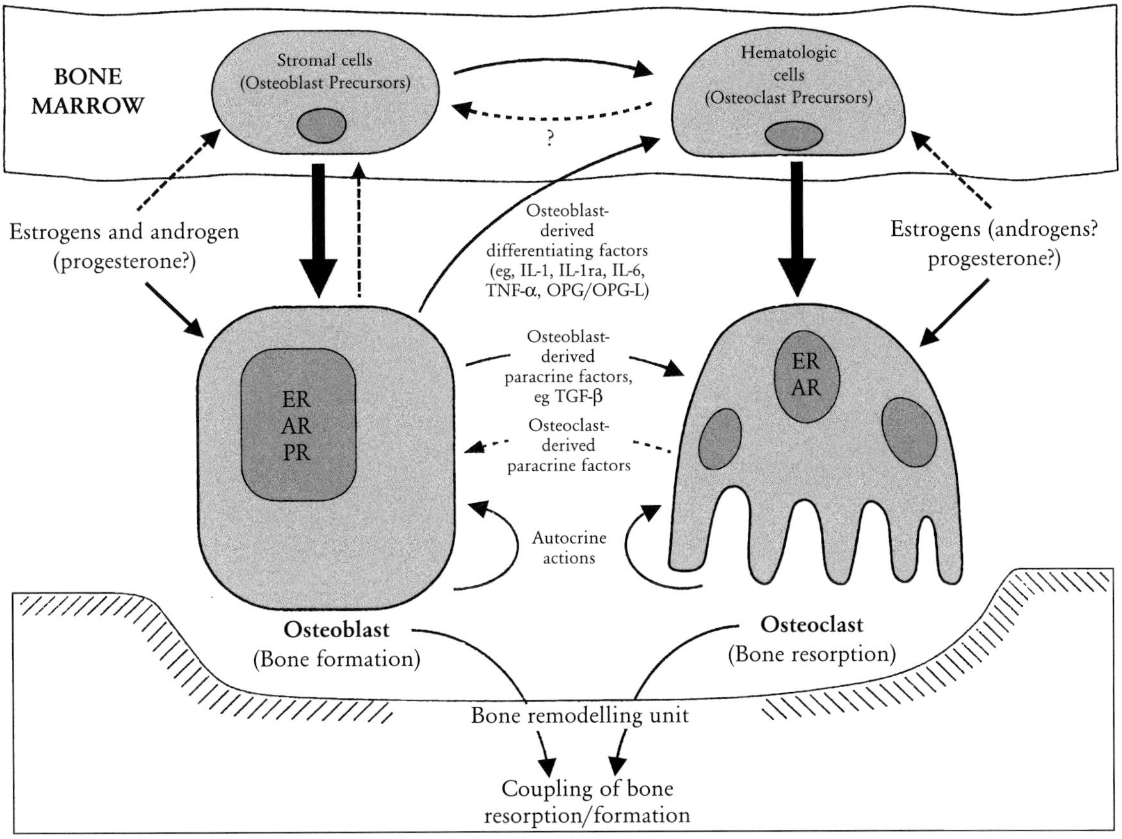

Figure 3 Schematic of the steroid actions and interactions with growth factors/cytokines in bone cells at bone resorption and formation site. This model is self-explanatory. The solid arrows represent pathways with significant support in the literature. The broken lines represent potential pathways not currently well identified or characterized. From reference 37, with permission. IL, interleukin; TNF, tumor necrosis factor; OPG, osteoprotegerin; OPG-L, osteoprotegerin ligand; TGF, transforming growth factor; ER, estrogen receptor; AR, androgen receptor; PR, progesterone receptor

primary, immortalized or transformed osteoblastic cells, particularly those of human origin (Table 1). This, in part, can be explained by the variable levels of estrogen receptors in osteoblasts (that may further diminish on culture), as well as to differences in cell source, methods of isolation, and culture. Since the expression level of endogenous ER in osteoblasts is limiting for estrogen responses[3,4,17,26], osteoblast lines, expressing artificially high levels of the receptor, have been generated by stable transfection of the ER-α gene. In these cell lines, the estrogen response is quantitatively and qualitatively dependent on the ER level, with a wider spectrum of responses produced by cells expressing the higher levels. Such cells have been valuable in identifying potential new estrogen regulated genes and the molecular mechanisms underlying the regulation.

Overexpression of the introduced ER gene may cause some spurious effects, believed to be due to the sequestering of common transcription factors by the exogenous receptor proteins. However, our laboratories and others have shown that immortalized human fetal osteoblast cell lines, stably transfected with ER-α expression vectors, elicit many of the responses to estrogen reported for osteoblasts with endogenous estrogen receptors[20,27,28]. As outlined in Figures 3 and 4, the best-understood mechanism of estrogen action on bone is the regulation of bone-resorptive cytokine synthesis by

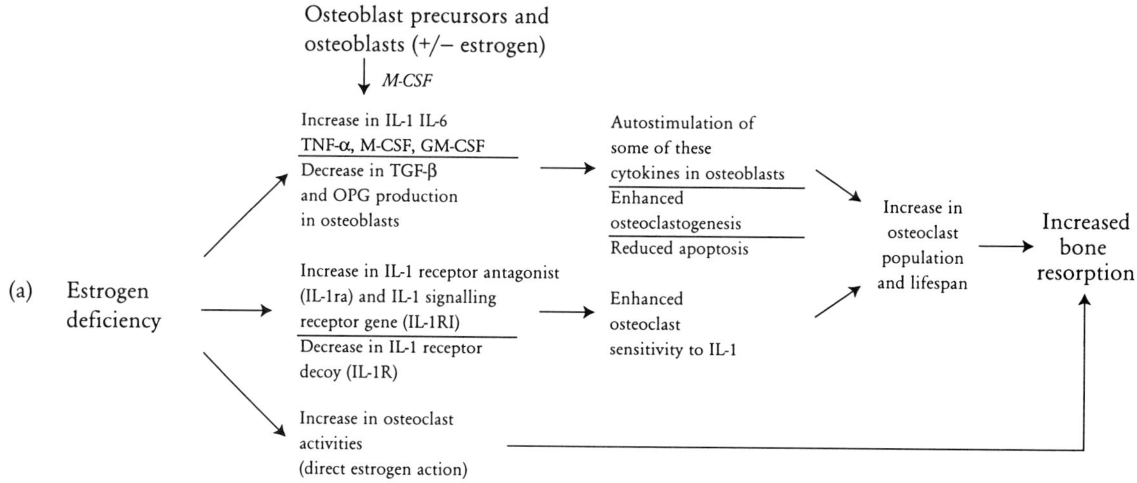

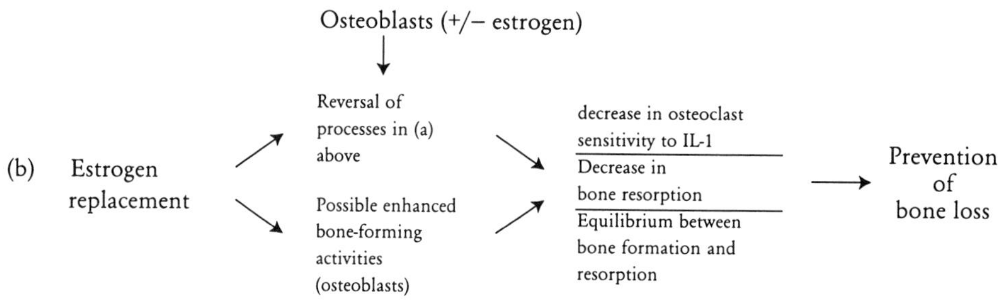

Figure 4 Potential pathways in the estrogen regulation of bone resorption. Interleukin (IL)-1, IL-6 and tissue necrosis factor (TNF)-α inhibit apoptosis and extend the lifespan of osteoclasts. In contrast, transforming growth factor (TGF)-β increases osteoclast apoptosis. From reference 37, with permission. M-CSF, macrophage colony-stimulating factor; GM-CSF, granulocyte-macrophage colony-stimulating factor; OPG, osteoprotegerin

cells of the osteogenic and monocyte/macrophage lineages. Estrogen has been reported to inhibit synthesis of interleukin (IL)-1, IL-6, IL-11, tumor necrosis factor, macrophage colony-stimulating factor and granulocyte-macrophage colony-stimulating factor, but increase the novel osteoprotegerin protein and transforming growth factor-β production in osteoblasts and their precursor cells. However, the debate continues as to which is the dominant cytokine(s) regulated by estrogen that is responsible for the increased bone resorption in estrogen-deficient conditions (for a review see references 3 and 4). As depicted in Figures 3 and 4, osteoprotegerin is produced by osteoblasts and is a major inhibitor of osteoclastogenesis. If the estrogen stimulation of osteoprotegerin synthesis observed in ER-transfected osteoblasts[29] is also found to occur *in vivo*, then inhibition of bone resorption by estrogen may in large part be mediated by a downregulation and mineralization of the two cytokines known to be essential for osteoclast formation, i.e. macrophage colony-stimulating factor and the osteoprotegerin ligand, respectively.

METHODS

The methods used in these studies have been previously described, including the development of the immortalized human cell lines (fetal osteoblast and fetal osteoblast/ER-α lines)[27,30,31], the analyses of bone matrix gene expression[28,30] and the more recent development of the fetal osteoblast/ER-β lines containing the new ER-β receptor species[32,33].

Table 1 Reported actions of estrogen on gene expression in osteoblast cells in culture. From reference 37, with permission

Gene	*Response*
Growth factors/cytokines	
IGF-I	↑
IGF-II	↔
IGF-BP-4	↑
TGF-β1	↑
BMP-6	↑
IL-1α, 1β	↓↓↔
IL-6	↓↓↔
TNF-α	↓
Osteoprotegerin	↑
Transcription factors	
c-fos	↑
TIEG	↑
NF-κβ	↑
c/EBP-β	↑
Bone matrix proteins	
Type I collagen	↑↑
Osteocalcin	↓↓
Alkaline phosphatase	↑↑
Receptors	
Progesterone	↑
1,25 vitamin D_3	↑
Parathyroid hormone	↓
Other	
Transferrin	↑
Protein kinase C	↓
Estrogen response element-CAT	↑
Various enzymes	↑
DNA replication	↑↓↔

↑↑↔ means there are conflicting data, but the evidence is stronger for induction; ↓↓↔ represents the same, but the evidence is stronger for a reduction. IGF, insulin-like growth factor; BP, binding protein; TGF, transforming growth factor; BMP, bone morphogenetic protein; IL, interleukin; TNF, tissue necrosis factor

RESULTS

Differential actions of ER-α and ER-β on human osteoblast cells

Our laboratories have developed immortalized cell lines of human fetal osteoblasts and have developed stably transfected ER-α- and ER-β-expressing cell lines from these parental lines[30-33]. The ER-α represents a human wild-type receptor and was stably transfected using the pHEGO-HYG vector, containing the hygromycin resistance gene. The ER-β represents a truncated version of the full-length ER-β, and was amplified by reverse-transcriptase polymerase chain reaction from ovary mRNA and cloned into a mammalian expression vector pZeo SV2. The latter contains a zeomycin resistance gene. All lines were cloned and the ER inserts verified using sequencing.

The lines produce a functional bone matrix with mineralized nodules in culture, synthesize all of the matrix proteins, growth factors/cytokines, and respond to hormones/growth factors/cytokines as reported for primary cultures of normal human and rodent osteoblasts[27-31,34-36]. Table 2 outlines the actions of estrogen on the fetal osteoblast/ER-α cells, as reported earlier, with references included. Recently, our laboratories have compared these results with fetal osteoblast/ER-β cells containing a comparable number of ER-β molecules per cell to the cells containing ER-α. As shown in Figure 5, panel C, in the fetal osteoblast/ER-α cell lines, estradiol inhibited bone matrix production (nodule appearance at 18 days post-confluence) compared to the fetal osteoblast cells or to untreated or ICI 182 780 (anti-estrogen)-treated fetal osteoblast/ER-α cells (nodule appearance at 8/10 days postconfluence). In the fetal osteoblast/ER-β cell lines, estradiol had little effect and often displayed enhanced matrix production and mineralization, i.e. increased the rate of nodule formation.

To determine the mechanism of this difference, we examined the regulation of extracellular matrix proteins by estradiol and tamoxifen in the human fetal osteoblast/ER-α and human fetal osteoblast/ER-β cells. Interestingly, differences in estrogen responses in the ER-α or ER-β cells in other parameters were observed. There were some added differences in response to estrogen by the ER-α and ER-β during the different cell states (matrix production versus mineralization). As outlined in Table 3, the ER-α cells displayed different responses than the ER-β cells with regard to the regulation of osteoblast gene expression. During matrix production, type I collagen production is directly proportional to nodule formation and moderately induced by steroid treatment in human fetal osteoblast/ER-α cells and with no effects in human fetal osteoblast/ER-β cells. Alkaline phosphatase is induced in estradiol-treated

Table 2 Summary of the actions of estrogens on the expression of bone matrix and growth factor genes in the fetal osteoblast/ER-α cell lines

Gene marker	*Changes in gene expression by estrogen*	*Changes in gene expression by tamoxifen*	*Reference*
PR	↑		27, 28
c-fos	↑		27
Alkaline phosphatase	↑	↔	28
OCLn	↓	↔	28
Cell proliferation	↓	↔	28
Type I collagen	↔	↑	28
Osteonectin	↔		28
IGF-I	↑		35
IGF-BP4	↑		36
Osteoprotegerin	↑		29
IL-6	↓		34
BMP-6	↑	↑	38
TIEG	↑		39
IL-11	↓		Waters (in preparation)
M-CSF	↑		Waters (in preparation)
TNF-α	↑	↓	Waters (in preparation)

The changes in gene expression were measured using one or more of the following parameters: mRNA, protein or biological activity. The methods and probes used to quantitate the levels of gene expression are described in the referenced source. PR, progesterone receptor; OCLn, osteocalcin; IGF, insulin-like growth factor; BP, binding protein; IL, interleukin; BMP, bone morphogenetic protein; M-CSF, macrophage colony-stimulating factor; TNF, tumor necrosis factor

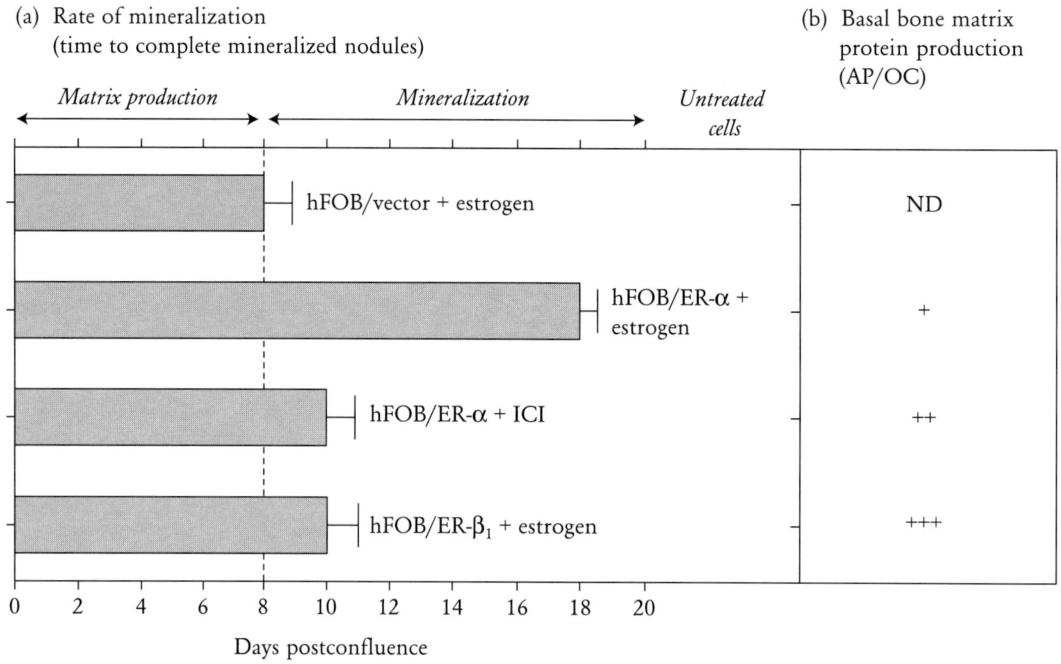

Figure 5 Actions of estrogen on the rate of bone matrix production and mineralization. The method for the analyses of bone matrix protein production and nodule formation have been reported previously[28,30–33]. hFOB, human fetal osteoblasts; ICI, ICI 182 780; AP, alkaline phosphatase; OC, osteocalcin

Table 3 Comparison of the estrogen regulation of bone matrix protein gene expression in osteoblast cells containing ER-α or ER-β*

Osteoblast cell line	*Rate of mineralization*	*Alkaline phosphatase*	*Osteocalcin*	*Type I coll*	*Osteonectin*
Estrogen					
Fetal osteoblast/ER-α	↓↓	↑↑	↓↓	↑	↔
Fetal osteoblast/ER-β	↑↑	↓↓	↔	↔	↔
Tamoxifen					
Fetal osteoblast/ER-α	↑↑	↑	↓↓	↑	↔
Fetal osteoblast/ER-β	↓	↓	↓	↔	↔

*The data represent comparisons of the levels of gene repression in fetal osteoblast/ER-α and fetal osteoblast/ER-β cell lines treated with estrogen or tamoxifen with those in the same cells treated with vehicle. The data on gene expression were collected from cells at the late stage of differentiation, at 17/18 days postconfluence during nodule formation (mineralization). The mineralization rate was measured at the midstage of differentiation, i.e. at 10/11 days postconfluence during matrix production and early mineralization. The bone matrix protein gene expression was measured at the level of secreted proteins. The mineralization rate (nodule formation) was measured using Alizarin Red and Von Kossa staining (K. Waters and colleagues, in preparation)

human fetal osteoblast/ER-α cells, even though they are not producing mineralized nodules, but is inhibited in human fetal osteoblast/ER-β cells. Osteocalcin is inhibited by estradiol in fetal osteoblast/ER-α cells, but is not regulated in ER-β cells. Tamoxifen behaves as a partial agonist in the human fetal osteoblast/ER-α cells, requiring higher doses than estradiol to achieve similar responses. Overall, estradiol has no effect on bone matrix proteins in the human fetal osteoblast/ER-β cells, with the exception of alkaline phosphatase, for which opposite actions by estrogen are observed, i.e. here estrogen inhibits alkaline phosphatase production. Conversely, tamoxifen moderately inhibits both alkaline phosphatase and osteocalcin secretion in the fetal osteoblast/ER-β cells. In summary, these data suggest that the presence of one or both of the estrogen receptor species in human osteoblast cells may determine osteoblast response and function by differentially modulating the actions on gene expression and ultimately bone matrix production and mineralization.

CONCLUSIONS

Recent advances in our understanding of the molecular mechanisms of estrogen action have revealed a higher level of complexity due to the identification of multiple ER isoforms and the ability of these isoforms to differentially modulate the activities of different estrogen responsive promoters. The differential promoter regulation occurs via interactions between the receptor and other families of transcription factors, enabling additional regulation of ERE-less promoters, and by interaction with co-activators and co-repressors that modify the transactivation activity of the ER. All of these processes may widen the spectrum of estrogen responses in target cells. A model simplifying the sequential steps of estrogen action in cells utilizing the two estrogen receptor species (α and β) is shown in Figure 1. Therefore, in a bone cell context, it will be possible to address some of the many important questions that remain. For example:

(1) Which ER isoform mediates the known cellular responses to estrogen;

(2) Do ER-α homodimers, ER-β homodimers and ER-α/β heterodimers produce similar or distinct effects on gene expression in bone cells;

(3) Does signalling through each receptor isoform influence the same panel of genes;

(4) What critical cytokines does estrogen regulate to ultimately affect osteoblastogenesis and osteoclastogenesis, and osteoblast–osteoclast coupling?

Identification of the ER-β isoform has opened up the field of research into the action of estrogen and the specificities of the isoforms. This research will be especially relevant to women's health issues, particularly estrogen replacement therapy. The potential to develop novel pharmaceutical agents to target specific receptors awaits further characterization of the ER isoforms.

ACKNOWLEDGEMENTS

The authors wish to thank Mr Larry Pederson and Ms Kay Rasmussen for their excellent technical assistance and Ms Jacquelyn House for her clerical assistance. This work was funded by NIH grant AG04875, The Mayo Foundation, and NIH training grant CA90441 (KW and MS).

References

1. Paganini-Hill A. The risks and benefits of estrogen replacement therapy: Leisure World. *Int J Fertil Menopausal Stud* 1995;40(Suppl 1):54–62
2. Riggs BL, Khosla S, Melton LJ. A unitary model for involutional osteoporosis: estrogen deficiency causes both type I and type II osteoporosis in postmenopausal women and contributes to bone loss in aging men. *J Bone Miner Res* 1998;13:763–73
3. Spelsberg TC, Subramaniam M, Riggs BL, *et al.* The actions and interactions of sex steroids and growth factors/cytokines on the skeleton. *Mol Endocrinol* 1999;13:819–28
4. Rickard DJ, Subramaniam M, Spelsberg TC. The molecular and cellular mechanisms of estrogen action on the skeleton. *J Cell Biochem* 2000;in press
5. Kuiper G, Gustafsson J-A. The novel estrogen receptor-β subtype: potential role in the cell- and promoter-specific actions of estrogens and anti-estrogens. *FEBS Lett* 1997;410:87–90
6. Paech K, Webb P, Kuiper GGJM, *et al.* Differential ligand activation of estrogen receptors ERα and ERβ at AP-1 sites. *Science* 1997;277:1508–10
7. Paige LA, Christensen DJ, Gron H, *et al.* Estrogen receptor (ER) modulators each induce distinct conformational changes in ERα and ERβ. *Proc Natl Acad Sci USA* 1999;96:3999–4004
8. Lu B, Leygue E, Dotzlaw H, *et al.* Estrogen receptor-β mRNA variants in human and murine tissues. *Mol Cell Endocrinol* 1998;138:199–203
9. Kuiper G, Carlquist M, Gustafsson J-A. Estrogen is a male and female hormone. *Sci Med* 1998;July/August:36–40
10. Wiegerinck M, Poortman J, Agema A, *et al.* Estrogen receptors in human vaginal tissue. *Maturitas* 1980;2:59–67
11. Galand P, Leroy F, Chretien J. Effect of oestradiol on cell proliferation and histological changes in the uterus and vagina of mice. *J Endocrinol* 1971;49:243–52
12. Stumpf W, Sar M. Autoradiographic localization of estrogen, androgen, progestin, and glucocorticosteriod in 'target tissues' and 'non-target tisssues'. In Pasqualini J, ed. *Receptors and Mechanisms of Action of Steriod Hormones.* New York: Marcel Dekker Inc., 1976:41–84
13. Couse J, Curtis S, Washburn T, *et al.* Analysis of transcription and estrogen insensitivity in the female mouse after targeted disruption of the estrogen receptor gene. *Mol Endocrinol* 1995;9:1441–54
14. Buchanan D, Kurita T, Taylor J, *et al.* Role of stromal and epithelial estrogen receptors in vaginal epithelial proliferation, stratification, and cornification. *Endocrinology* 1998;139:4345–52
15. Chen G, Oliver R, Leung B, *et al.* Estrogen receptor alpha and beta expression in the vaginal walls and uterosacral ligaments of premenopausal and postmenopausal women. *Fertil Steril* 1998;71:1099–102
16. Maclean A, Nicol L, Hodgins M. Immunohistochemical localization of estrogen receptors in the vulva and vagina. *J Reprod Med* 1990;35:1015–16
17. Eriksen EF, Colvard DS, Berg NJ, *et al.* Evidence of estrogen receptors in human osteoblast-like cells. *Science* 1988;241:84–6
18. Komm BS, Terpening CM, Benz DJ, *et al.* Estrogen binding, receptor mRNA, and biologic response in osteoblast-like osteosarcoma cells. *Science* 1988;241:81–4
19. Hoyland JA, Mee AP, Baird P, *et al.* Demonstration of estrogen receptor mRNA in bone using *in situ* reverse-transcriptase polymerase chain reaction. *Bone* 1997;20:87–92
20. Bodine PVN, Green J, Harris HA, *et al.* Functional properties of a conditionally phenotypic, estrogen-responsive, human osteoblast cell line. *J Cell Biochem* 1997;65:368–87

21. Bodine PVN, Henderson RA, Green J, *et al.* Estrogen receptor-α is developmentally regulated during osteoblast differentiation and contributes to selective estrogen responsiveness of gene expression. *Endocrinology* 1998;139:2048-57
22. Arts J, Kuiper GGJM, Janssen JMMF, *et al.* Differential expression of estrogen receptors α and β mRNA during differentiation of human osteoblast SV-HFO cells. *Endocrinology* 1997;138:5067-70
23. Lim SK, Won YJ, Lee HC, *et al.* A PCR analysis of ERα and ERβ mRNA abundance in rats and the effect of ovariectomy. *J Bone Miner Res* 1999;14: 1189-96
24. Turner RT, Kidder LS, Zhang M, *et al.* Estrogen has rapid tissue-specific effects on rat bone. *J Appl Physiol* 1999;86:1950-8
25. Turner RT, Riggs BL, Spelsberg TC. Skeletal effects of estrogen. *Endocr Rev* 1994;16:275-300
26. Ernst M, Parker MG, Rodan GA. Functional estrogen receptors in osteoblastic cells demonstrated by transfection with a reporter gene containing an estrogen response element. *Mol Endocrinol* 1991;5: 1597-606
27. Harris SA, Tau KR, Enger RJ, *et al.* Estrogen response in the hFOB1.19 human fetal osteoblast cell line stably transfected with the human estrogen receptor gene. *J Cell Biochem* 1995;59:193-201
28. Robinson JA, Harris SA, Riggs BL. Estrogen regulation of human osteoblastic cell proliferation and differentiation. *Endocrinology* 1997;138:2919-27
29. Hofbauer LC, Khosla S, Dunstan CR, *et al.* Estrogen stimulates gene expression and protein production of osteoprotegerin by human osteoblastic cells. *Endocrinology* 1999;140:4367-70
30. Harris SA, Enger RJ, Riggs BL, *et al.* Development and characterization of a conditionally immortalized human fetal osteoblastic cell line. *J Bone Miner Res* 1995;10:178-86
31. Spelsberg TC, Harris SA, Riggs BL. Immortalized osteoblast cell systems (new human fetal osteoblast systems). *Calcif Tiss Int* 1995;56:S18-21
32. Waters KM, Subramaniam M, Riggs BL, *et al.* Contrasting roles of estrogen receptor α and estrogen receptor β on human osteoblast differentiation phenotype. *J Bone Miner Res* 1998;23(Suppl): S266
33. Waters KM, Subramaniam M, Moore J, *et al.* Differentiation regulation of bone matrix proteins and cytokines by estrogen and SERMs through estrogen receptor α and estrogen receptor β in human osteoblast cells. *J Bone Miner Res* 1999;14(Suppl 1):S450
34. Kassem M, Harris SA, Spelsberg TC, *et al.* Estrogen inhibits interleukin-6 production and gene expression in a human osteoblastic cell line with high levels of estrogen receptors. *J Bone Miner Res* 1996; 11:193-9
35. Kassem M, Okazaki R, Harris SA, *et al.* Estrogen effects on insulin-like growth factor gene expression in a human osteoblastic cell line with high levels of estrogen receptor. *Calcif Tiss Int* 1997;62: 60-6
36. Kassem M, Okazaki R, De Leon D, *et al.* Potential mechanism of estrogen-mediated decrease in bone formation: estrogen increases production of inhibitory insulin-like growth factor-binding protein-4. *Proc Assoc Am Physicians* 1996;108:155-64
37. Spelsberg TC, Subramaniam M, Riggs BL, *et al.* The actions and interactions of sex steroids and growth factors/cytokines on the skeleton. *Mol Endocrinol* 1999;13:819-28
38. Rickard DJ, Hofbauer LC, Bonde SK, *et al.* Bone morphogenetic protein-6 production in human osteoblastic cell lines: selective regulation by estrogen. *J Clin Invest* 1998;101:413-22
39. Tau KR, Hefferan TE, Waters KM, *et al.* Estrogen regulation of a TGF-β inducible early gene that inhibits DNA synthesis in human osteoblasts. *Endocrinology* 1998;139:1346-53

Treatment of osteoporosis with antiresorptive drugs: facts and controversies 50

E. F. Eriksen and T. H. Sørensen

INTRODUCTION

All drugs (estrogen, selective estrogen receptor modulators (SERMs), bisphosphonates and calcitonin) currently used for the treatment of osteoporosis target the osteoclast. They are so-called antiresorptive regimens. Antiresorptive drugs are thought to mainly lower bone remodelling activity, thereby preserving cancellous bone structure and thickness of cortical bone. Recent results obtained with the various antiresorptive regimens have, however, pointed towards other mechanisms (e.g. changes in matrix structure and mineralization) being important too (see below).

This chapter will review the use of antiresorptive drugs for secondary and tertiary prophylaxis of osteoporosis. Secondary prophylaxis is defined as the initiative to prevent fractures in individuals with increased risk identified by screening, while tertiary prophylaxis is the initiative to prevent fractures in individuals with preexisting fractures.

SECONDARY PROPHYLAXIS

Estrogen

Effect of estrogen treatment on bone mass

A large number of short-term studies (2–3 years) have demonstrated that estrogen effectively reduces bone loss after the menopause[1–5]. Just after the initiation of treatment, the bone mineral content in the spine increases by about 3–6% in most studies, while cortical bone mainly shows preservation of bone mass or smaller increases[5]. The effect can be elicited irrespective of time after menopause.

In a case-control study, Ettinger and colleagues[4] reported a 19% increase in bone mineral content of the forearm in postmenopausal women on long-term estrogen/gestagen for at least 5 years (mean 17.8 years), as compared to age-matched controls. This study also reported an increase in spinal bone mineral density of 54%. Eiken and co-workers[6] recently reported results obtained in a randomized 10-year study on hormone replacement therapy (HRT) and bone mass. After 10 years, bone mass in the spine was found to be significantly higher in HRT-treated women than in those who remained untreated (14.5%; $p < 0.001$). Forearm bone mineral content decreased by 0.7% over the 10-year period in the HRT treatment groups, compared with a reduction of 17.6% in untreated women ($p < 0.001$). Mean forearm bone mineral content was 20.3% higher in women who had received HRT than in those who had not received therapy at the end of the 10-year follow-up[6].

Effects of estrogen treatment on bone remodelling

Numerous studies have demonstrated that estrogen treatment of normal and osteoporotic women reduces serum levels of alkaline phosphatase, osteocalcin and collagen propeptides, and urinary hydroxyproline and collagen cross-link excretion by about 50%[7,8]. Histomorphometric studies corroborate these findings. In a clinical controlled study, performed on 12 osteoporotic women after 150 weeks of estrogen/gestagen treatment, Steiniche[9] found that the balance between the thickness of bone resorbed and the thickness of bone formed per remodelling cycle was unchanged, but bone turnover went down by 50%.

In a randomized, double blind, clinical prospective trial, comprising 35 women treated with either HRT (cyclic estradiol/norethisterone acetate) or placebo, Eriksen and colleagues[10] investigated the effects of a cyclic estrogen/progestagen regimen on bone remodelling by bone histomorphometry. Bone biopsies were obtained before and after 2 years of treatment. Untreated women developed a progressively more negative balance of bone resorption and formation, while women on HRT displayed preservation of bone balance (Figure 1). The untreated women developed a pronounced increase in erosion depth over 2 years, while the HRT group revealed no change. Thus, bone remodelling in early postmenopausal women is characterized by progressive osteoclastic hyperactivity, which is reduced by cyclic HRT. This reduction of resorptive activity at the bone multicellular unit (BMU) level after HRT seems to precede the reduction in activation frequency demonstrated in older postmenopausal women by Steiniche[9].

Effect of estrogen prophylaxis on fracture risk

There are no long-term, randomized prospective studies that demonstrate a reduction in fracture risk in women on estrogen replacement therapy (ERT) after the menopause. Several retrospective and cohort studies, however, support this concept, showing about a 50% reduction in hip fractures[11-15]. Grady and associates[16] performed a

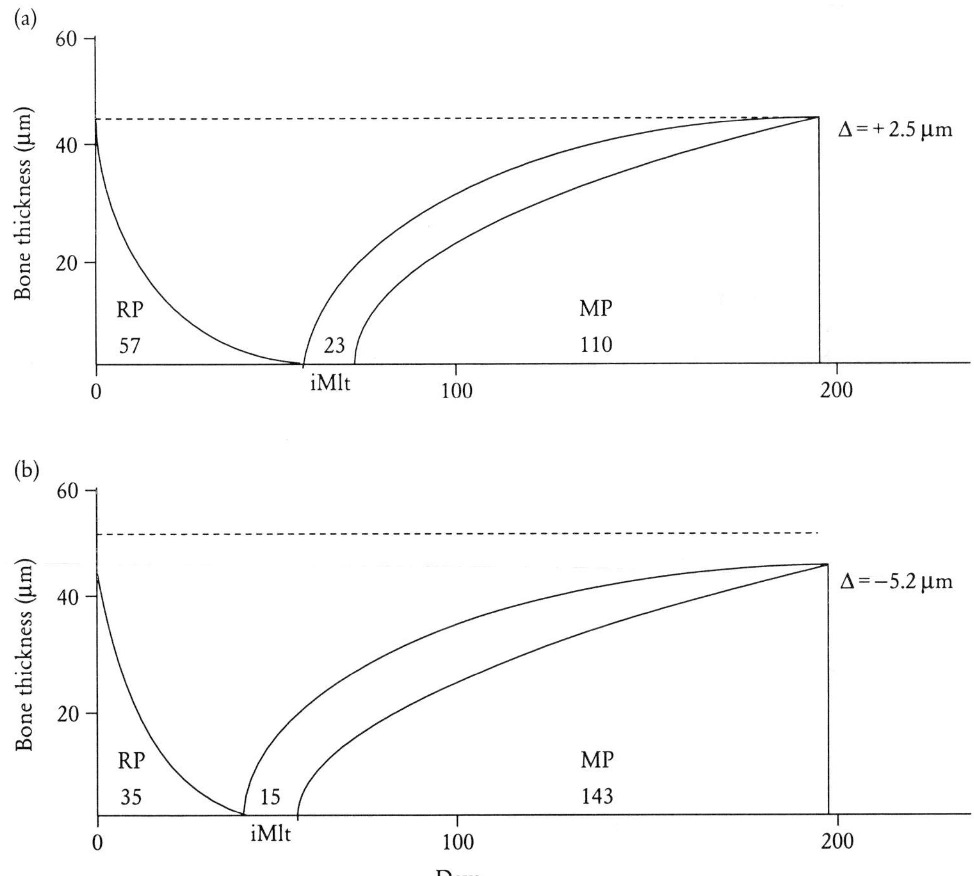

Figure 1 Effects of a 2-year regimen with estradiol (2 mg) and norethisterone acetate (1 mg) on bone remodelling in early postmenopausal women. The graphs display reconstructed remodelling cycles showing the thickness of bone resorbed and subsequently formed (*y* axis) in the hormone replacement therapy (HRT) (a) and placebo (b) groups. Note the slightly positive balance between resorption and formation in the the treatment group, compared to the profound negative balance in the placebo group. The *x* axis shows the duration of the different time periods during bone remodelling: resorption period (RP), initial mineralization lag time (iMlt) and mineralization period (MP). From reference 10 with permission

meta-analysis on all published fracture studies and calculated a relative risk of 0.75 for hip fracture after estrogen treatment.

Ettinger and co-workers[4] compared the occurrence of fractures in different parts of the skeleton in 245 postmenopausal Caucasian females on long-term ERT (more than 5 years, average 14 years) with matched controls. The two groups were comparable with respect to menopausal age, height, body weight, parity, smoking, education and occupation. The observation period was 17.6 years and the mean age at the end of the study was 69 years. The investigation showed a marked reduction in the overall fracture rate in the ERT group. The reduction was only related to the occurrence of osteoporotic fractures, which was reduced to 54% in controls. The number of vertebral compression fractures was 34 in the control group, compared to 11 in the estrogen group ($p < 0.001$). In a 10-year prospective study, Al Azzawi and colleagues[17] reported a reduced fracture rate in oophorectomized women on ERT compared to untreated women. In the ERT group, 4% of the women had infractions in the vertebral bodies, compared to 38% in the untreated group. After 10 years, crush fractures were observed in 1.7% of the estrogen-treated group, compared to 8.5% in the controls. The patients were, however, not randomized to the two groups. Thus, differences in lifestyle may have played a role.

Low-dose estrogen/progestogen HRT

In older women, the 2 mg estrogen doses elicit side-effects to a degree that may impair compliance. Therefore, trials using lower doses of estrogen and progestogen have been carried out. McClung and co-workers[18] tested the effects of various doses of estradiol (0.25, 0.5, 1 and 2 mg) combined with corresponding lower doses of norethisterone acetate (0.25, 0.5, 1 and 2 mg). They found that all combinations, even 0.25 mg estradiol plus 0.25 mg norethisterone acetate, preserved bone mass in early postmenopausal women, but that increasing doses improved bone mass in a dose-dependent fashion up to the maximal effect of 2 mg (increase in spinal bone mineral density of 5.0%). A halving of the steroid dose (1 mg estradiol and 1 mg norethisterone acetate) resulted in an increase in the spinal bone mineral density of 3.8%. The addition of norethisterone acetate to estradiol resulted in more pronounced increases than those seen with estradiol alone. Thus, progestogens exert additive effects when combined with a lower dose of estradiol. These doses form the basis for a new low-dose combination, Activelle®. In a European study on postmenopausal women[19], Activelle was found to increase the spinal bone mineral density by 5.4% and return biochemical markers of bone turnover to premenopausal levels.

Other regimens for secondary prophylaxis

Drugs primarily used for tertiary prophylaxis will, of course, also exert effects on the bone mass in younger women. Their effects in the early menopause are summarized below, but the detailed mode of action will be dealt with in the section on tertiary prophylaxis.

SERMs

Selective estrogen receptor modulators, such as tamoxifen and raloxifene, preserve bone mass in women after the menopause. Raloxifene increases bone mass by 1–2%, which is less than the increases of 4–10% seen with HRT and bisphosphonates[20]. This smaller increase in bone mass is probably due to the less pronounced reduction in turnover (30% versus 50–80% for HRT and bisphosphonates) seen with these drugs[20].

Other steroids

Certain progestins and anabolic steroids may produce effects on the skeleton similar to those of estrogen. Significant increases in bone mineral content in postmenopausal women have been demonstrated after a daily dose of 5 mg norethisterone alone[21]. Progesterone will also retard bone loss in the postmenopausal period[22].

Tibolone is a drug with mixed estrogenic, androgenic and gestagenic effects. In a randomized prospective trial, spinal trabecular bone mineral density was measured with quantitative computed tomography[23]. In the placebo group, the 2-year change versus baseline for the trabecular bone mineral density was –6.4%. Cortical bone mineral density did not change significantly. At 24 months, both tibolone groups showed a statistically significantly higher trabecular bone mineral density: 9.4% for the 1.25 mg group and 14.7% for the 2.5 mg group.

Anabolic steroids have been used previously and exert effects similar to those of other sex steroids[24]. Due to their masculinizing effects, however, they have become obsolete in most countries.

Bisphosphonates

Only a few studies have investigated the effects of bisphosphonates on early postmenopausal women, but generally the effects of these drugs are less pronounced than those seen in older women. Herd and associates[25] tested the effects of cyclic etidronate over a period of 2 years on women within 10 years of the menopause. The increases in bone mineral density were 1.7% 1–3 years after the menopause, 1.4% 4–6 years after the menopause and 3.4% 7–10 years after the menopause. Thus, bisphosphonates exert smaller effects on bone mass in early postmenopausal women than HRT. In another study, the effects of alendronate and HRT on bone mass were compared. HRT caused 1–2% higher bone mass than the 3.4% seen for 5 mg of alendronate[26].

TERTIARY PROPHYLAXIS

HRT

Estrogen is able to slow down bone loss, even in established osteoporosis in both the spine and the hip, as demonstrated by Lindsay and Tohme[27]. The changes in bone mass are similar to those obtained in postmenopausal women in some studies, while others have shown the skeleton in older women to be more responsive, resulting in bone mass changes of 9–10% over 2 years[28]. Kleis Møller and colleagues[29] tested the effects of combined estradiol (2 mg) and norethisterone acetate (1 mg) (Kliogest®) on the bone mass in women with severe osteoporosis. The bone mass increased by 9.0%, again a more pronounced increase than that seen in early menopausal women. Other studies have, however, demonstrated significant effects of calcium supplementation in women after the menopause[30,31]. Estrogen therapy is therefore also effective in the treatment of manifest osteoporosis.

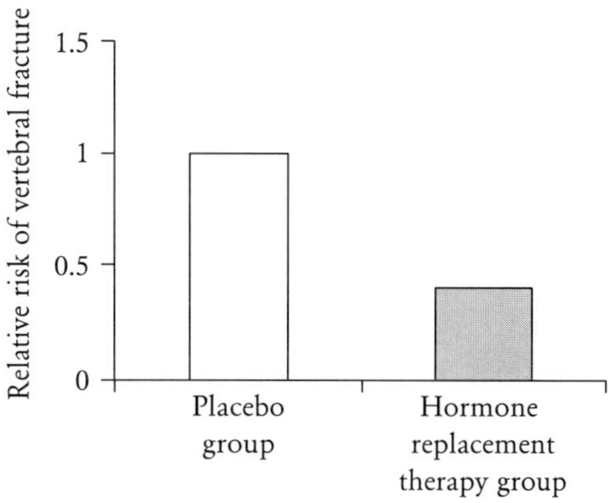

Figure 2 Effects of a 1-year treatment with transdermal estradiol combined with medroxyprogesterone acetate on fractures in osteoporotic women. From reference 32

Lufkin and co-workers[32] studied 75 postmenopausal women, 47–75 years of age, with one or more vertebral fractures due to osteoporosis. Thirty-nine women received dermal patches delivering 0.1 mg of 17β-estradiol for days 1–21 and oral progestogen (medroxyprogesterone acetate). Eight new fractures occurred in seven women in the estrogen group, whereas 20 occurred in 12 women in the placebo group, yielding a lower vertebral fracture rate in the estrogen group (relative risk 0.39, 95% confidence interval (CI) 0.16–0.95) (Figure 2).

Continuous combined HRT is the treatment of choice in older women due to the absence of cyclic bleeding. Older women are, however, more sensitive to the side-effects associated with HRT, especially breast tenderness. This can be overcome to some degree by starting with lower doses, before increasing to 2 mg of estradiol. Another approach is to administer lower doses in a continuous combined regimen, containing only 1 mg estradiol (e.g. Activelle).

SERMs

Raloxifene has been tested in a large-scale study comprising 7705 women. The women had to have a lumbar spine or hip *t* score < -2.5 and/or a vertebral fracture to be included in the study, and were treated with 60 or 120 mg of raloxifene for 2 years. About one-third of the women had pre-existing vertebral fractures. After 3 years, the bone mass

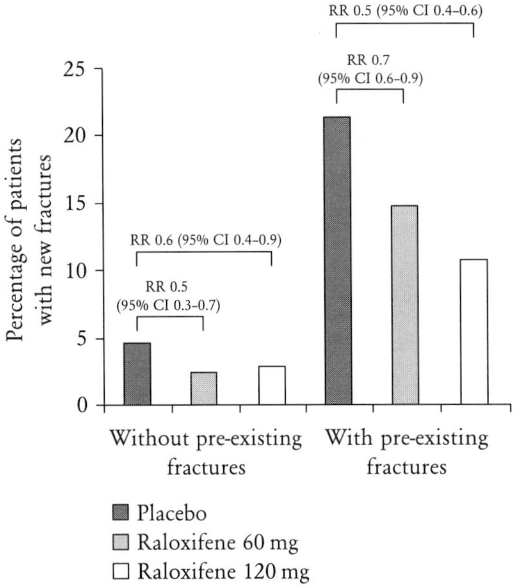

Figure 3 The effects of a 3-year regimen with raloxifene on new vertebral fractures in the study period. The results have been grouped according to the presence or absence of incident vertebral fractures before inclusion. RR, relative risk; CI, confidence interval. From reference 33 with permission

only went up by 2–3%. In the group of women without pre-existing fractures, 60 mg of raloxifene caused a significant reduction of 50% in vertebral fractures[33]. For patients with prevalent spinal fractures, the reduction was 30% in the 60 mg group and 50% in the 120 mg group[33] (Figure 3). Women treated with raloxifene did not have more bleeding disturbances than those given a placebo (3%). They did not experience breast tenderness and exhibited a reduced risk for breast cancer (1.7/1000 versus 3.2/1000 in the placebo group after 3.5 years, $p < 0.001$)[20,34]. A slight increase in the number of hot flushes was seen and a significant three-fold increase in the relative risk for deep venous thrombosis, similar to that seen for HRT, was found[20,34].

Bisphosphonates

Mode of action

The pharmacokinetic properties of bisphosphonates are characterized by bad absorption (< 1%) and pronounced selectivity for binding to hydroxyapatite. After having ingested a bisphosphonate, the former property necessitates a fasting condition lasting for at least 30 min, otherwise complexing with calcium will cause the drug to pass through the gut without any absorption.

The drugs inhibit osteoclast recruitment and activity by various mechanisms, but the common denominator seems to be increased osteoclast apoptosis. Some bisphosphonates form toxic complexes by binding to adenosine triphosphate, while others, especially aminobisphosphonates, exert an increase in osteoclast apoptosis by interference with the anchoring of membrane proteins in the cell membrane. They are able to inhibit the process called geranylation, which binds membrane proteins to fatty acids, thus securing the anchoring of the membrane protein in the cell membrane[35]. Recent results also suggest that bisphosphonates may exert positive effects on osteoblastic bone formation by inhibiting osteoblast apoptosis[36].

At the tissue level, bisphosphonates reduce bone turnover (activation frequency) by 50–90% and decrease erosion depth[37,38]. These effects explain part of the positive balance demonstrated using histomorphometric analysis. With the pronounced reduction of bone turnover, secondary mineralization of the bone matrix increases, which further contributes to the increase in bone mass[39].

Effects on bone mass and fracture

The first bisphosphonate to show antifracture efficacy was etidronate. This drug is given in a cyclic fashion for 2 weeks every 3 months. For the remaining period, the patients are given 500–1000 mg calcium. Two studies independently demonstrated a 50% reduction in spinal fractures in patients treated with cyclic etidronate and calcium[40,41]. Later, a British study demonstrated effects on non-vertebral fractures (wrist, hip and others)[42]. Furthermore, the drug has been shown to induce a continuous increase in bone mass over a 7-year period[43].

Alendronate, a newer, more potent aminobisphosphonate, has been tested in two very big, randomized, placebo-controlled studies. Liberman and co-workers[44] studied the effects of a 3-year course of alendronate (5, 10 and 20 mg) in 994 women with a bone mass t score < -2.5. Bone

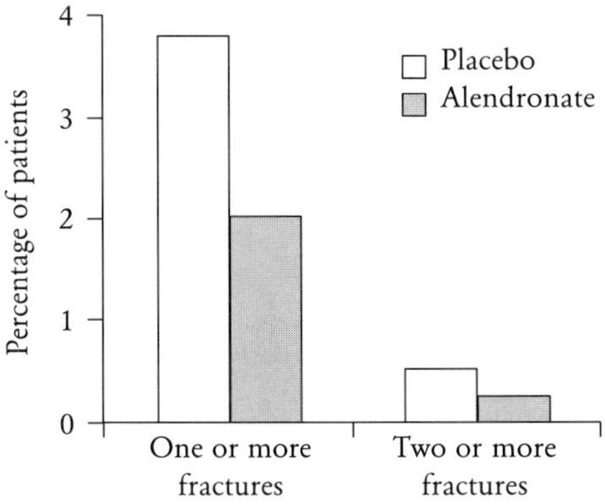

Figure 4 Effects of alendronate on fractures in women without pre-existing fractures. The number of individuals with one or more fractures was reduced by 44% and the number of individuals with two or more fractures by 60%. From reference 50

mineral density of the spine increased by 8.8% and that of the femoral neck by 5.9%. A 48% reduction in new vertebral fractures and significantly less reduction in height in the alendronate-treated women was demonstrated[44]. Black and associates[45] studied 2000 women aged 55–81 years with low femoral bone mass and at least one vertebral fracture. Eight per cent of women in the alendronate group had one or more new morphometric vertebral fractures, compared to 15.0% in the placebo group (relative risk 0.53, 95% CI 0.41-0.68). For clinically apparent vertebral fractures, the corresponding figures were 2.3% in the alendronate group and 5.0% in the placebo group (relative risk 0.45, 95% CI 0.27–0.72). The relative risks for hip fracture and wrist fracture for alendronate versus placebo were 0.49 (95% CI 0.23–0.99) and 0.52 (95% CI 0.31–0.87), respectively. In women without pre-existing fractures, significant antifracture efficacy has also been demonstrated (Figure 4).

Both alendronate and etidronate have also been shown to be effective against corticosteroid-induced osteoporosis. Two other bisphosphonates, risedronate and ibandronate, are currently being tested. So far, risedronate has shown antifracture efficacy similar to that of alendronate and etidronate. No fracture data have yet been provided for ibandronate, which is given intravenously every 3 months.

Calcitonin

Calcitonin can be used to slow down bone loss in osteoporotics, and significant increases in total body calcium have been reported after long-term injections of calcitonin[46,47]. Small, but significant, increases in spinal and proximal forearm bone mass (0.8–1.4%) have also been reported after intranasal application of calcitonin[48].

Significant effects on spinal fractures have been reported in two studies. Overgaard and colleagues[48] reported a relative risk reduction to 0.23 in a pooled group of patients treated with either 50, 100 or 200 IU of calcitonin. In a larger study of 1255 postmenopausal women with pre-existing vertebral fractures, Chestnut and co-workers[49] reported a significant reduction of 36% in the incidence of vertebral fractures in women receiving 200 IU of salmon calcitonin via nasal spray. The bone mineral density increased by 1.2% in that group. Two other subgroups receiving 100 IU and 400 IU of calcitonin did not exhibit significant fracture reduction.

CONCLUSION

Theoretically, the decrease in resorption depth and the reduction in bone remodelling activity caused by antiresorptive drugs should reduce the risk of perforative reduction and thus the disintegration of the trabecular network, resulting in reduced biomechanical strength and increased propensity for fracture. If this hypothesis were the sole explanation for the antifracture efficacy of antiresorptive drugs, a clear correlation between increase in bone mass and reduction in fractures should be demonstrable. From the data summarized above, this is clearly not the case. Two regimens causing very different changes in bone mineral density (e.g. raloxifene and alendronate) yield about the same antifracture efficacy. Furthermore, the fact that antiresorptive drugs, such as alendronate and raloxifene, show greater antifracture efficacy in more severely affected patients (i.e. the patients with pre-existing fractures) also demands an explanation. If the main action of antiresorptive drugs were preservation of trabecular architecture, one would expect a lower level of efficacy in individuals with more severe

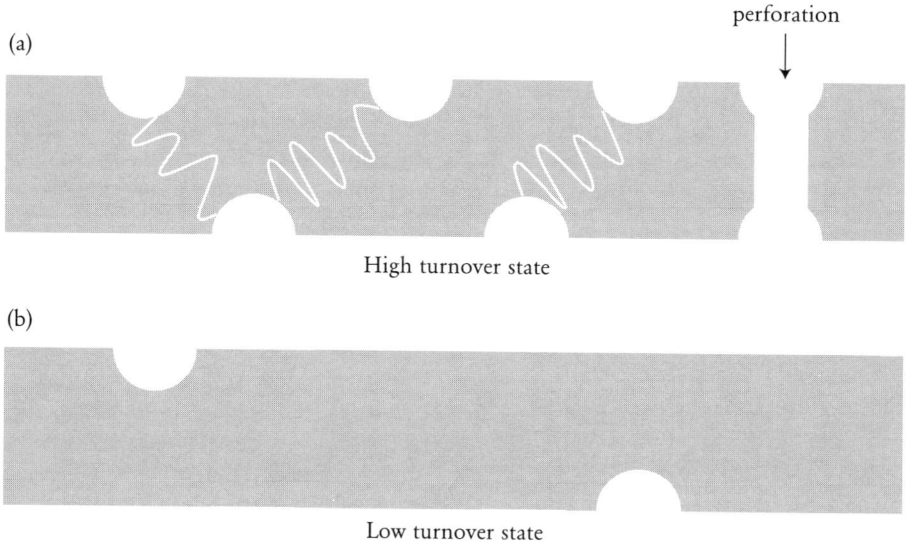

Figure 5 During high turnover states, the risk for trabecular perforations increases. Moreover, the high number of resorptive sites on trabecular surfaces cause structural instabilities ('stress risers'), which may further predispose to microfracture (a). Treatment with antiresorptive drugs (b) lowers the number of active resorption sites on the trabecular surface, thus increasing structural stability

osteoporosis, because the trabecular network has already undergone significant deterioration. This is certainly not the case. In the two studies where discrimination between patients with and without pre-existing fractures was possible (i.e. the raloxifene and alendronate studies), the patients with previous fractures exhibited more pronounced reductions in fracture incidence than the group as a whole.

Several alternative modes of action could be involved:

(1) Antiresorptive drugs reduce the number of resorptive sites per unit trabecular surface. This reduces the emergence of stress risers (i.e. structural instabilities due to close apposition of resorption lacunae) (Figure 5).

(2) Antiresorptive drugs may cause changes in bone matrix quality due to changes in matrix constituents such as type I collagen and non-collagenous proteins.

(3) Antiresorptive drugs may cause alterations in matrix mineralization, thereby improving matrix properties.

(4) Antiresorptive drugs may sensitize the osteocyte network to mechanical or other stimuli, resulting in increased bone mass.

(5) Antiresorptive drugs may increase cortical thickness.

(6) Antiresorptive drugs may exert anabolic actions on osteoblasts by reducing osteoblast apoptosis.

References

1. Horsman A, Gallagher JC, Simpson M, Nordin BEC. Prospective trial of estrogen and calcium in postmenopausal women. *Br Med J* 1977;2:789–92
2. Christiansen CC, Christensen MS, McNair P, Transbol I. Bone mass in postmenopausal women after withdrawal of oestrogen/gestagen replacement therapy. *Lancet* 1981;1:459–61
3. Lindsay R, Hart DM, Forest C, Baird C. Prevention of spinal osteoporosis in oophorectomized women. *Lancet* 1980;2:1151–4

4. Ettinger B, Genant HK, Cann CE. Long-term estrogen replacement therapy prevents bone loss and fractures. *Ann Intern Med* 1985;102:319–24
5. Munk Jensen N, Pors Nielsen S, Obel EB, Bonne Eriksen P. Reversal of postmenopausal vertebral bone loss by oestrogen and progestagen: a double blind placebo controlled study. *Br Med J* 1988; 296:1150–2
6. Eiken P, Kolthoff N, Nielsen SP. Effect of 10 years' hormone replacement therapy on bone mineral content in postmenopausal women. *Bone* 1996;19: 191S–3S
7. Hasling C, Eriksen EF, Melkko J, *et al.* Effects of a combined estrogen–gestagen regimen on serum levels of the carboxy-terminal propeptide of human type I procollagen in osteoporosis. *J Bone Miner Res* 1991;6:1295–300
8. Chen JT, Hosoda K, Hasumi K, Ogata E, Shiraki M. Serum *N*-terminal osteocalcin is a good indicator for estimating responders to hormone replacement therapy in postmenopausal women. *J Bone Miner Res* 1996;11:1784–92
9. Steiniche T. Bone histomorphometry in the pathophysiological evaluation of primary and secondary osteoporosis and various treatment modalities. *APMIS* 1995;51(Suppl):1–44
10. Eriksen EF, Langdahl B, Rungby J, Kassem M. Estrogen prevents osteoclastic hyperactivity around menopause: a histomorphometric study. *J Bone Miner Res* 1999;14:1217–21
11. Weiss NS, Ure CL, Ballard JH, Williams AR, Daling JF. Decreased risk of fractures of the hip and lower forearm with postmenopausal use of estrogen. *N Engl J Med* 1980;303:1195–7
12. Hutchinson TA, Polansky SM, Feinstein AR. Postmenopausal oestrogen protects against fractures of hip and distal radius: a case control study. *Lancet* 1979;2:705–9
13. Johnson RE, Specht EE. The risk of hip fracture in postmenopausal females with and without estrogen exposure. *Am J Public Health* 1981;71:139–44
14. Krieger NS, Kelsey JL, Holford TR, O'Connor T. An epidemiologic study of hip fracture in postmenopausal women. *Am J Epidemiol* 1978;116: 141–8
15. Paganini-Hill A, Ross RK, Gerkins VR, Henderson BE, Arthur M, Marci TM. Menopausal estrogen therapy and hip fractures. *Ann Intern Med* 1981; 95:28–31
16. Grady D, Rubin SM, Petitti DB, *et al.* Hormone therapy to prevent disease and prolong life in postmenopausal women. *Ann Intern Med* 1992;117: 1016–37
17. Al Azzawi F, Hart DM, Lindsay R. Long term effect of oestrogen replacement therapy on bone mass as measured by dual photon absorptiometry. *Br Med J Clin Res Educ* 1987;294:1261–2
18. McClung M, Greenwald M, Gluck O, Nanavati N, Huang W. Efficacy of Activelle to increase bone mineral density in postmenopausal women. *Bone* 1998;23:S465
19. Delmas PD, Confavreaux E, Fardellone P, De Vernejoul MC, Cormier C, Arce JC. Combinations of 1 mg of 17beta estradiol and low doses of norethisterone acetate prevent bone loss in postmenopausal women. Presented at the *26th European Symposium on Calcified Tissues*, Maastricht, The Netherlands, 1999
20. Delmas PD, Bjarnason NH, Mitlak BH, *et al.* Effects of raloxifene on bone mineral densiy, serum cholesterol concentrations, and uterine endometrium in postmenopausal women. *N Engl J Med* 1997;337:1641–7
21. Abdalla H, Hart DM, Lindsay R, Leggate I, Hooke A. Prevention of bone loss in postmenopausal women by norethisterone. *Obstet Gynecol* 1985;6: 789–92
22. Lindsay R, Hart DM, Purdie DW, Ferguson MM, Clark AC, Kraszewski A. Comparative effects of oestrogen and progestogen on bone loss in postmenopausal women. *Clin Sci Mol Med* 1978;54: 193–5
23. Berning B, Kuijk CV, Kuiper JW, Bennink HJ, Kicovic PM, Fauser BC. Effects of two doses of tibolone on trabecular and cortical bone loss in early postmenopausal women: a two-year randomized, placebo-controlled study. *Bone* 1996;19: 395–9
24. Riggs BL, Jowsey J, Goldsmith R, Kelly PJ, Hoffman DL, Arnaud CD. Short and long term effects of estrogens and synthetic anabolic steroids in postmenopausal osteoporosis. *J Clin Invest* 1959; 51:1972
25. Herd RJ, Balena R, Blake GM, Ryan PJ, Fogelman I. The prevention of early postmenopausal bone loss by cyclical etidronate therapy: a 2-year double blind, placebo controlled study. *Am J Med* 1997; 103:91–9
26. Hosking D, Chilvers CE, Christiansen C, *et al.* Prevention of bone loss with alendronate in postmenopausal women under 60 years of age. Early Postmenopausal Intervention Cohort Study Group. *N Engl J Med* 1998;338:485–92
27. Lindsay R, Tohme JF. Estrogen treatment of patients with established postmenopausal osteoporosis. *Obstet Gynecol* 1990;76:290–5
28. Christiansen C, Riis BJ. 17 Beta-estradiol and continuous norethisterone: a unique treatment for established osteoporosis in elderly women. *J Clin Endocrinol Metab* 1990;71:836–41
29. Kleis Moeller M, Brixen K, Andresen J, Eriksen EF. Combined HRT and cyclic growth hormone therapy for osteoporosis: results of a 2 year randomized, controlled trial. *Bone* 1998;25:S466
30. Elders PJ, Netelenbos JC, Lips P, *et al.* Calcium supplementation reduces vertebral bone loss in perimenopausal women: a controlled trial in 248

women between 46 and 55 years of age. *J Clin Endocrinol Metab* 1991;73:533–40
31. Reid IR, Ames RW, Evans MC, Gamble GD, Sharpe SJ. Effect of calcium supplementation on bone loss in postmenopausal women. *N Engl J Med* 1993;328:460–4
32. Lufkin EG, Wahner HW, O'Fallon WM, *et al.* Treatment of postmenopausal osteoporosis with transdermal estrogen. *Ann Intern Med* 1992;117:1–9
33. Ettinger B, Black DM, Mitlak B, *et al.* Reduction of vertebral fracture risk in postmenopausal women with osteoporosis treated with raloxifene. *J Am Med Assoc* 1999;282:637–45
34. Cummings SR, Eckert S, Krueger KA, *et al.* The effect of raloxifene on risk of breast cancer in postmenopausal women: results from the MORE randomized trial. Multiple Outcomes of Raloxifene Evaluation [see comments]. *J Am Med Assoc* 1999;281:2189–97
35. Luckman SP, Hughes DE, Coxon FP, Graham R, Russell G, Rogers MJ. Nitrogen-containing bisphosphonates inhibit the mevalonate pathway and prevent post-translational prenylation of GTP-binding proteins, including Ras. *J Bone Miner Res* 1998;13:581–9
36. Plotkin LI, Bellido T, Bonewald L, Papapoulos SE, Jilka RL, Manolagas SC. Bisphosphonates prevent glucocorticoid-induced apoptosis of osteocytes *in vitro*: a putative mechanism influencing mechanosensing. *Bone* 1998;23:S157
37. Steiniche T, Hasling C, Charles P, Eriksen EF, Melsen F, Mosekilde L. The effects of etidronate on trabecular bone remodeling in postmenopausal spinal osteoporosis: a randomized study comparing intermittent treatment and an ADFR regime. *Bone* 1991;12:155–63
38. Chavassieux PM, Arlot ME, Reda C, Wei L, Yates AJ, Meunier PJ. Histomorphometric assessment of the long-term effects of alendronate on bone quality and remodeling in patients with osteoporosis. *J Clin Invest* 1997;100:1475–80
39. Meunier PJ, Boivin G. Bone mineral density reflects bone mass but also the degree of mineralization of bone: therapeutic implications. *Bone* 1997;21:373–7
40. Storm T, Thamsborg G, Steiniche T, Genant HK, Sorensen OH. Effect of intermittent cyclical etidronate therapy on bone mass and fracture rate in women with postmenopausal osteoporosis [see comments]. *N Engl J Med* 1990;322:1265–71
41. Harris ST, Watts NB, Jackson RD, *et al.* Four-year study of intermittent cyclic etidronate treatment of postmenopausal osteoporosis: three years of blinded therapy followed by one year of open therapy [see comments]. *Am J Med* 1993;95:557–67
42. Van Staa TP, Abenhaim L, Cooper C. Use of cyclical etidronate and prevention of non-vertebral fractures. *Br J Rheumatol* 1998;37:87–94
43. Miller PD, Watts NB, Licata AA, *et al.* Cyclical etidronate in the treatment of postmenopausal osteoporosis: efficacy and safety after seven years of treatment. *Am J Med* 1997;103:468–76
44. Liberman UA, Weiss SR, Broll J, *et al.* Effect of oral alendronate on bone mineral density and the incidence of fractures in postmenopausal osteoporosis. The alendronate Phase III Osteoporosis Treatment Study Group. *N Engl J Med* 1997;333:1437–43
45. Black DM, Reiss TF, Nevitt MC, Cauley J, Karpf D, Cummings SR. Design of the Fracture Intervention Trial. *Osteoporos Int* 1993;3(Suppl 3):S29–39
46. Gruber HE, Ivey JL, Baylink DJ, *et al.* Long term calcitonin therapy in postmenopausal osteoporosis. *Metabolism* 1984;33:295–303
47. Mazzuoli GF, Passeri YM, Gennari C, *et al.* Effects of salmon calcitonin in postmenopausal osteoporosis: a controlled double blind clinical study. *Calcif Tiss Int* 1986;38:3–8
48. Overgaard K, Riis B, Christiansen C, Pødenphant J, Johansen JS. Nasal calcitonin for treatment of established osteoporosis. *Clin Endocrinol (Oxford)* 1989;30:435–42
49. Chestnut C, Baylink D, Doyle DV, *et al.* Salmon calcitonin nasal spray prevents vertebral fractures in established osteoporosis. Further interim results of the PROOF study. *Osteoporos Int* 1999;8:13
50. Cummings SR, Black DM, Thompson DE, *et al.* Effect of alendronate on risk of fracture in women with low bone density but without vertebral fracture: results from the Fracture Intervention Trial. *J Am Med Assoc* 1998;280:2077–82

Bisphosphonates in prevention and treatment of osteoporosis: state of the art 51

J.-Y. Reginster, A. Biermans and J.-F. Monville

INTRODUCTION

The historical background of bisphosphonates, previously called diphosphonates, is closely linked to the history of inorganic pyrophosphates. Inorganic pyrophosphate is the simplest of the polyphosphates, a family of compounds characterized by the existence of at least one phosphorus-oxygen-phosphorus bridge. Polyphosphates prevent precipitation of calcium carbonate in solution, which is the main reason for their long-lasting marketing as additives that prevent calcium carbonate scaling in salt water[1]. Noting the interest in the physicochemical properties of pyrophosphates, in 1970 Russell and Fleisch investigated the development of analogs that were stable *in vivo* and resisted enzymatic hydrolysis: bisphosphonates, in which a stable phosphorus-carbon-phosphorus bridge replaced the former phosphorus-oxygen-phosphorus bridge[2]. Bisphosphonates *in vitro*, prevent the precipitation of calcium and phosphorus in solution, block transformation of amorphous calcium phosphates in hydroxyapatite and inhibit aggregation of hydroxyapatite crystals[3]. Bisphosphonates are extremely potent inhibitors of bone resorption[4]. They interfere with several stages of the osteoresorption process. Different mechanisms of action, acting simultaneously and synergistically, are likely to be involved, including an acute phenomenon, mainly physicochemical, and a cellular and/or biochemical effect, which has a longer latency[5]. The relative contribution of each of them depends on the nature of the respective bisphosphonate. The anti-resorptive action of bisphosphonates has been widely used in human patients. Several bisphosphonates were tested in various clinical situations related to an increase of osteoclastic resorption, including Paget's disease of bone, tumor- and non-tumor-induced hypercalcemia, primary hyperthyroidism, osteoporosis of hypodynamism, glucocorticoid-induced osteoporosis, juvenile idiopathic osteoporosis and primary involutional osteoporosis[6]. Postmenopausal osteoporosis is a disorder characterized by an increase in bone resorption relative to bone formation, consistently linked to an increased rate of bone turnover[7]. Therefore, it was rather logical to consider bisphosphonates, which are selective inhibitors of osteoclastic bone resorption, as a potential preventive and therapeutic approach to postmenopausal osteoporosis[8].

ETIDRONATE

Etidronate has been widely investigated as a monotherapy for postmenopausal osteoporosis given either continuously[9] or intermittently[10]. This bisphosphonate has already been used in several protocols based on the concept of a 'coherence therapy' of osteoporosis[11,12]. Discrepant outcomes resulted from the various therapeutic regimens[9,12,13]. Storm and colleagues[10], when giving etidronate intermittently (400 mg/day for 14 days every 4 months over 3 years) to osteoporotic women, observed a significant increase (1.8% per year) in bone mineral density at the spine without any concomitant loss of cortical bone. Notwithstanding, the rate of new vertebral fractures observed in the treated group during the 3 years of the trial was not significantly different from that observed in the control group (treated with placebo). A separate analysis of the second and third years (excluding the first year) of treatment was the only way to show a significant ($p = 0.023$) reduction of fracture incidence in the group treated with etidronate. In a multicenter North American trial[11], during which etidronate was administered following a similar regimen (400 mg/day for 14 days every 3 months for 2 years), although in half of the patients this was after the administration over 3 days of 1 g/day phosphorus, patients who received etidronate had a significant increase in spinal bone density (2.6–2.1% per year for etidronate/phosphorus and etidronate/placebo) with no cortical loss. The incidence of new fractures was identical in the four groups involved in the trial (etidronate/phosphorus, etidronate/placebo, phosphorus/placebo, placebo/placebo) but, when pooling patients treated with etidronate, independently of the former intake of phosphorus, the authors reported a slightly significant reduction in the incidence of vertebral fractures ($p = 0.043$) compared with the two other therapeutic groups. The follow-up of this trial for another year revealed an increase in the rate of vertebral fractures in the group treated with etidronate so that, at the end of the global period of 3 years, there was no more significant difference in the overall population between patients treated with placebo and those treated with etidronate. A *post-hoc* analysis revealed, however, that patients whose spinal bone mineral density (BMD) was below the 50th centile of the distribution of BMD in osteoporotic patients, and who concomitantly had more than two prevalent fractures at the start of the trial (17% of the population), experienced a significant reduction in the rate of vertebral fractures when treated with etidronate compared with those treated with placebo. These results suggested a plausible role for etidronate in the treatment of severe osteoporosis[14]. No effect of etidronate on non-vertebral fracture rates was demonstrated in a prospective controlled trial. In a study collecting information from 550 general practices in the UK that provide a medical record to the general practice research database, a total of 7977 patients undergoing cyclical etidronate treatment and 7977 age- and practice-matched control patients with a diagnosis of osteoporosis were analyzed. People taking cyclical etidronate had a significantly reduced risk of non-vertebral fracture (by 20%) and of hip fracture (34%) relative to the osteoporosis control patients. Once fracture incidence rates were compared between the two groups, the rate of non-vertebral, hip and wrist fractures decreased significantly with increasing etidronate exposure[15]. Intermittent administration of etidronate, at the above-mentioned doses for 2–3 years, appears to be related to an increased prevalence of histological abnormalities, characterized by histological osteomalacia and mineralization impairments[16,17], but these abnormalities have not been shown to have clinical significance[16–18]. The absence of a relationship between these histological changes and the clinical pattern of patients treated with cyclical etidronate is in accordance with further results which show normal histological features and an absence of, and increase in, vertebral fracture incidence when cyclical administration of etidronate was prolonged for 4 or 5 years[19,20].

In a subset of osteoporotic women treated for up to 7 years with cyclical etidronate, results from transiliac crest bone biopsy samples suggested that, after 3 years of treatment, bone turnover returned towards baseline levels, whereas bone mineralization remained within normal limits by histological and histomorphometric assessment[21].

CLODRONATE

Clodronate has been exhaustively investigated and prescribed in several disorders characterized by an enhanced bone resorption[22]. However, limited data are available concerning the use of this bisphosphonate in osteoporosis. Administration of intermittent oral clodronate (200–600 mg/day for 3 months followed by a similar wash-out period) to a small cohort of patients with osteoporosis yielded a significant increase in total body calcium (8%) after 20 months[23]. Oral clodronate (400 mg daily for 30 days every 3 months) with or without concomitant calcitriol was also associated with a significant increase in lumbar bone density (+3.88% and +3.21% without and with calcitriol, respectively) after 12 months, while untreated patients lost 2.34% of their spinal bone during the same period[24]. Recently, the oral administration for 3 years of 800 mg/day of clodronate to elderly women (mean age 80 years) recruited from general practice registers was reported significantly to prevent decreases in hip (+0.44% vs. –2.8% with placebo) and distal forearm BMD (0.0% vs. –1.6% with placebo). This effect was linked to a reduction in bone turnover evidenced by a significant decrease in serum carboxyterminal telopeptide of type I collagen (CrossLaps™)[25]. Intramuscular clodronate (100 mg every week) given to women with osteoporosis (spinal BMD *T* score less than –2.5) induced a significant increase in spinal BMD (+4.5%) after 2 years with no significant changes at the femoral neck level, and a transient increase at the trochanter and Ward's triangle[26]. Monthly intravenous infusion of 200 mg clodronate for 2 years to women with low lumbar BMD prevented further bone loss to a similar extent as transdermal 17β-estradiol (50 μg/day)[27]. In a long-term study evaluating the effects of intravenous infusion of 200 mg of clodronate every 3 weeks for 6 years to osteoporotic patients (*T* score less than –2.5 for spinal BMD), lumbar BMD increased significantly and the upward trend persisted for all 6 years of therapy (5.69%) compared with controls (–1.47%)[28]. In a subset of patients monitored for 3 years, clodronate was reported to reduce with borderline significance ($p = 0.067$) the number of patients experiencing new vertebral fractures, while the total number of vertebral fractures was significantly reduced ($p = 0.0013$)[29]. Oral clodronate (2400 mg/day) was tested in patients with glucocorticosteroid-induced osteoporosis. After 12 months of this regimen, a significant increase was reported for BMD of the spine (3.0%), femoral neck (4.3%) and trochanteric regions (2.8%), while lower doses were either effective only at the spine (1600 mg/day) or ineffective at the spine and hip (800 mg/day)[30]. However, no studies have been conducted with the adequate methodology to demonstrate convincingly the antifracture efficacy of this bisphosphonate in postmenopausal osteoporosis.

PAMIDRONATE

Administration of 150 mg/day of pamidronate for 2 weeks was reported to normalize calcium balance, while such a treatment given for up to 6.2 years (mean 3.7 years) was associated with a significant and sustained 3% annual increase in lumbar BMD[31]. However, this study was subject to major methodological flaws, which preclude the reaching of any significant conclusion.

More recently, a similar regimen (150 mg/day continuously) was investigated in a prospective, double-blind, placebo-controlled study where 48 postmenopausal women with established osteoporosis were followed for 2 years. Significant increases in BMD were observed in patients treated with pamidronate for total body (+1.9%), lumbar spine (+7%) and femoral trochanter (+5.4%), while the significant decrease observed for the placebo group at the femoral neck and Ward's triangle did not occur in the pamidronate group. Vertebral fracture rates were non-significantly ($p = 0.07$) reduced in the pamidronate group[32].

However, the development of the oral form of pamidronate has been jeopardized by the report of erosive esophagitis, which seems to be a common feature of all amino biphosphonates[33], while its intravenous administration has yielded only transient positive results in terms of BMD[34].

ALENDRONATE

Exhaustive preclinical assessment of alendronate evaluated the effects of this bisphophonate on the biomechanical properties of the skeleton. Globally, results obtained in both rats[35] and baboons[36] concluded that alendronate significantly improves both bone mineral content and biomechanical resistance of trabecular and cortical bone. In early-postmenopausal women, 2.5 or 5 mg/day of alendronate prevented cortical and trabecular bone loss over 2 years, in a similar way to conjugated equine estrogens (0.625 mg/day) and medroxyprogesterone acetate (5 mg/day) or 17β-estradiol (1–2 mg/day) and norethisterone acetate (0–1 mg/day). The 5-mg/day dose gave better results than the 2.5-mg/day dose at all measured sites including spine (+3.46% vs. +2.28%), total hip (+1.85% vs. +1.06%) and total body (+0.67% vs. –0.03%)[37]. Dose-dependent effects of alendronate to reduce bone turnover and increase spinal bone mass were reported in postmenopausal women with low BMD. In this population, the 10-mg/day dose, suggested to correspond to the best risk/benefit ratio for treatment of osteoporosis, induced significant increases in BMD after 2[38] and 3 years[39]. In the 2-year study, mean changes in BMD with 10 mg/day alendronate were +7.21% at the spine, +5.27% for total hip and +2.53% for total body, while biochemical markers of bone remodelling declined about 50% after 3 months for resorption markers and 6 months for formation markers[38].

The 3-year study showed similar results with increases of 2.4%, 5.5% and 7.2% for lumbar spine, femoral neck and trochanter BMD, respectively[39].

The results were pooled from two studies in which three doses of alendronate were given for 3 years (5, 10 and 20 mg/day for 2 years followed by 5 mg/day for 1 year) to women with low BMD (including a 20% subset with prevalent fractures)[40]. Compared to the placebo group, a significant reduction in the proportion of women with new vertebral fractures (3.2% vs. 6.2%; $p = 0.03$) and a decreased progression of vertebral deformities (33% vs. 41%; $p = 0.028$) were observed. Significant reduction of the risk of vertebral (relative risk, RR = 0.54), hip (RR = 0.49), wrist (RR = 0.56) and all clinical fractures (RR = 0.72) was also reported in the Fracture Intervention Trial, among women who had low BMD and vertebral fractures[41]. In women with low BMD but without vertebral fracture, 4 years of alendronate treatment safely increased BMD and decreased the risk of first vertebral deformity. This antifracture efficacy was documented only in women whose baseline BMD *T* score at the femoral neck was below 2.5 standard deviations below the normal young adult mean[42]. In patients participating in the Fracture Intervention Trial[41,42], women who had larger increases in total hip BMD during the first 12 months had a lower incidence of new vertebral fractures during the 3-year follow-up period. Only 3.2% of women with increases of more than 3% in total hip BMD experienced new vertebral fractures, whereas 6.3% of women whose BMD declined or remained stable experienced new fractures (odds ratio 0.45; 95% confidence interval 0.27–0.72)[43].

Esophageal erosion and ulcerative esophagitis have been reported in association with the use of alendronate[44,45]. However, particular recommendations for alendronate intake (swallowing alendronate with 180–240 ml water on arising in the morning and remaining upright for at least 30 min after swallowing the tablet and until the first food of the day has been ingested) reduces this risk to the background incidence observed in an age-matched population. This was recently reported from a survey of 13 placebo-controlled studies which together enrolled 14 000 postmenopausal women. In this survey, the incidence of upper gastrointestinal adverse reactions was not increased in women receiving alendronate, even in high-risk subgroups. Esophagitis was rare, although a slightly higher incidence (alendronate 0.7% vs. placebo 0.4%) was seen in the Fracture Intervention Trial ($n = 6049$)[46].

A combination of alendronate (10 mg/day) and raloxifene (60 mg/day) given for 12 months to postmenopausal women with low femoral density induced a greater reduction in bone turnover and a higher increase in femoral neck BMD than either alendronate or raloxifene alone. Whether this combination may provide relevant benefits in terms of fracture reduction remains to be investigated[47].

IBANDRONATE

Ibandronate is a new bisphosphonate which is two, ten, 50 and 500 times more potent than risedronate, alendronate, pamidronate and clodronate, respectively, as inhibitor of the retinoid-induced bone resorption in the thyroparathyroidectomized rat model[48]. Both oral and intravenous routes of administration of ibandronate have been investigated in postmenopausal osteoporosis. Continuous daily oral intake of 2.5 mg ibandronate for 12 months induced recorded BMD increases of 4.8% (spine), 2.0–3.3% (hip), 2.0% (total skeleton) and 0.9% (forearm)[49]. In a population of postmenopausal women with osteoporosis, intravenous ibandronate was investigated in a randomized, partly double-blinded, placebo-controlled study. Women received either a placebo or ibandronate (0.25, 0.5, 1 or 2 mg) every 3 months. Lumbar spine BMD did not change in the placebo group, but increased by 2.4%, 3.5%, 3.7% and 5.2%, respectively, at 12 months for the dose-ranging groups. The increase was statistically significantly different from placebo for the 0.5-, 1- and 2-mg groups, whereas with 0.25 mg no significant differences occurred. After 1 year, total hip and trochanter BMD increased significantly by 1.8% and 2.9% for total hip and 2.7% and 4.2% for trochanter in the 1- and 2-mg groups, respectively. There was no significant difference in the overall number of adverse events in the ibandronate groups compared with the placebo group.

Considering specific adverse event, no dose dependency and difference from placebo could be observed, apart from an acute reaction that occurred in 7% of the patients[50].

If these extremely promising results are confirmed in terms of antifracture efficacy, intermittent parenteral administration of ibandronate should become a first-choice alternative to solve the problem linked with poor compliance with or tolerance to oral medications of the bisphosphonates family.

NERIDRONATE

Neridronate was recently shown selectively to suppress peptide-bound deoxypyridinoline excretion in postmenopausal women with low BMD[51]. Further investigations into the effects and mechanisms of action of this bisphosphonate have been requested and are in progress.

TILUDRONATE

Preclinical studies evaluating the effects of tiludronate on skeletal metabolism were of particular interest. They demonstrated a dose-dependent inhibition of osteoclastic resorption in several models of rodent[52] or non-rodent[53] mammals (in accordance with results obtained with other bisphosphonates), and they confirmed the harmlessness of this compound to the biomechanical resistance of trabecular and cortical bone[53]. The most original features of these investigations comprised the observation of an increase in the mineralization rate and an improvement of bone mechanical properties in a callus from dogs having been exposed to hemiosteotomy of the ulna[54]. These results were in agreement with previous reports of the efficacy of tiludronate in Paget's disease of the bone[55,56], where the proportion of responders to tiludronate was twice as high as that observed with etidronate. Tiludronate, given for 6 months to healthy, early-postmenopausal women, prevented spinal bone loss for up to 12 months compared with women who received placebo for the same duration[57]. This early report was later confirmed in a multicenter trial where women treated with oral tiludronate 200 mg/day continuously for 6 months lost significantly ($p = 0.016$) less femoral bone after 18 months than those receiving placebo (–1% vs. –2.8%). Results at the level of the lumbar spine showed a similar trend which was borderline significant ($p = 0.065$)[58,59].

However, the results of two large, prospective, double-blind, randomized controlled trials evaluating the effect of tiludronate in the treatment of established osteoporosis, including women with either low BMD or prevalent vertebral fractures, failed to demonstrate any significant antifracture effect. This negative conclusion is likely to be related to the use of a largely suboptimal dose of tiludronate, i.e. 200 mg daily for 7 days per month[60,61].

RISEDRONATE

In rats, subcutaneous injection of risedronate 5 μg/kg per day significantly reduced histological parameters reflecting osteoclastic resorption, without interaction with bone formation or mineralization[62]. Similarly, the biochemical properties of vertebrae and femoral neck obtained from dogs treated with risedronate for 2 years at doses from 0.2 to 2 mg/kg per day were not significantly modified. In women with breast cancer and chemotherapy-induced menopause, risedronate was given intermittently (10–30 mg/day for 2 weeks every 3 months) for 2–3 years[63]. These doses of risedronate prevented the bone loss observed in the control population. A dose of 5 mg risedronate given either continuously or intermittently (2 weeks of risedronate followed by 2 weeks of placebo) for 2 years was evaluated in early-postmenopausal women with normal bone mass. At the end of the trial, a significant difference ($p < 0.0001$) appeared between the three groups in the evolution of lumbar spine bone mass. At the trochanteric level, bone mass increased (+2.3%) in the group treated with the continuous regimen, was maintained (+0.5%) with the intermittent regimen and decreased (–1%) in the placebo arm[64]. This effect was mediated by a decreased bone resorption, as confirmed by a drastic reduction in urinary deoxypyridinoline (–31% and –15% for continuous and intermittent risedronate regimens, respectively)[64]. Paired bone biopsies obtained before and after 1 year of treatment revealed no signs of osteomalacia[65].

In severe osteoporosis (low bone mass and prevalent fractures), risedronate (two periods of 20 mg/day for 7 days each, followed by 14 days of calcium) decreased collagen cross-links urinary excretion significantly by more than half and for up to 3 months[66]. Daily administration of 2.5 mg risedronate to osteoporotic women with prevalent spinal fractures at baseline resulted in a significant trend towards an increased bone mass at the spine and trochanter, but no reduction of new vertebral fractures[67]. The recommended daily dose of 5 mg/day of risedronate was tested in women with low BMD of the spine and women with prevalent vertebral fractures. In postmenopausal women with lumbar spine BMD *T* score less than –2, 5 mg of daily risedronate increased BMD by 4.06%, 1.31% and 2.72% at the lumbar spine, femoral neck and femoral trochanter, respectively, after 24 months. All these values were significantly different from the changes observed in the placebo group[68]. Three-year administration of risedronate (5 mg/day) to women with established postmenopausal osteoporosis (prevalent vertebral fractures and low BMD) resulted in a significant decrease in the incidence of new vertebral fractures (risk reduction of 41–49%), with bone biopsy samples indicating that risedronate produced moderate (50%) suppression of bone turnover and that bone formed during risedronate treatment was of normal structure and mineralization[69–71]. In this population, spinal antifracture efficacy of risedronate appears to occur as soon as the first year of treatment[72]. When pooling results from two double-blind studies enrolling 3684 postmenopausal women with prevalent vertebral fractures and isolating, in a *post-hoc* analysis, a subpopulation of patients with at least two vertebral fractures at baseline, treatment with 5 mg of risedronate daily reduced the incidence of new vertebral fractures by 47% compared with controls (95% confidence interval 31–59%) over 3 years. Over the same period, the incidence of non-vertebral fractures in the risedronate 5-mg group was 36% lower than that in the controls (95% confidence interval 13–53%) ($p < 0.005$)[73]. However, since the prolonged use of risedronate in women with established osteoporosis was recently consistently linked with a statistically significant increase in the occurrence of pulmonary cancer (3.9/1000 patient-years of exposure and 1.9/1000 patient-years of exposure for 2.5 and 5 mg/day, respectively, compared to 1.2/1000 patient-years of exposure with placebo, based on the results from ten phase III studies involving approximately 30 000 patient-years of exposure), the role of risedronate in the treatment of postmenopausal osteoporosis will have to be assessed on the basis of a large and extensive review of its risk/benefit ratio.

CONCLUSION

Over recent years, bisphosphonates have emerged as the first-line treatment of postmenopausal and senile osteoporosis. In the past, etidronate demonstrated a positive effect on BMD of the lumbar spine, without harmful effect at the level of the hip. However, the antifracture efficacy of this compound has been repeatedly challenged. Owing to this weak efficacy and the risk of inducing focal osteomalacia after prolonged use, this molecule is now considered as obsolete and cannot any longer be recommended. Clodronate and pamidronate were shown to have promising effects on spinal or appendicular BMD, but the appropriate studies to demonstrate their antifracture efficacy were never conducted. Tiludronate had a highly promising risk/benefit ratio. Unfortunately, the dose selected for the pivotal trials was likely to be largely suboptimal, and this mistake jeopardized the development of this bisphosphonate in osteoporosis. Alendronate has been the center of the largest-ever performed development program in osteoporosis. From all double-blind, placebo-controlled studies, the coherent evidence emerged that 10 mg/day of alendronate is a safe and efficient treatment of osteoporosis, in women with low mineral density (*T* score ≤ –2.5) or with prevalent fractures. In this population, daily administration of alendronate significantly reduces the risk of vertebral and non-vertebral fractures. Concerns were expressed about the upper gastrointestinal safety of alendronate. These problems can be solved if the patients are fulfilling particular recommendations for alendronate intake. Risedronate was recently shown significantly to reduce vertebral fractures in women with established osteoporosis. This effect appears to occur as soon as the first year of treatment. In a *post-hoc* analysis investigating a population of women with at least two vertebral fractures at the beginning of the trial, an effect was also observed on extravertebral fractures. This awaits confirmation by the results of ongoing prospective studies with hip fracture reduction as a primary end-point. When comparing alendronate and risedronate, it appears that neither of these two bisphosphonates emerges significantly in terms of spinal fracture reduction. Today, alendronate has the advantage of having unequivocally demonstrated its anti-fracture efficacy at the level of the hip and the forearm, which is not the case for risedronate. Furthermore, prolonged use of risedronate in women with established osteoporosis has been consistently linked to a statistically significant increase in the occurrence of pulmonary cancer. Notwithstanding that no definite conclusion can be drawn regarding the causality of risedronate in the occurrence of these pulmonary cancers, it is now reasonable, owing to the clinical relevance of this adverse reaction, to limit the use of risedronate to women who are either non-responders or intolerant to other treatments, including alendronate. Ibandronate, a new bisphosphonate currently under development, has the characteristic of being able to be given intravenously. If the promising data observed on BMD are confirmed in terms of fracture reduction, the possibility of improving the compliance of patients by by-passing the oral route might become a breakthrough in the race to determine the optimal bisphosphonates treatment.

References

1. Fleisch H. *Bisphosphonates in Bone Disease. From the Laboratory to the Patient.* Carnforth, UK: Parthenon Publishing, 1995
2. Russell RGG, Fleisch H. Inorganic pyrophosphate and pyrophosphatases in calcification and calcium homeostasis. *Clin Orthop* 1970;69:101–7
3. Fleisch H. Diphosphonates: history and mechanisms of action. *Metab Bone Dis Relat Res* 1981;3: 279–88
4. Treschel U, Strutrer A, Fleisch H. Hypercalcaemia induced with an arotinoid in thyroparathyroidectomized rats. New model to study bone resorption *in vivo. J Clin Invest* 1986;80:1979–86
5. Fleisch H. Experimental basis for the use of bisphosphonates in Paget's disease of bone. *Clin Orthop Relat Res* 1987;217:72–8
6. Reginster J-Y. *Ostéoporose Postménopausique. Traitement Prophylactique.* Paris: Masson, 1993
7. Riggs BL, Melton LJ. Involution osteoporosis. *Am J Med* 1986;314:1676–84
8. Reginster J-Y. Les bisphosphonates constituent-ils un réel progrès thérapeutique dans l'ostéoporose? *Méd Hyg* 1996;54:1497–501
9. Heaney RP, Saville PD. Etidronate disodium in postmenopausal osteoporosis. *Clin Pharm Ther* 1976;20:593–604
10. Storm T, Thamsborg G, Steinich T, Genant HK, Sorensen OH. Effect of intermittent cyclical etidronate therapy on bone mass and fracture rate in women with postmenopausal osteoporosis. *N Engl J Med* 1990;322:1265–71
11. Watts NB, Harris ST, Genant HK, *et al.* Intermittent cyclical etidronate treatment of postmenopausal osteoporosis. *N Engl J Med* 1990;323:73–9
12. Pacifici R, MacMurtry C, Vered I, Rupich R, Avioli LV. Coherence therapy does not prevent axial bone loss in osteoporotic women: a preliminary comparative study. *J Clin Endocrinol Metab* 1988;66:747–53
13. Smith ML, Fogelman I, Hart DM, Scott E, Bevan I, Leggate I. Effect of etidronate disodium on bone turnover following surgical menopause. *Calcif Tissue Int* 1989;44:74–9
14. Harris ST, Watts NB, Jackson RD, *et al.* Four years of intermittent cyclical etidronate treatment of postmenopausal osteoporosis: three years of blinded therapy followed by one year of open therapy. *Am J Med* 1993;95:557–67
15. Van Staa TP, Abenhaim L, Cooper C. Use of cyclical etidronate and prevention of non-vertebral fractures. *Br J Rheumatol* 1998;37:1253–4
16. Axelrod DW, Teitelbaum SL. Results of long-term cyclical etidronate therapy: bone histomorphometry and clinical correlates. *J Bone Miner Res* 1994;9(Suppl 1):136
17. Thomas T, Lafage MH, Alexandre C. Atypical osteomalacia after 2 years etidronate intermittent cyclic administration in osteoporosis. *J Rheumatol* 1995;22:11

18. Storm T, Thamsborg G, Kollerup G, Sorensen HA. Five years of intermittent cyclical etidronate therapy increases bone mass and reduces vertebral fracture rates in postmenopausal osteoporosis. *Bone Miner* 1992;17(Suppl 1):24
19. Jackson RD, Harris ST, Genant HK, *et al.* Cyclical etidronate treatment of postmenopausal osteoporosis: 4-year experience. *Bone Miner* 1992;17 (Suppl 1):154
20. Miller P, Huffer W, MacIntyre D, *et al.* Bone histomorphometry after long-term treatment with cyclical phosphorus and etidronate. *Bone Miner* 1992;17(Suppl 1):23
21. Storm T, Sorensen HA, Thamsborg G, *et al.* Bone histomorphometric changes after up to seven years of cyclical etidronate treatment. *J Bone Miner Res* 1996;11(Suppl 1):151
22. Plosker GL, Goa KL. Clodronate. A review of its pharmacological properties and therapeutic efficacy in resorptive bone disease. *Drugs* 1994; 47:945–82
23. Chesnut CH. Synthetic calcitonin, diphosphonates and anabolic steroids in the treatment of postmenopausal osteoporosis. In Christiansen C, Arnaud CD, Nordin BEC, *et al.*, eds. *Osteoporosis 1984.* Copenhagen: Osteopress Publishers, 1984: 594–655
24. Giannini S, D'Angelo A, Malvasi L, *et al.* Effects of one-year cyclical treatment with clodronate on postmenopausal bone loss. *Bone* 1993;14:137–41
25. McCloskey EV, de Takats D, Pande K, *et al.* Oral clodronate prevents bone loss in elderly women over 3 years of treatment. *J Bone Miner Res* 1999;14 (Suppl 1):525
26. Rossini M, Braga V, Gatti D, Gerardi D, Zamberlan N, Adami S. Intramuscular clodronate therapy in postmenopausal osteoporosis. *Bone* 1999;24:125–9
27. Filipponi P, Pedetti M, Fedell L, *et al.* Cyclical clodronate is effective in preventing postmenopausal bone loss: a comparative study with transcutaneous hormone replacement therapy. *J Bone Miner Res* 1995;10:697–703
28. Filipponi P, Cristallini S, Rizzello E, *et al.* Cyclical intravenous clodronate in postmenopausal osteoporosis: results of a long-term clinical trial. *Bone* 1996;18:179–84
29. Filipponi P, Cristallini S, Rizzello E, Policani G, Gregorio F, Boldrini S. 6-year cyclical intravenous clodronate in postmenopausal osteoporosis: effect on bone mass and vertebral fractures. *Osteoporosis Int* 1996;6(Suppl 1):260
30. Herrala J, Puolijoki H, Liipo K, *et al.* Clodronate is effective in preventing corticosteroid-induced bone loss among asthmatic patients. *Bone* 1998;22: 577–82
31. Valkema R, Vismans FJE, Papapoulos SE, Pauwels EKJ, Bijvoet OLM. Maintained improvement in calcium balance and bone mineral content in patients with osteoporosis treated with the bisphosphonate APD. *Bone Miner* 1989;5:183–92
32. Reid IR, Wattie DJ, Evans MC, Gamble GD, Stapleton JP, Cornish J. Continuous therapy with pamidronate, a potent bisphosphonate, in postmenopausal osteoporosis. *J Clin Endocrinol Metab* 1994;79:1595–9
33. Lufkin EG, Argueta R, Whitaker MD, *et al.* Pamidronate: an unrecognized problem in gastrointestinal tolerability. *Osteoporosis Int* 1994;4:320–2
34. Devogelaer JP, Esselinckx W, Nagant de Deuxchaisnes CA. A randomized, controlled trial of APD (disodium pamidronate) given intravenously with and without sodium fluoride in involutional osteoporosis. *J Bone Miner Res* 1992;5 (Suppl 2):252
35. Toolan BC, Shea M, Myers ER, *et al.* Effects of 4-amino-1-hydroxybutylidene bisphosphonate on bone biomechanisms in rats. *J Bone Miner Res* 1992;7:1399–406
36. Balena R, Toolan BC, Shea M, *et al.* The effects of 2-year treatment with the aminobisphosphonate alendronate on bone metabolism, bone histomorphometry, and bone strength in ovariectomized nonhuman primates. *J Clin Invest* 1993;92: 2577–86
37. Hosking DJ, McClung MR, Ravin P, *et al.* Alendronate in the prevention of osteoporosis: EPIC study two-year results. *J Bone Miner Res* 1996;11(Suppl 1):133
38. Chesnut CH, McClung MR, Ensrud KE, *et al.* Alendronate treatment of the postmenopausal osteoporotic woman: effect of multiple dosages on bone mass and bone remodeling. *Am J Med* 1995; 99:144–52
39. Devogelaer JP, Broll H, Correa-Rotter R, *et al.* Oral alendronate induces progressive increases in bone mass of the spine, hip, and total body over 3 years in postmenopausal women with osteoporosis. *Bone* 1996;18:141–50
40. Liberman U, Weiss SR, Broll J, *et al.* Effect of oral alendronate on bone mineral density and the incidence of fractures in postmenopausal osteoporosis. *N Engl J Med* 1995;333:1437–43
41. Black DM, Cummings SR, Thompson D. Alendronate reduces the risk of vertebral and clinical fractures in women with existing vertebral fractures: results of the Fracture Intervention Trial. *Lancet* 1996;348:1535–41
42. Cummings SR, Black DM, Thompson EE, *et al.* Effect of alendronate on risk of fracture in women with low bone density but without vertebral fractures. *J Am Med Assoc* 1998;280:2077–82
43. Hochberg M, Ross P, Black D, *et al.* for the Fracture Intervention Trial Research Group. Larger increases in bone mineral density during alendronate therapy are associated with a lower risk of new vertebral fractures in women with

postmenopausal osteoporosis. *Arthritis Rheum* 1999;42:1246–54
44. De Groen PC, Lubbe DF, Hirsch LJ, *et al.* Esophagitis associated with the use of alendronate. *N Engl J Med* 1996;335:1016–21
45. Maconi G, Porro GB. Multiple ulcerative esophagitis caused by alendronate. *Am J Gastroenterol* 1995; 90:1889–90
46. Leung A, Heyden N, Czachur M, Gilbert J, Daifotis A, Yates AJ. Update of alendronate safety in clinical trials. *J Bone Miner Res* 1999;14(Suppl 1):525
47. Johnell O, Scheele W, Lu Y, Lakshmanan M. Effects of raloxifene (RLN), alendronate (ALN) and RLX + ALN on bone mineral density (BMD) and biochemical markers of bone turnover in postmenopausal women with osteoporosis. *J Bone Miner Res* 1999;14(Suppl 1):157
48. Muhlbauer RC, Bauss F, Schenk R, *et al.* Ibandronate, a potent new bisphosphonate to inhibit bone resorption. *J Bone Miner Res* 1991;6:1003–11
49. Ravin P, Clemmensen B, Riis J, Christiansen C. The effect on bone mass and bone markers of different doses of ibandronate - a new bisphosphonate for prevention and treatment of postmenopausal osteoporosis. A 1-year, randomized, double-blind, placebo-controlled dose-finding study. *Bone* 1996; 19:527–33
50. Thiebaud D, Burckhardt P, Kriegbaum H, *et al.* Three monthly intravenous injections of ibandronate in the treatment of postmenopausal osteoporosis. *Am J Med* 1997;103:298–307
51. Tobias JH, Laversuch CV, Wilson N, Robins P. Neridronate preferentially suppresses the urinary excretion of peptide-bound deoxypyridinoline in postmenopausal women. *Calcif Tissue Int* 1996;59: 407–9
52. Ammann P, Rizzoli R, Caverzasio J, Shigematsu T, Slosman D, Bonjour J-P. Effects of the bisphosphonate tiludronate on bone resorption, calcium balance, and bone mineral density. *J Bone Miner Res* 1993;8:1491–8
53. Geusens P, Nijs J, Van Der Perre G, *et al.* Longitudinal effect of tiludronate on bone mineral density, resonant frequency, and strength in monkeys. *J Bone Miner Res* 1992;7:599–609
54. Chastagnier D, Barbier A, de Vernejoul MC, Geusens P, Lacheretz F. Effects of two bisphosphonates (tiludronate and etidronate) on bone healing. *J Bone Miner Res* 1993;8(Suppl 1):236
55. Reginster JY, Colson F, Morlock G, Combe B, Ethgen D, Geusens P. Evaluation of the efficacy and safety of oral tiludronate in Paget's disease of bone. A double-blind, multiple-dosage, placebo-controlled study. *Arthritis Rheum* 1992;35:967–74
56. Roux C, Gennari C, Farrerons J, *et al.* Comparative, prospective, double-blind, multicenter study of the efficacy of tiludronate and etidronate in Paget's disease of bone. *Arthritis Rheum* 1995;38:851–8
57. Reginster JY, Lecart MP, Deroisy R, *et al.* Prevention of postmenopausal bone loss by tiludronate. *Lancet* 1989;2:1469–71
58. Roux C, Deroisy R, Basse-Cathalinat B, *et al.* Prevention of early postmenopausal bone loss with oral tiludronate. *Osteoporosis Int* 1996;6(Suppl 1):249
59. Chappard D, Miner P, Privat C, *et al.* Effects of tiludronate on bone loss in paraplegic patients. *J Bone Miner Res* 1995;10:112–18
60. Reginster JY, Roux C, Christiansen C, Rouillon A, Tou C. Intermittent cyclical low dose tiludronate in treatment of postmenopausal osteoporosis. Report of two phase III European studies (2305 patients). *Bone* 1998;23:S594
61. Genant HK, Chesnut CH, Eisman JA, *et al.* Chronic intermittent cyclical administration of tiludronate in postmenopausal osteoporosis: report of two multicenter studies in 2316 patients. *Bone* 1998;23:S175
62. Wronski TJ, Yen CF, Scott KS. Estrogen and disphosphonate treatment provide long-term protection against osteopenia in ovariectomized rats. *J Bone Miner Res* 1991;6:387–94
63. Ettinger B, Genant H, Bekker P, Shen I, Axelrod D. A pilot three-year of risedronate in women with breast cancer and chemotherapy-induced menopause. *J Bone Miner Res* 1995;10(Suppl 1):198
64. Mortensen L, Charles P, Bekker P, Digennaro J, Johnston C. Risedronate increases bone mass in an early postmenopausal population: two years of treatment plus one year of follow up. *J Clin Endocrinol Metab* 1998;83:396–402
65. Langdahl B, Eriksen EF, Mortensen L, Charles P, Bekker P, Axelrod D. Histomorphometry from a three-year risedronate bone loss prevention study. *J Bone Miner Res* 1995;10(Suppl 1):199
66. Zegels B, Balena R, Eastell R, Russell RGG, Pack SE, Reginster JY. Effect of risedronate on collagen cross links in postmenopausal osteoporosis. *J Bone Miner Res* 1995;10(Suppl 1):455
67. Clemmensen B, Ravin P, Zegels B, Taquet AN, Christiansen C, Reginster JY. A two-year phase II study with 1-year of follow-up of risedronate (NE58095®) in postmenopausal osteoporosis. *Osteoporosis Int* 1997;7:488–95
68. Ribot C, Smith R, Fogelman I, *et al.* Risedronate increases bone mineral density and is well-tolerated in postmenopausal women with low bone mineral density. *J Bone Miner Res* 1999;14(Suppl 1):136
69. Watts N, Hangartner C, Chestnut C, *et al.* Risedronate treatment prevents vertebral and non vertebral fractures in women with postmenopausal osteoporosis. *Calcif Tissue Int* 1999;64:S98
70. Eastell R, Minner H, Sorensen O, *et al.* Risedronate reduces fracture risk in women with established postmenopausal osteoporosis. *Calcif Tissue Int* 1999; 64:S99

71. Eriksen E, Melsen F, Brown J, *et al.* Three years of risedronate treatment significantly decreases bone turnover without impairing mineralization. *J Bone Miner Res* 1999;14(Suppl 1):404
72. Watts N, Roux C, Genant H, *et al.* Risedronate reduces vertebral fracture risk after the first year of treatment in postmenopausal women with established osteoporosis. *J Bone Miner Res* 1999;14(Suppl 1):136
73. Vieth R, Chan PC, MacFarlane GD. Randomized, prospective evaluation of effectiveness and safety of vitamin D_3 intake exceeding the lowest observed adverse effect level. *J Bone Miner Res* 1999;14(Suppl 1):538

Effects of menopause and estrogen replacement therapy on cerebral blood flow in women

52

T. Ohkura

INTRODUCTION

Estrogen influences hemodynamics to increase cardiac output and decrease peripheral vascular resistance in women taking oral contraceptives[1], in those undergoing ovulation induction[2] and in pregnant women[3]. Doppler studies have revealed that estrogen replacement therapy (ERT) reduces the pulsatility index in the internal carotid[4] and middle cerebral arteries[5]. However, little information is available concerning the effect of ERT on cerebral and cerebellar blood flows. Furthermore, there are no reports on the effect of the menopause on cerebral and cerebellar blood flows.

The present studies were designed to investigate the effect of the menopause on cerebral and cerebellar blood flows in women (Study I) and the effect of ERT alone or ERT with short-term administration of medroxyprogesterone acetate (MPA) on cerebral and cerebellar blood flows in postmenopausal women (Study II). The cerebral and cerebellar blood flows were measured quantitatively using the technetium-99m-ethylcysteinate dimer (^{99m}Tc-ECD) and single photon emission computed tomography (SPECT).

Data are presented as means ± SD. Statistical analyses were carried out using a paired or unpaired Student's *t* test.

STUDY I

The cerebral and cerebellar blood flows were measured using ^{99m}Tc-ECD and SPECT in 39 women aged 43–50 years, of whom 17 were premenopausal with a mean age of 47.4 ± 2.4 years and 22 were postmenopausal with a mean age of 47.3 ± 2.4 years. The mean cerebral blood flow of 43.7 ± 4.1 ml/100 g per min in the postmenopausal women was significantly lower than that of 48.0 ± 2.4 ml/100 g per min in the premenopausal women ($p < 0.001$). The mean cerebellar blood flow of 47.5 ± 4.7 ml/100 g per min in the postmenopausal women was also significantly lower than that in the premenopausal women ($p < 0.0001$). The serum estradiol level was taken to be 10 pg/ml when it was < 10pg/ml. The mean serum estradiol levels were 86.8 ± 60.3 pg/ml in the premenopausal women ($n = 17$) and 10.0 ± 0.0 pg/ml in the postmenopausal women ($n = 22$). There were no significant differences in the mean values of mean blood pressure, hemoglobin levels and hematocrit between pre- and postmenopausal women. These results suggest that both the cerebral blood flow and the cerebellar blood flow decrease after the menopause.

STUDY II

Short-term ERT alone or ERT with short-term administration of MPA

Forty-five postmenopausal women were divided into three groups (groups A, B and C). Each group consisted of 15 women. Another 11 women were recruited as a control group (group D). Their treatment and mean age are shown in Table 1. The cerebral and cerebellar blood flows were measured before and on the 21st day of treatment. Subjects in the control group received neither conjugated equine estrogen nor placebo and their cerebral and cerebellar blood flows were measured twice at intervals of 3 weeks. The cerebral and cerebellar blood flows in group A were significantly increased during ERT ($p < 0.0001$), and the percentage

Table 1 Treatment of subjects with estrogen replacement therapy (ERT) alone or ERT combined with short-term administration of medroxyprogesterone acetate (MPA)

Group	*ERT/HRT*	*Patients (n)*	*Duration of treatment*	*Mean age (± SD) of patients* (years)
A	CEE 0.625 mg/day	15	3 weeks	52.5 ± 4.4
B	CEE 1.25 mg/day	15	3 weeks	51.4 ± 4.5
C	CEE 0.625–1.25 mg/day combined with MPA 5–10 mg/day	15	CEE for 3 weeks and MPA for 8–12 days	50.9 ± 7.8
D	Control*	11	(3 weeks)*	53.1 ± 5.4
E	CEE with or without MPA	21	HRT for > 1 year†	50.8 ± 5.1

*Subjects in the control group received neither conjugated equine estrogen (CEE) nor placebo, and their cerebral and cerebellar blood flows were measured twice at intervals of 3 weeks; †a mean duration of 14.0 ± 2.2 months; HRT, hormone replacement therapy

increases were 7.4 ± 5.4% and 6.5 ± 4.9%, respectively. The cerebral and cerebellar blood flows in group B were significantly increased during ERT ($p < 0.001$), the percentage increases being 7.7 ± 5.4% and 6.0 ± 4.5%, respectively. The cerebral and cerebellar blood flows in group C were also significantly increased during ERT ($p < 0.001$ and $p < 0.0001$, respectively), and the percentage increases were 7.2 ± 5.5% and 6.4 ± 4.1%, respectively.

Long-term ERT/hormone replacement therapy (HRT)

At a mean duration of 14.0 ± 2.2 months after the first cerebral and cerebellar blood flow measurements, the third cerebral and cerebellar blood flow measurements were performed on 21 out of 45 women in groups A, B and C in the same way as in the above-mentioned Study I. They received HRT for more than 1 year following treatment in Study I (group E) (Table 1). Our HRT regimen consisted of sequential conjugated equine estrogen and MPA therapy: the subjects received 0.625–1.25 mg/day of conjugated equine estrogen from days 1 to 25 and 5–10 mg/day of MPA from days 14 to 25 of estrogen treatment.

The cerebral and cerebellar blood flows in group E were also significantly increased at more than 1 year ($p < 0.001$ and $p < 0.0002$, respectively), the percentage increases being 6.2 ± 5.9% and 7.6 ± 7.5%, respectively.

The results of Study I and Study II revealed that there were no significant differences in the percentage increases in cerebral blood flow between ERT with conjugated equine estrogen 0.625 mg/day and ERT with conjugated equine estrogen 1.25 mg/day, and that short- and long-term ERT, as well as sequential conjugated equine estrogen and MPA therapy, significantly increased the cerebral and cerebellar blood flows in postmenopausal women.

DISCUSSION

Study I may be the first report demonstrating the effect of the menopause on the cerebral and cerebellar blood flows. However, the number of premenopausal women was smaller than that of postmenopausal women. Furthermore, the study was only cross-sectional. A further investigation including a longitudinal study is needed.

We have previously reported that ERT increases the cerebral and cerebellar blood flows[6] and the regional cerebral blood flow[7] in nine postmenopausal women (mean age ± SE: 43.7 ± 2.5 years), including young prematurely menopausal women and those who have undergone surgical menopause. Both cerebral and cerebellar blood flows were significantly increased during ERT, and the mean percentage increases in cerebral blood flow and cerebellar blood flow were 29.5 ± 10.2% and 29.3 ± 10.4%, respectively[7].

In Study II, the cerebral and cerebellar blood flows were significantly increased by 3 weeks of ERT in postmenopausal women without premature menopause. There were no significant differences between the two doses used (0.625 mg/day and 1.25 mg/day) and sequential conjugated equine estrogen and MPA therapy in the percentage increases in cerebral or cerebellar blood flow. The cerebral and cerebellar blood flows were also significantly increased with long-term ERT/HRT for more than 1 year. The percentage increases in the cerebral and cerebellar blood flows with long-term ERT/HRT were as high as those with 3 weeks of ERT. Furthermore, the percentage increases in the cerebral and cerebellar blood flows with sequential conjugated equine estrogen and MPA therapy were as high as those with conjugated equine estrogen alone. However, changes in the cerebral and cerebellar blood flows during combined, continuous conjugated equine estrogen and MPA therapy remain to be determined.

The mechanisms by which estrogen causes systemic vasodilatation have not been clarified sufficiently, but the following possible mechanisms may be considered. Estrogen affects endothelium-derived vasodilators such as prostacyclin[8] and nitric oxide[9]. Another possible mechanism is that estrogen exerts a direct effect on arterial tone because vascular smooth muscle cells possess estrogen receptors and respond to estrogen[10]. Furthermore, estrogen demonstrates calcium-antagonistic properties by blocking voltage-sensitive calcium channels in human aortic smooth muscle[11].

In the present study, the percentage increases in the cerebral and cerebellar blood flows were much bigger in younger postmenopausal women, including prematurely menopausal women[6], than in postmenopausal women without premature menopause. The reasons why the percentage increases in young postmenopausal women were bigger have not been well elucidated, but the following possible reasons may be considered. First, the cerebral blood flow in both men and women decreases with age[12]. The cerebral blood flow may have responded to ERT better in younger postmenopausal women than in older postmenopausal women. Second, the first brain blood flow measurements were performed on younger postmenopausal women 4 weeks after HRT had been discontinued. In contrast, most of the postmenopausal women in the present study received ERT/HRT for the first time. The cerebral and cerebellar blood flows before ERT may have been decreased 4 weeks after discontinuation of HRT in younger postmenopausal women.

In summary, the results of Study I suggest that cerebral and cerebellar blood flows decrease after the menopause, and the results of Study II have revealed that ERT or HRT increases the cerebral and cerebellar blood flows in postmenopausal women. However, the effect of combined, continuous, conjugated equine estrogen and MPA therapy remains to be determined. Further investigations are needed to replicate these findings and to elucidate the effect of a continuous, combined regimen of estrogen and progestogen.

ACKNOWLEDGEMENTS

The studies were supported by Grants-in-Aid for Scientific Research from the Ministry of Education and Culture (No. 08671920) and by Health Sciences Research Grants from the Ministry of Health and Welfare (Comprehensive Research on Aging and Health; H10-Choju-007).

References

1. Lehtovirta P. Haemodynamic effects of combined oestrogen-progestogen oral contraceptives. *Obstet Gynaecol Br Commonw* 1974;81:517-25
2. Veille JV, Morton MJ, Burry K, Nemethy M, Speroff L. Estradiol and hemodynamics during ovulation induction. *J Clin Endocrinol Metab* 1986; 63:721-4
3. Mashini IS, Albazzaz SJ, Fadel HE, *et al.* Serial noninvasive evaluation of cardiovascular hemodynamics during pregnancy. *Am J Obstet Gynecol* 1987;156:1208-13
4. Gangar KF, Vyas S, Whitehead M, Crook D, Meire H, Campbell S. Pulsatility index in internal carotid

artery in relation to transdermal oestradiol and time since menopause. *Lancet* 1991;338:839–42

5. Penotti M, Nencioni T, Gabrielli L, Farina M, Castiglioni E, Polvani F. Blood flow variations in internal carotid and middle cerebral arteries induced by postmenopausal hormone replacement therapy. *Am J Obstet Gynecol* 1993;169:1226–32
6. Ohkura T, Teshima Y, Isse K, *et al.* Estrogen increases cerebral and cerebellar blood flows in postmenopausal women. *Menopause* 1995;2:13–18
7. Ohkura T, Matsuda H, Iwasaki N, *et al.* Effect of estrogen on regional cerebral blood flow in postmenopausal women. *J Jpn Menopause Soc* 1996;4: 254–61
8. Mueck AO, Seeger H, Korte K, Lippert TH. The effect of 17β-estradiol and endothelin 1 on prostacyclin and thromboxane production in human endothelial cell cultures. *Clin Exp Obstet Gynecol* 1996;20:203–6
9. Rosselli M, Imthurn B, Keller PJ, Jackson EK, Dubey RK. Circulating nitric oxide (nitrite/nitrate) levels in postmenopausal women substituted with 17β-estradiol and norethisterone acetate: a two-year follow-up study. *Hypertension* 1995;25: 848–53
10. Orimo A, Inoue S, Ikegami A, *et al.* Vascular smooth muscle cells as target for estrogen. *Biochem Biophys Res Commun* 1993;195:730–6
11. Mueck AO, Seeger H, Hanke H, Lippert TH. Calcium-antagonistic effect of estradiol compared with nifedipine, verapamil, and diltiazem – *in vitro* investigations in human aortic smooth muscle cells [Abstract]. *Menopause* 1995;2:262–3
12. Rodriguez G, Warkentin S, Risberg J, Rosadini G. Sex differences in regional cerebral blood flow. *J Cereb Blood Flow Metab* 1988;8:783–9

Phytoestrogens and cardiovascular risk 53

A. Pines

INTRODUCTION

On the verge of the new millennium, growing numbers of women seek traditional (so-called 'natural') remedies for the relief of various menopause-related symptoms. Recent studies showed that about 50% of postmenopausal women used at least one non-medically prescribed alternative medicine preparation[1,2]. This in part is due to the belief that natural substances are healthier and safer, but it also results from fears concerning breast cancer risk and other adverse effects of hormone replacement therapy (HRT). One of the most discussed issues relating to alternative medicine and the menopause is the alleged effects of phytoestrogens as a substitute for estrogen. Phytoestrogens have many favorable points to start with: they are abundant in nature, they have been well known for almost 5000 years and regular ingestion of a phytoestrogen-rich diet in early menopause has been linked with a lower frequency of acute menopausal symptoms[3,4]. Japanese women with their high intake of soy - a rich source of phytoestrogen - have a low incidence of breast cancer and few menopausal symptoms. However, while circumstantial evidence for the beneficial effects of phytoestrogens are increasing, large-scale, well-designed, definitive clinical trials on these issues are lacking, mainly because it is difficult to obtain funding for trials of an unpatentable product. Therefore, the effects of phytoestrogens on various organs and metabolic pathways await further verification and documentation.

Before discussing in detail the issue of phytoestrogens and cardiovascular risk, one should start with some introductory information on this group of substances[4-7]. Phytoestrogen is a general name that represents several chemical classes, among which the most important ones are the isoflavones and the lignans. After consumption, complex enzymatic metabolic conversions occur in the gastrointestinal tract; the metabolites enter the enterohepatic circulation and are excreted in the bile, feces and urine. Isoflavones that display estrogenic activity occur almost exclusively in legumes and beans. The structure of soy isoflavones (genistein (trihydroxyisoflavone) and daidzein (dihydroxyisoflavone)) is similar to that of estradiol; thus they have the capability of binding to the estrogen receptor. The reaction to this binding is tissue specific, varying from agonistic to antagonistic. Results from animal and human studies indicate that isoflavones may be defined as selective estrogen receptor modulators (SERMs), having an estrogenic effect at some sites (liver/lipoprotein metabolism, coronary arteries, bones and brain), but being antiestrogenic at other sites (endometrium and breast). The recent identification of two types of estrogen receptor (ER) makes this situation even more complex, since it was found that the affinity of isoflavones to ERβ was much greater than to ERα, although any reaction to isoflavones is only 1‰ of that caused by estradiol[7]. The anti-proliferative effects of phytoestrogen have also been described in estrogen receptor-negative cell lines, which raises the possibility that isoflavones may work through other mechanisms that are not related to estrogen.

CHOLESTEROL AND ISOFLAVONES

The association between isoflavones and the lipid profile is well documented. Studies in male and female monkeys showed that supplementation of intact soy protein had a hypocholesterolemic effect, while feeding with soy protein depleted of isoflavones was less effective[8]. In another monkey study[9], the soy plus isoflavones diet was indeed superior to soy protein alone with regard to lowering lipid levels; however, the soy itself had more effect than another source of protein - caseine/lactoalbumin. This raises the question of whether some of the beneficial effect is related to the soy protein itself or to traces of isoflavones left after extraction.

Studies in humans have been less conclusive, perhaps because of the variety of sources and amounts of soy protein consumed, as well as different selection of subjects and different protocols employed. A meta-analysis of 38 studies on the effect of soy protein on lipid levels concluded that ingestion of such diets (average 47 g/day) resulted in a net decrease of 23 mg/dl in serum cholesterol, a decrease of 22 mg/dl in low-density lipoprotein (LDL)-cholesterol, a minor but not significant increase in high-density lipoprotein (HDL)-cholesterol and a decrease of 13 mg/dl in triglycerides[10]. The benefit was marginal for persons with a normal baseline lipid profile, while those in the higher quartiles of cholesterol concentrations at baseline showed the most remarkable results. Recent studies referred to the lipid-lowering effect of isoflavones *per se* rather than soy protein. In a short-term clinical trial in perimenopausal women aged 45–55 years, three diet supplements were tested[11]. The study had a cross-over design consisting of 6-week intervention periods. Participants had a supplement of 20 g of carbohydrates, or 20 g of soy protein which included 34 mg of phytoestrogen on a once daily regimen, or the same soy protein but in divided portions to be consumed twice daily. This particular soy supplement contained about half of the average daily intake of phytoestrogens in a Japanese diet. In both soy groups total cholesterol declined by 6% and the LDL fraction was 7% lower by the end of 6 weeks. There were no significant changes in HDL-cholesterol or in triglycerides.

There have been several recent small-scale studies, however, which concluded that there was no effect of phytoestrogen on lipids. In the study of Nestel and colleagues[12] only 21 women participated; some were still perimenopausal, some had discontinued HRT just 6 weeks prior to the beginning of the study and some were vegetarians. This was a placebo-controlled cross-over trial, using isoflavones 80 mg daily for 5 or 10 weeks. The study of Hodgson and co-workers[13] included mainly men, with only 13 postmenopausal women, of whom only six received isoflavones and seven were in the placebo group. Participants received one tablet daily containing 55 mg isoflavones for 8 weeks. It is important to note that in both the above studies the mean baseline cholesterol levels were normal, which may be consistent with the earlier mentioned data suggesting that the lipid-lowering effect of phytoestrogen is more evident in hypercholesterolemic persons. In a single study lipoprotein (a) levels remained unchanged with isoflavones[13]. No alterations in the ability of LDL to be oxidized *in vitro* were noted in one clinical trial[12], although few laboratory studies claimed that isoflavones possess anti-oxidant properties[14,15].

Other cardiovascular risk factors were rarely investigated in the context of isoflavone supplementation. There are scarce data on diabetes mellitus and isoflavones. In one study in monkeys, soy protein improved insulin sensitivity and glucose effectiveness, as determined by minimal model analyses[16]. No changes in serum glucose were noted in the aforementioned study of Nestel and associates[12]. As for the soy protein itself, unlike animal protein it is probably not harmful to renal function or to the extent of proteinuria in diabetics[17].

ISOFLAVONES AND BLOOD PRESSURE

One study mentioned a 5-mmHg drop in diastolic blood pressure in a small group taking isoflavones[11], yet Nestel and co-workers[12] found no difference between women on isoflavones and those on placebo, although for both groups there was a decrease in mean, systolic and diastolic pressures at the end of the study compared to baseline values.

ISOFLAVONES AND VASOMOTION

Several studies have investigated the effects of isoflavones on arterial tone, elasticity and compliance. A dilator response to acetylcholine was demonstrated in the atherosclerotic coronary arteries of female monkeys fed a diet high in isoflavones[18]. Nestel and colleagues reported two studies: the first[12] included peri- and postmenopausal women taking 80 mg isoflavones for 10 weeks. Systemic arterial compliance improved by 26% compared to the compliance in those taking placebo. No differences were recorded in brachial blood flow following a challenge with nitroprusside or acetylcholine, or after artery occlusion, but these parameters were measured in only a few women. In the second study[19], after 5 weeks of ingestion of 40 or 80 mg isoflavones derived from red clover, there was a 20% rise in arterial compliance as compared to the compliance after 5 weeks of placebo.

COAGULATION, ATHEROSCLEROSIS AND ISOFLAVONES

Genistein was found to have several anti-atherogenic properties. The most intriguing was its effect as a potent inhibitor of tyrosine kinase activity. Many growth factors work through the cellular receptors that increase the activity of tyrosine kinase. Genistein was able to reduce the action of those growth factors, among which were platelet-derived growth factor and fibroblast growth factor, which have an important role in vascular smooth muscle proliferation and atherosclerosis[4,20]. Genistein also interferes with thrombin-induced platelet activation, aggregation and deposition, and with thromboxane-induced platelet aggregation[21].

A more important issue, of course, is the possible association between isoflavones and coronary artery disease. Age-adjusted cardiac mortality rates are six-fold lower in Japan than in the USA in men aged 40–69 years, and eight-fold lower in women of similar ages[22]. Data suggest that, beside genetic and lifestyle differences between these populations which could contribute to coronary artery disease rates, a diet rich in soy protein could play a role in the reduction of atherosclerosis[23]. In a study on monkeys fed for 14 months with casein-lactalbumin as control, soy protein from which isoflavones were extracted, or isoflavone-intact soy protein, not only was the expected beneficial effect on the lipid profile recorded, but also the extent of atherosclerosis in the carotid artery was 85% lower in animals given isoflavones than in those given casein[9]. The group on soy protein from which isoflavones were extracted showed only a 50% decrease in plaque size and a small degree of lipid lowering, suggesting that either some isoflavones remained despite extraction or that the soy protein itself had an effect.

In conclusion, despite a vast amount of data on phytoestrogens, it is still not clear whether plant-derived estrogens are an adequate substitute for regular estrogens. A recent Editorial in the journal *Climacteric* had the title: 'Is there a proven place for phytoestrogens in the menopause?'[24]. The authors thought that currently there is no reliable evidence confirming a substantial role for phytoestrogens in the treatment of postmenopausal women. Another recent Editorial in *The Lancet* briefly discussed the use of phytoestrogens in menopausal women, but did not make any solid recommendations[25]. In the meantime, another concept has been developed, the essence of which is to combine low-dose estradiol and phytoestrogens for use in later stages of the menopause[16,26]. The role of phytoestrogen in this context would be two-fold: it might increase the beneficial effects of estrogen in certain organs and tissues, but hopefully would obviate the need for adding a progestagen, because of its anti-estrogenic effect on the endometrium and possible protective effects on the breast. The study of Wagner and colleagues[16] is encouraging, since the combined anti-atherosclerotic effect of estradiol and phytoestrogen was found to be greater than that of each compound alone. Another issue that is still open is the contribution of the soy protein itself to the attributed effects of phytoestrogen. Since the phytoestrogen market is evolving rapidly, I believe that in the next few years more data will be published that will clarify these unresolved questions.

References

1. Stadberg E, Mattsson L, Milsom I. The prevalence and severity of climacteric symptoms and the use of different treatment regimens in a Swedish population. *Acta Obstet Gynecol Scand* 1997;76:442-8
2. MacLennan AH, Wilson DH, Taylor AW. Prevalence and cost of alternative medicine in Australia. *Lancet* 1996;347:569-73
3. Barnes S. Evolution of the health benefits of soy isoflavones. *Proc Soc Exp Biol Med* 1998;217:386-92
4. Setchell KDR. Phytoestrogens: the biochemistry, physiology, and implications for human health of soy isoflavones. *Am J Clin Nutr* 1998;68(suppl): 1333S-46S
5. Bingham SA, Atkinson C, Liggins J, Bluck L, Coward A. Phyto-oestrogens: where are we now? *Br J Nutr* 1998;79:393-406
6. Murkies AL, Wilcox G, Davis SR. Phytoestrogens. *J Clin Endocrinol Metab* 1998;83:297-303
7. Cassidy A, Milligan S. How significant are environmental estrogens to women? *Climacteric* 1998;1: 229-42
8. Anthony MS, Clarkson TB, Hughes CL Jr, Morgan TM, Burke GL. Soybean isoflavones improve cardiovascular risk factors without affecting the reproductive system of peripubertal rhesus monkeys. *J Nutr* 1996;126:43-50
9. Anthony MS, Clarkson TB, Bullock BC, Wagner JD. Soy protein versus soy phytoestrogen in the prevention of diet-induced coronary artery atherosclerosis of male cynomolgus monkeys. *Arterioscler Thromb Vasc Biol* 1997;17:2524-31
10. Anderson JW, Johnstone BM, Cook-Newell ME. Meta-analysis of the effects of soy protein intake on serum lipids. *N Engl J Med* 1995;333:276-82
11. Washburn S, Burke GL, Morgan T, Anthony M. Effect of soy protein supplementation on serum lipoproteins, blood pressure, and menopausal symptoms in perimenopausal women. *Menopause* 1999;6:7-13
12. Nestel PJ, Yamashita T, Sasahara T, *et al.* Soy isoflavones improve systemic arterial compliance but not plasma lipids in menopausal and perimenopausal women. *Arterioscler Thromb Vasc Biol* 1997;17:3392-8
13. Hodgson JM, Puddey IB, Beilin LJ, Mori TA, Croft KD. Supplementation with isoflavonoid phytoestrogens does not alter serum lipid concentration: a randomized controlled trial in humans. *J Nutr* 1998;128:728-32
14. Wei H, Bowen R, Cai Q, Barnes S, Wang Y. Antioxidant and antipromotional effects of the soybean isoflavone genistein. *Proc Soc Exp Biol Med* 1995; 208:124-30
15. Tikkanen M, Wahala K, Ojala S, Vihma V, Aldercreutz H. Effect of phytoestrogen intake on low density lipoprotein oxidation resistance. *Proc Natl Acad Sci* 1998;95:3106-10
16. Wagner JD, Cefalu WT, Anthony MS, Litwak KN, Zhang L, Clarkson TB. Dietary soy protein and estrogen replacement therapy improve cardiovascular risk factors and decrease aortic cholesteryl ester content in ovariectomized cynomolgus monkeys. *Metabolism* 1997;46:698-705
17. Anderson JW, Blake JE, Turner J, Smith BM. Effects of soy protein on renal function and proteinuria in patients with type 2 diabetes. *Am J Clin Nutr* 1998;68(suppl):1347S-53S
18. Honore EK, Williams JK, Anthony MS, Clarkson TB. Soy isoflavones enhance coronary vascular reactivity in atherosclerotic female macaques. *Fertil Steril* 1997;67:148-54
19. Nestel PJ, Pomeroy S, Kay S, *et al.* Isoflavones from red clover improve systemic compliance but not plasma lipids in menopausal women. *J Clin Endocrinol Metab* 1999;84:895-8
20. Kim H, Peterson TG, Barnes S. Mechanisms of action of the soy isoflavone genistein: emerging role for its effects via transforming growth factor β signaling pathways. *Am J Clin Nutr* 1998;68(suppl): 1418S-25S
21. Wilcox JN, Blumenthal BF. Thrombotic mechanisms in atherosclerosis: potential impact of soy proteins. *J Nutr* 1995;125:631S-8S
22. Beaglehole R. International trends in coronary heart disease mortality, morbidity, and risk factors. *Epidemiol Rev* 1990;12:1-15
23. Anthony MS, Clarkson TB, Williams JK. Effects of soy isoflavones on atherosclerosis: potential mechanisms. *Am J Clin Nutr* 1998;68(suppl):1390S-3S
24. Ginsburg J, Prelevic GM. Is there a proven place for phytoestrogens in the menopause? *Climacteric* 1999; 2:75-8
25. Finkel E. Phyto-oestrogens: the way to postmenopausal health? *Lancet* 1999;352:1762
26. Clarkson TB, Anthony MS, Williams JK, Honore EK, Cline JM. The potential of soybean phytoestrogen for postmenopausal hormone replacement therapy. *Proc Soc Exp Biol Med* 1998;217:365-8

The role of bone turnover measurement in the management of osteoporosis

54

C. Christiansen

INTRODUCTION

The understanding of the pathophysiology of postmenopausal bone loss has improved significantly during the past decade and has placed the role of bone turnover in focus as an independent risk factor for osteoporosis. Increased bone turnover results in bone loss and perhaps a deterioration of bone structure. Bone turnover is reflected by the concentration in serum and urine of enzymes involved in the turnover processes or by products that are released during bone formation or bone degradation. Assessment of these so-called 'biochemical markers of bone turnover' has rapidly improved in specificity and sensitivity within the past 5 years. Furthermore, the understanding of the indication for use and the interpretation of results are evolving. The potential roles of these markers are discussed in this paper.

BONE TURNOVER: MODELLING AND REMODELLING

Bone is continuously being turned over by the two processes of modelling and remodelling. In the former, which takes place principally in the child, new bone is formed at a location different from the one destroyed. This results in a change in the shape of the skeleton. In remodelling, which is the main process in the adult, resorption and formation occur in the same place, so that no change occurs in the shape of the bone. Both modelling and remodelling, however, result in the replacement of old bone by new bone. This allows the mechanical integrity of the skeleton to be maintained. The turnover also allows the bone to play its role as an ion bank.

As mentioned, bone remodelling consists of two processes: bone resorption and bone formation and the sequence is always the same. The process is performed by small, geographically defined assemblies of cells, the basic multicellular units (BMUs). In response to stimulation by unknown factors, a number of osteoclasts gather and start to resorb bone, thus producing minute resorption lacunae (Howship's lacunae). This resorption phase is followed by a formation phase, in which a group of osteoblasts lay down organic bone matrix (osteoid) in the resorption lacunae. Eventually the osteoid is mineralized. Resorption is always followed by formation - a phenomenon called 'coupling'.

There are several ways in which the remodelling system can change or fail. The number of (active) BMUs throughout the skeleton may vary, the speed at which each BMU works may vary and an imbalance between the resorption and formation processes may occur.

The remodelling rate is between 2 and 10% of the skeletal mass per year. It is increased by parathyroid hormone, thyroxine, growth hormone and 1,25-$(OH)_2$ vitamin D, and it is decreased by calcitonin, estrogen and glucocorticosteroids. It is also modulated by mechanical conditions. The cancellous bone, which represents about 20% of the skeletal mass, makes up 80% of the turnover, while the cortex, which represents 80% of the bone, makes up only 20% of the turnover.

For some years after cessation of growth, bone mass probably increases to consolidate the skeleton. At skeletal maturity, men have 50% more skeletal mass than women. It is not certain at what age peak bone mass is achieved, and it may vary from one society to another according to many different factors. At a certain point thereafter, the skeletal mass will start to decrease, i.e. bone density decreases whereas bone size and shape stay more or less the same (with a few exceptions). The bone loss in men seems to follow a linear function. This age-related loss of bone has been compared to the loss of other functions with age, e.g. that of muscle mass. The bone loss in men is low, probably in the order of 3–5% per decade, which explains the rather low incidence of osteoporotic fractures in men.

In women the process is more complicated. Bone loss before the menopause is small and probably parallels that in men. However, significant premenopausal bone loss may occur in women with conditions that affect estrogen production. It is not known how large a proportion of premenopausal women have relative estrogen deficiency, and whether this proportion increases/changes with changing life style, habits, stress, birth rate, etc. Around the menopause, however, bone loss accelerates, averaging 2% per year. This bone loss continues for many years after the menopause and is still present in elderly and old women[1]. The accelerated postmenopausal bone loss and the relatively lower peak bone mass explains why osteoporosis is much more common in women than in men. The rate of loss in the postmenopausal years varies from one woman to another, ranging from less than 1% to more than 5% per year.

The bone turnover in postmenopausal women is characterized by increased bone resorption and bone formation. The postmenopausal bone loss implies that there is more bone resorption than bone formation (Figure 1). Women have increased bone turnover for many years after the menopause - probably for the rest of their lives - and therefore also increased bone loss. The higher the bone turnover, the larger the difference between bone resorption and bone formation, and the larger the resulting rate of bone loss.

THE BIOCHEMISTRY OF BONE TURNOVER

The rate of formation and degradation of the bone tissue can be assessed in blood and urine by measuring enzymatic activity or bone matrix components released into the circulation during formation or resorption. The measured parameters have been separated into markers of formation and resorption, but in disease states where both events are coupled and change in the same direction,

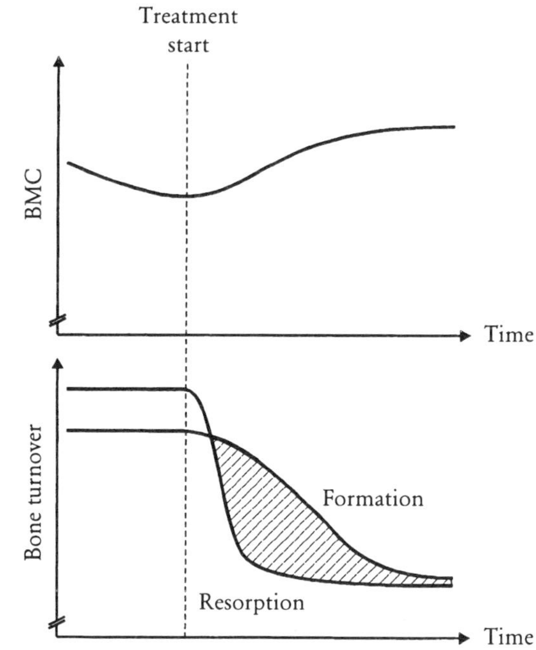

Figure 1 Changes in bone mineral content (BMC) and bone turnover with age

either of these markers will reflect the overall rate of bone turnover. Bone markers cannot discriminate between turnover changes of a specific skeletal envelope, i.e. trabecular versus cortical, but reflect the overall net changes of resorption and formation. These markers are of unequal specificity and sensitivity, which implies that it is not yet possible to estimate the net excess of resorption over formation by comparing the relative increase of a resorption marker over a formation marker. Circulating levels of these markers can be influenced by factors other than bone turnover such as their metabolic clearance (liver uptake, renal excretion and/or trapping on bone hydroxyapatite), and by the pattern of immunoreactive moieties recognized by a given antibody. Thus, each of these assays has to be carefully validated in a specific clinical situation before conclusions about its clinical utility can be drawn.

In contrast to metabolic bone diseases such as Paget's disease of bone or renal osteodystrophy, which are both characterized by dramatic changes of bone turnover, the postmenopausal bone turnover is a condition where moderate modifications of the bone remodelling activity can lead to a substantial loss of bone mass after a long period of time. Consequently, there have been efforts to develop specific and sensitive biochemical markers of bone turnover that are able to detect such moderate changes in bone remodelling. Table 1 gives a list of available markers.

POTENTIAL USE OF BIOCHEMICAL MARKERS

Below is listed a number of diagnostic potentials for the assessment of biochemical markers of bone remodelling:

Table 1 Biochemical markers of bone turnover

Markers of bone resorption	*Markers of bone formation*
CTX (CrossLaps)	total alkaline phosphatase
NTX (Osteomark)	bone alkaline phosphatase
Pyridinolone and Deoxy-Pyr	osteocalcin
Calcium	free bone Gla protein
Hydroxyproline	P1CP and P1NP
TRAP	
Hydroxylysine	
1CTP	

(1) What effect do the menopause and therapy have on bone turnover?

(2) What is the rate of bone loss?

(3) Does an instituted therapy have the expected effect?

The effect of menopause and therapy

Figure 2a shows the effect of the menopause on several parameters of bone formation and resorption. The menopause has a substantial effect on most of the markers. There are differences in terms of percentage increase and variation including biological variation (the scatter around the mean). Often, the markers increase to a level reaching the upper end of the normal premenopausal range. The parameters of bone degradation generally increase mostly as a response to the menopause, when compared to the other markers. However, these markers also showed a relatively large scatter around the mean.

Figure 2b shows the effect of hormone replacement therapy (HRT) on the different biochemical markers. Again, generally all markers decrease in

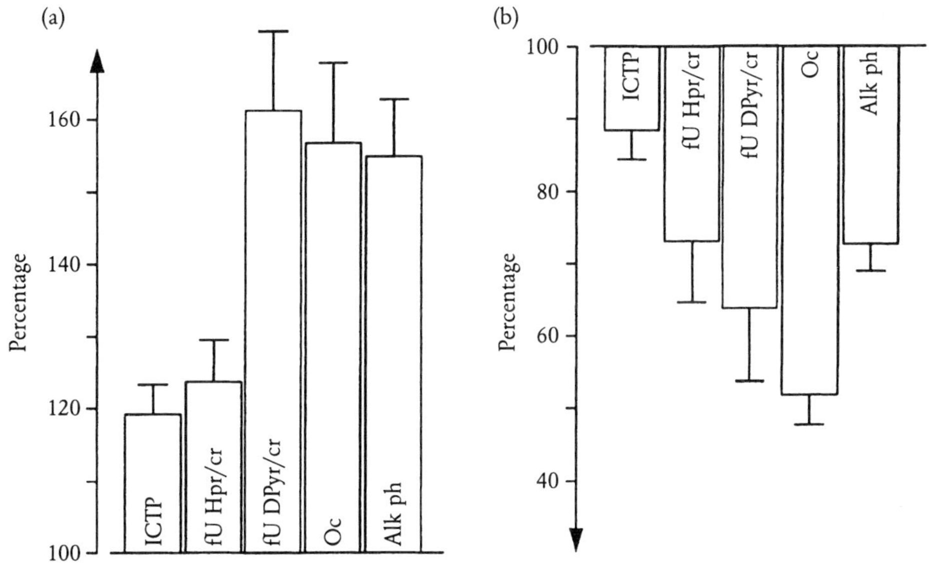

Figure 2 The effect of the menopause (a) and hormone replacement therapy (b) on biochemical markers of bone resorption and bone formation. (a) Mean ± SEM of measurements in 44 postmenopausal women given as a percentage of mean premenopausal values. (b) Changes after 1 year of hormone replacement therapy in 20 postmenopausal women (mean ± SEM, percentage of initial values). ICTP, serum carboxy-terminal telopeptide of type I collagen; fU Hpr/cr and fU DPyr/cr, fasting urinary excretion of hydroxyproline and deoxypyridinoline corrected for creatinine; Oc, serum osteocalcin; Alk ph, serum total alkaline phosphatase

response to therapy - some decreases are more pronounced than others.

Rate of bone loss

Decreased bone mass is the main risk factor for sustaining a fracture as a result of minor trauma or even no trauma. This has been supported by several retrospective and longitudinal studies[1,2]. Bone loss, by simply decreasing the bone mass, is probably an important determinant of fracture risk, but other factors associated with bone loss such as development of micro-architectural abnormalities and micro-damage could also contribute[3].

Some individuals lose bone at a more rapid rate than others, and this rapid rate may persist in some of these individuals over a period of years[4-6]. Such rapid loss could result in trabecular damage and additional risk of fracture above that contributed by the loss of bone alone. It is also possible that even a relatively short period (2-3 years) of rapid bone loss might contribute to perforation of trabecular bone and thus to increased fracture incidence.

Long-term prospective studies of bone loss from the spine and hip have yet to be published, owing primarily to the more recent availability of techniques to measure these sites. However, the same group of women was followed from the menopause (range: 6 months to 3 years after the last menstruation) prospectively for 15 years[5]. At baseline, the women were stratified according to the rate of bone loss[6]. Those women with an estimated rate of loss above 3% per year in the first 2 following years were called fast bone losers and those with a bone loss below this were called normal bone losers. The bone mineral density was similar in the two groups at baseline.

At 15 years, determination of biochemical markers of bone resorption (CrossLaps) and formation (osteocalcin) revealed that the fast bone losers had significantly higher bone turnover than the normal bone losers (Table 2). Furthermore, the fast bone losers had lower bone mineral density at all sites of the skeleton (forearm, spine, hip), when compared to the normal bone losers. The difference was approximately 10%, which is equivalent to approximately one standard deviation. The role of baseline bone mass and rate of loss on fracture

Table 2 Biochemical markers of bone turnover at 15 years in the groups of fast and normal bone losers, as they were defined 15 years ago

	Fast bone losers (n = 49)	*Normal bone losers* (n = 133)
Height (cm)	161.6 5.8	160.2 5.6
Weight (kg)	62.9 12.5*	67.3 12.7
CrossLaps/Cr (nmol/mol)	0.43 0.17**	0.33 0.14
Osteocalcin (ng/ml)	11.0 4.8**	9.0 4.8

* $p < 0.01$; ** $p < 0.001$

risk was evaluated. The data showed that a low baseline bone mass (below −1SD) and a fast rate of loss predisposed to fracture to the same extent (odds ratio 1.9 and 2.0, respectively, both $p < 0.05$). A combination of a low baseline bone mass and a fast rate of loss increased the odds ratio of suffering a fracture to 3.0.

Another more recent prospective study of risk factors for hip fractures conducted in a large cohort of healthy elderly women in France supports this hypothesis[7]. In those women who had a hip fracture within a 2-year follow-up, baseline measurements of urinary CrossLaps and Pyrilinks-D (an immunoassay of D-pyr) were higher than in non-fractured controls; increased CrossLaps above the normal range of premenopausal women was associated with an 80% increase in the risk of hip fracture.

The biochemical markers of bone turnover reflect bone loss: the higher the markers the higher the rate of loss. A recent study[8,9] showed that CrossLaps correlated with the rate of bone loss with r values of 0.75 (forearm) and 0.79 (spine) (Table 3). If a bone loss of more than 3.0% per year is defined to be a risk factor, the use of a CrossLaps cut-off limit of 600 μg/mmol creatinine gave a diagnostic sensitivity of 73% and a specificity of 79%. Another group[10] found that levels of hydroxyproline, pyridinoline and deoxypyridinoline correlated with the spinal rate of loss, with r values of 0.66, 0.63 and 0.66, respectively (Table 3).

What should the clinician use now as criteria for preventive intervention against osteoporosis? A practical approach may be suggested. A measurement of bone mass should be made only when

Table 3 The correlation between a baseline value of a biochemical marker of bone turnover and the bone loss in the following 2 years in early postmenopausal women

Marker	*Forearm r value*	*Spine r value*
Urinary calcium	0.33	0.48
Urinary hydroxyproline	–	0.66
Urinary Pyr	–	0.63
Urinary D-Pyr	–	0.66
Osteocalcin	0.52	0.48
T-AP	0.28	0.25

intervention to prevent bone loss can be prescribed and will be accepted. Most commonly such a measurement would take place at the menopause, when intervention with HRT is considered, but other forms of therapy are under development for which similar criteria could be applied. If the measurement was greater than 1SD above the mean for normal young women, no further measurement would be needed and no intervention undertaken. If the measurement was lower than −1SD below the mean for normal young women, intervention would be recommended (provided no contraindications were present). For those within ± 1SD, the bone mass measurement could be repeated in 1-5 years. A measurement at 1 year would probably detect the extremely fast bone losers, but a clinically relevant bone loss of 3% per year could often be within the error of the method used to measure bone density[11]. Waiting for 5 years could thus result in a 15-30% loss of bone mass before treatment was instituted. Alternatively, a determination of one of two biochemical markers of bone turnover could reveal the rate of loss.

Does the intervention have the expected effect?

There have been some indications that the biochemical markers may aid in choosing the treatment that will yield the best result.

In a study by Civitelli and associates[12], elderly women with osteoporotic fractures were treated with salmon calcitonin. A retrospective analysis of the data showed that the women with baseline high bone turnover had the highest response to treatment in bone mineral density. Corresponding results have been reported by Overgaard and colleagues[13], but the area needs further investigation.

It is a common request from physicians and patients that an instituted therapy should be proved to be effective. The efficacy of prevention and treatment of bone loss and osteoporosis may be followed up by serial bone mass measurements. Because of the relatively small changes in bone mass and the precision of the bone mass measurement methods, which is of a magnitude comparable to the changes in bone mass, this procedure may take an unacceptably long time. It is possible, however, that the biochemical markers may be useful to predict the effect of therapy. The advantage of using the biochemical markers is that they change 50–100% in response to HRT within a few months, whereas the precision of the methods is in the area of 5%. This gives a beneficial change : precision ratio when compared to bone mass measurements. Preliminary data show that the change in biochemical markers from baseline to 6 months' treatment correlates with the change in bone mass with an *r* value of 0.67 (data not shown). The data indicate that there is a large potential here for biochemical markers.

References

1. Gärdsell P, Johnell O, Nilsson BE. The predictive value of bone loss for fragility fractures in women: a longitudinal study over 15 years. *Calcif Tissue Int* 1991;49:90–4
2. Melton JL, Atkinson EJ, O'Fallon WM, Wahner HW, Riggs BL. Long-term fracture prediction by bone mineral assessed at different skeletal sites. *J Bone Miner Res* 1993;8:1227–33
3. Parfitt AM, Kleerekoper M, Villaneuva AR. Increased bone age: mechanisms and consequences. In Christiansen C, Jensen J, Riis BJ, *et al.*, eds. *Osteoporosis 1987. Proceedings of the International Symposium on Osteoporosis.* Copenhagen: Osteopress, 1987:301–8
4. Christiansen C, Riss BJ, Rødbro P. Prediction of rapid bone loss in postmenopausal women. *Lancet* 1987;1:1105–8
5. Hansen MA, Overgaard K, Riis BJ, Christiansen C. Role of osteoporosis; 12 year study. *Br Med J* 1991;303:961–4
6. Christiansen C, Riis BJ, Rødbro P. Screening procedure for women at risk of developing postmenopausal osteoporosis. *Osteoporosis Int* 1990;1:35–40
7. Garnero P, Hauscher E, Chapuy MC, *et al.* Markers of bone resorption predict hip fractures in elderly women: the EPIDOS prospective study. *J Bone Miner Res* 1995;10:1531–8
8. Qvist P, Bonde M, Rosenqvist C, Christiansen C. Use of a new biochemical marker (CrossLaps™) for the estimation of rate of postmenopausal bone loss. *J Bone Miner Res* 1994;9(Suppl 1):S334
9. Bonde M, Qvist P, Fledelius C, Riis BJ, Christiansen C. Applications of an enzyme immunoassay for a new marker of bone resorption (CrossLaps™) – follow up on hormone replacement therapy and osteoporosis risk assessment. *J Clin Endocrinol Metab* 1995;80:864–8
10. Kraenzlin ME, Kraenzlin CA, Haas HG. Comparison of the utility of various biochemical markers to predict bone loss in clinical practice. *J Bone Miner Res* 1994;9(Suppl 1):S157
11. Heaney RP. En recherche de la différence ($p < 0.05$). *Bone Miner* 1986;1:99–114
12. Civitelli R, Gonnelli S, Zacchei F, *et al.* Bone turnover in postmenopausal osteoporosis. Effect of calcitonin treatment. *J Clin Invest* 1988;82:1268–74
13. Overgaard K, Hansen MA, Herss Nielsen V-A, Riis BJ, Christiansen C. Discontinuous calcitonin treatment of established osteoporosis – effect of withdrawal of treatment. *Am J Med* 1990;89:1–6

Assessment of cortical and trabecular bone mass by pQCT

55

T. Sone and M. Fukunaga

INTRODUCTION

Osteoporosis is a disease characterized by a low bone mass and microarchitectural deterioration of the bone tissue, with a consequent increase in bone fragility and susceptibility to fracture[1]. A technique that measures information about the bone mass and microarchitecture should therefore provide the most accurate assessment of fracture risk. Currently, however, no validated technique to measure bone microarchitecture non-invasively exists and a bone mineral measurement has been shown to be the most important determinant of fracture risk. A variety of techniques are currently available to measure bone mass non-invasively: radiographic absorptiometry, single photon and single-energy X-ray absorptiometry, dual photon and dual-energy X-ray absorptiometry, standard quantitative computed tomography (QCT) and peripheral QCT (pQCT). Of these techniques, only QCT has the potential to measure true volumetric bone mineral density (BMD; g/cm^3), separating cortical and trabecular BMD. Since pQCT allows the assessment of purely trabecular bone, which has a greater metabolic activity than cortical bone, it may theoretically provide a more sensitive measure of fracture risk. In this article we will review the capabilities of pQCT in assessing the densitometric and architectural properties of the skeleton, and discuss the usefulness of pQCT in the diagnosis of postmenopausal osteoporosis.

pQCT INSTRUMENTS

Since 1976, pQCT has been used on a research basis[2], and it has recently become commercially available for measuring the radius, tibia and femur[3-6]. In Japan, more than 50 of the two different pQCT systems were installed by January 1998: the XCT-960 (Stratec, Birkenfeld, Germany) and the Densiscan-1000 (ScancoMedical, Zurich, Swizerland). The XCT-960 (or the new version, XCT-2000, which is now available) is based on a single-slice technique, while the Densiscan-1000 is based on a multi-slice technique to minimize sampling errors. Using the procedures recommended by the individual equipment manufacturer, regions of interest are automatically defined after identifying the appropriate external landmarks (Figure 1). Both machines measure equivalent sites in the distal radius. However, because of the different modes of operation (the Densiscan averages the results of ten contiguous slices over 14.5 mm thickness, whereas the Stratec measures a single slice of 2.5 mm thickness), the density values are not exactly comparable between the two machines. Unlike the Stratec machine, the Densiscan machine makes additional measurements at a more proximal site and also provides high-resolution images.

After the scan, the radius is segmented from the surrounding soft tissue using a thresholding algorithm (the Stratec machine) or using the contour detection algorithm (the Densiscan machine). The mean density of this area is defined as total bone density. Subsequently, 55% (the Stratec) or 50% (the Densiscan) of the area for the total BMD is peeled off concentrically. The mean density within the remaining 45 or 50% core area is defined as trabecular bone density. In the Stratec machine, the BMD of the cortical and subcortical region is also calculated using a thresholding algorithm, whereas the Densiscan utilizes total BMD at a more proximal site as a measure of the cortical bone density.

The cortical geometrical parameters are calculated using the pQCT images. These include cortical thickness, cross-sectional area and moment of

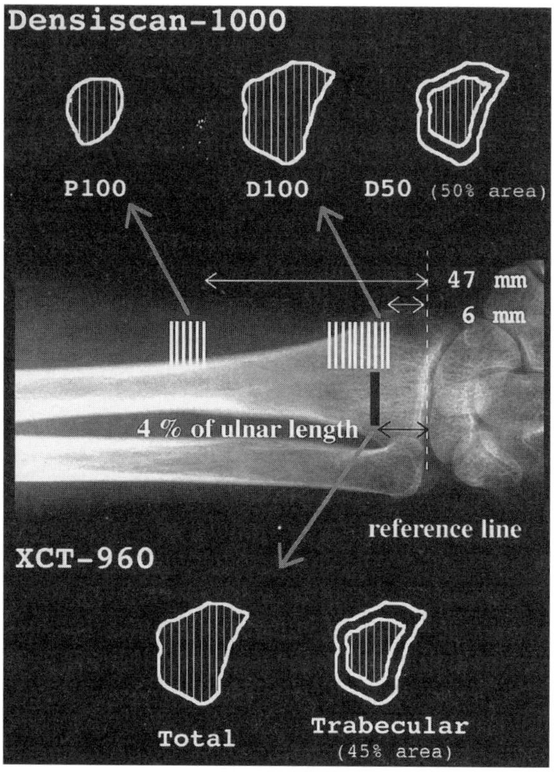

Figure 1 Coronal scout view of the forearm showing measurement sites. Using the Densiscan-1000, two stacks of computed tomography scans are taken. The distal stack is used for the determination of the total bone mineral density (BMD) (D100) and the trabecular BMD (D50). The proximal stack yields the diaphysis BMD (P100). Using the XCT-960, a single slice is used. Shaded areas are the regions for BMD determination

inertia of cortical bone. The compact bone density of the cortex is determined by defining the region of measurement precisely within the compact bone[7]. Finally, high-resolution pQCT has the potential to provide quantitative information regarding the trabecular structure, and several investigational works using thin-slice high-resolution tomography have been reported[8-11].

ACCURACY AND PRECISION

The assessment of precision errors in measurement is very important for the characterization of a technique's ability to detect longitudinal changes. The major source of imprecision in radial pQCT is the variability of positioning. Published short-term precision errors of a single-slice pQCT system for determining the radial BMD range between 1 and 2%[12,13]. Using a highly precise pQCT system, a precision error of 0.3% has been reported[14]. We found the precision error to be 1.76% (0.027 mm) when assessing the cortical thickness of the radial diaphysis.

Accuracy errors in bone measurement are of clinical importance when the patient value is compared with a reference population. The reliability of a diagnostic test depends on the accuracy error of the test and the biological variation of the variable in the population to which the test is applied. The accuracy errors of pQCT mainly depend on the amount of marrow fat and on beam hardening, and have been reported to be between 7 and 18% for the BMD in the distal radius[14-16].

pQCT VALUES IN NORMAL JAPANESE WOMEN

Hasegawa and colleagues[17] measured 617 normal Japanese women by Stratec XCT-960 and showed a linear postmenopausal decline of BMD averaging 1.1% per year. The overall decreases in total BMD and trabecular BMD from the young adult peak values to those at 70–79 years of age were 34% and 32%, respectively. The postmenopausal bone loss occurred nearly at the same rate in the trabecular bone and the endocortical area in the radius. We evaluated the age-related changes in cortical thickness and density in the radius by thin-slice and high-resolution pQCT scans[18]. The cortical thickness was calculated using the thresholding algorithm and a circular ring model assumption. The most dramatic percentage decrease in age-related change was found in the cortical thickness (Table 1). More than 80% of age-related bone loss in the radius is caused by a decreased thickness of the cortical bone. These results suggest the importance of the endocortical change in evaluating postmenopausal bone loss.

DIAGNOSIS OF OSTEOPOROSIS BY pQCT

We have studied 48 Japanese women by pQCT (the Densiscan-1000) and dual X-ray absorptiometry (DXA), and compared the ability of radial pQCT and DXA to discriminate women with osteoporotic vertebral fractures from those without[19]. The radial BMDs measured by pQCT correlated moderately well with the BMDs in the lumbar spine, radius and femoral neck measured by DXA ($r = 0.470–0.855$) (Table 2). The lumbar BMD measured by DXA showed the highest correlation to trabecular BMD measured by pQCT. The diagnostic ability of pQCT and DXA to detect vertebral osteoporosis was determined by comparing BMD measurements. Kappa statistics showed that, in general, the diagnostic agreement between these measurements was fair or moderate (Table 3). The discriminative ability of these methods for vertebral fracture was assessed by receiver operating characteristic (ROC) analysis. The areas under the ROC curves were 0.68, 0.71, 0.69 and 0.78 for trabecular, total and cortical BMD by pQCT, and lumbar BMD by DXA, respectively (Figure 2). These results suggest that the fracture risk assessment could be best made by lumbar DXA.

There have been several reports regarding the comparison of the diagnostic efficacy for primary osteoporosis between pQCT and other densitometric techniques. Grampp and co-workers[20,21] demonstrated that the measurement of bone mass using pQCT weakly discriminated between women with fractures and age-matched

Table 1 Age-related changes in cortical parameters of the radius evaluated by thin-slice and high-resolution pQCT scan

	Percentage decrease in BMD from 40 to 70 years of age	
	Linear regression model	*Square regression model*
Cortical density	4.9	5.0
Cortical area	29.3	38.1
Cortical thickness	29.3	55.9
Total density	21.7	38.7

BMD, bone mineral density

Table 2 Correlations (r values) between radial bone mineral density (BMD) measured by the Densiscan-1000 and BMD measured by dual X-ray absorptiometry (DXA) in 48, 22–75-year-old Japanese women

	Correlation value (r)		
DXA measurement	*D50 (trabecular BMD by Densiscan-1000)*	*D100 (total BMD by Densiscan-1000)*	*P100 (diaphysis BMD by Densiscan-1000)*
Mid-radial BMD	0.741	0.723	0.855
Lumbar spine BMD	0.688	0.523	0.470
Femoral neck BMD	0.715	0.639	0.699

D50, D100 and P100 are defined in Figure 1

Table 3 Diagnostic agreement of vertebral osteoporosis between different bone mineral density (BMD) measurements

DXA measurement	*pQCT measurement*	*Percentage agreement*	*Kappa score*	*95% confidence interval for Kappa score*
Lumbar spine BMD	D50	77.1	0.53	0.29–0.76
	D100	79.2	0.57	0.34–0.81
	P100	64.6	0.31	0.08–0.55
Mid-radial BMD	D50	79.2	0.58	0.36–0.80
	D100	77.1	0.54	0.30–0.77
	P100	79.2	0.59	0.38–0.80
Femoral neck BMD	D50	64.6	0.35	0.15–0.56
	D100	66.7	0.37	0.15–0.60
	P100	72.9	0.40	0.13–0.67

D50, D100 and P100 are defined in Figure 1. DXA, dual X-ray absorptiometry; pQCT, peripheral quantitative computed tomography

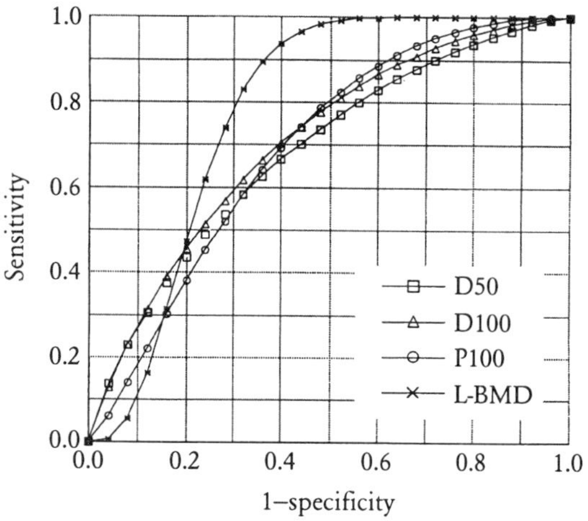

Figure 2 Receiver operating characteristic curves for radial peripheral quantitative computed tomography (D50, D100 and P100 (defined in Figure 1)) and lumbar dual X-ray absorptiometry (L-BMD) in discriminating women with vertebral fractures from non-fractured controls

non-fractured controls. In comparison, bone mass at the lumbar spine, measured using DXA or lumbar QCT, showed a stronger capability for discriminating between women with fractures and non-fractured controls. Similarly, Formica and colleagues[22] reported that pQCT showed a poor ability to identify prevalent fractures compared with axial bone measurement by DXA.

Based on our observations and other reports, current pQCT parameters, such as pure trabecular bone volumetric density, do not appear to be accurate discriminators of prevalent fractures.

THE USE OF pQCT IN MONITORING SKELETAL CHANGES

Because of its high precision, pQCT could be suited to monitoring therapeutic interventions. Dambacher and associates[23] reported the clinical utility of the highly precise pQCT system in differentiating between fast and slow bone losers and in monitoring the response to treatment in postmenopausal osteoporosis. However, concern has been expressed regarding the use of peripheral measurements for evaluating the efficacy of therapeutic interventions. It has been demonstrated that a greater response to the administration of therapeutic agents is observed with the axial compared to the appendicular skeleton.

SUMMARY

The measurements made by pQCT can provide precise information regarding trabecular BMD, cortical BMD, cortical geometry and trabecular structure. According to the results of recent clinical studies, however, bone mass measurement by pQCT does not appear to surpass the measurement of axial bone mass by DXA in assessing fracture risk. Cortical geometry and trabecular structure, in addition to bone mass, may contribute to a more comprehensive understanding of bone strength. Additional clinical applications of pQCT, specifically the assessment of rates of change for monitoring disease progression or response to treatment, require further investigation.

References

1. Anonymous. Consensus development conference: diagnosis, prophylaxis and treatment of osteoporosis. *Am J Med* 1993;94:646–50
2. Rüegsegger P, Elsasser U, Anliker M, *et al.* Quantification of bone mineralization using computed tomography. *Radiology* 1976;121:93–7
3. Müller A, Rüegsegger E, Rüegsegger P. Peripheral QCT: a low-risk procedure to identify women predisposed to osteoporosis. *Phys Med Biol* 1989;34: 741–9
4. Schneider P, Borner W. Peripheral quantitative computed tomography for bone mineral measurement using a new special QCT-scanner. Methodology, normal values, comparison with manifest osteoporosis. *Fortschr Rontgenstr* 1991;154: 292–9

5. Sievanen H, Koskue V, Rauhio A, *et al.* Peripheral quantitative computed tomography in human long bones: evaluation of *in vitro* and *in vivo* precision. *J Bone Miner Res* 1998;13:871–82
6. Braun MJ, Meta MD, Schneider P, *et al.* Clinical evaluation of a high-resolution new peripheral quantitative computerized tomography (pQCT) scanner for the bone densitometry at the lower limbs. *Phys Med Biol* 1998;43:2279–94
7. Rüegsegger P, Durand EP, Dambacher MA. Differential effects of aging and disease on trabecular and compact bone density of the radius. *Bone* 1991;12: 99–105
8. Gordon CL, Webber CE, Nicholson PS. Relation between image-based assessment of distal radius trabecular structure and compressive strength. *Can Assoc Radiol J* 1998;49:390–7
9. Jiang Y, Zhao J, Augat P, *et al.* Trabecular bone mineral and calculated structure of human bone specimens scanned by peripheral quantitative computed tomography: relation to biomechanical properties. *J Bone Miner Res* 1998;13:1783–90
10. Laib A, Hildebrand T, Hauselmann HJ, *et al.* Ridge number density: a new parameter for *in vivo* bone structure analysis. *Bone* 1997;21:541–6
11. Genant HK, Lang TF, Engelke K, *et al.* Advances in the noninvasive assessment of bone density, quality, and structure. *Calcif Tiss Int* 1996;59: S10–15
12. Genant HK, Engelke K, Fuerst T, *et al.* Noninvasive assessment of bone mineral and structure: state of the art. *J Bone Miner Res* 1996;11:707–30
13. Rüegsegger P. The use of peripheral QCT in the evaluation of bone remodelling. *Endocrinologist* 1994;4:167–76
14. Imai Y, Sone T, Mikawa Y, *et al.* Precision and accuracy for peripheral quantitative computed tomography evaluated using cadaveric radii. *J Clin Densitom* 1998;1:165–72
15. Takada M, Engelke K, Hagiwara S, *et al.* Accuracy and precision study *in vitro* for peripheral quantitative computed tomography. *Osteoporos Int* 1996;6: 207–12
16. Louis O, Soykens S, Willnecker J, *et al.* Cortical and total bone mineral content of the radius: accuracy of peripheral computed tomography. *Bone* 1996; 18:467–72
17. Hasegawa Y, Kushida K, Yamazaki K, *et al.* Volumetric bone mineral density using peripheral quantitative computed tomography in Japanese women. *Osteoporos Int* 1997;7:195–9
18. Sone T, Imai Y, Tomomitsu T, *et al.* Age-related rarefaction and bone loss of cortical bone: study with high-resolution pQCT instrument [in Japanese]. *Osteoporos Jpn* 1997;5:194–6
19. Imai Y. Bone mineral density measurements using peripheral quantitative computed tomography: an evaluation of its clinical utility [in Japanese]. *Kawasaki Igakkaishi* 1999;25:25–33
20. Grampp S, Lang P, Jergas M, *et al.* Assessment of the skeletal status by peripheral quantitative computed tomography of the forearm: short-term precision *in vivo* and comparison to dual X-ray absorptiometry. *J Bone Miner Res* 1995;10:1566–76
21. Grampp S, Jergas M, Lang P, *et al.* Quantitative CT assessment of the lumbar spine and radius in patients with osteoporosis. *Am J Roentgenol* 1996; 167:133–40
22. Formica CA, Nieves JW, Cosman F, *et al.* Comparative assessment of bone mineral measurements using dual X-ray absorptiometry and peripheral quantitative computed tomography. *Osteoporos Int* 1998;8:460–7
23. Dambacher MA, Neff M, Kissling R, *et al.* Highly precise peripheral quantitative computed tomography for the evaluation of bone density, loss of bone density and structures. Consequences for prophylaxis and treatment. *Drugs Aging* 1998;1:15–24

The combination of low bone mineral density and other risk factors in osteoporosis 56

J. A. Kanis, O. Johnell, A. Oden, B. Jonsson, A. Dawson, D. Muchmore and W. Dere

INTRODUCTION

A large number of risk factors have been identified for osteoporotic fractures. Strong risk factors include old age, low body mass index, a maternal family history of hip fracture, prior fragility fractures and, in particular, low bone mineral density (BMD). This paper describes how these factors can be used in combination to estimate long-term risks of hip fracture, one of the most serious complications of osteoporosis[1].

BONE MINERAL DENSITY

Many prospective studies have shown that BMD measurements provide prognostic information on fracture risk[1]. A recent meta-analysis estimates that the risk of hip fracture is increased 2.6-fold for each standard deviation decrease in BMD at the hip[2]. Indeed, bone mineral assessments are at least as good for predicting hip fracture as blood pressure measurements are for predicting stroke, and considerably better than cholesterol measurements for predicting myocardial infarction in men[1,2]. Despite this, the accuracy of bone mineral measurement is considered to be insufficient for use as a screening tool[1].

A problem with the use of BMD alone is that, whereas specificity is high over a range of assumptions, sensitivity is low[1]. This means that many individuals who will fracture in their lifetime will not be identified to be at high risk on the basis of their assessment (Figure 1). Moreover, the relative risk of fracture determined by bone mineral density in short-term studies is likely to overestimate the risk many years later[3], particularly in the case of hip fracture, which has a long latency between the onset of bone loss and the clinical event.

OTHER RISK FACTORS

Whereas the assessment of BMD forms the cornerstone for the diagnosis of osteoporosis, other risk factors have been identified that contribute to risk independently of low BMD. The attenuation of ultrasound[4] may give information on skeletal risk over and above that provided by absorptiometric techniques. Other examples (Table 1)[5] include biochemical indices of bone resorption where prospective studies suggest that increased values are associated with an approximately two-fold increase in fracture risk in women independently of bone mineral density[6,7]. Low body weight, smoking, a family history of fragility fracture, and a prior osteoporotic fracture are additive factors[8,9], some of which have been incorporated into practice guidelines[10,11]. In women, the geometry of the hip also appears to be a BMD-independent factor for hip fracture risk. The risk increases approximately two-fold in women for each standard deviation increase in the length of the femoral neck after adjustment for BMD[12]. Density-independent components of fracture risk such as falls are clearly important for hip fracture. A variety of simple tests have been devised to assess postural stability and visual acuity, and poor postural stability and poor visual acuity have been shown to be associated with increased risk of hip fracture independently of BMD[13,14]. Finally, the risk of hip fracture is substantially increased in the presence of a prior Colles' fracture[15], fragility or other fracture[9,16]. In the case of a prior hip fracture, the risk of a repeat fracture is approximately doubled after adjusting for BMD[9].

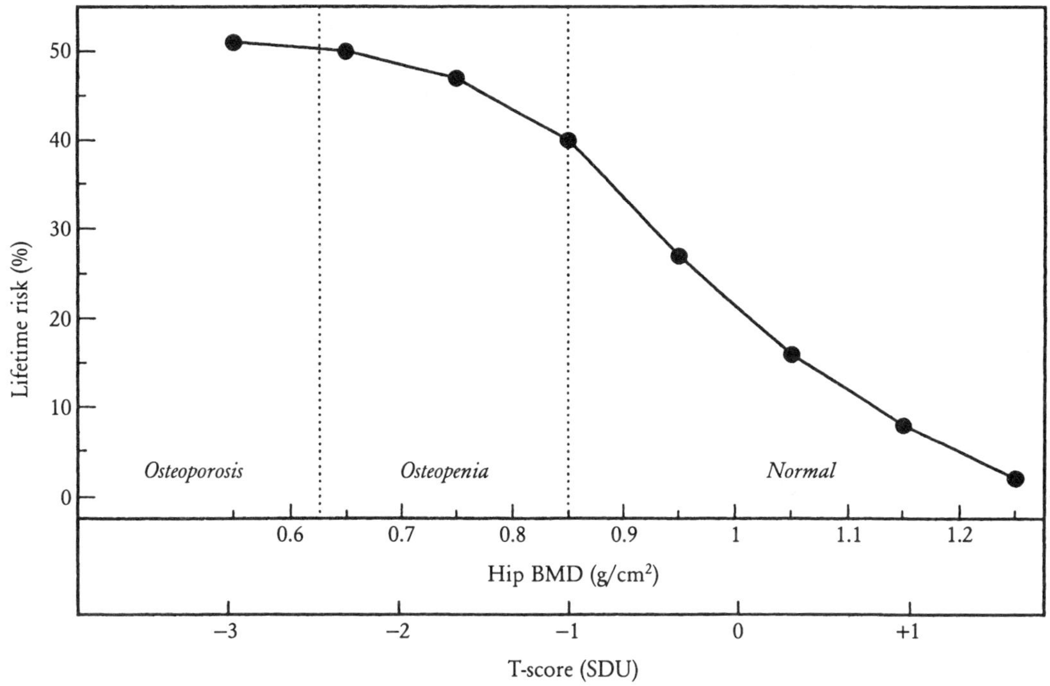

Figure 1 Lifetime risk of hip fracture in women at the age of 50 years in Sweden according to bone mineral density (BMD) measurements at the hip. Note that many fractures will occur in women with low bone mass (osteopenia) or normal bone density

Table 1 Examples of relative risks of hip fracture in women with and without adjustment for bone mineral density (BMD). From reference 5

	Relative risk	
	Crude	*Adjusted*
Hip BMD 1 SD below mean population value	2.6	
Non-carboxylated osteocalcin about normal	2.0	1.8
Biochemical index of bone resorption above premenopausal range	2.2	2.0
Prior fragility fracture after the age of 50 years	1.4	1.3
Body weight below 57.8 kg	1.8	1.4
Hip axis length 1 SD above population mean value	2.7	1.9
First-degree relative aged 50 years or more with a history of fragility fractures	1.7	1.5
Maternal family history of hip fracture	2.0	1.9
Current cigarette smoking	1.9	1.2
Poor visual acuity (<2/10)	2.0	2.0
Low gait speed (1 SD decrease)	1.4	1.3
Increase in body sway (1 SD)	1.9	1.7

LONG-TERM RISK

The assessment of absolute risk rather than relative risk is appropriate for the assessment of patients. In this context, long-term risks are useful, since they depend upon age and life expectancy as well as the current absolute risk. Absolute risks of hip fracture have been well characterized in Sweden.

The average lifetime risk for hip fracture in Swedish women at the age of 50 years is 22.7%, and this decreases with age to 18.9% at the age of 85 years[17]. The average lifetime risk in men is approximately half that of women over the same age range (9.6–11.1%), owing to the lower absolute risk and lower life expectancy (Figure 2). As expected, lifetime risks increase progressively with relative risk over all ages in both men and women.

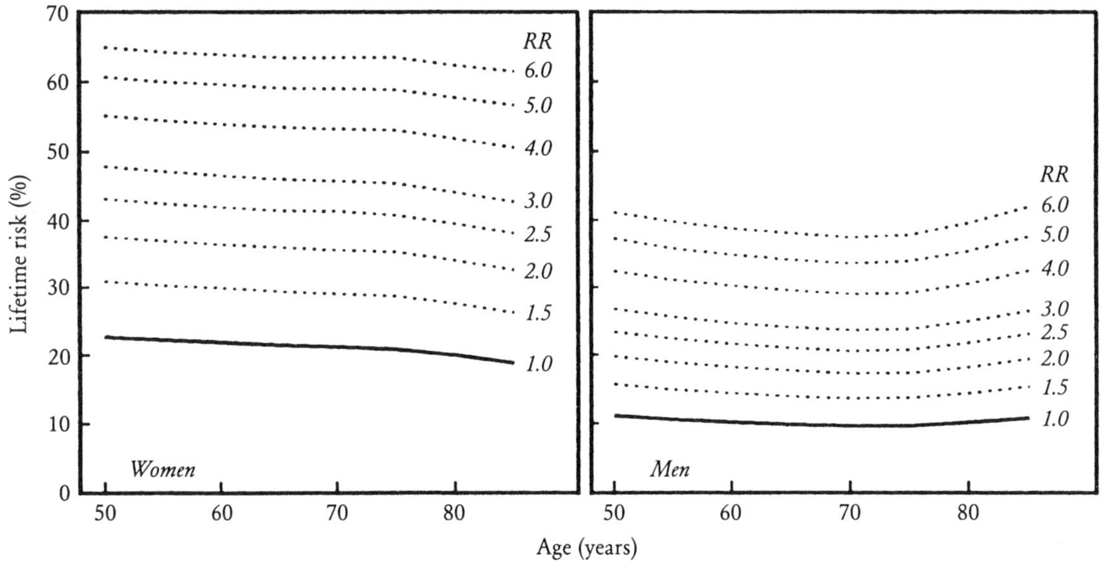

Figure 2 Lifetime risk of hip fracture in Swedish men and women according to age and relative risk[5]. The solid line shows average lifetime risk at the ages shown and the dotted lines the risk according to relative risk (RR)

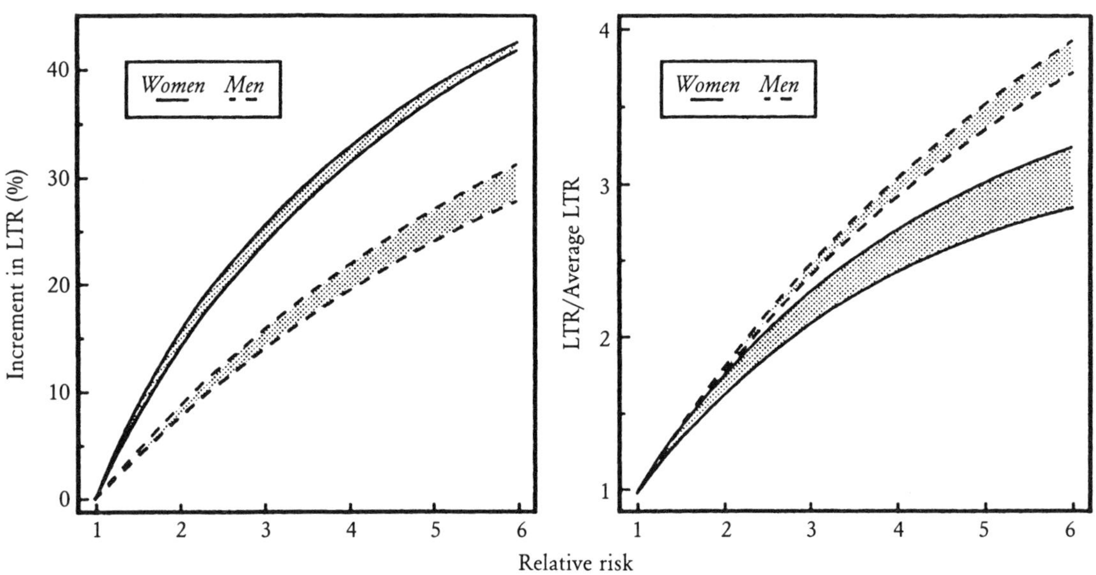

Figure 3 Effect of increases in relative risk on lifetime risk (LTR) of hip fracture in men and women expressed as the increment (left panel) or the increase over average lifetime risk (right panel)[5]. The shaded areas shown for each sex denote the range according to age (between the ages of 50 and 85 years)

With progressive increases in relative risk, the increment in lifetime risk is stable across all ages in both sexes, permitting the calculation of added risk irrespective of age (Figure 3). The absolute increment in lifetime risk is greater in women than in men. The increase in lifetime risk over baseline risk is, however, greater in men than in women over all ages. In women, a relative risk of 6.0 is associated with a tripling in lifetime risk. In men, however, the increment is greater, with a nearly four-fold increase in risk compared to the average risk for men.

It is important to recognize, however, that the relationship of lifetime risk with age may not be so constant in other communities, where there might be differences in current mortality, mortality trends, or the slope of hip fracture risk with age[18]. Mortality varies widely between countries as does the slope of the risk of hip fracture with age[19,20]. For this reason, it will be important to assess lifetime risks in different communities. Lifetime risks of hip fracture appear, however, to be relatively stable with age in Argentina and Hong Kong, which have lower risks than that in Sweden (Table 2). It is also important to recognize that the algorithm is based on hip fracture risk and may not be appropriate for other fragility fractures. This is particularly likely for forearm fractures, for which in many countries the incidence reaches a plateau with age or falls after the age of 60 or 70 years[1,21,22].

Table 2 Lifetime risk of hip fracture (computed from changes in mortality expected from 1995) in women according to relative risk and age in Hong Kong and Argentina. From reference 5

Relative risk	*Age* (years)	*Argentina*	*Hong Kong*
1.0	50	17.4	15.6
	80	18.4	14.1
5.0	50	48.7	51.7
	80	53.3	48.9

IMPLICATIONS OF MULTIPLE RISK ASSESSMENT

The effect of selecting segments of the population with different relative risks on the sensitivity and specificity of the assessment is shown in Table 3 for women at the age of 50 years[5]. Specificity and sensitivity are defined in terms of 15-year risks. Thus, specificity is defined as the proportion of women who would not sustain a fracture within 15 years with assessment values above the cut-off level. Conversely, sensitivity is defined as the proportion of women who will sustain a hip fracture with a positive test result.

Sensitivity and specificity were calculated assuming that the high-risk category is 15% of the population with the lowest BMD at the hip, which is the range that might be contemplated with a screening strategy. The specificity remained high over all ranges of risk assumptions (over 85%). In contrast, the sensitivity varied between 25 and 70% depending on the assumptions made (see Table 3). Sensitivity increased the higher the gradient of risk assumed.

The positive predictive value of the test (the proportion of detected individuals who sustained a hip fracture) increased markedly with increasing relative risk. Thus, the positive predictive value increased from 2.2 to 5.8% where 15% of the population would be considered to be at risk.

Table 3 Estimates of positive predictive value (PPV), sensitivity and specificity of measurements to predict hip fracture over 15 years or to death in women aged 50 years or 65 years, assuming that 15% of the population at highest risk would be identified. From reference 5

Gradient of risk (RR/SD)	*Women aged 50 years*			*Women aged 65 years*		
	PPV (%)	*Sensitivity* (%)	*Specificity* (%)	*PPV* (%)	*Sensitivity* (%)	*Specificity* (%)
1.5	2.2	26.5	85.1	12.8	25.7	85.9
2.0	3.1	36.4	85.3	17.0	34.1	86.5
2.5	3.8	44.5	85.4	20.1	40.4	87.0
3.0	4.3	51.1	85.5	22.3	44.8	87.4
4.0	5.1	60.6	85.6	24.7	49.7	87.8
5.0	5.6	66.1	85.7	25.6	51.4	87.9
6.0	5.8	69.0	85.7	25.6	51.4	87.9

The effect of targeting assessment at later life is shown in Table 3. Sensitivity was lower and specificity higher at each gradient of risk than at the age of 50 years, but the effect was small. As expected, there was a large effect of age on positive predictive value which increased five- to six-fold at the age of 65 years compared to estimates at the age of 50 years.

APPLICATION OF RISK FACTORS

The parallel assessment of a number of risk factors with or without BMD assessment permits the identification of groups or individuals at highest risk. The multiple factors available to contribute to risk more or less independently indicate that the gradient of risk between those characterized at high or low risk can be increased by multiple assessments which contribute to risk independently. For example, a woman with a BMD 1 SD below the population average with poor visual acuity would have a relative risk and remaining lifetime risk of hip fracture that would be greater than that expected from either factor alone[14]. The true relative risk is not, however, a multiple of the risks given in Table 1 (i.e. $2.6 \times 2.0 = 5.2$).

Some downward adjustment of the relative risks is required since, apart from low BMD, the risks are relative to those without the risk factor rather than the risks being relative to the general population. In the example above, poor visual acuity ($\leq 2/10$) is associated with a relative risk of 2.0 compared to individuals with better acuity. Poor visual acuity was found in 7.3% of the population. The adjusted relative risk approximates to:

$$RR/(p \times RR + (1 - p))$$

where p is the prevalence of the risk factor and RR the unadjusted value. In the example above, the relative risk with poor visual acuity adjusted to the general population is:

$$2.0 / (0.073 \times 2.0 + (1 - 0.073)) = 1.86$$

Downward adjustment of the risk associated with a low BMD is also required[5]. Hip fracture rates increase logarithmically with decreasing BMD, but BMD is normally distributed. For this reason, individuals with a BMD equal to the mean have a risk of hip fracture that is lower than the average risk. On the assumption that risk increases 2.6-fold for each standard deviation decrease in BMD, the risk of hip fracture of an individual with a T-score of −1 would be:

$$2.6 \times \exp(-\ln(2.6)^2/2) = 1.65$$

Thus, in the woman with poor visual acuity and a BMD 1 SD below average, the relative risk of hip fracture is $1.65 \times 1.86 = 3.07$, corresponding to a lifetime risk of 43–48% (depending on age; see Figure 2).

The examples given in Table 1 are risk estimates adjusted for BMD, but are not otherwise adjusted. For example, the increase in risk associated with low body mass index is not adjusted for postural instability. It will be necessary to make such adjustments from several large population studies before these can be utilized as independent and additive risk functions.

CONCLUSIONS

As shown in this paper, the use of multiple risk factors increases the sensitivity of assessment substantially without trading off the specificity, and thus performs better than the use of BMD assessments alone. Indeed, it is possible that the sensitivity of assessments might be improved sufficiently to allow screening rather than case-finding strategies to be adopted in the future. For example, if 15% of the female population at the age of 50 years could be found with a relative risk for hip fracture of 6.0, this would be expected to save 16.3% of all hip fractures over the lifetime of the cohort with a treatment that had an effectiveness of 50%. The gains would be greater in more elderly populations.

Similar approaches have been used in the management of cardiovascular diseases[23]. The consideration of smoking, blood pressure, diabetes and serum cholesterol permit the identification of patients at high risk (> 20% 5-year risk), whereas the use of serum cholesterol alone has a low gradient of risk, significantly poorer than the assessment of BMD alone to predict hip fracture[1,2]. It is of interest that the combination of relatively few risk factors can yield relative risks of 5 or more and that the gains in sensitivity are modest above this risk. It is likely, therefore, that relatively few risk factors will need to be identified to optimize risk assessment. Indeed, it is possible that screening strategies could be devised for osteoporosis once the inter-relationships between risks have been adequately characterized.

The level of risk that demands intervention or further assessment depends upon many factors, including the risks and benefits of intervention. If a lifetime risk of, for example, 40% were unacceptable, then a relative risk of 2.4 would exceed this threshold in women. The threshold relative risk in men would be 6.0. The setting of such thresholds will in part depend on health economic considerations. Such studies will be important for optimizing the selection of individuals for treatment and in the development of screening strategies.

References

1. World Health Organization. *Assessment of Fracture Risk and its Application to Screening for Postmenopausal Osteoporosis*, WHO Technical Report Series. Geneva: WHO, 1994:843
2. Marshall D, Johnell O, Wedel H. Meta-analysis of how well measures of bone mineral density predict occurrence of osteoporotic fractures. *Br Med J* 1996;312:1254–9
3. Johnell O, Kanis JA, Oden A, Jonsson B, *et al.* Prediction of fracture from bone mineral density measurements overestimates risk. *J Bone Miner Res* 1998;8(suppl 3):29
4. Hans D, Dargent P, Schott AM, *et al.* Ultrasound heel measurements to predict hip fracture in elderly women: the EPIDOS prospective study, for the EPIDOS prospective study group. *Lancet* 1996;348: 511–14
5. Kanis JA, Johnell O, Oden A, *et al.* Risk of hip fracture derived from relative risks: an analysis applied to the population of Sweden. *Osteoporosis Int* 1999;in press
6. Riis BJ. The role of bone loss. *Am J Med* 1995;98 (suppl 2A):29–32
7. Garnero P, Hauser E, Chapuy MC, *et al.* Markers of bone turnover predict hip fractures in elderly women. The EPIDOS prospective study. *J Bone Miner Res* 1996;11:1531–8
8. Gardsell P, Johnell O, Nilsson BE. Predicting fractures using forearm bone densitometry. *Calcif Tissue Int* 1989;44:235–42
9. Cummings SR, Nevitt MC, Browner WS, *et al.* Risk factors for hip fracture in white women. *N Engl J Med* 1995;332:767–73
10. Kanis JA, Delmas P, Burckhardt P, *et al.*, on behalf of the European Foundation for Osteoporosis and Bone Disease. Guidelines for diagnosis and management of osteoporosis. *Osteoporosis Int* 1997; 7:390–406
11. Eddy D, Lindsay R, Cummings SR, *et al.* Osteoporosis: review of the evidence for prevention, diagnosis and cost-effectiveness analysis. *Osteoporosis Int* 1998;(suppl 4):1–88
12. Faulkner KG, Cummings SR, Black D, *et al.* Simple measurement of femoral geometry predicts hip fracture: the study of osteoporotic fractures. *J Bone Miner Res* 1993;8:1211–17
13. Nguyen T, Sambrook P, Kelly P, *et al.* Prediction of osteoporotic fractures by postural instability and bone density. *Br Med J* 1993;307:1111–15
14. Dargent-Molina P, Favier F, Grandjean H, *et al.* Fall-related factors and risk of hip fracture: the EPIDOS prospective study, for the EPIDOS group. *Lancet* 1996;348:145–9
15. Mallmin H, Ljunghall S, Persson I, *et al.* Fracture of the distal forearm as a forecaster of a subsequent hip fracture. A population based cohort study with 24 years follow-up. *Calcif Tissue Int* 1993;52:269–72
16. Lauritzen JB, Schwartz P, McNair P, *et al.* Radial and humeral fractures as predictors of subsequent hip, radial or humeral fractures in women and their seasonal variation. *Osteoporosis Int* 1993;3:133–7
17. Oden A, Dawson A, Dere W, *et al.* Lifetime risk of hip fracture is underestimated. *Osteoporosis Int* 1998;8:599–603
18. Suman VJ, Atkinson EJ, O'Fallon WM, *et al.* A nomogram for predicting lifetime hip fracture risk from radius bone mineral density and age. *Bone* 1993;14:843–6
19. Elffors I, Allander E, Kanis JA, *et al.* The variable incidence of hip fracture in southern Europe: the MEDOS Study. *Osteoporosis Int* 1994;4:253–63
20. Johnell O, Gullberg B, Allander E, *et al.* The apparent incidence of hip fracture in Europe: a study of national register sources. *Osteoporosis Int* 1992;2: 298–302

21. Bengner U, Johnell O. Increasing incidence of forearm fractures. *Acta Orthop Scand* 1985;56:158–60
22. Falch JA. Epidemiology of fracture of the distal forearm in Oslo, Norway. *Acta Orthop Scand* 1983; 54:291–5
23. Dyslipidaemia Advisory Group on behalf of the National Heart Foundation of New Zealand. National Heart Foundation clinical guidelines for the assessment and management of dyslipidaemia. *NZ Med J* 1996;109:224–32

Options for the prevention and treatment of osteoporosis 57

M. McClung

INTRODUCTION

As we have learned from previous papers in this symposium, osteoporosis is a disorder of increased fracture risk by virtue of low bone density and the architectural changes that accompany bone loss. The skeleton becomes more fragile and the probability of fractures increases. Significant skeletal risk factors for fracture include low bone mass, high bone turnover and the presence of previous fragility fractures. The consequences of osteoporosis, both in personal and in population terms, are related solely to the occurrence of fractures[1]. The excess mortality, morbidity and health-care costs are sustained only after fractures occur. For these reasons, the foremost objective of therapy in treating women with osteoporosis is to reduce the incidence of new fractures. The treatment and prevention of osteoporosis is thus directed at normalizing bone turnover, preserving or increasing bone mass and improving bone strength, the ultimate objective being a reduction in fracture risk. We now have an impressive set of options for accomplishing these objectives, many of which have been shown in appropriate clinical studies to reduce fracture risk in carefully selected sets of patients.

CALCIUM AND VITAMIN D

The bone loss that occurs in older individuals is the consequence of high rates of bone turnover. This is largely due to an inadequate intake of calcium and vitamin D and the resultant secondary hyperparathyroidism that drives osteoclastic bone resorption. Providing adequate calcium and vitamin D intake reduces bone turnover and slows bone loss in older postmenopausal women. Several studies have demonstrated a beneficial effect of calcium, with or without vitamin D, in reducing the fracture risk in older adults[2-4]. Except for patients with hyperparathyroidism and renal stones, an adequate intake of calcium and vitamin D is indicated in all women over the age of 65 years. The target doses of calcium and vitamin D are stated to be 1200–1500 mg per day and 400 IU per day, respectively. The effect of estrogen on bone density seems to be impaired in the setting of low calcium intake. Calcium and vitamin D may have additional beneficial effects on muscle function, strength and perhaps fall frequency. This body of evidence supports the tenet that providing adequate intake of calcium and vitamin D is an important component of osteoporosis treatment, especially in older women. The role of calcium and vitamin D therapy in the first few years after the menopause is less clear. Furthermore, bone loss has been consistently observed in the calcium-treated control groups of several clinical trials in younger postmenopausal women[5-8], suggesting that calcium alone does not prevent early menopausal bone loss.

ACTIVE METABOLITES OF VITAMIN D

The renal activation to calcitriol (1,25-$(OH)_2$ vitamin D) is required for the effects of vitamin D on gastrointestinal calcium absorption. Renal 1-hydroxylase activity decreases with age, increasing the frequency of vitamin D insufficiency in older adults. Several studies have evaluated the effects of active forms of vitamin D (calcitriol, alphacalcidol) in treating osteoporosis. Improvements in bone density and fracture reduction have been seen in some studies[9,10]. The frequency of hypercalcemia and hypercalciuria has often been quite high. Whether active forms of vitamin D are more effective than simply providing higher doses of standard vitamin D is uncertain.

ESTROGEN THERAPY

Bone turnover increases and bone loss begins in earnest at the time of the menopause. The route of administration of estrogen seems to be unimportant for skeletal effects. Both oral and transdermal estrogen preparations provide skeletal benefits. Estrogen replacement therapy (ERT) restores bone turnover to normal premenopausal levels and is effective in preserving or increasing bone density in both young and older postmenopausal women[5,6,11]. Acceptance of ERT is limited by side-effects such as bleeding and breast pain, as well as concern about the potential association with increased breast cancer risk. The tolerability of ERT is improved with lower doses. Recent studies in both older and younger women demonstrate that 0.3 mg of conjugated equine estrogen[12] or 0.5 mg of 17β-estradiol (McClung, unpublished data) is effective in preventing bone loss.

Estrogen therapy is often taken with a progestogen to reduce the risk of endometrial hyperplasia and cancer. Pure progestogens, such as medroxyprogesterone acetate or micronized progesterone, are skeletally neutral and do not alter the bone density response to ERT[5]. Progestogens such as norethindrone acetate, a derivative of 19-nortestosterone, are skeletally active and may have an additive effect on bone density when combined with estrogen[13].

The skeletal effects of estrogen fade quickly when therapy is discontinued. Bone turnover increases and bone loss resumes within a few months of stopping therapy. It is unlikely that the beneficial effect of estrogen is sustained for more than a few years after its use is stopped. This is consistent with case-control studies in which bone density is preserved and fracture risk reduced in women currently on estrogen therapy, but not in women who took estrogen in the remote past. It appears that it is never too late to begin ERT, and benefit is observed in women who began treatment in later life, although the optimal effect on fracture reduction is observed in women who take estrogen continuously from the menopause onward.

The antifracture efficacy of estrogen therapy is derived almost entirely from case-control studies. Reduced risks of spinal, hip and other fractures have been observed in older women who were taking estrogen, compared to those who never took estrogen. In a recent randomized trial, estrogen therapy for 4 years did not reduce the overall fracture risk[14]. However, the women in this study were selected on the basis of heart disease rather than fracture risk. These results are similar to studies with other antiresorptive agents in which fracture reduction was not observed in women at low fracture risk[15]. Randomized clinical trials are needed to evaluate both the skeletal and extraskeletal effects of estrogen therapy.

Estrogen therapy is accepted as long-term treatment for only a small proportion of postmenopausal women. For those few women who cannot take estrogen and for the many women who choose not to take hormones, effective alternatives are desirable.

ESTROGEN-LIKE DRUGS

The ideal therapy for postmenopausal women would be an agent possessing the full spectrum of beneficial effects of estrogen, without adverse effects on the uterus, breast or coagulation parameters. The realizations that estrogen acts through at least two different intracellular receptors and that the receptors differ in their tissue distribution provide a potential mechanism for selective estrogen modulation of tissue responses. Tamoxifen and raloxifene are drugs with demonstrated tissue selectivity. Tamoxifen has modest estrogen-like effects on the skeleton in postmenopausal women, while being an antagonist in the breast. Its estrogen-like action in the endometrium limits its usefulness as a long-term treatment for osteoporosis. Raloxifene has the advantage of not promoting endometrial proliferation or vaginal bleeding. Although less potent than both estrogen or bisphosphonates, raloxifene therapy preserves bone density in both young and older postmenopausal women[7,16]. At a dose of 60 mg daily, raloxifene reduces the incidence of new vertebral fractures by 30–50% in older postmenopausal women with very low bone density or previous spinal fractures[16]. An effect on non-spinal fracture incidence has not been demonstrated. The risk for breast cancer in older women with osteoporosis was decreased 61% over 3 years with raloxifene therapy[17], but the effect on breast cancer risk in younger women is not yet known. The role of raloxifene in treating women with a previous history of breast cancer is currently being evaluated.

Vasomotor symptoms in young women and symptoms of urogenital atrophy in older women are not responsive to raloxifene therapy. Women with a history of previous thromboembolic events may not be candidates for estrogen, tamoxifen or raloxifene therapy because of an increased incidence of deep vein thrombosis and pulmonary embolism with each of these agents. The important effects of raloxifene on cardiovascular disease and cognition remain to be understood.

Tibolone is a steroid drug with true tissue specificity. The drug itself has little activity, but is metabolized into either estrogen or progestogenic metabolites in different tissues. In the uterus, the progestational metabolite predominates, while in the liver and bone, tibolone has predominantly estrogen-like effects. At a dose of 2.5 mg daily, tibolone maintains bone density, reduces vasomotor symptoms and is associated with a low incidence of vaginal bleeding in young postmenopausal women[18]. A recent unpublished study demonstrated that doses as low as 0.625 mg daily are effective in preventing bone loss in both the hip and spine. Our understanding of the effects of tibolone on fracture reduction, breast cancer, cardiovascular end-points and thromboembolic events awaits further studies.

NON-ESTROGEN THERAPIES

Bisphosphonates are analogs of pyrophosphate that are potent inhibitors of bone resorption. Several bisphosphonates are now in clinical use[19]. The various members of this class of drugs differ in their mechanism of action, potency and side-effect profiles. Bisphosphonates are poorly absorbed and must be administered on an empty stomach. The safety of bisphosphonate use in patients with renal insufficiency or in pregnancy has not been adequately evaluated. Calcium and vitamin D deficiencies should be corrected before beginning treatment with alendronate or other bisphosphonates.

Etidronate prevents bone loss in early postmenopausal women and reduces the vertebral fracture risk in patients with severe osteoporosis. The drug is well tolerated, but must be given intermittently (e.g. 2 weeks every 3 months) to avoid an impairment of bone mineralization.

Alendronate is a more potent bisphosphonate that normalizes bone turnover within 1 month of beginning therapy and increases bone density in important skeletal sites[20,21]. Several large and independent studies, as well as a meta-analysis of smaller studies, have documented the antifracture efficacy of alendronate. The incidence of both spinal and non-spinal fractures, including hip and wrist fractures, is reduced by approximately 50% in women with osteoporosis or with previous vertebral fractures[15,22]. Despite similar changes in bone turnover and bone density, no effect on non-vertebral fractures has been observed in women without osteoporosis[15]. This observation, similar to that seen with estrogen in the Heart and Estrogen/progestin Replacement Study (HERS)[14], underscores the point that the antifracture efficacy of treatment is most evident in patients at high current fracture risk. The effect of preventive therapy to reduce the incidence of fractures will require treatment over a much longer interval of time.

Discontinuation of alendronate therapy results in a return of bone turnover toward baseline and a gradual resumption of bone loss[23]. Thus, as with estrogen, long-term treatment will be required for optimal benefit. The current studies with alendronate have assessed daily dosing. Intermittent dosing regimens should be effective and are now being evaluated. The major side-effect of alendronate in clinical practice is esophageal erosion and ulceration due to the direct irritating effect of alendronate on the esophageal mucosa in an acidic environment. The frequency of upper gastrointestinal tract symptoms was similar in alendronate- and placebo-treated patients in clinical trials (30–40%)[24]. About 10% of patients in clinical practice are unable to take alendronate because of the gastrointestinal side-effects. The frequency of upper gastrointestinal tract intolerance is minimized with proper dosing. Alendronate is contraindicated in patients with significant disorders of esophageal motility.

Risedronate is also a potent bisphosphonate shown to normalize bone turnover, increase bone density and reduce both spinal and non-spinal fractures[25]. In women with a low bone mass and previous vertebral fractures, the incidence of new vertebral fractures is reduced by 40–50% in 3 years. In a recently reported study, risedronate significantly reduced hip fracture risk in older women selected to be at high risk for hip fracture on the basis of very low hip bone mineral density. No difference has been observed in gastrointestinal side-effects between risedronate and placebo-treated patients in clinical trials. The tolerability of this drug in clinical practice awaits further experience.

Ibandronate is a very potent bisphosphonate with skeletal effects when given by daily oral dosing or by short intravenous infusion every 3 months. The effects on fracture reduction are currently being evaluated. The intermittent intravenous dosing will be very attractive for older, institutionalized patients, and will minimize or eliminate gastrointestinal intolerance, improper dosing and perhaps poor compliance.

Calcitonin is a calcium-regulating hormone that directly inhibits osteoclastic bone resorption[26]. Given either by subcutaneous injection or by nasal spray, calcitonin has very small effects on reducing bone turnover or increasing bone density. Small clinical trials have suggested a reduction in vertebral fracture frequency. The preliminary report of the major clinical trial of nasal calcitonin in women with prevalent vertebral fractures describes a 36% reduction in the incidence of new vertebral fractures at a dose of 200 IU, daily given for 5 years. No effect on spinal fracture frequency was noted with lower or higher doses. The effect of calcitonin therapy on non-vertebral fractures remains unproven in prospective trials. No serious safety concerns exist with calcitonin therapy, especially with the nasal spray preparation. The use of calcitonin therapy in early postmenopausal women has not been adequately evaluated.

OTHER OPTIONS

Phytoestrogen

Isoflavones and other phytoestrogens have weak estrogen-like effects on the skeleton. They may be used in preventing bone loss in postmenopausal women, but probably would not be as effective as estrogen or bisphosphonates in reducing the fracture risk in older women who have already developed osteoporosis.

Fluoride

Unlike previously discussed agents, fluoride activates bone formation without increasing bone resorption. High doses of fluoride increase bone density substantially, but do not decrease the fracture risk. The results of studies of the effects of lower doses of fluoride on fracture incidence are inconclusive. The response to a combination of low-dose fluoride and potent antiresorptive agents has theoretical appeal, but has not been adequately explored.

Parathyroid hormone and its analogs

Parathyroid hormone (PTH) activates bone turnover and appears to be anabolic to the trabecular compartment of the skeleton. Administration of PTH to women receiving estrogen results in a substantial increase in bone mass in the spine[27]. A recent study by Roe and colleagues[28] confirmed this finding and also noted an increase in bone volume and an increase in bone mass in the proximal femur. The effects on fracture incidence have not yet been assessed. It is possible that PTH may augment the antifracture efficacy of potent antiresorptive agents.

Androgen

In combination with estrogen, oral testosterone therapy increases bone mass more than does estrogen alone, and, in older adults, it increases muscle mass and strength. Masculinizing side-effects limit the use of higher androgen doses in women. More studies are needed to evaluate the use of low-dose androgen therapy alone and in combination with estrogen-like drugs or bisphosphonates.

NON-PHARMACOLOGICAL THERAPY

Fractures in patients with osteoporosis most often appear after trauma, including falls and lifting injuries. It is unproven that therapy for osteoporosis will have a major effect on fracture incidence in patients whose major risk for fracture is weakness or frailty. Correcting fall-related risk factors with exercise, the use of ambulatory supports, avoidance of sedative medications, and providing a safe home environment may be of value in treating patients with osteoporosis to reduce fracture risk[29]. The use of hip protectors may be beneficial in older patients at high risk for falling.

INDICATIONS FOR THERAPY

The provision of adequate calcium and vitamin D through the dietary supplements is reasonable for all older adults. Non-pharmacological therapy is indicated for patients in whom risk factors for falls are evident. Pharmacological therapy is effective in reducing fracture risk in patients with previous fragility fractures or with osteoporosis diagnosed by bone density testing (T score < -2.5). It is these patients who clearly should be identified and encouraged to begin therapy with an agent proven to reduce fracture risk[30]. The indications for pharmacological therapy to prevent bone loss and osteoporosis are less clear. The use of drugs such as estrogen, raloxifene and tibolone is strongly influenced by their perceived extraskeletal effects. The decision to use agents such as bisphosphonates and calcitonin, whose effects are limited to the skeleton, for osteoporosis prevention is more difficult. Therapy for many years will be required before antifracture efficacy will be observed, and it is not clear that early treatment with such agents will be more efficacious or cost-effective than waiting to begin therapy in women with osteoporosis prior to their first fracture. None of the options for treating osteoporosis will be effective unless strategies to improve long-term adherence to therapy are developed.

SUMMARY

Osteoporosis can no longer be considered an inevitable consequence of aging. We now have tools to identify patients with osteoporosis and to assess fracture risk. For patients found to be at high current fracture risk, several pharmacological agents, in addition to calcium and vitamin D, are known to reduce fracture incidence. With our expanding menu of effective treatment options, therapy should be considered in all patients with osteoporosis or prior fragility fractures. The specific indications for pharmacological therapy to prevent osteoporosis await further studies.

References

1. Lindsay R. The burden of osteoporosis: cost. *Am J Med* 1995;98(Suppl 2A):9S–11S
2. Chapuy MC, Arlot ME, Duboeuf F, *et al.* Vitamin D3 and calcium to prevent hip fractures in elderly women. *N Engl J Med* 1992;327:1637–42
3. Recker RR, Hinders S, Davies KM, *et al.* Correcting calcium nutritional deficiency prevents spine fractures in elderly women. *J Bone Miner Res* 1996;11: 1961–6
4. Dawson-Hughes B, Harris SS, Krall EA, *et al.* Effect of calcium and vitamin D supplementation on bone density in men and women 65 years of age or older. *N Engl J Med* 1997;337:670–6
5. The Writing Group for the PEPI Trial. Effects of hormone therapy on bone mineral density. Results from the Postmenopausal Estrogen/Progestin Interventions (PEPI) trial. *J Am Med Assoc* 1996; 276:1389–96
6. Speroff L, Rowan J, Symons J, *et al.* The comparative effect on bone density, endometrium, and lipids of continuous hormones as replacement therapy (CHART study). A randomized controlled trial. *J Am Med Assoc* 1996;276:1397–403

7. Delmas P, Bjarnason NH, Mitlak BH, *et al.* Effects of raloxifene on bone mineral density, serum cholesterol concentrations, and uterine endometrium in postmenopausal women. *N Engl J Med* 1997;337:1641–7
8. McClung MR, Clemmesen B, Daifotis A, *et al.* Alendronate prevents postmenopausal bone loss in women without osteoporosis. *Ann Intern Med* 1998; 128:253–61
9. Tilyard MW, Spears GF, Thomson J, *et al.* Treatment of postmenopausal osteoporosis with calcitriol or calcium. *N Engl J Med* 1992;326:357–62
10. Orimo H, Shiraki M, Hayashi Y, *et al.* Effect of 1 alpha-hydroxyvitamin D-3 on lumbar spine bone mineral density and vertebral fractures in patients with postmenopausal osteoporosis. *Calcif Tissue Int* 1994;54:370–6
11. Hosking D, Chilvers CED, Christiansen C, *et al.* Prevention of bone loss with alendronate in postmenopausal women under 60 years of age. *N Engl J Med* 1998;338:485–92
12. Recker RR, Davies KM, Dowd RM, *et al.* The effect of low-dose continuous estrogen and progesterone therapy with calcium and vitamin D on bone in elderly women. *Ann Intern Med* 1999;130:897–904
13. Christiansen C, Riis BJ. 17-Beta-estradiol and continuous norethisterone: a unique treatment for established osteoporosis in elderly women. *J Clin Endocrinol Metab* 1990;71:836–41
14. Hulley S, Grady D, Bush T, *et al.* Randomized trial of estrogen plus progestin for secondary prevention of coronary heart disease in postmenopausal women. *J Am Med Assoc* 1998;280:605–13
15. Cummings SR, Black DM, Thompson DE, *et al.* Effect of alendronate on risk of fracture in women with low bone density but without vertebral fractures. *J Am Med Assoc* 1998;280:2077–82
16. Ettinger B, Black DM, Mitlak BH, *et al.* Reduction of vertebral fracture risk in postmenopausal women with osteoporosis treated with raloxifene. *J Am Med Assoc* 1999;282:637–45
17. Cummings SR, Eckert S, Krueger KA, *et al.* The effect of raloxifene on risk of breast cancer in postmenopausal women. *J Am Med Assoc* 1999;281: 2189–244
18. Moore RA. Livial: a review of clinical studies. *Br J Obstet Gynaecol* 1999;106(Suppl):1–21
19. Watts NB. Treatment of osteoporosis with bisphosphonates. In Watts NB, ed. *Endocrinology and Metabolism Clinics of North America.* Philadelphia: WB Saunders, 1998;27:419–39
20. Chesnut CH, McClung MR, Ensrud K, *et al.* Alendronate treatment of the postmenopausal osteoporotic woman: effect of multiple dosages on bone mass and bone remodeling. *Am J Med* 1995;99: 144–52
21. Liberman UA, Weiss SR, Broll J, *et al.* Effect of oral alendronate on bone mineral density and the incidence of fractures in postmenopausal osteoporosis. *N Engl J Med* 1995;333:1437–43
22. Black DM, Cummings SR, Karpf DB, *et al.* Randomised trial of effect of alendronate on risk of fracture in women with existing vertebral fractures. *Lancet* 1996;348:1535–41
23. Stock JL, Bell NH, Chesnut CH, *et al.* Increments in bone mineral density of the lumbar spine and hip and suppression of bone turnover are maintained after discontinuation of alendronate in postmenopausal women. *Am J Med* 1997;103:291–7
24. Watts N, Freedholm D, Daifotis A. The clinical tolerability profile of alendronate. *Int J Clin Pract* 1999;April(Suppl 100):51–61
25. Harris ST, Watts NB, Genant HK, *et al.* Effects of risedronate treatment on vertebral and non-vertebral fractures in women with postmenopausal osteoporosis. A randomized clinical trial. *J Am Med Assoc* 1999;282:1344–52
26. Lindsay R, Nieves J, Formica C, *et al.* Randomised controlled study of effect of parathyroid hormone on vertebral-bone mass and fracture incidence among postmenopausal women on oestrogen with osteoporosis. *Lancet* 1997;350:550–5
27. Silverman SL. Calcitonin. *Am J Med Sci* 1997;313: 17–22
28. Roe EB, Sanchez SD, del Puerto GA, *et al.* Parathyroid hormone 1-34 (hPTH1-34) and estrogen produce dramatic bone density increases in postmenopausal osteoporosis – results from a placebo-controlled randomized trial. *J Bone Miner Res* 1999;14(Suppl 1):S137
29. McClung MR, Spencer K. Nonpharmacologic therapy for osteoporosis. In Rosen CJ, ed. *Osteoporosis: Diagnostic and Therapeutic Principles.* Totowa, NJ: Humana Press Inc., 1996:189–99
30. Kanis JA, Delmas P, Burckhardt P, *et al.* Guidelines for diagnosis and management of osteoporosis. *Osteoporosis Int* 1997;7:390–406

Food components and menopausal health 58

M. L. Wahlqvist and F. S. Dalais

NEW-GENERATION NUTRITIONAL SCIENCE

Most of the 20th century has seen nutritional scientists focus on, at first, disorders of energy and nutrient deficiency and, in the latter part, disorders of what has been termed macronutrient excess. The critical concern for most of the world's population during this century has been having enough food and, in relation to this, the notion of protective foods has emerged from time to time. Both the concepts of deficiency and protection have taken on new meaning in the last decade of this century because of important advances in the integrative sciences and in food chemistry, at a time when biomedical science has exploded.

Basic population health statistics of life expectancy from different age starting points and major cohort studies of populations with defined food cultures have drawn attention to the potential for the human diet to confer substantial advantage in both morbidity and mortality. Notable among these food cultures are those in countries with the longest life expectancies: the studies of Yamori in Okinawa and of migrant Okinawans in Hawaii and Brazil[1], the NHANES study (National Health and Nutrition Examination Study) in the USA[2], and the study in western Sweden of cardiovascular disease in women[3]. Taken together, these studies have underscored the important interplay between gender, socioeconomic status, physical activity and food culture. It is fascinating to see the commonality of food diversity and regular fish consumption in Japanese, Hong Kong, Mediterranean, North American and Scandinavian cultures in relation to their relative longevities. However, even though it is becoming apparent that women and men can achieve optimal health in different ecological settings, if there is compromise on food diversity, it may need to be matched by the regular consumption of foods of high nutritional quality. Nutritional quality is defined as 'food component density' and is measured as the mass of food components per unit energy content of food. Examples of nutritious foods, so defined, are fish, lean meat, eggs, liver, yeast or wheat germ. The counterpart nutrition index of problematic human diets is that of energy density, defined as the energy value (calories or kJ) per unit mass of food. The higher the energy density, the greater the propensity to positive energy balance and obesity with its sequelae.

Nutritional science has also begun to focus on aging. When these studies are of women, they can shed light on nutrition and the menopause. There are three major international studies underway of this type. The first is the SENECA study of the European Union[4]; the second is the Food Habits in Later Life (FHILL) of the International Union of Nutritional Sciences (IUNS), which includes Europe, Asia, Australia, Meso-America and Africa[5]; and the third is the CRONOS study[6] in urban settings of developing countries. After 5 years of follow-up, it is apparent that integrative indices of food culture can predict survival better than any food or nutrient alone; this is particularly so for the Greek diet, at its most traditional, even if it is the mode of analysis for other European style food cultures[7,8]. Given the differences, as well as the commonalities, between food culture associated with successful aging, the question is whether 'fusion cultures' might out-perform the individual contributory cultures. This possibility is now emerging in culturally pluralistic societies such as Canada, the USA and Australia. We still do not know the limits of health advancement among older women, whose life expectancy continues to exceed that of men and in some developed countries, such as Japan, Hong Kong, and

Australia, has been increasing by 1 year every 3 years for the past 30 years. At present, it is generally agreed that the maximal human lifespan is about 120 years, but the number of centenarians in some countries has now reached 0.1% of the entire population. Ongoing improvements in human biology and the likelihood that much of this is due to food availability and variety holds promise for active inquiry about the benefits of food patterns and food components for menopausal women.

A notable turning point in the enquiry about nutrition and the menopause occurred when our research group asked the question in the late 1980s as to whether food intake could account for differences in the experience of the menopause between food cultures. To address this question, we gave soy flour, linseed as seeds, or red clover sprouts to postmenopausal women in a Latin square design and found that the foods were estrogenic[9]. As phytochemical levels in the blood increased, so vaginal cytology, assessed in a blinded design, improved, and the blood levels of the gonadotropin, follicle stimulating hormone, fell[10]. The era of phytoestrogens and the menopause had begun!

NEW-GENERATION FOOD SCIENCE

It was previously thought that the components of food with biological activity in humans were simply classifiable into the macronutrients (protein, fat, carbohydrate, dietary fiber and water), which, with the exception of water, had an energy value, and the micronutrients (vitamins and the major and minor elements). It is now recognized that the chemicals that characterize the food by color, taste and smell, and protect it in life against other organisms, are natural antioxidants and have many more functions that are of relevance to human biology. When these chemicals are found in plants they are referred to as 'phytochemicals' and in animals they are known as 'zoochemicals'. The greatest interest is currently being shown in phytochemicals from fruits, vegetables, grains, nuts and other seeds. Many of the compounds in question are multifunctional compounds with antimutagenic, antiangiogenic, antioxidant, antimicrobial and estrogenic properties, among others[11]. The more the function of these compounds is understood in human biological systems, the more some are likely to be regarded as necessary for optimal health, with little distinction, apart from the time course over which they operate, from other nutrients regarded as essential.

At the same time as new food components are being discovered beyond the macro- and micronutrients, new functions of known food nutrients are being described. Important examples are the functions of vitamin D other than in bone health, including cellular differentiation, immune function and muscle strength; the role of omega-3 polyunsaturated fatty acids in cell regulatory pathways through prostaglandins, and in membrance functions for receptors and myocardial electrical activity; and the functions of certain water-soluble vitamins in cardiovascular disease prevention.

The role of the water-soluble vitamins folic acid, vitamin B_6 and vitamin B_{12} in protecting against atherosclerotic vascular disease has been becoming increasingly clear[12]. The mechanism appears to be mediated through the lowering of plasma homocysteine, which is vascular toxic and promotes thrombotic events.

GENDER, FOOD AND SURVIVAL

Wherever there is not an exceptional maternal mortality rate, and as long as girls are not selectively maltreated, women's life expectancy at birth exceeds that of men. The reasons for this are not well known, but they may be genetic, reside in endogenous factors such as immune function and hormonal profiles, or reflect different lifestyles between the genders.

In so far as exogenous factors are concerned, food knowledge, choice and skill may often give women a biological advantage. One of the best examples of this food intake difference by gender is the greater food diversity that women consume[13]. The greater the food diversity score, the longer women or men live, but since women have the more diverse diets in general, as a group they have less to gain than men. Thus, for further optimization of women's health and optimization at older ages, it is possible to explore the role of particular foods within this diversity for women.

NUTRITION AND THE MENOPAUSE

Immunodeficiency

Protein energy malnutrition is the best-studied nutritional situation that contributes to immunodeficiency. It is the basis of the world-wide nexus between malnutrition and infection, and is probably a contributor to certain forms of neoplastic disease as well.

There has been particular interest in certain amino acids (glutamine and the tripeptide glutathione) and essential fatty acids (omega-3 and omega-6 polyunsaturated fatty acids) as determinants of immune status.

Among the micronutrients of particular interest are pyridoxine (vitamin B_6) and zinc[14]. The role of macrophages in converting 25-hydroxy- to 1,25-dihydroxyvitamin D to act locally is also now appreciated.

Certain phytochemicals, such as the flavonoids in blackcurrants and berries, are notable for their immunomodulatory properties.

Sarcopenia

Progressive reduction in skeletal muscle mass with age (sarcopenia) is a major health risk for older women[15]. The reasons for this are that lean mass is the basis for strength and locomotion, a reserve of nutrients in time of metabolic stress, and a large contributor to basal metabolic rate and overall energy balance. Sarcopenia may occur with advancing years for a variety of reasons, including inadequate or inappropriate food intake, physical inactivity, wasting disease or as part of the underlying aging process. To some extent, it is likely to be preventable and reversible. Sarcopenia is partly recognized by the World Health Organization (WHO) analysis of body mass index (BMI (kg/m^2), see below) as a criterion for chronic energy deficiency. Stage 1 chronic energy deficiency is defined as a BMI of 17 kg/m^2 to < 18.5 kg/m^2, stage 2 as 16 $kg/m^2 < 17$ kg/m^2 and stage 3 as < 16 kg/m^2.

Overfatness, general obesity and abdominal obesity

BMI is the currently accepted way of classifying degrees of overfatness and, indeed, chronic energy deficiency. Even though, for a given BMI, women have more body fat than men, the same BMI has similar predictive power, all other things being equal, for survival in men and women. It is appropriate for women to have more fat than men during their reproductive years. However, this is less certain for the menopausal years. Young adults whose BMI is between 19 and 24.9 kg/m^2 are regarded as having an acceptable weight to height relationship. However, there is concern that BMIs greater than 22.5 kg/m^2 may increase the risk for diabetes and cardiovascular disease in women[16]. The risk for premature death increases substantially once the BMI is ≥ 30.0 kg/m^2 and increases dramatically at ≥ 40.0 kg/m^2. Much of the predictive power of BMI for health outcome is located in abdominal fatness, which may be assessed by abdominal circumference (waist at the umbilicus or, by WHO criteria, midway between the lower bony rib cage and the iliac crest) or by an abdominal : hip ratio. In Caucasian populations, the abdominal circumference should definitely be < 100 cm for men and < 95 cm for women although there is no international agreement on this. Most experts suggest that the abdominal : hip ratio in men should be less than 0.85 and in women less than 0.80. There are now studies showing that, in Asian populations with a low BMI, an increased abdominal : hip ratio is associated with the manifestation of cardiovascular risk[17,18]; both papers cited are relevant to menopausal women.

Higher BMIs (between 25.0 kg/m^2 and 30.0 kg/m^2) in older individuals are a health conundrum. This is because there is ample evidence that they are associated with an increased risk of diabetes, but, in terms of life expectancy, older individuals tolerate these BMIs better than younger individuals.

The stage may be set for abdominal obesity and general obesity in later life by events occurring as early as in fetal life and may be dependent on maternal nutrition[19]. There is a higher prevalence of diabetes and cardiovascular risk among adults who were born with low birth weights and then exposed, later in life, to a more affluent diet and lower levels of physical activity than those for which their genetic programming took place as fetuses of mothers who suffered nutritional deprivation. Thus, nutritional status during the menopause may depend on a whole life of nutrition.

Diabetes

World-wide, impaired glucose tolerance and type II diabetes are increasing in prevalence among menopausal women. How much this is related to the menopause or estrogen deficiency and how much to age-related changes in body composition is uncertain. A Melbourne prospective study of menopausal women indicates that about 10% may develop impaired glucose tolerance and 2–3% diabetes over 5 years[20], and this is dependent on the degree and distribution of body fatness. The question is to what extent age and estrogen deficiency contribute independently to glycemic status and insulin resistance.

It is theoretically possible that either endogenous estrogen deficiency or phytoestrogen deficiency could contribute to the development of abdominal fatness in menopausal women and, in turn, insulin resistance.

Intervention studies in Sweden and in China demonstrate the great importance of regular physical activity in reducing the progression of impaired glucose tolerance to diabetes; furthermore, nutritional intervention can also play a role, although the best nutritional interventions are yet to be devised and tested[21,22].

Contrary to popular practice, evidence points to snacking rather than large meals as being a way of minimizing insulin resistance and hyperglycemia, as well as other cardiovascular factors. Such an approach to eating would also allow for the use of nutritious snacks, such as fruit, without an adverse effect on glycemic status, while retaining the health-protective role of such foods in the diet.

Obesity and even diabetes in elderly Greek women appears not to be associated with the expected levels of morbidity and mortality found in their non-Greek counterparts. It has been postulated by Kouris-Blazos and colleagues[23] that this paradox is attributable to the protective consumption of an array of plant foods, such as lentils, herbs and spices, in the traditional Greek diet.

Cardiovascular disease

The impact of cardiovascular risk for cardiovascular disease in women becomes more apparent at a later stage than in men, in the menopausal years. One reason for this might be that the abdominal : hip ratio of such women begins to approximate to that of men at this stage of life[24]. Another might be that estrogen deficiency plays a role in the pathogenesis of cardiovascular disease. In this respect, phytoestrogen intake is likely to be relevant; as evidence increases for soy-derived isoflavones preventing the expression of cardiovascular risk, the case can be made for cardiovascular disease being, in part, an isoflavone deficiency disorder.

Yet another intriguing possibility is that, once menstruation has ceased, women store iron to a greater extent and begin to behave like men in relation to iron status[25]. The mechanism proposed is that iron acts as an oxidant and damages the vasculature and myocardium.

Foods that lower plasma homocysteine are likely to be very important in a cardioprotective diet. Good food sources of folate include liver, citrus fruits, green leafy vegetables and nuts, those of vitamin B_6 include liver, fish and bananas, and sources of vitamin B_{12} are animal-derived foods, such as liver and lean meat, together with fish and eggs.

For cardioprotective carotenoids, lycopene, the red color in tomatoes, is attracting attention[26]. Food vitamin E has been shown to be protective against cardiovascular disease in the Iowa Women's study and similar results have been obtained for supplementary vitamin E in the US Nurses Study.

Osteoporosis

When considering diet, most attention has been directed towards calcium intake as a contributor to osteoporosis in estrogen-deficient postmenopausal women[25]. However, there is growing evidence that, in Europe and Asia, the women with the lower calcium intakes can have the better bone mineral density. This is not to say that calcium is not important for bone, but what it does say is that there are bound to be other important nutritional and associated lifestyle factors which determine calcium accretion in bone.

One important nutritional factor is sodium intake, which, through increased excretion stimulates urinary calcium excretion[27]. Therefore, high sodium intakes from salt, monosodium glutamate and sodium bicarbonate, which is used to keep vegetables green and as a leavening agent in breads and cakes, needs to be evaluated at the time of assessing calcium balance.

Vitamin D deficiency is becoming more prevalent among older people, especially those who spend most time indoors without sunlight exposure to stimulate vitamin D synthesis in the skin. In this respect, the winter months are those where vitamin D deficiency is most likely. Older individuals also synthesize less vitamin D in the skin and need more than the 20 min of sunlight that younger people require to make adequate quantities of vitamin D. Older people may also be resistant to vitamin D because of impaired synthesis of 1,25-dihydroxyvitamin D caused by renal impairment. Dietary intake of vitamin D is often precarious because good food sources are usually limited to fish and, to a lesser extent, eggs. Unless fortified, milk is not a good source of vitamin D, although it is a good source of calcium. Vitamin D supplementation by way of fish liver oils has been shown to decrease fracture rates markedly within 18 months in menopausal women[28]. This effect may reflect the combined value of vitamin D in influencing bone health and muscle strength and therefore proneness to fall.

One of the most attractive candidates for bone protection in Oriental women must be their consumption of isoflavones from soy. In short-term human studies of menopausal women, these phytoestrogenic compounds have been shown to stop bone loss and actually increase it[29,30]. Of even greater cultural interest, some Chinese food subcultures and the Okinawan food culture combine the intakes of isoflavones from soy as tofu, of vitamin D and calcium from fish, and of calcium from green vegetables at one and the same meal, if not in the same recipe - the synergy of such food components in a food culture is potentially considerable for bone health.

There is also evidence that fruits and vegetables, perhaps because of their phytochemical content, may protect against osteoporosis[31]. Another possibility is that vitamin K-rich vegetables might favorably affect the vitamin K-dependent protein osteocalcin.

Neoplastic disease

The most consistent finding in nutritional studies of cancer is the protective role of fruit and vegetables[32]. It is likely that a range of phytochemicals from fruit and vegetables offer this protection through various mechanisms.

In the case of grains, the strongest evidence is in the prevention of large bowel cancel[33], but there is also a protective effect for other cancers.

The cancer-protective properties of soy-containing diets, such as those of China, Japan and Java, are consistently associated with low incidence rates for breast cancer in women and prostate cancer in men[34]. The best candidates for this relationship are the isoflavone (daidzein and genistein) content of soy and products such as tofu and tempeh[35]. The growing consumption of soy-based products, such as breads and drinks, in Western food culture holds promise for a reduction in these otherwise intransigent neoplasias.

There is a body of evidence that supports the role of omega-3 polyunsaturated fatty acids, from a gene regulatory point of view, in reducing cancer incidence, notably bowel cancer. It has already been noted that vitamin D, whose best food source is fish, induces cell differentiation and therefore reduces the risk of certain neoplastic diseases.

Therefore, there is a growing case for menopausal women to regularly include fruit and vegetables, soy and fish in their diets to reduce their risks for various cancers.

Cognitive function

Although most of the investigations of omega-3 polyunsaturated fatty acids and cognitive function have been in neonates and infants, the previously unexpected plasticity of the adult central nervous system (CNS) makes it likely that cognitive function in later life could be favorably affected by intakes of omega-3 polyunsaturated fatty acids at the upper end of the range of human intakes. There is an abundance of long-chain omega-3 polyunsaturated fatty acids in the CNS, whose precursors must be obtained from the diet.

At the same time, the need to protect a CNS rich in polyunsaturated fatty acids against oxidation indicates a high requirement for effective antioxidants. It appears that the most important antioxidant in the CNS is the tripeptide glutathione. Although glutathione is synthesized *in vivo*, its formation can be stimulated by the ingestion of whey proteins rich in the dipeptide precursor of glutathione. There is evidence that supplementation with the antioxidant vitamin E can retard the development of cognitive impairment manifest as Alzheimer's disease[36].

The lipid transport apoprotein, apo E, has three isoforms, apo E2, apo E3 and apo E4. Apo E4 predisposes to Alzheimer's disease; one reason for this might be its role in the transport of amyloid precursor protein. Apo E4 production can be stimulated by high-fat diets, which raises the possibility that dietary fat intervention in people with the apo E4 allele might reduce the risk of Alzheimer's disease. This is an area of considerable interest at the present time.

The work of Masters[37] suggests that, in people with marginal cognitive function, excessive zinc intake leads to cognitive decompensation. If this is the case, it would be a difficult situation to manage in the aged, since older people tend to have poor zinc nutrition. The safety margin for zinc is, in any case, narrow, because to increase zinc intake is to decrease copper absorption.

An area of emerging interest is the role of vitamin K in CNS function by way of vitamin K-dependent proteins. For the CNS, menaquinone (vitamin K_2), rather than phylloquinone (vitamin K_1), is the more relevant. A good source of menaquinone is the dairy product cheese, and it is presumably produced by the bacterial cultures used in cheese manufacture. An adequate intake of menaquinone may be necessary to maintain optimal cognitive function.

The evidence for estrogens playing a role in cognitive function is increasingly strong. It is uncertain how they might act, but one suggestion is that, through a vasodilatory function, they improve cerebral blood flow and decrease the patchy plaque formation of Alzheimer's disease. There is preliminary evidence that isoflavones from soy may decrease the deposition of amyloid, the hallmark of Alzheimer's disease[38].

Although at the moment these are no more than clues to the nutritional prevention of cognitive impairment with age, they do hold out some interesting prospects.

Mood

It looks as though a subgroup of people with depression may benefit from an increased intake of omega-3 polyunsaturated fatty acids[39]. The correction of hypertriglyceridemia with omega-3 polyunsaturated fatty acids supplementation has also been associated with mood improvement in some individuals.

Appetite, taste and smell

Generally, impairment of taste and smell develops with advancing years[40,41]. This means that elderly people may lose interest in food or seek ways of increasing flavor. Higher caffeine intakes can lower the taste threshold in older people and explain some of the interest in caffeine-containing beverages. The corollary is that more salt (sodium) may be added to food in a way that is detrimental for blood pressure and cardiac failure.

When zinc status is marginal on account of a poor intake of zinc-rich foods, such as meat, or because of increased zincuria with the use of diuretics, not only is taste impaired, but appetite is adversely affected.

Thus, in elderly women, there is an important interplay between appetite, taste and smell on the one hand and nutritional status on the other.

Water balance

Thirst in older people in less well tuned to fluid balance[42]. Thus, the risk of dehydration is greater than in their younger counterparts.

AVOIDING DISABILITY AND FRAILTY

One of the greatest challenges during the menopause is to minimize disability and avoid frailty.

Trends in disability scores

There have been promising improvements in age-adjusted disability scores in the UK over the past 20 years and a tapering off of these scores with advancing years in North America[43]. This is encouraging for the quest to compress morbidity towards the end of life.

Role of physical activity

Fries[44] has demonstrated that regular physical activity from the age of 50 years can defer the onset of disability by 15–20 years. We also know that physical activity can prolong life and that strength training decreases the likelihood of nutritional and metabolic disease[45,46].

Nature of frailty

Frailty is a condition or syndrome that results from a multisystem reduction in reserve capacity to the extent that a number of physiological systems are close to, or past, the threshold of symptomatic clinical failure. As a consequence, the frail person is at an increased risk of disability and death from minor external stresses.

Avoiding frailty

The best prospects for avoiding frailty are to be physically active, so as to maintain muscle strength and mass, and therefore decrease the risk of falls, to eat nutritious food, so as to obtain the wide range of food components conducive to health, and to be socially active, to make physical activity and healthy eating more likely[47].

HEALTHY AGING AND WOMEN

By bringing the available evidence together, and allowing for a measure of uncertainty in the evidence, it can still be argued that a combination of social activity, physical activity (both aerobic and strength training) and a consumption of a variety of foods, with an emphasis on plant-derived foods and some fish, eaten in small amounts across the day, is the way most older women can optimize their health.

References

1. Mizushima S, Moriguchi EH, Ishikawa P, *et al.* Fish intake and cardiovascular risk among middle-aged Japanese in Japan and Brazil. *J Cardiovasc Risk* 1997;4:191–9
2. Marwick C. NHANES III health data relevant for aging nation. *J Am Med Assoc* 1997;277:100–2
3. Lapidus L, Andersson H, Bengtsson C, Bosaeus I. Dietary habits in relation to incidence of cardiovascular disease and death in women: a 12-year follow-up of participants in the population study of women in Gothenburg, Sweden. *Am J Clin Nutr* 1986;44:444–8
4. SENECA. Nutrition and the elderly in Europe. Follow-up study and longitudinal analysis. *Eur J Clin Nutr* 1996;50:S1–127
5. Wahlqvist ML, Hsu-Hage BHH, Kouris-Blazos A, Lukito W, IUNS Study Investigators. The IUNS cross-cultural study of 'Food Habits In Later Life' – an overview of key findings. *Asia Pacific J Clin Nutr* 1995;4:233–43
6. Gross R, ed. *CRONOS (Cross-Cultural Research on the Nutrition of Older Subjects)*, 3rd edn. *Food Nutr Bull* 1997;18:267–303
7. Trichopoulou A, Kouris-Blazos A, Wahlqvist ML, *et al.* Diet and overall survival in elderly people. *Br Med J* 1995;311:1457–60
8. Schroll M, Bjornsbo-Scroll K, Ferrt N, Livingstone MB. Health and physical performance of elderly Europeans. SENECA Investigators. *Eur J Clin Nutr* 1996;50:S105–11
9. Wilcox G, Wahlqvist ML, Burger HG, Medley G. Oestrogenic effects of plant foods in postmenopausal women. *Br Med J* 1990;301:905–6
10. Morton MS, Wilcox G, Wahlqvist ML, Griffiths K. Determination of lignans and isoflavonoids in human female plasma following dietary supplementation. *J Endocrinol* 1994;142:251–9

11. Wahlqvist ML, Dalais FS. Phytoestrogens: emerging multifaceted plant compounds. *Med J Aust* 1997;167:119-20
12. Rimm EB, Willett WC, Hu FB, *et al.* Folate and vitamin B6 from diet and supplements in relation to risk of coronary heart disease among women. *J Am Med Assoc* 1998;279:359-64
13. Kant AK, Schatzkin A, Ziegler RG. Dietary diversity and subsequent cause-specific mortality in the NHANES I epidemiologic follow-up study. *J Am Coll Nutr* 1995;14:233-8
14. Lukito W, Boyce NW, Chandra RK. Nutrition and immunity. In Wahlqvist ML, Vobecky JS, eds. *Medical Practice of Preventive Nutrition.* London: Smith-Gordon, 1994
15. Heymsfield SB, Wang J, Lichtman S, Kamen Y, Kehayias J, Pierson RN Jr. Body composition in elderly subjects: a critical appraisal of clinical methodology. *Am J Clin Nutr* 1989;50:1167-75
16. Carey VJ, Walters EE, Colditz GA, *et al.* Body fat distribution and risk of non-insulin-dependent diabetes mellitus in women. The Nurses' Health Study. *Am J Epidemiol* 1997;145:614-19
17. Durenberg-Yap M, Yian TB, Kai CS, Deurenberg P, Van Staveren WA. Manifestation of cardiovascular risk factors at low levels of body mass index and waist-to-hip ratio in Singaporean Chinese. *Asia Pacific J Clin Nutr* 1999;8:177-83
18. Tam TT, Gross R, Lukito W, Rumawas JSP. Chronic energy deficiency and relative abdominal overfatness coexist in free-living elderly individuals in Ho Chi Minh City, Vietnam. *Asia Pacific J Clin Nutr* 1999;8:129-35
19. Wilson J. The Barker hypothesis. An analysis. *Aust NZ J Obstet Gynaecol* 1999;39:1-7
20. Garamszegi CV, Guthrie JR, Dennerstein L, Wahlqvist ML, Burger HG. Impaired glucose tolerance in mid-aged women: a prospective study. *Climacteric* 1999;2:300
21. Eriksson KF, Lindgarde F. No excess 12-year mortality in men with impaired glucose tolerance who participated in the Malmo Preventive Trial with diet and exercise. *Diabetologia* 1998;41:1010-16
22. Pan XR, Li GW, Hu YH, *et al.* Effects of diet and exercise in preventing NIDDM in people with impaired glucose tolerance. The Da Qing IGT and Diabetes Study. *Diabetes Care* 1997;20:537-44
23. Kouris-Blazos A, Wahlqvist ML, Trichopoulou A, Polychronopoulos E, Trichopoulos D. Health and nutritional status of elderly Greek migrants to Melbourne, Australia. *Age Ageing* 1996;25:177-89
24. Lapidus L, Bengtsson C, Larsson B, Pennert K, Rybo E, Sjostrom L. Distribution of adipose tissue and risk of cardiovascular disease and death in women: a 12-year follow-up of participants in the population study of women in Gothenburg, Sweden. *Br Med J* 1984;289:1257-61
25. Horwath C, Kouris-Blazos A, Savige GS, Wahlqvist ML. Eating your way to a successful old age, with special reference to older women. *Asia Pacific J Clin Nutr* 1999;8:216-25
26. Kohlmeier L, Kark JD, Gomez-Gracia E, *et al.* Lycopene and myocardial infarction risk in the EURAMIC Study. *Am J Epidemiol* 1997;146:618-26
27. Goulding A, Campbell D. Dietary NaCl loads promote calciuria and bone loss in adult oophorectomized rats consuming a low calcium diet. *J Nutr* 1983;113:1409-14
28. Chapuy MC, Arlot ME, Duboeuf F, *et al.* Vitamin D3 and calcium to prevent hip fractures in elderly women. *N Engl J Med* 1992;327:1637-42
29. Dalais FS, Rice GE, Wahlqvist ML, *et al.* Effects of dietary phytoestrogens in postmenopausal women. *Climacteric* 1998;1:124-9
30. Potter SM, Baum JA, Teng H, Stillman RJ, Shay NF, Erdman JW Jr. Soy protein and isoflavones: their effects on blood lipids and bone density in postmenopausal women. *Am J Clin Nutr* 1998;68: S1375-9
31. Wattanapenpaiboon N, Lukito W, Wahlqvist ML, Hsu-Hage BH-H, Strauss BJG, The Anglo-Celtic Study Investigators. Contribution of food intake to bone mineral density in Anglo-Celtic Australians [Abstract]. Presented at the *7th Asian Congress of Nutrition*, Beijing, China, 7-11 October 1995:480
32. World Cancer Research Fund and American Institute for Cancer Research. *Food, Nutrition and the Prevention of Cancer: A Global Perspective.* Washington DC: American Institute for Cancer Research, 1997
33. MacLennan R, Macrae F, Bain C, *et al.* Randomized trial of intake of fat, fiber, and beta carotene to prevent colorectal adenomas. The Australian Polyp Prevention Project. *J Natl Cancer Inst* 1995;87: 1760-6
34. Messina MJ, Persky V, Setchell KD, Barnes S. Soy intake and cancer risk: a review of the *in vitro* and *in vivo* data. *Nutr Cancer* 1994;21:113-31
35. Wang H, Murphy PA. Isoflavone content in commercial soybean foods. *J Agricult Food Chem* 1994; 42:1666-73
36. Sano M, Ernesto C, Thomas RG, *et al.* A controlled trial of selegiline, alpha-tocopherol, or both as treatment for Alzheimer's disease. The Alzheimer's Disease Co-operative Study. *N Engl J Med* 1997; 336:1216-22
37. Masters CL, Beyreuther K. Environmental and nutritional clues to the etiology of Alzheimer's disease through the study of the amyloid precursor protein. *Proc Nutr Soc Aust* 1998;22:223
38. Kim H, Xia H, Li L, Gewin J. Modulation of neurodegeneration markers by dietary soy in a primate model of menopause [Abstract]. Presented at the *3rd International Symposium on the Role of Soy in Preventing and Treating Chronic Disease*, Washington, DC, USA, 31 October-3 November 1999
39. Adams PB, Lawson S, Sanigorski A, Sinclair AJ. Arachidonic acid to eicosapentaenoic acid ratio in

blood correlates positively with clinical symptoms of depression. *Lipids* 1996;31:S157-61
40. Schiffman SS. Taste and smell in disease. Part I. *N Engl J Med* 1983;308:1275-9
41. Schiffman SS. Taste and smell in disease. Part II. *N Engl J Med* 1983;308:1337-43
42. Rolls BJ, Phillips PA. Aging and disturbances of thirst and fluid balance. *Nutr Rev* 1990;48:137-44
43. Khaw KT. Healthy aging. *Br Med J* 1997;315:1090-6
44. Fries JF. Physical activity, the compression of morbidity, and the health of the elderly. *J R Soc Med* 1996;89:64-8
45. Paffenbarger RS Jr, Hyde RT, Wing AL, Hsieh CC. Physical activity, all-cause mortality, and longevity of college alumni. *N Engl J Med* 1986;314:605-16
46. Fiatarone MA, Evans WJ. The etiology and reversibility of muscle dysfunction in the aged. *J Gerontol* 1993;48:77-83
47. Lapidus L, Bengtsson C. Socioeconomic factors and physical activity in relation to cardiovascular disease and death. A 12-year follow-up of participants in a population study of women in Gothenburg, Sweden. *Br Heart J* 1986;55:295-301

Soy foods, soy phytoestrogens and bone health

59

M. J. Messina and F. S. Dalais

INTRODUCTION

Osteoporosis, which is a world-wide problem of immense magnitude, is a multifactorial condition of the skeleton in which skeletal strength is reduced by such an extent that fractures occur on minor trauma. Individuals with osteoporosis frequently have both reduced bone mass and microstructural disturbances of the bone architecture. In 1990, there were 1.66 million hip fractures world-wide[1]. However, the world population is aging, so morbidity and mortality resulting from osteoporosis will increase markedly within the next 50 years, especially in Asia, Latin America, the Middle East and Africa[2].

Approximately twice as many women as men develop osteoporosis, with fracture rates also being twice as high in women[3]. Furthermore, on average, men develop fractures approximately 5 years later than women[4]. The longer lifespan of women further increases their osteoporosis burden.

The role of estrogen in bone health is apparent from the marked loss in bone mass during the years immediately prior to and following the menopause and from the reduction in fracture risk associated with the use of estrogen replacement therapy. Estrogen exerts several bone-protective actions, including increasing the synthesis of 1,25-dihydroxyvitamin D, controlling the production of bone-resorbing cytokines and decreasing the sensitivity of bone to parathyroid hormones[5]. Despite the potential value of estrogen replacement in reducing the burden of osteoporosis, the public health impact of estrogen is in question, because many women are unwilling to use long-term estrogen replacement therapy[6]. Thus, there is a need for more acceptable alternative approaches for reducing fracture risk. Soy foods and soybean isoflavones are increasingly being viewed as such alternatives.

EMERGING INTEREST IN SOY FOODS IN RELATION TO BONE HEALTH

During the past several years, soy foods and soybean constituents have come under investigation for their role in chronic disease prevention, especially heart disease and cancer[7-9]. However, the most natural role for soy may be its role in reducing the risk for osteoporosis.

Two factors in particular provided the basis for the initial speculation that soy might contribute to bone health. These are the estrogenic properties of soybean isoflavones[10,11] and the effectiveness of the synthetic isoflavone, ipriflavone, in reducing bone loss in perimenopausal and postmenopausal women[12-14]. In addition, as discussed below, several human studies have shown that soy protein, when substituted for animal protein, decreases calcium excretion[15,16].

This brief review highlights key animal and human research relevant to the effects of both soy protein and soybean isoflavones on bone health. In addition, general background information on isoflavones is provided.

ISOFLAVONES: GENERAL OVERVIEW

The basic structural feature of flavonoid compounds is the flavone nucleus, which is comprised of two benzene rings linked through a heterocyclic pyran ring. The position of the benzenoid B ring divides the flavonoid class into flavonoids (2-position) and isoflavonoids (3-position). The primary isoflavones in soybeans are genistein (4′,5,7-trihydroxyisoflavone) and daidzein (4′,7-dihydroxyisoflavone) and their respective β-glycosides, genistin and daidzin. Typically, there is somewhat more genist(e)in than daidz(e)in in soybeans and soy foods[17-22]. There are also small amounts of a third isoflavone in soybeans, glycitein (7,4′-dihydroxy-6-methoxyisoflavone), and its glycoside, glycitin.

However, unlike flavonoids, isoflavones have an extremely limited distribution in nature. Only in soybeans are isoflavones present in nutritionally relevant amounts. The United States Department of Agriculture and several other groups have published values for the isoflavone content of a variety of soy products[23-25]. One serving of a traditional soy food, such as a cup of soy milk or 85–115 g of tofu, contains about 30 mg of isoflavones. Isolated soy protein (< 90% protein) and defatted soy flour (about 50% protein) contain about 0.5–2 mg and 2–3 mg isoflavones/g protein, respectively. Isoflavones are quite heat stable. Baking or frying does not alter the total isoflavone content[26].

Recent data indicate that the isoflavone intake of Japanese adults in Japan is about 30 mg/day[27]. Not unexpectedly, intake in the USA is likely to be no more than a few mg/day, with the exception of certain subpopulations, such as vegetarians and Asian Americans[28].

Isoflavones bind to estrogen receptors and affect estrogen-regulated gene products[10,11] and, for this reason, are often referred to as phytoestrogens (plant estrogens). Depending upon the assay employed, on a molar basis, isoflavones possess between 1×10^{-4} and 1×10^{-2} times the activity of 17β-estradiol[11,25,29]. The finding that genistein binds with much greater affinity to estrogen receptor-β than estrogen receptor-α[30,31] may be particularly relevant to effects on bone tissue, since estrogen receptor-β is present in bone cells[32,33]. However, isoflavones are more than just phytoestrogens, and many of the most important physiological effects of isoflavones, especially of genistein, are likely to be only partially related to direct interaction with, or binding to, estrogen receptors. Genistein influences signal transduction through a variety of mechanisms and therefore affects the growth and regulation of many different cell types[34-39].

EFFECTS OF SOY/ISOFLAVONES

In vitro studies

Yamaguchi and Gao have examined the effects of genistein on femoral metaphyseal bone tissue from older female Wistar rats in culture in several studies. They found that, over the concentration range of 10^{-7}–10^{-5} mol/l, genistein inhibited bone loss induced by parathyroid hormone and prostaglandin E_2[40] and, at concentrations of 10^{-5} and 10^{-4} mol/l in the absence of parathyroid hormone and prostaglandin E_2, genistein caused a significant increase in bone calcium content[40,41]. These findings are similar to the results of their cell work[42], although genistein concentrations of 10^{-4} mol/l would not be expected to occur *in vivo*. 17β-Estradiol (10^{-9} mol/l) also inhibited bone loss in their study, although, in combination with genistein, no additive responses were observed. This may have been because maximal stimulatory concentrations of estrogen were used. Genistein prevented parathyroid hormone-induced increases and decreases in bone acid phosphatase and bone alkaline phosphatase, respectively, and, by itself, significantly increased bone alkaline phosphatase activity. This suggests that genistein was stimulating bone formation. Interestingly, tamoxifen (10^{-6} mol/l) by itself had no effect on bone tissue, but completely inhibited the effects of both genistein and 17β-estradiol.

Other research has similarly shown that genistein (10^{-5} mol/l) increases the calcium content of femoral metaphyseal and diaphyseal bone tissue in culture. Furthermore, the effect of genistein on calcium content and bone alkaline phosphatase activity was synergistically enhanced by the addition of zinc (10^{-5} mol/l), an effect that was completed inhibited by the addition of cycloheximide (10^{-6} mol/l), an inhibitor of protein synthesis, to the culture medium[43]. In both studies, genistein was found to increase bone DNA content, suggesting that genistein increased bone cell proliferation[43].

In culture, daidzein has a very similar effect to that of genistein on femoral diaphyseal (cortical bone) tissue from older female Wistar rats[44]. Research indicates that maximal stimulatory effects of genistein and daidzein on bone calcium content and bone alkaline phosphatase activity are similar to those of 17β-estradiol, but much higher concentrations of isoflavones are required (10^{-5} versus 10^{-8} mol/l)[44]. As was shown for genistein, zinc synergistically enhances the effect of daidzein on bone calcium content[43], although, unlike in the previously cited study, zinc did not enhance the effect of isoflavones on either bone DNA or alkaline phosphatase activity. Furthermore, at maximal concentrations, neither additive nor synergistic effects between daidzein and genistein were noted[44]. However, this may have been because maximal stimulatory concentrations of each isoflavone were used. The combined effects using lower concentrations were not studied.

Finally, in contrast to these favorable effects of daidzein, daidzein (10^{-8}–10^{-10} mol/l), but not genistein or ipriflavone, stimulated bone resorption in a pit formation assay[45]. The authors of this study speculated that daidzein induced osteoclast differentiation by inhibiting the casein kinase II activity of its progenitors.

Animal studies

The ovariectomized rat model is accepted by the US Food and Drug Administration as a model for studying osteoporosis[17]. Within the past few years, several investigators have found that isolated isoflavones are quite effective in this model. For example, Ishida and colleagues[18] found that daidzin (the glycoside form of daidzein), when orally administered immediately after surgical removal of the ovaries, retarded femoral bone loss in a dose-dependent manner. Genistin (the glycoside form of genistein) had a similar effect to daidzin at the one dose studied and both isoflavones were almost, but not quite, as effective as estrone[37]. Both Blair and co-workers[19] and Fanti and associates[20] also found that genistein was effective in retarding bone loss in ovariectomized rats.

Soy protein has also been shown by several investigators to retard bone loss in ovariectomized rats[21,22,46]. With one exception, these studies were not designed to determine whether soy protein *per se*, or some other component associated with soy protein, such as isoflavones, was responsible for the effects on bone tissue. However, Arjmandi and colleagues fed ovariectomized rats two different types of soy protein: one naturally high in isoflavones (soy+) and the other (soy–) low in isoflavones as a result of alcohol extraction. Diets containing soy+, but not soy–, retarded bone loss in the femur and spine[46]. Thus, it would appear that isoflavones contribute significantly to the effects of soy protein on bone tissue.

Human feeding studies

Human research on the effects of soy foods or soy protein on bone health is limited. Furthermore, all studies conducted thus far were of a fairly short duration, generally between 3 and 6 months. Nevertheless, these studies are consistent in showing, based on urinary markers, that soy inhibits bone turnover and/or stimulates bone formation in postmenopausal women[47-51]. More importantly, three[52-54] of four studies[55] have found that soy favorably affects bone mineral density in perimenopausal or postmenopausal women. However, positive effects were noted only at the spine and not at other bone sites, such as the hip[53,54].

Although no human studies have used isolated isoflavones, three human studies do suggest that isoflavones are the bone-protective components of soy foods. Potter and co-workers[54] found that, in postmenopausal women, favorable effects on the spine were observed in women fed soy protein containing 90 mg of isoflavones, but not 60 mg of isoflavones. Similarly, in perimenopausal women, Alekel and Peterson[53] found that isoflavone-rich soy protein, but not isoflavone-poor soy protein, was protective against spinal bone loss. Finally, in an open-group longitudinal study, Scheiber and associates[50] noted that serum isoflavone levels were correlated with a reduction in bone resorption and an increase in bone formation in postmenopausal women fed soy foods. To date, these studies have included a small number of subjects over a short duration. The effects of soy and its components should hopefully become clearer with a recently completed 2-year study of 241 perimenopausal women by Burke and colleagues (personal communication).

PROTEIN AND CALCIUM EXCRETION

In 1968, Wachman and Bernstein proposed that a high protein intake, by increasing urinary calcium excretion, could lead to osteoporosis[56]. The hypercalciuric effect of protein is primarily attributed to the metabolism of the sulfur-containing amino acids methionine and cysteine[57,58]. This suggests that, because proteins differ markedly in their sulfur amino acid content, their effects on calcium excretion should also differ. Furthermore, since soybeans are relatively low in sulfur amino acids, this suggests that soy protein is less hypercalciuric than animal protein. In fact, several human studies have demonstrated this to be the case[15,16]. For example, Breslau and co-workers[15] fed subjects, in random order, each of three different diets containing similar amounts of protein and calcium for 12-day periods, but found that subjects excreted 150, 121, and 103 mg of calcium/24 h when on the animal protein, soy and animal protein, and soy protein diets, respectively.

The clinical significance of substituting soy foods for animal foods on calcium balance and hence bone health will, of course, depend upon the relative level of intake. Each gram of protein is thought to increase calcium excretion by about 1-2 mg[59,60]. Since net calcium absorption is only about 10%, the hypercalciuric effect of protein is certainly not trivial[59,61]. All other things being equal, one might expect that substituting 20 g of soy protein for animal protein would decrease calcium loss by as much as 10 mg, which would, in theory, reduce dietary calcium requirements by as much as 100 mg/day.

SOY INTAKE AND OSTEOPOROSIS IN JAPAN

Asian hip fracture rates are about 50% lower than those of Western Caucasians[62,63]. Some have speculated that soy intake contributes to this lower rate. However, the lower rate is more likely to stem from the short hip axis length of Japanese women[64,65] and the lower incidence of falls among older Japanese women (relative to Caucasian women)[66,67]. Furthermore, thus far, human studies indicate that soy only has effects on the spine, and the amount of isoflavones shown to be effective in the dose-response study by Potter and colleagues[54] greatly exceeds typical Asian isoflavone intake. Nevertheless, several studies that were recently presented at an international symposium on soy reported that isoflavone intake was correlated with higher femoral bone mineral density in Asian women[68-70]. However, results from other studies do not agree with these findings (references 71-73 and personal communication).

CONCLUSIONS

Overall, the evidence that soy protein favorably affects bone health is quite encouraging. Of course, because of the limited data, no firm conclusions can be made at this time. Thus far, studies have only been conducted in women. Nevertheless, the strength of the evidence clearly justifies conducting long-term studies using either isolated isoflavones or soy foods. Arguments can be made in favor of each approach. Should longer-term studies show that soy/isoflavones favorably affect bone mineral density, studies comparing fracture incidence will be needed. The results of these studies will probably not be known for at least 5-10 years. However, because of the many hypothesized health benefits of soy foods, and their nutrient profile, the public should be encouraged to incorporate soy foods into their diet. Those individuals replacing dairy milk with soy milk should be advised to consume calcium-fortified products. Calcium bioavailability from soy foods is equal to that from dairy milk[74].

Since few dose-response studies have been conducted, estimating the amount of soy protein or isoflavones required for beneficial effects on bone health is difficult, but, based on the work of Alekel and Peterson[53] and Potter and co-workers[54], 60-90 mg of isoflavones/day may be needed. This amount of isoflavones would require consuming two or three servings of traditional soy foods. From a practical perspective, incorporating this amount of soy into the diet will be a challenge for many consumers. Of course, some consumers may use supplements as a means of acquiring isoflavones. However, it is also important to recognize that the food industry is developing new soy products that should make such dietary changes more feasible. The recent approval of a new health claim by the US Food and Drug Administration, stating that the daily consumption of 25 g of soy protein may reduce the risk of cardiovascular disease, will further facilitate the incorporation of soy into the diet. Furthermore, it may be that lesser amounts of soy/isoflavones consumed over the course of a lifetime will also exert favorable effects on bone tissue. However, this remains to be determined.

References

1. Cooper C, Campion G, Melton LJ III. Hip fractures in the elderly: a worldwide projection. *Osteoporos Int* 1992;2:285–9
2. Melton LJ III. Epidemiology of hip fractures: implications of the exponential increase with age. *Bone* 1996;18:121S–5S
3. Melton LJ III, Chrischilles EA, Cooper C, *et al.* Perspective. How many women have osteoporosis? *J Bone Miner Res* 1992;7:1005–10
4. De Laet CE, van Hout BA, Burger H, *et al.* Bone density and risk of hip fracture in men and women: cross sectional analysis. *Br Med J* 1997;315:221–5
5. Riggs BL, Khosla S, Melton LJ III. A unitary model for involutional osteoporosis: estrogen deficiency causes both type I and type II osteoporosis in postmenopausal women and contributes to bone loss in aging men. *J Bone Miner Res* 1998;13:763–73
6. Faulkner DL, Young C, Hutchins D, *et al.* Patient noncompliance with hormone replacement therapy: a nationwide estimate using a large prescription claims database. *Menopause* 1998;5:226–9
7. Adlercreutz H, Mazur W. Phyto-oestrogens and western diseases. *Ann Med* 1997;29:95–120
8. Cassidy A. Physiological effects of phytooestrogens in relation to cancer and other human health risks. *Proc Nutr Soc* 1996;55:399–417
9. Messina MJ, Persky V, Setchell KD, *et al.* Soy intake and cancer risk: a review of the *in vitro* and *in vivo* data. *Nutr Cancer* 1994;21:113–31
10. Markiewicz L, Garey J, Adlercreutz H, *et al. In vitro* bioassays of non-steroidal phytoestrogens. *J Steroid Biochem Mol Biol* 1993;45:399–405
11. Mayr U, Butsch A, Schneider S. Validation of two *in vitro* test systems for estrogenic activities with zearalenone, phytoestrogens and cereal extracts. *Toxicology* 1992;74:135–49
12. Valente M, Bufalino L, Castiglione GN, *et al.* Effects of 1-year treatment with ipriflavone on bone in postmenopausal women with low bone mass. *Calcif Tiss Int* 1994;54:377–80
13. Brandi ML. Flavonoids: biochemical effects and therapeutic applications. *Bone Miner* 1992;19:S3–64
14. Civitelli R. *In vitro* and *in vivo* effects of ipriflavone on bone formation and bone biomechanics. *Calcif Tiss Int* 1997;61:S12–14
15. Breslau NA, Brinkley L, Hill KD, *et al.* Relationship of animal protein-rich diet to kidney stone formation and calcium metabolism. *J Clin Endocrinol Metabol* 1988;66:140–6
16. Anderson JJB, Thomsen K, Christiansen C. High protein meals, insular hormones and urinary calcium excretion in human subjects. In Christiansen C, Johansen JS, Riis BJ, eds. *Osteoporosis*. Viborg, Denmark: Nørhaven A/S, 1987
17. Thompson DD, Simmons HA, Pirie CM, *et al.* FDA guidelines and animal models for osteoporosis. *Bone* 1998;17:125S–33S
18. Ishida H, Uesugi T, Hirai K, *et al.* Preventive effects of the plant isoflavones, daidzin and genistin, on bone loss in ovariectomized rats fed a calcium-deficient diet. *Biol Pharm Bull* 1998;21:62–6
19. Blair HC, Jordan SE, Peterson TG, *et al.* Variable effects of tyrosine kinase inhibitors on avian osteoclastic activity and reduction of bone loss in ovariectomized rats. *J Cell Biochem* 1996;61:629–37
20. Fanti P, Monier-Faugere MC, Geng Z, *et al.* The phytoestrogen genistein reduces bone loss in short-term ovariectomized rats. *Osteoporos Int* 1998;8:274–81
21. Harrison E, Adjel A, Ameho C, *et al.* The effect of soybean protein on bone loss in a rat model of postmenopausal osteoporosis. *J Nutr Sci Vitaminol* 1998;44:257–68
22. Omi N, Aoi S, Murata K, *et al.* Evaluation of the effect of soybean milk and soybean milk peptides on bone metabolism in the rat model with ovariectomized osteoporosis. *J Nutr Sci Vitaminol* 1994;40:201–11
23. Coward L, Barnes NC, Setchell KDR, *et al.* Genistein, daidzein, and their β-glycoside conjugates: antitumor isoflavones in soybean foods from American and Asian diets. *J Agricult Food Chem* 1993;41:1961–7

24. Reinli K, Block G. Phytoestrogen content of foods - a compendium of literature values. *Nutr Cancer* 1996;26:123-48
25. Murphy PA, Song T, Buseman G, *et al.* Isoflavones in retail and institutional soy foods. *J Agricult Food Chem* 1999;47:2697-704
26. Coward L, Smith M, Kirk M, *et al.* Chemical modification of isoflavones in soyfoods during cooking and processing. *Am J Clin Nutr* 1998;68:1486S-91S
27. Nagata C, Takatsuka N, Kurisu Y, *et al.* Decreased serum total cholesterol concentration is associated with high intake of soy products in Japanese men and women. *J Nutr* 1998;128:209-13
28. Juturu V, Hsheih G, Kris-Etherton PM. Soy consumption and nutrient intakes of American adults based on the CSFII data base 1994-1996. Presented at the *3rd International Symposium on the Role of Soy in Preventing and Treating Chronic Disease*, Washington, DC, October 1999
29. Nagel SC, vom Saal FS, Welshons WV. Developmental effects of estrogenic chemicals are predicted by an *in vitro* assay incorporating modification of cell uptake by serum. *J Steroid Biochem Mol Biol* 1999;69:343-57
30. Kuiper GG, Lemmen JG, Carlsson B, *et al.* Interaction of estrogenic chemicals and phytoestrogens with estrogen receptor beta. *Endocrinology* 1998;139: 4252-63
31. Kuiper GG, Carlsson B, Grandien K, *et al.* Comparison of the ligand binding specificity and transcript tissue distribution of estrogen receptors alpha and beta. *Endocrinology* 1997;138:863-70
32. Oursler MJ, Osdoby P, Pyfferoen J, *et al.* Avian osteoclasts as estrogen target cells. *Proc Natl Acad Sci USA* 1991;88:6613-17
33. Eriksen EF, Colvard DS, Berg NJ, *et al.* Evidence of estrogen receptors in normal human osteoblast-like cells. *Science* 1988;241:84-6
34. Akiyama T, Ishida J, Nakagawa S, *et al.* Genistein, a specific inhibitor of tyrosine-specific protein kinases. *J Biol Chem* 1987;262:5592-5
35. Thorburn J, Thorburn T. The tyrosine kinase inhibitor, genistein, prevents α-adrenergic-induced cardiac muscle cell hypertrophy by inhibiting activation of the Ras-MAP kinase signalling pathway. *Biochem Biophys Res Commun* 1994;202:1586-91
36. Constantinou A, Kiguchi K, Huberman E. Induction of differentiation and DNA strand breakage in human HL-60 and K-562 leukemia cells by genistein. *Cancer Res* 1990;50:2618-24
37. Imoto M, Yamashita T, Sawa T, *et al.* Inhibition of cellular phosphatidylinositol turnover by psitectorigenin. *FEBS Lett* 1988;230:43-6
38. Linassier C, Pierre M, Le Peco J-B, *et al.* Mechanism of action in NIH-3T3 cells of genistein, an inhibitor of EGF receptor tyrosine kinase activity. *Biochem Pharm* 1990;39:187-93
39. Kim H, Peterson TG, Barnes S. Mechanisms of action of the soy isoflavone genistein: emerging role for its effect via transforming growth factor b signalling pathways. *Am J Clin Nutr* 1998;68: 1418S-25S
40. Yamaguchi M, Gao YH. Inhibitory effect of genistein on bone resorption in tissue culture. *Biochem Pharmacol* 1998;55:71-6
41. Yamaguchi M, Gao YH. Anabolic effect of genistein on bone metabolism in the femoral-metaphyseal tissues of elderly rats is inhibited by the anti-estrogen tamoxifen. *Res Exp Med (Berlin)* 1997;197:101-7
42. Gao YH, Yamaguchi M. Inhibitory effect of genistein on osteoclast-like cell formation in mouse marrow cultures. *Biochem Pharmacol* 1999;58: 767-72
43. Gao YH, Yamaguchi M. Zinc enhancement of genistein's anabolic effect on bone components in elderly female rats. *Gen Pharmacol* 1998;31:199-202
44. Gao YH, Yamaguchi M. Anabolic effect of daidzein on cortical bone in tissue culture: comparison with genistein effect. *Mol Cell Biochem* 1999;194:93-7
45. Tobe H, Komiyama O, Komiyama Y, *et al.* Daidzein stimulation of bone resorption in pit formation assay. *Biosci Biotechnol Biochem* 1997; 61:370-1
46. Arjmandi BH, Birnbaum R, Goyal N, *et al.* Bone-sparing effect of soy protein in ovarian hormone deficient rats is related to its isoflavone content. *Am J Clin Nutr* 1998;68:1364S-8S
47. Murkies AL, Lombard C, Strauss BJG, *et al.* Dietary flour supplementation decreases post-menopausal hot flushes: effect of soy and wheat. *Maturitas* 1995;21:189-95
48. Washburn S, Burke G, Morgan T, *et al.* Effect of soy protein supplementation on serum lipoproteins, blood pressure, and menopausal symptoms in perimenopausal women. *Menopause* 1999;6:7-11
49. Pansini F, Bonaccorsi G, Albertaza P, *et al.* Soy phytoestrogens and bone [Abstract 97, 061] *North Am Menopause Soc Meetings* 1997:44
50. Scheiber MD, Liu JH, Subbiah MTR, *et al.* Dietary soy isoflavones favorably influence lipids and bone turnover in healthy postmenopausal women. Presented at the *3rd International Symposium on the Role of Soy in Preventing and Treating Chronic Disease*, Washington, DC, October 1999
51. Wong WW. Effects of soy isoflavones on blood lipids, blood pressure, and biochemical markers of bone metabolism in postmenopausal women. Presented at the *3rd International Symposium on the Role of Soy in Preventing and Treating Chronic Disease*, Washington, DC, October 1999
52. Dalais FS, Rice GE, Wahlqvist ML, *et al.* Effects of dietary phytoestrogens in postmenopausal women. *Climacteric* 1998;1:124-9
53. Alekel DL, Peterson CT. Isoflavone-rich soy protein isolate exerts significant bone-sparing in the lumbar spine of perimenopausal women. Presented at the *3rd International Symposium on the Role of Soy in*

Preventing and Treating Chronic Disease, Washington, DC, October 1999

54. Potter SM, Baum JA, Teng H, *et al.* Soy protein and isoflavones: their effects on blood lipids and bone density in postmenopausal women. *Am J Clin Nutr* 1998;68:1375S-9S
55. Gallagher JC, Rafferty K, Haynatzka V, *et al.* The effect of soy protein on bone metabolism. Presented at the *3rd International Symposium on the Role of Soy in Preventing and Treating Chronic Disease*, Washington, DC, October 1999
56. Wachman A, Bernstein DS. Diet and osteoporosis. *Lancet* 1968;1:958-9
57. Hunt JN. The influence of dietary sulphur on the urinary output of acid in man. *Clin Sci* 1956;11: 119-36
58. Remer T, Manz F. Estimation of the renal net acid excretion by adults consuming diets containing variable amounts of protein. *Am J Clin Nutr* 1994; 59:1356-61
59. Nordin BEC. Calcium and osteoporosis. *Nutrition* 1997;13:664-86
60. Heaney RP. Nutrient interactions and the calcium economy. *J Lab Clin Med* 1994;124:15-16
61. Heaney RP. Nutrition: a whole-organism science. *Nutrition* 1997;13:689-90
62. Ho SC, Bacon E, Harris T, *et al.* Hip fracture rates in Hong Kong and the United States, 1988 through 1989. *Am J Public Health* 1993;83:694-7
63. Ross PD, Norimatsu H, Davis JW, *et al.* A comparison of hip fracture incidence among native Japanese, Japanese Americans, and American Caucasians. *Am J Epidemiol* 1991;133:801-9
64. Cummings SR, Cauley JA, Palermo L, *et al.* Racial differences in hip axis lengths might explain racial differences in rates of hip fracture. *Osteoporos Int* 1994;4:226-9
65. Faulkner KG, Cummings SR, Black D, *et al.* Simple measurement of femoral geometry predicts hip fracture: the study of osteoporotic fractures. *J Bone Miner Res* 1993;8:1211-17
66. Aoyagi K, Ross PD, Davis JW, *et al.* Falls among community-dwelling elderly in Japan. *J Bone Miner Res* 1998;13:1468-74
67. Davis JW, Ross PD, Nevitt MC, *et al.* Incidence rates of falls among Japanese men and women living in Hawaii. *J Clin Epidemiol* 1997;50:589-94
68. Sung CJ, Choi SH, Ko BS. Urinary isoflavone levels and several factors that influence bone metabolism in postmenopausal women. Presented at the *3rd International Symposium on the Role of Soy in Preventing and Treating Chronic Disease*, Washington, DC, October 1999
69. Fukui Y, Miura A, Nara Y, *et al.* Relationship between urinary isoflavones and bone metabolism in postmenopausal Japanese women. Presented at the *3rd International Symposium on the Role of Soy in Preventing and Treating Chronic Disease*, Washington, DC, October 1999
70. Rice MM, LaCroix AZ, Lampe JW, *et al.* Soy consumption and bone mineral density in older Japanese American women in King County, Washington. Presented at the *3rd International Symposium on the Role of Soy in Preventing and Treating Chronic Disease*, Washington, DC, October 1999
71. Fujiwara S, Kasagi F, Yamada M, *et al.* Risk factors for hip fracture in a Japanese cohort. *J Bone Miner Res* 1997;12:998-1004
72. Lacey JM, Anderson JJB, Fujita T, *et al.* Correlates of cortical bone mass among premenopausal and postmenopausal Japanese women. *J Bone Miner Res* 1991;6:651-9
73. Dennison E, Yoshimura N, Hashimoto T, *et al.* Bone loss in Great Britain and Japan: a comparative longitudinal study. *Bone* 1998;23:379-82
74. Weaver CM, Plawecki KL. Dietary calcium: adequacy of a vegetarian diet. *Am J Clin Nutr* 1994;59(Suppl):1238-41

Efficacy and tolerance of different kinds of ERT

60

J. Donát

INTRODUCTION

The aim of this study was to compare three ways of administering 17β-estradiol, applied as estrogen replacement therapy (ERT), to three compatible groups of women.

OBJECTIVES

(1) To evaluate over 4 weeks the influence of different kinds of parenteral ERT in dyslipidemic women who had undergone surgical menopause on:

(a) The Kupperman index (the parameter of clinical efficacy on acute symptomatology);

(b) Plasma levels of luteinizing hormone (LH), follicle stimulating hormone (FSH), estrone and estradiol;

(c) Tolerance and side-effects.

(2) To evaluate over 12 months:

(a) The influence of different kinds of estradiol therapy on plasma levels of estrone, estradiol and essential parameters of lipid metabolism;

(b) The changes of mammary density;

(c) Patient compliance and tolerance.

(3) To appreciate:

(a) The advantages and disadvantages of various kinds of estradiol therapy;

(b) The possibility of mutual substitution of three kinds of ERT in the prevention and treatment of estrogen deficiency syndrome.

SUBJECTS AND METHODS

Subjects

There were quite rigid limits to selecting the women: the first condition for participation was a past hysterectomy, most often for uterine myomatosis. In some cases, a hysterectomy had been performed together with an adnexectomy to deal with a pathological finding in the ovaries. Only in one case was the surgery performed for malignancy (a Wertheim–Meigs operation for cancer of the cervix).

The second prerequisite for participation was a postmenopausal hormone status in women with intact ovaries, i.e. the FSH levels had to be over 40 IU/l. The final prerequisite called for abnormal levels of cholesterol and low-density lipoprotein (LDL), with normal high-density lipoprotein (HDL) cholesterol and triglyceride levels.

A total of 55 patients took part in the study. The patients were divided into three groups (Table 1): group A received transdermal ERT (Climara®); group B received percutaneous ERT (Estrogel®); and group C received vaginal ERT (Vagifem®).

Methods

The following laboratory examinations were carried out:

(1) Serum LH, FSH, estrone and estradiol levels;

(2) Total cholesterol, HDL cholesterol, LDL cholesterol, triglyceride levels and the LDL/HDL ratio.

The following clinical examinations were performed:

(1) Kupperman index;

(2) Mammography.

The following statistical analyses were performed:

(1) Non-parametric Wilcoxon test (for paired t test);

(2) Mann–Whitney test (for unpaired t test).

RESULTS

Four-week ERT analysis

In the 4-week analysis of ERT, we found:

(1) A statistically significant increase in the serum estradiol level with each type of therapy (Figures 1, 2 and 3). In groups A and B, the increase in the serum estradiol level was apparent after the first week of estradiol administration ($p < 0.01$ and $p < 0.05$, respectively), while in group C, the increase was seen after the second week of estradiol administration ($p < 0.05$).

(2) A statistically significant increase ($p < 0.01$) in the serum estrone level with percutaneous therapy. This was apparent after the first week of estradiol administration (Figure 2).

(3) Statistically significant decreases ($p < 0.01$) in serum LH and FSH levels with both transdermal and percutaneous therapy. These decreases were apparent after the first week of estradiol administration (Figures 4 and 5).

(4) No statistically significant differences in serum LH and FSH levels with vaginal therapy (Figure 6).

Table 1 Division of patients by method of estrogen replacement therapy (ERT)

Group	*Method of ERT*	*No. of patients*	*Mean age* (years)	*Mean time after hysterectomy with or without ovariectomy* (years)
A	transdermal (Climara)	23	54.9	7.0
B	percutaneous (Estrogel)	16	53.8	10.1
C	vaginal (Vagifem)	16	52.7	7.5

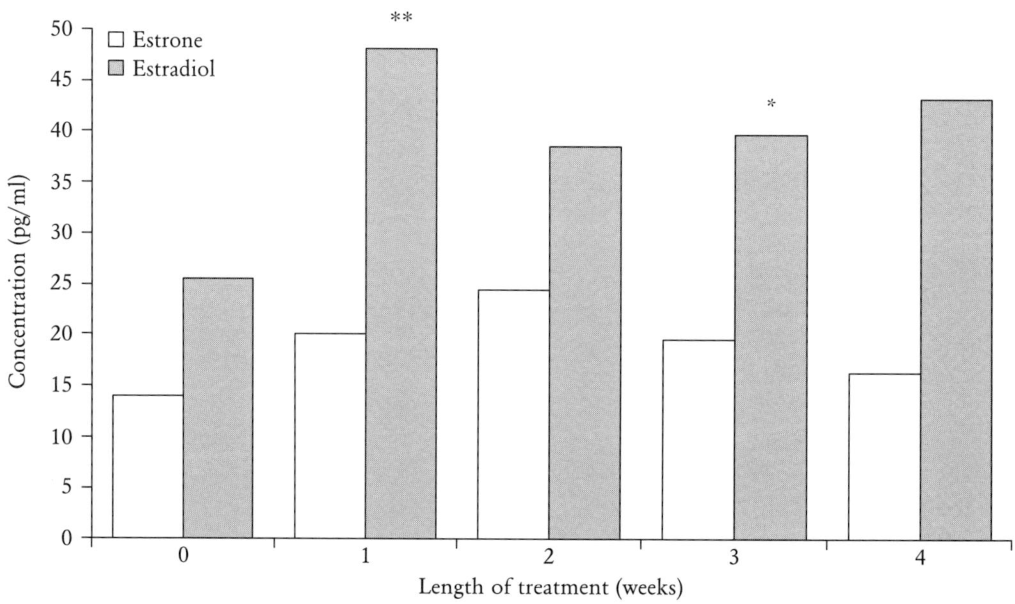

Figure 1 Changes in estrone and estradiol serum levels over 4 weeks of treatment with transdermal estrogen replacement therapy. $^{**}p < 0.01$; $^{*}p < 0.05$

(5) A significant decrease in the Kupperman index with each type of therapy (Figure 7). On average, the Kupperman index decreased from 28.2 to 6.4 (decrease of 77%) in group A, from 25.3 to 10.0 (decrease of 60%) in group B and from 21.8 to 8.0 (decrease of 63%) in group C.

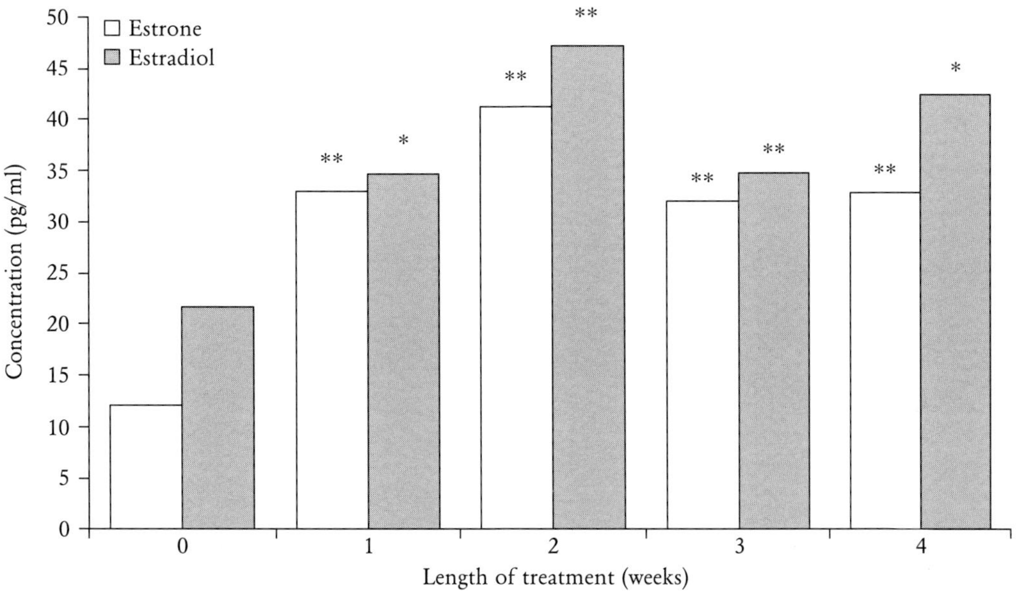

Figure 2 Changes in estrone and estradiol serum levels over 4 weeks of treatment with percutaneous estrogen replacement therapy. $^{**}p < 0.01$; $^{*}p < 0.05$

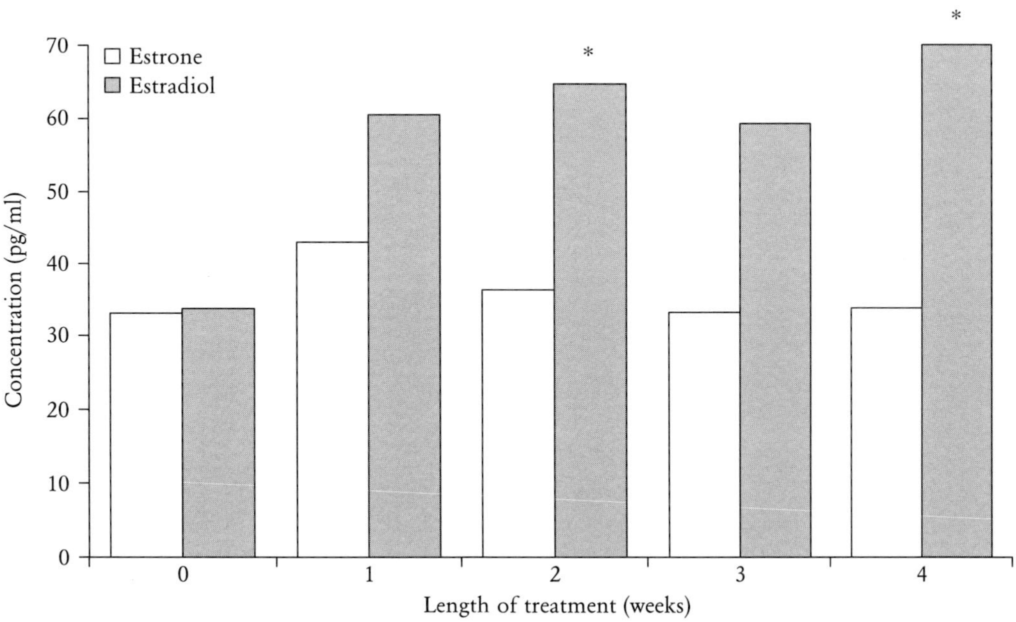

Figure 3 Changes in estrone and estradiol serum levels over 4 weeks of treatment with vaginal estrogen replacement therapy. $^{*}p < 0.05$

Twelve-month ERT analysis

In the 12-month analysis of ERT, we found:

(1) A statistically significant increase (at the 5% level of significance) in the serum estradiol level with each type of therapy (Figure 8).

(2) A statistically significant decrease (at the 5% level of significance) in the LDL/HDL ratio

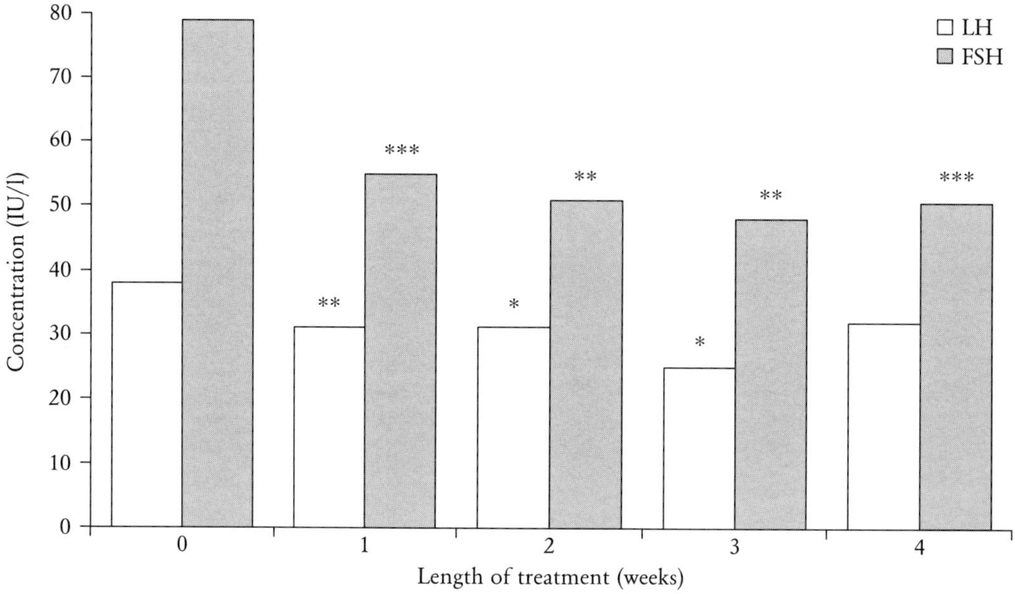

Figure 4 Changes in luteinizing hormone (LH) and follicle stimulating hormone (FSH) serum levels over 4 weeks of transdermal estrogen replacement therapy. $^{***}p < 0.001$; $^{**}p < 0.01$; $^{*}p < 0.05$

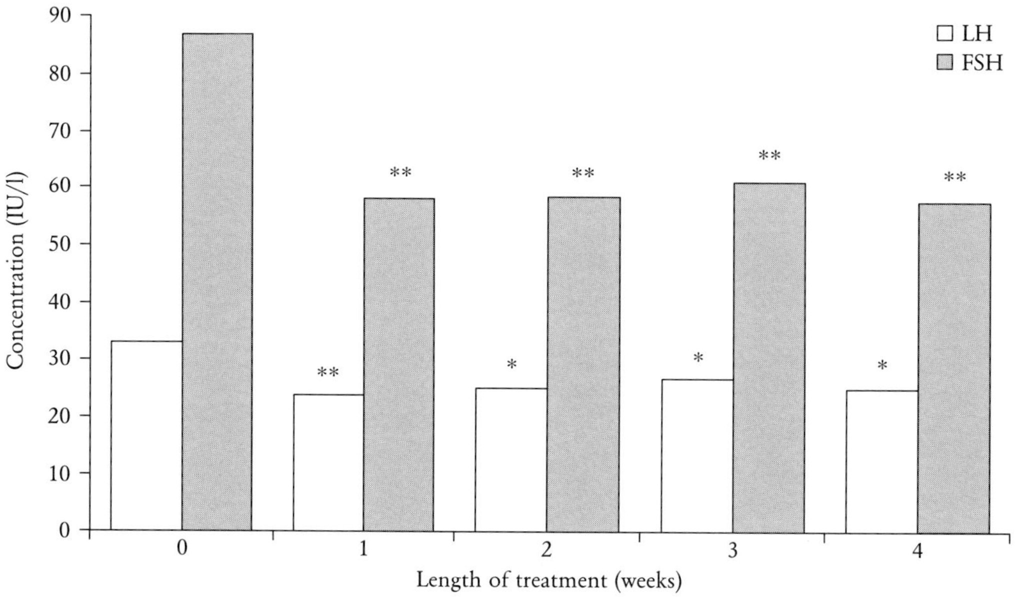

Figure 5 Changes in luteinizing hormone (LH) and follicle stimulating hormone (FSH) serum levels over 4 weeks of percutaneous estrogen replacement therapy. $^{**}p < 0.01$; $^{*}p < 0.05$

with both transdermal and vaginal estradiol administration (Figures 9 and 10).

(3) No statistically significant changes in the lipid profile with estradiol applied percutaneously (Figure 11).

(4) A slight positive effect on other lipid parameters, but no statistically significant changes in any group (Figures 9, 10 and 11).

(5) No statistically significant changes in any of the lipid profile parameters evaluated for each

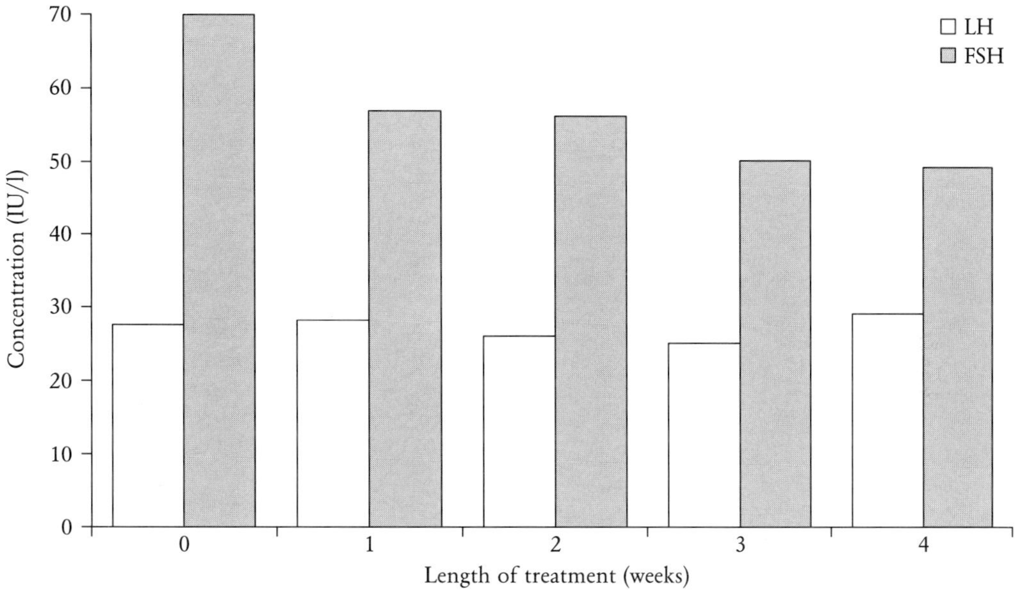

Figure 6 Changes in luteinizing hormone (LH) and follicle stimulating hormone (FSH) serum levels over 4 weeks of vaginal estrogen replacement therapy

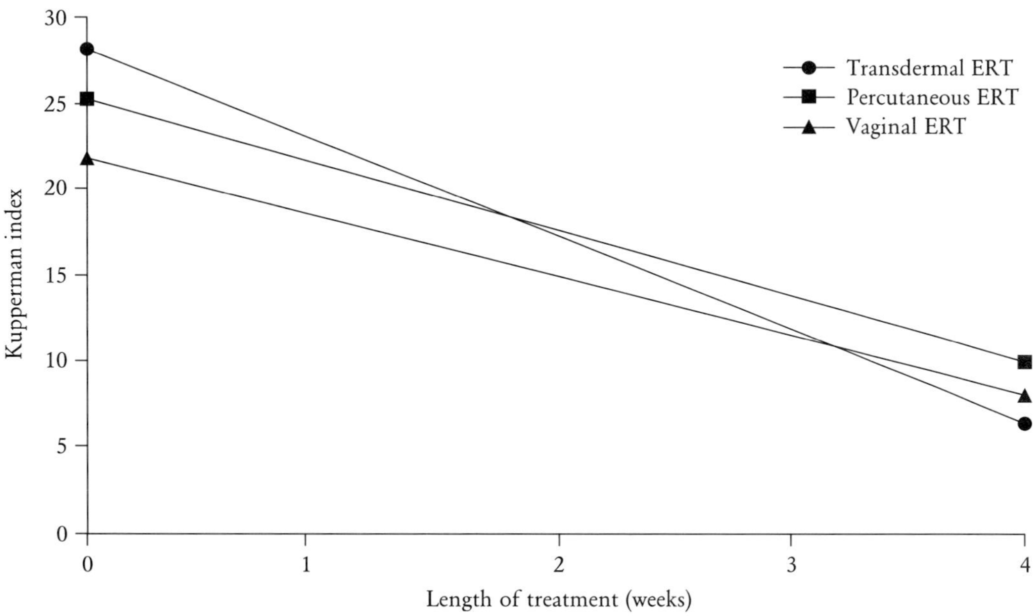

Figure 7 Changes in the Kupperman index over 4 weeks of treatment with transdermal, percutaneous and vaginal estrogen replacement therapy (ERT)

type of ERT before and after the 12 months of therapy (Figures 12 and 13).

(6) Mammography demonstrated normal findings in 64.8% and slight dysplasia (1st grade) in 35.2% of patients before ERT. No substantial changes in mammary density were found after 12 months with any type of ERT.

(7) Due to adverse side-effects or other reasons, the 12-month therapy was not finished by two patients (8.7%) in group A (one for

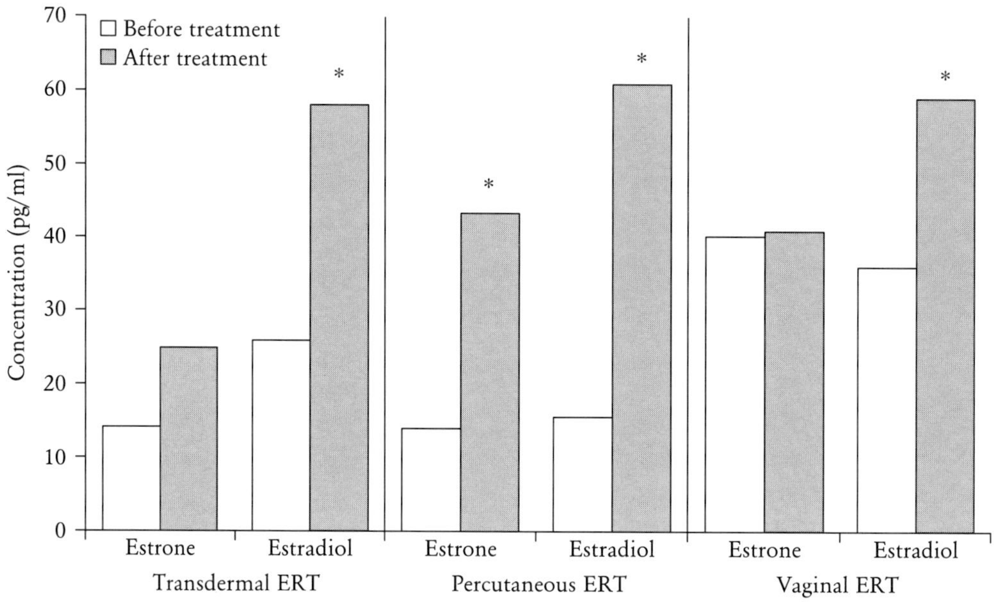

Figure 8 Estrone and estradiol serum levels before and after 12 months of treatment with transdermal, percutaneous and vaginal estrogen replacement therapy (ERT). $^*p < 0.05$

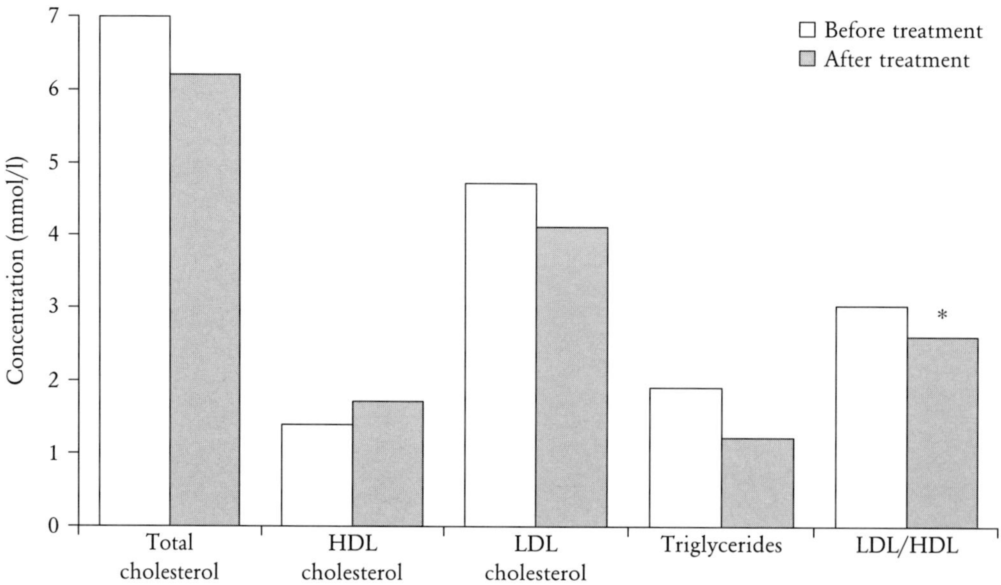

Figure 9 Lipid parameters before and after 12 months of treatment with transdermal estrogen replacement therapy. HDL, high-density lipoprotein; LDL, low-density lipoprotein; $^*p < 0.05$

skin complaints (pruritus) and the other for an allergic reaction on the face), one patient (6.25%) in group B (for a benign breast disease) and one patient (6.25%) in group C (for unsatisfactory effect of the therapy).

DISCUSSION

Side-effects of percutaneous and vaginal estradiol therapy were not found and the treatment was terminated in only one patient on percutaneous ERT and one patient on vaginal ERT. However, the reason for the termination of treatment in the

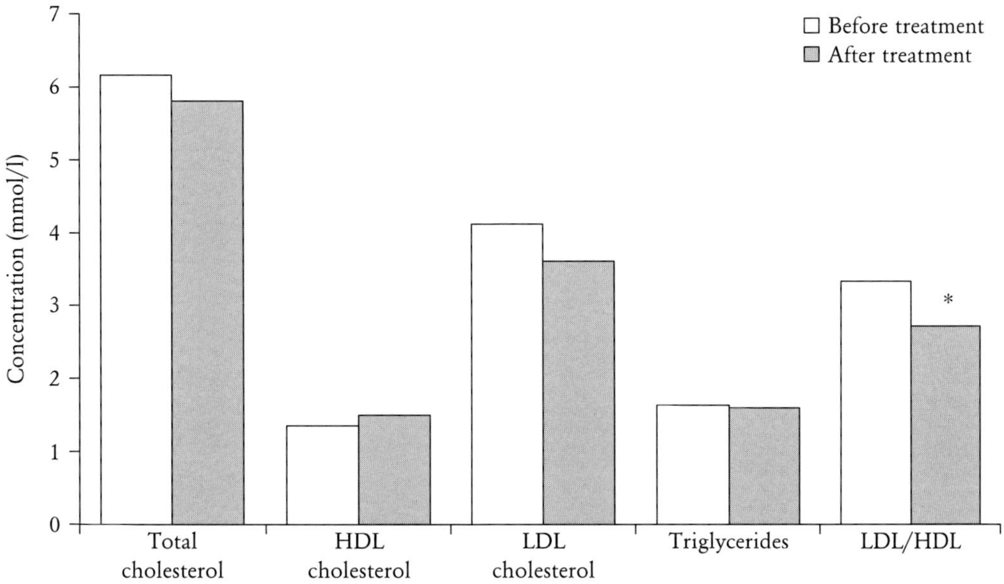

Figure 10 Lipid parameters before and after 12 months of treatment with vaginal estrogen replacement therapy. HDL, high-density lipoprotein; LDL, low-density lipoprotein; $^{*}p < 0.05$

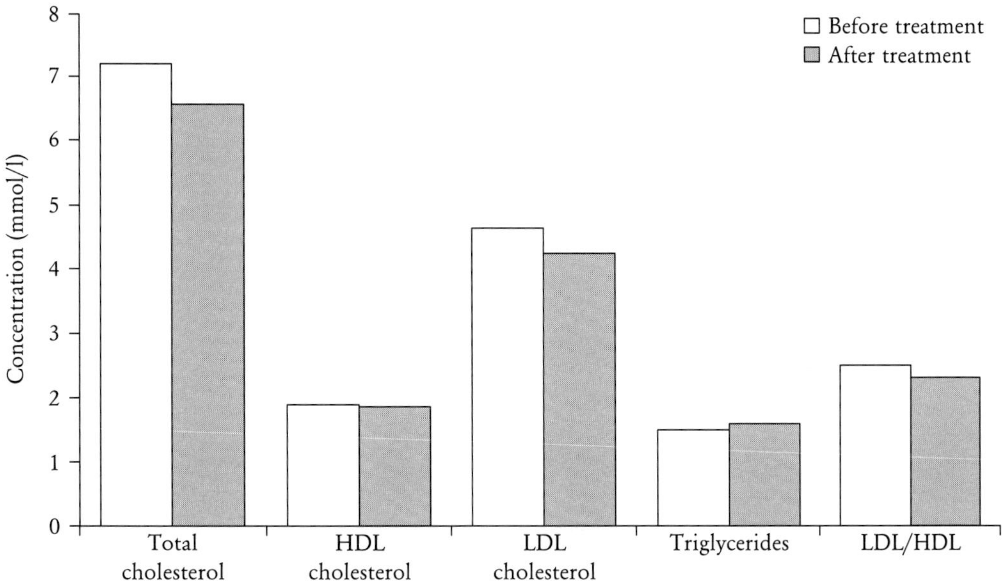

Figure 11 Lipid parameters before and after 12 months of treatment with percutaneous estrogen replacement therapy. HDL, high-density lipoprotein; LDL, low-density lipoprotein

patient on percutaneous estradiol therapy was the patient's fear of breast cancer caused by the inadequate information given to her by her general practitioner. The vaginal administration of estradiol was terminated in one patient since it was not efficient due to acute symptoms of the climacteric syndrome. Vaginal treatment was recommended, not only because the patient experienced hot flushes, but also because of vaginal and urological symptoms. The complaints decreased or disappeared in the course of 2–4 weeks of therapy. The sharp drop in the Kupperman index indicated an immediate effect of estrogen on the acute symptoms of the climacteric syndrome in all groups. In fact, all

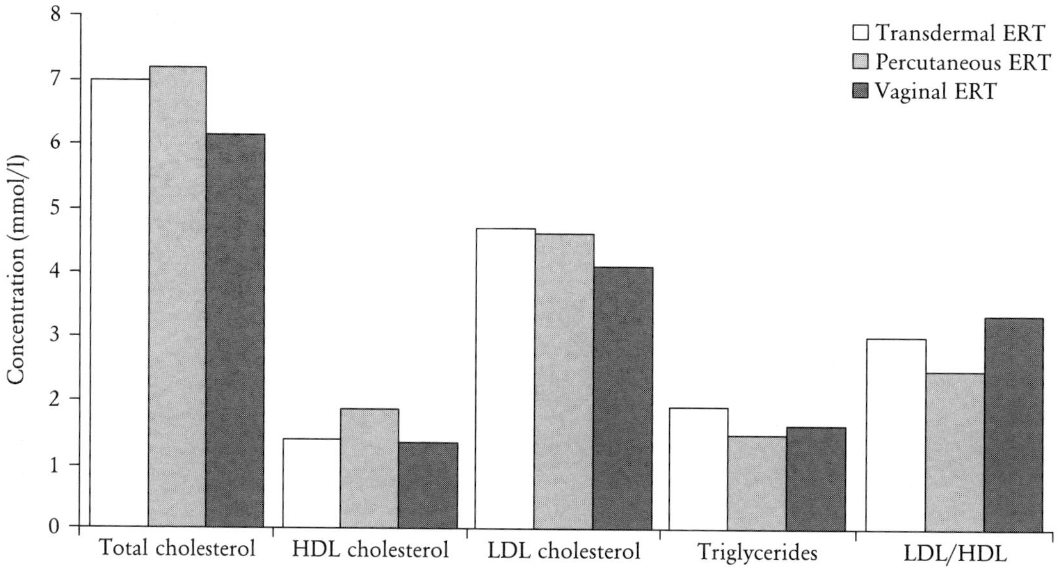

Figure 12 Lipid parameters at baseline with transdermal, percutaneous and vaginal estrogen replacement therapy (ERT). HDL, high-density lipoprotein; LDL, low-density lipoprotein

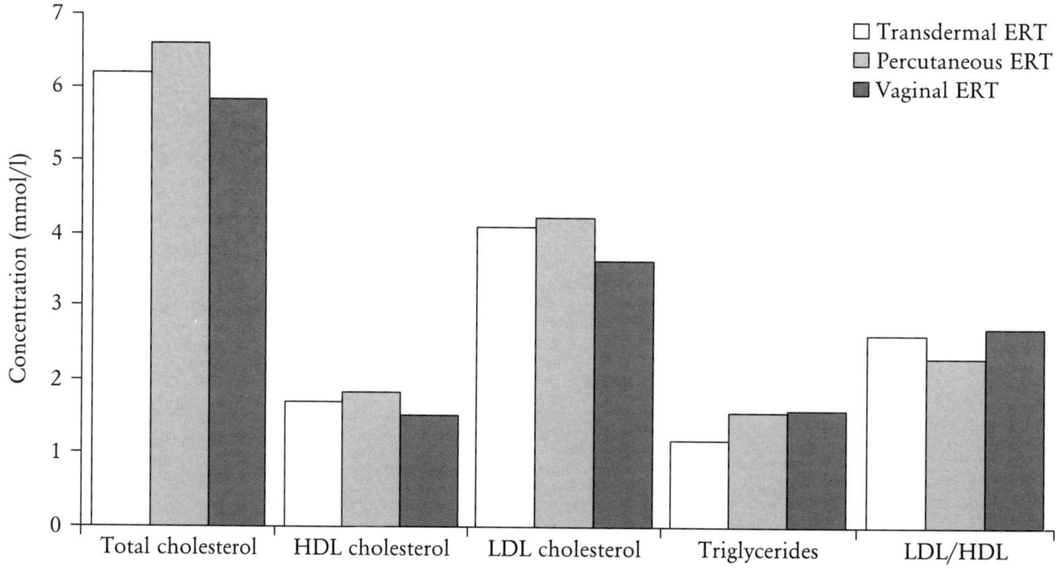

Figure 13 Lipid parameters after 12 months of treatment with transdermal, percutaneous and vaginal estrogen replacement therapy (ERT). HDL, high-density lipoprotein; LDL, low-density lipoprotein

patients showed a medium degree of the climacteric syndrome (classification 20–35). The sharpest drop of 77% in 4 weeks was found with the transdermal application of estradiol, followed by a 63% drop with the vaginal therapy and a 60% drop with the percutaneous ERT. Our results for percutaneous estradiol administration are comparable with the results of Huber[1]. He found a considerable reduction in perimenopausal symptoms assessed by the Kupperman index and also good efficacy and tolerability in a group of patients who received Estrogel.

Estradiol absorption from the vagina depends on several factors: vaginal wall atrophy, possible secondary infections, the question of blood supply and the individual capacity of the vagina to absorb medicaments. In any case, vaginal forms of hormone application seem to work well and their benefical effects have recently been emphasized, for both hormonal contraception and hormone replacement therapy.

Bachmann and colleagues[2] compared Vagifem with placebo and their results showed a significant improvement in vaginal health with vaginal estradiol administration, but Notelovitz and coworkers[3] found no significant absorption of estrogen from vaginal tablets (Vagifem) during 12 weeks of treatment in healthy postmenopausal women with atrophic vaginitis.

In an analysis of ERT performed over a short time, most changes were brought about by transdermal or percutaneous treatment, a statistically significant fall in FSH and LH and an increase in estradiol levels being evident after the first week of ERT. The hormonal changes indicated certain variability, but the clinical effect assessed by the basic Kupperman index was satisfactory. It is necessary to stress at this point that the Kupperman index assesses only acute symptoms, which means the quality of life at a given moment. It can also help to judge the effects of treating acute symptoms such as hot flushes, perspiration, psychological discomfort, paresthesia, dizziness and palpitations. However, it cannot estimate the risk of estrogen deficiency syndromes: the organic syndrome, when mucous membranes are affected, and the metabolic syndrome, when the cardiovascular system, the skeleton or the brain is affected. Our patients showed slight dyslipidemia, together with increased LDL cholesterol levels, but normal HDL cholesterol and triglyceride levels. During the 12-month treatment period, the index of LDL/HDL improved significantly in the patients being treated with transdermal or vaginal ERT. The patients being treated with percutaneous ERT demonstrated an improvement in most indicators, but these changes were not statistically significant. It is necessary to emphasize again that the triglyceride levels were normal in all patients of the observed groups even after 12 months of treatment. The statistically significant increase in estradiol levels was maintained. Parenteral forms of therapy applied either percutaneously or vaginally seem to be effective and some of them are mutually interchangeable when side-effects appear.

CONCLUSIONS

(1) All three types of ERT produce a quick increase in serum estradiol levels to premenopausal values;

(2) Estradiol levels are well balanced with all kinds of estradiol therapy;

(3) Estrone levels do not change with transdermal and vaginal therapies;

(4) The estrone level becomes three times greater with percutaneous therapy;

(5) All three types of ERT demonstrate good clinical effects, are well tolerated and have minimal side-effects.

References

1. Huber J. A percutaneous estrogen gel (Estrogel) is effective to reduce perimenopausal symptoms. Presented at the symposium *Percutaneous estrogen - a new way of therapy for postmenopausal syndrome, IV European Congress on Menopause*, Vienna, Austria, 1997
2. Bachmann G, Notelovitz M, Nanavati N, Mazzeo M. Safety and efficacy of a low-dose estrogen intravaginal tablet (Vagifem) to treat estrogen-deficiency derived atrophic vaginitis. Presented at the *9th Annual North American Menopause Society*, Toronto, Canada, 1998
3. Notelovitz M, Funk S, Nanavati N, Mazzeo M. Systemic absorption of 17beta-estradiol (E2) during treatment with vaginal E2: 10 μg and Vagifem 25 μg tablets. Presented at the *9th Annual North American Menopause Society*, Toronto, Canada, 1998

Effects of oral and transdermal HRT in relation to serum estrogen levels

61

T. Aono, T. Yasui, H. Uemura and M. Irahara

INTRODUCTION

An estrogen threshold hypothesis has been proposed by Barbieri[1], which suggests that different tissues have different sensitivities to estradiol. A decrease in urinary calcium excretion is very sensitive to an estradiol level as low as 20 pg/ml, and estradiol levels between 35 and 70 pg/ml effectively relieve vasomotor symptoms, whereas an estradiol level of more than 70 pg/ml is needed to change the serum lipid profile[1,2]. Furthermore, breast cancer can be very sensitive to the growth-promoting effects of estradiol concentrations as low as 10–20 pg/ml, and estradiol levels in the region of 30 pg/ml produce regression of endometriotic lesions[1]. Therefore, it is necessary to assess the combined effects of serum estrogen levels and estrogenic preparations in postmenopausal women treated with hormone replacement therapy (HRT). In the present study, we measured the serum levels of estrone and 17β-estradiol precisely in postmenopausal Japanese women receiving HRT, and clarified the relationship between estrogen levels and the effects on vasomotor symptoms, bone mineral density, lipid metabolism and breakthrough bleeding.

PATIENTS AND METHODS

Eighty-four postmenopausal or bilaterally ovariectomized women aged 30–64 years, who suffered from vasomotor symptoms such as hot flushes or atrophy of the vagina, were treated with three kinds of HRT as follows. Thirty-three patients received oral administration of 0.625 mg conjugated equine estrogen (CEE; Premarin®, Wyeth, Newbridge, Ireland) and 2.5 mg medroxyprogesterone acetate (MPA; Provera®, Upjohn, MI, USA) every other day, 37 patients received oral administration of 0.625 mg CEE and 2.5 mg MPA every day, and 14 patients received 25μg/day transdermal estradiol (Estraderm TTS®, Novartis, Basel, Switzerland) and daily oral 2.5 mg MPA. All women were in good health, as shown by medical history, physical examination and blood chemistry profile, and had not received any hormonal therapy previously. The mean levels of 17β-estradiol in the three groups before treatment were 3.7, 4.4 and 5.2 pg/ml, respectively. We measured the serum levels of estrone and 17β-estradiol, bone mineral density of the lumbar spine, total cholesterol, triglyceride, high-density lipoprotein (HDL) cholesterol, and apolipoproteins A1, B and E before and 12 months after treatment. All subjects were reclassified into three groups according to the estradiol levels after 12 months of treatment:

(1) Low estradiol group (< 15 pg/ml; $n = 28$);

(2) Middle estradiol group (≥ 15 and < 25 pg/ml; $n = 28$);

(3) High estradiol group (≥ 25 pg/ml; $n = 28$).

The relationships between serum estradiol levels and vasomotor symptoms, bone mineral density, lipid metabolism and unscheduled bleeding were examined. Age, years since menopause, body mass index and bone mineral density of the lumbar spine (L2–L4) (Table 1), and lipid profile before treatment were not significantly different among the three groups. In studying the lipid profile, we divided the subjects into four groups: low-, middle- and high-estradiol groups with oral CEE and MPA, and a transdermal-estradiol group, because the effects of transdermal estradiol, which has no hepatic first-pass effect, on the lipid profile were different from those of oral CEE by hepatic first-pass effect.

Table 1 Baseline characteristics of patients. Values are mean ± SE where appropriate

	Low-estradiol group ($E_2 < 15$ pg/ml)	*Middle-estradiol group ($15 \leq E_2 < 25$ pg/ml)*	*High-estradiol group ($E_2 \geq 25$ pg/ml)*
No. of patients	28	28	28
Age (years)	51.9 ± 1.1	51.2 ± 0.8	51.0 ± 1.5
Years since menopause	5.2 ± 0.9	3.3 ± 0.7	4.7 ± 0.9
BMI	23.5 ± 0.6	22.7 ± 0.5	21.7 ± 0.4*
Spine BMD (g/cm^2)	0.919 ± 0.027	0.897 ± 0.024	0.900 ± 0.027
Estrone (pg/ml)	12.5 ± 1.4	18.3 ± 1.9*	17.8 ± 2.5*
17β-estradiol (pg/ml)	3.0 ± 0.3	4.4 ± 0.7	5.2 ± 0.6

*$p < 0.05$ versus low-estradiol group; E_2, 17β-estradiol; BMI, body mass index; BMD, bone mineral density

Measurements of estrone and 17β-estradiol

We have developed a highly sensitive and specific assay for estrone and 17β-estradiol in the serum. Estrone and estradiol, obtained by solid-phase extraction using a Sep pak tC18 cartridge (Waters Co., MA, USA), were purified by high-performance liquid chromatography (HPLC). The quantitation of estrone and 17β-estradiol was carried out by specific radioimmunoassay. The minimum detectable doses for estrone and 17β-estradiol were 1.05 pg/ml and 0.65 pg/ml, respectively. The serum levels of 17β-estradiol using this method strongly correlated with those by gas chromatography-mass spectrometry. In our preliminary work, serum levels of estrone and 17β-estradiol with a single oral administration of CEE reached peaks of 125.9 and 13.7 pg/ml, respectively, after 12 h of administration. Based on the results, which showed that levels of estrone and 17β-estradiol plateaued and were not significantly different between 12 and 18 h, blood samples were drawn at 12–18 h after the ingestion of CEE during HRT. The blood was centrifuged at 4 °C and the serum samples obtained were frozen until analysis.

Statistical analysis

Results were expressed as mean ± SE. Statistical differences between baseline and treatment values within the groups were determined by the two-sided paired *t* test, and differences between the groups determined by analysis of variance were assessed by Student's *t* test. Values of *p* less than 0.05 were considered to be statistically significant.

RESULTS

The mean levels of estrone and 17β-estradiol 12–18 h after the administration of CEE and MPA every other day were 71.7 and 14.9 pg/ml at 12 months, respectively, whereas these levels with daily CEE and MPA were 139.8 and 22.8 pg/ml, respectively. On the other hand, the mean levels of estrone and 17β-estradiol with transdermal estradiol and MPA were 51.7 and 40.5 pg/ml, respectively.

The Kupperman index was determined every 3 months for the study of vasomotor symptoms. As shown in Figure 1, a significant ($p < 0.01$) decrease in the Kupperman index was recognized in the three groups after 3 months of treatment. The incidence of breakthrough bleeding during treatment in the low-estradiol group was less than that in the middle- and high-estradiol groups during treatment, and there was no unscheduled bleeding after 12 months of treatment in the low-estradiol group (Figure 2).

Bone mineral density of the L2–L4 vertebral bodies was measured by dual energy X-ray absorptiometry (Hologic QDR 2000, Hologic Corp, MA, USA) before the initiation of treatment and 12 months later. Data were expressed as bone mineral density in g/cm^2. As shown in Figure 3, there were significant percentage increases in the bone mineral density of the lumbar spine in the middle- and high-estradiol groups (3.2 ± 0.9%, $p < 0.01$; 4.0 ± 0.6%, $p < 0.001$, respectively), but not in the low-estradiol group.

Serum total cholesterol, triglyceride and HDL cholesterol were analyzed using an enzymatic colorimetric method. The low-density lipoprotein (LDL) cholesterol level was calculated according to

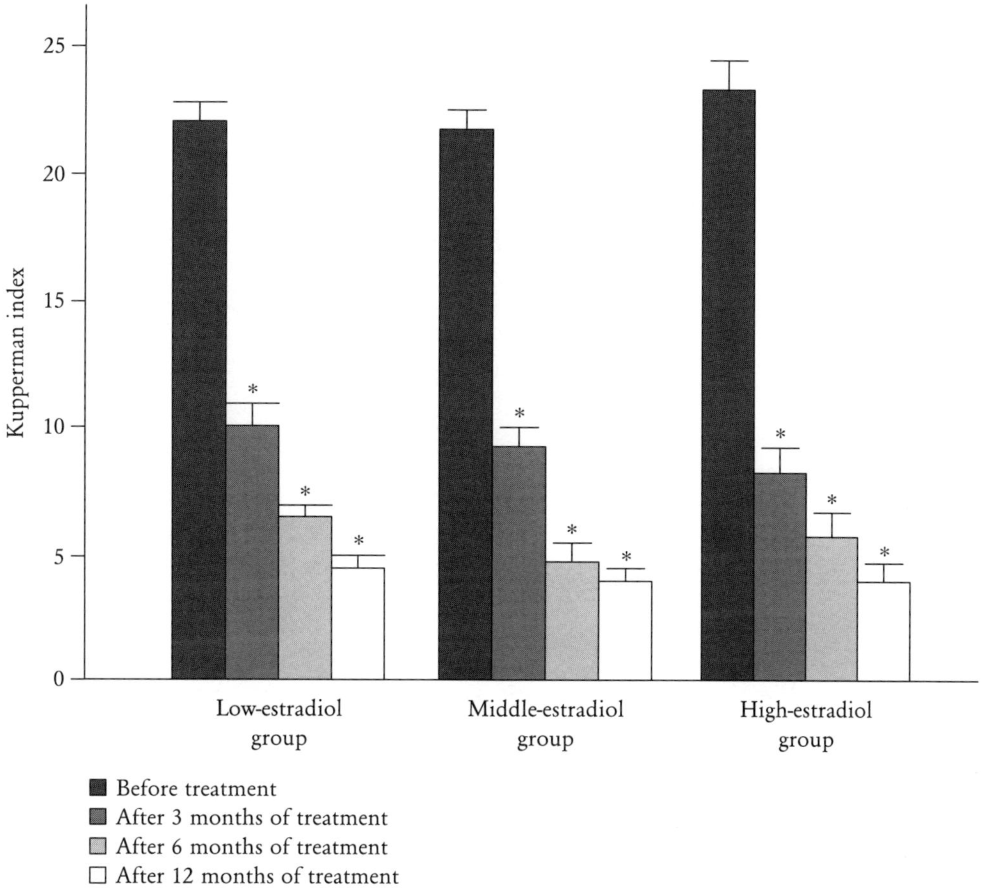

Figure 1 Changes in the Kupperman index in postmenopausal women before and during hormone replacement therapy. Values represent the mean ± SE. *$p < 0.01$ versus before treatment

the Friedewald formula. Apolipoprotein A1 (Apo A1), B (Apo B) and E (Apo E) levels were estimated by an immunoturbidimetric method. Levels of total cholesterol in the high- and transdermal-estradiol groups decreased significantly (−8.0 ± 2.4%, $p < 0.01$; −7.2 ± 2.5%, $p < 0.05$, respectively), whereas those in the other two groups decreased slightly. Changes in the levels of LDL cholesterol were similar to those of total cholesterol. HDL cholesterol levels rose significantly in the middle-, high- and transdermal-estradiol groups (14.4 ± 3.7%, $p < 0.01$; 12.9 ± 3.6%, $p < 0.01$; 12.4 ± 5.6%, $p < 0.05$, respectively). The treatment in all groups caused a significant increase in the level of apolipoprotein A1 (9.4 ± 2.6%, $p < 0.01$; 9.0 ± 2.6%, $p < 0.01$; 13.6 ± 4.3%, $p < 0.01$; 8.1%, $p < 0.05$, respectively). The levels of apolipoprotein B decreased significantly ($p < 0.01$) in the high-estradiol group (−11.2 ± 3.8%), but no significant changes were found in the other groups. The levels of apolipoprotein E decreased significantly ($p < 0.01$) in the middle- and high-estradiol groups (−13.8 ± 4.6%, $p < 0.01$; −15.9 ± 6.7%, $p < 0.01$, respectively) (Figure 4).

DISCUSSION

HRT can benefit postmenopausal women by reducing the frequency of hot flushes, improving vulvovaginal atrophy, preventing bone loss and protecting against cardiovascular disease. Recently, a low daily dose of 0.31 mg CEE has been used for preventing postmenopausal bone loss to avoid adverse effects such as unscheduled bleeding

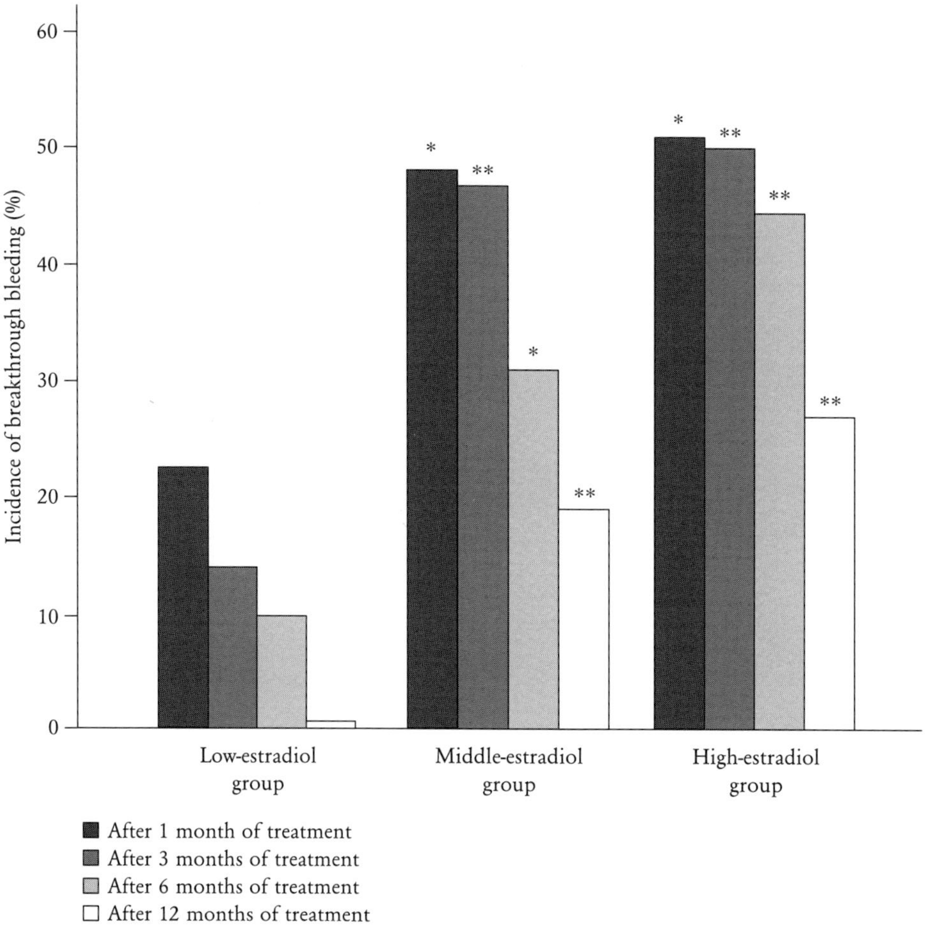

Figure 2 Incidence of breakthrough bleeding in oral hormone replacement therapy. $^{*}p < 0.05$ versus low-estradiol group; $^{**}p < 0.01$ versus low-estradiol group

and breast tenderness [3-5]. However, the precise level of estradiol to be used in HRT with CEE and MPA has not been clarified, because it is very difficult to measure the precise serum estrogen levels in women receiving oral CEE. This preparation, derived from pregnant mares' urine, is a mixture of estrogens, estrone sulfate being the major component, and the other estrogens, such as sodium equilin sulfate, are converted to unconjugated estrone and estradiol. Therefore, it is difficult to measure the estrogen level precisely. We developed a highly sensitive and specific assay for serum estrone and estradiol using HPLC and radioimmunoassay, and could detect the precise levels of estrone and estradiol after 12 months of treatment.

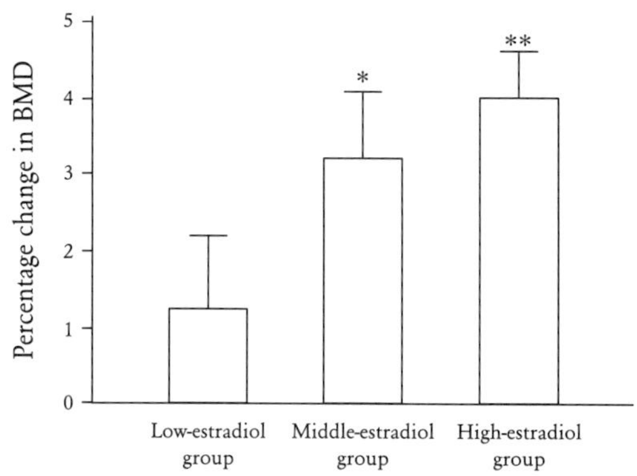

Figure 3 Mean percentage change from baseline in bone mineral density (BMD) of the lumbar spine after 12 months of treatment. Values represent the mean ± SE. $^{*}p < 0.01$ versus baseline values; $^{**}p < 0.001$ versus baseline values

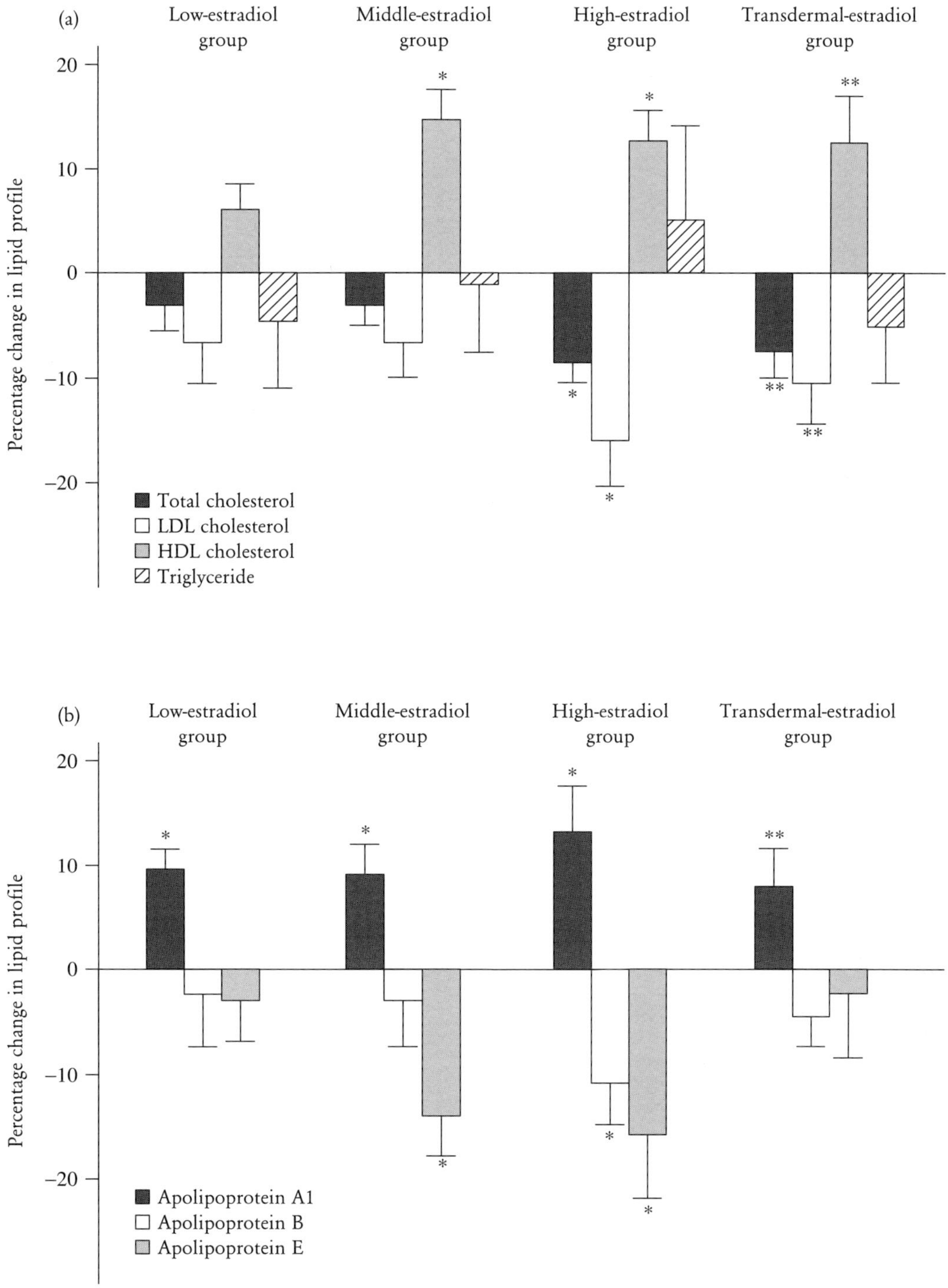

Figure 4 Mean percentage change from baseline in lipid profile (total cholesterol, low-density lipoprotein (LDL) cholesterol, high-density lipoprotein (HDL) cholesterol and triglyceride (a), and apolipoproteins (b)) after 12 months of treatment. Values represent the mean ± SE. $^{*}p < 0.01$ versus baseline values. $^{**}p < 0.05$ versus baseline values

Our results clearly indicate that vasomotor symptoms can be relieved if the estradiol level is less than 15 pg/ml, which results in less breakthrough bleeding, while more than 15 pg/ml of estradiol is required to increase bone mineral density. Furthermore, the levels of estradiol required to decrease total cholesterol and LDL cholesterol are more than 25 pg/ml, whereas those needed to increase HDL cholesterol are more than 15 pg/ml. Thus, low doses of HRT, such as a daily dose of CEE of 0.31 mg or 0.625 mg every other day, are successful in preventing bone loss and relieving vasomotor symptoms. In addition, an estradiol level of more than 25 pg/ml, using a daily dose of 0.625 mg CEE and transdermal estradiol 25 μg/day, is necessary to decrease total and LDL cholesterol in hypercholesterolemic women. In the present study, we determined the precise estradiol level during HRT and clarified that each tissue has a certain threshold to estradiol. From these results, it is advisable to select a suitable HRT regimen in order to maintain appropriate estradiol levels in accordance with the purpose of the therapy in postmenopausal women.

ACKNOWLEDGEMENT

The authors wish to thank Mitsubishi Kagaku of Bio-Clinical Laboratories, Tokyo, Japan for measuring the serum levels of estrone and estradiol.

References

1. Barbieri RL. Hormone treatment of endometriosis: the estrogen threshold hypothesis. *Am J Obstet Gynecol* 1992;166:740–5
2. Nichols KC, Schenkel L, Benson H. 17β-estradiol for postmenopausal estrogen replacement therapy. *Obstet Gynecol Surv* 1984;39:230–45
3. Ettinger B, Genant HK, Cann CE. Postmenopausal bone loss is prevented by treatment with low-dosage estrogen with calcium. *Ann Int Med* 1987;106:40–5
4. Webber CE, Blake JM, Chambers LF, *et al.* Effects of 2 years of hormone replacement upon bone mass, serum lipids and lipoproteins. *Maturitas* 1994;19: 13–23
5. Mizunuma H, Okano H, Soda M, *et al.* Prevention of postmenopausal bone loss with minimal uterine bleeding using low dose continuous estrogen/ progestin therapy: a 2-year prospective study. *Maturitas* 1997;27:69–76

Aerodiol: estrogen replacement therapy via the nasal route for the treatment of menopausal symptoms

62

J. Studd

The efficacy of hormone replacement therapy (HRT) in reducing the incidence of menopausal symptoms in women is now well established[1,2]. Estrogen supplementation also offers mid- to long-term benefits, reducing postmenopausal bone loss and the incidence of fractures[3] and cardiovascular disease[4].

However, to cope with the forecast increase in the number of women requiring estrogen replacement, new treatment choices are welcome, particularly if they bring additional clinical and/or practical benefits.

THE RATIONALE FOR ESTROGEN REPLACEMENT THERAPY VIA THE NASAL ROUTE

The two most widely used forms of estrogen for the treatment of postmenopausal symptoms are conjugated equine extracts and 17β-estradiol (E2). Such estrogens are most frequently administered orally[5], a delivery route which, although effective, is associated with a number of disadvantages, including variable bioavailability and significant intestinal and hepatic first-pass effects[6]. The oral route necessitates the administration of high doses to achieve therapeutic activity.

Although transdermal patches have overcome some of the drawbacks of oral therapy, they present additional problems, including wide interindividual variation in absorption rate (including the presence of poor absorbers[7]), the loss of 4–9% of patches due to poor adhesion, and local dermatological reactions[8,9].

Aerodiol is the first medication to introduce the nasal route of administration for HRT[10–14]. The nasal system offers benefits such as easy dosage titration, greater consistency of absorption and a user-friendly administration (in terms of rapidity, discretion and the absence of skin trace), at physiological doses.

Aerodiol capitalizes on the excellent absorption capacity of the nasal mucosa. Incorporation of a cyclodextrin solubilizing agent, randomly methylated β-cyclodextrin (RAMEB)[15,16] (Figure 1), into the spray formulation facilitates the production of an aqueous solution of 17β-estradiol, one which is both effectively absorbed and well tolerated by the nasal mucosa.

Intranasal absorption is facilitated by the highly vascularized, microvillous nature of the nasal mucosa, which has been estimated to present 160 cm^2 for absorption[17]. The pharmacokinetics of Aerodiol differs from that of estradiol taken orally or transdermally, intranasally administered estradiol having a very rapid uptake, and achieving maximal plasma levels within 10–30 min. Plasma

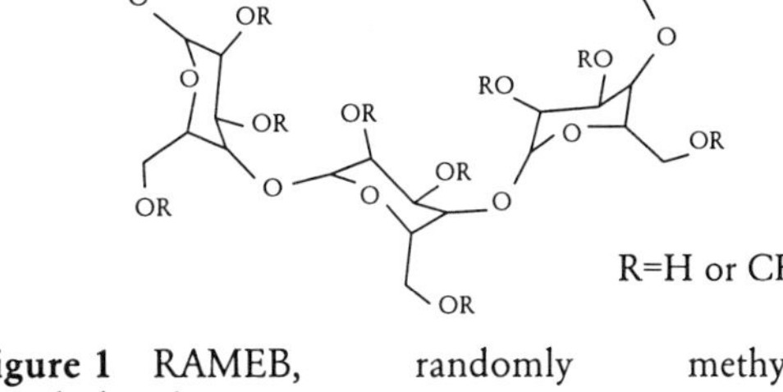

R=H or CH

Figure 1 RAMEB, randomly methylated β-cyclodextrin

levels return to 10% of the maximal value approximately 2 h after administration, and to levels of untreated postmenopausal women within 12 h. Consequently, daily administration of Aerodiol produces a 'pulsed estrogen' profile, as opposed to the relatively sustained serum levels seen with oral and transdermal therapy[18].

Only in recent years has the mechanism of action of estrogens become more clearly understood[19]. Estrogen activity is linked to the presence of nuclear receptors, found for the most part in the main genital target tissues as well as in bone, the cardiovascular system and the brain. Once estradiol penetrates the cell, it binds to a specific site on the nuclear receptor. The activation of the ligand receptor complex triggers a series of events leading to the synthesis of different proteins. The estrogenic effects induced by exogenous administration are directly related to the amount of these activated receptors, rather than to the estradiol plasma levels. The long half-life of these receptors ensures prolonged activity over time with intermittent administration, thus explaining why Aerodiol's pulsed estrogen profile achieves therapeutic estrogenization of target tissues and effective, sustained, symptom control from once-daily dosing.

RELIABLE AND CONSISTENT ESTROGEN ABSORPTION

Clinical studies confirm that Aerodiol facilitates effective and consistent absorption of estrogen[20] – no women have been classified as 'non-absorbers' throughout clinical development. The dose administered is reproducible from one woman to another and from one day to the next, unlike transdermal therapies, for example. For one woman in four or five using patches, estradiol absorption is insufficient, necessitating the use of higher doses or a switch of treatment.

EASY DOSE ADAPTATION

A potentially important benefit of Aerodiol's nasal system is its ease of dose titration. The 300-μg daily dose (one spray in each nostril in the morning or evening), appropriate for around 80% of women, can be adapted easily according to a woman's needs, without change of pack presentation, up to a maximum of 600 μg, i.e. one spray in each nostril, morning and evening.

Evidence suggests that as many as one in five women will need to adapt the dose of their estrogen replacement therapy in order to achieve the desired symptom control. In a study demonstrating Aerodiol's efficacy equivalence to oral estradiol in over 600 women, 22% of women required dose adaptation in the Aerodiol group and 20% in the oral estradiol group[21].

CLINICAL VALIDATION OF THE NASAL CONCEPT

Aerodiol has been shown to be significantly more effective than placebo in a specific 'validation of the concept' trial conducted internationally in a randomized population of 420 recently menopausal women aged between 45 and 60 years[14].

At its recommended starting dose of 300 μg daily (one spray in each nostril once daily), Aerodiol reduces the Kupperman index (a weighted mean of the main climacteric symptoms), hot flushes and markers of bone resorption (urinary pyridinolines, CrossLaps) from the 4th week of treatment, to a significantly greater extent than placebo.

AS EFFECTIVE AS REFERENCE ORAL THERAPY

Aerodiol 300 μg daily has been shown to be as effective as reference oral estradiol 2 mg (the most commonly used tablet form of estradiol in Europe) in an international, multicenter, randomized, double-blind trial of 659 women aged between 40 and 60 years, postmenopausal for less than 10 years[21].

Climacteric symptoms

Aerodiol reduced Kupperman index scores by more than 65% relative to baseline, a reduction statistically equivalent to that of oral estradiol 2 mg (Figure 2).

Moreover, Aerodiol eliminated hot flushes (mild, moderate and severe) in the majority of women presenting with such symptoms, the mean

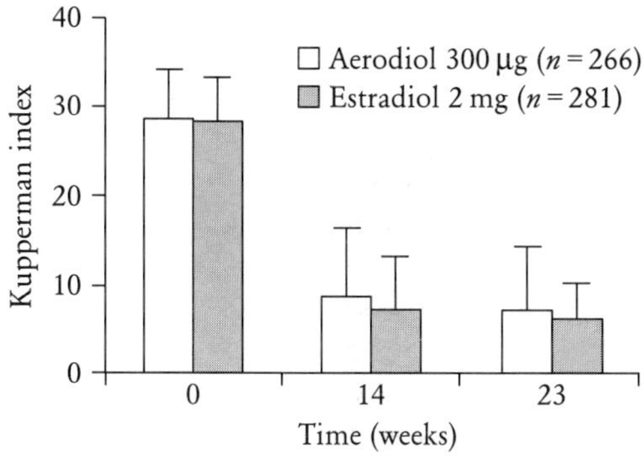

Figure 2 Reduction in Kupperman index, equivalent to reference estradiol tablet therapy. Reproduced from reference 21

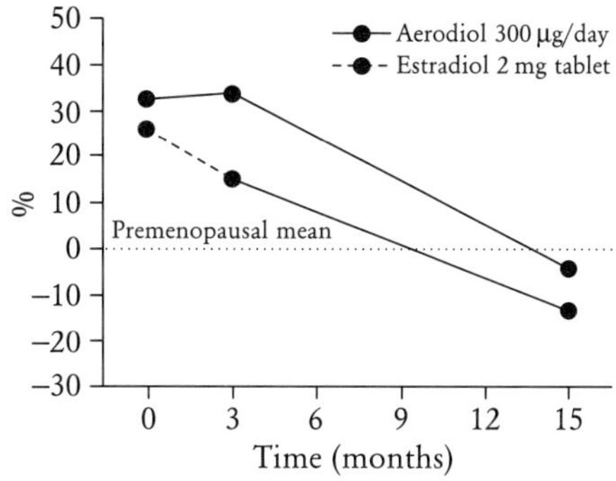

Figure 3 Serum osteocalcin. Values are expressed as percentage of premenopausal mean. Source: reference 23

number of hot flushes decreasing by 87% from baseline after 14 weeks of treatment.

Such improvement in Kupperman index and in the incidence of hot flushes with Aerodiol 300 µg daily is comparable to that observed with transdermal estradiol 50 µg therapy[22].

The efficacy of Aerodiol and oral estradiol 2 mg is similar regarding other clinical parameters, i.e. a similar decrease is seen in the number of patients with atrophic or subatrophic vaginal mucosa, and a decrease in the number of patients reporting genitourinary symptoms (dysuria, stress incontinence, urgency, dyspareunia). Aerodiol's efficacy seems to be unaffected in women who smoke.

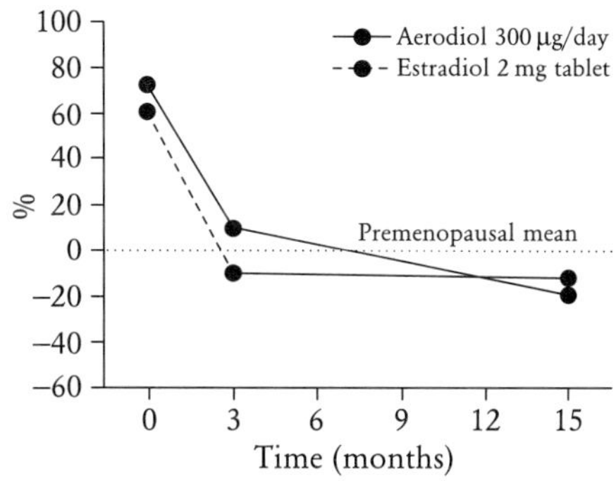

Figure 4 Urinary CTX (CrossLaps®). Values are expressed as percentage of premenopausal mean. Reproduced from reference 23. Copyright © 1999, The Endocrine Society

Bone metabolism

Large prospective studies conducted with oral and transdermal therapies show that changes in bone markers correlate closely with changes in bone mass: a normalization of bone markers with estrogen replacement is predictive of treatment efficacy for the prevention of postmenopausal bone loss. Urinary CrossLaps (a marker of bone resorption) decreases markedly after 4 weeks' treatment with Aerodiol, with a further significant decrease after 12 weeks (reaching premenopausal values)[23]. Interestingly, markers of bone formation (e.g. osteocalcin) initially increase with Aerodiol over the first 4 weeks of treatment and thereafter reduce to premenopausal values after 12 months (Figure 3). No such initial increase is seen with oral estrogen therapy. A possible explanation lies in the difference between the effects of oral and nasal administration on insulin growth factor type I (IGF-I), a protein synthesized by the liver, which stimulates osteoformation, which seems to be very much reduced by oral therapy and not so by nasal therapy.

Both bone resorption markers (urinary CrossLaps) and bone formation markers (osteocalcin, bone alkaline phosphatase, *N*-terminal propeptide of procollagen type I (PINP)) are significantly decreased (to premenopausal values) after 1 year's treatment with Aerodiol, indicative of a normalization of bone turnover (Figures 3 and 4)[23].

LONG-TERM EFFICACY

Clinical studies of 1 year and beyond confirm that Aerodiol is effective in the long term[24].

Throughout the first 12 months of treatment, further reductions in Kupperman index and in the number of hot flushes are seen, without resurgence of symptoms.

AERODIOL IS WELL TOLERATED

A new form of HRT must, of course, be well tolerated if it is to be considered as a viable treatment option. Throughout Aerodiol's clinical development, the nasal system has shown itself to be well tolerated - gynecologically, metabolically and locally[24].

Gynecological tolerance

General gynecological effects observed with estrogen therapy such as mastalgia and irregular bleeds seem to occur less frequently with Aerodiol than with reference oral estradiol 2 mg therapy[24]. Evidence suggests that severe mastalgia is significantly less frequent with Aerodiol than with oral estradiol 2 mg (Figure 5)[21].

Moreover, fewer episodes of breakthrough bleeding are reported with Aerodiol 300 µg than with oral estradiol 2 mg (23% with Aerodiol 300 µg vs 27% with oral estradiol 2 mg).

No cases of endometrial hyperplasia have been reported (in over 400 women using Aerodiol for at least 1 year).

Metabolic tolerance

Aerodiol demonstrates good metabolic tolerance, with a profile rather typical of an administration route that avoids hepatic first-pass metabolism[21]. In practice, this means that Aerodiol does not disturb lipids, and reduces total cholesterol, lipoprotein(a) and apolipoprotein B. Unlike tablet therapies (which are metabolized in the liver), Aerodiol does not increase triglycerides.

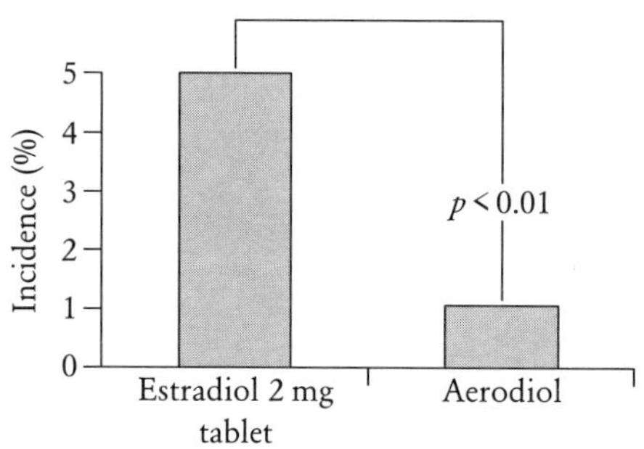

Figure 5 Reduced incidence of severe mastalgia with Aerodiol vs. reference estradiol tablet therapy. Reproduced from reference 21

Nasal tolerance

Aerodiol is well tolerated by the nasal mucosa. The most frequently reported symptoms are a prickling sensation, a runny nose or sneezing, such symptoms being, in the majority of cases, mild and occurring with only slightly higher frequency than in control groups. Such symptoms prompt less than 3.5% of women to stop therapy, a dropout rate which compares favorably with the 5–8% of women who stop transdermal therapy due to adverse skin reactions.

ACCEPTABILITY AND PREFERENCE

The fact that 85% of women are still taking Aerodiol at 1 year is a good indicator that Aerodiol is well accepted. Women find the nasal spray discrete, easy and pleasant to use.

Women prefer Aerodiol to transdermal therapy

When asked to choose between Aerodiol's nasal system and transdermal (patch) therapy, women seem to prefer Aerodiol. Some women find patches esthetically unpleasant and adapting the dose can be difficult.

An international cross-over open study conducted in seven countries[22] (in a total of 361 women) compared the therapeutic benefit of 12 weeks of treatment of Aerodiol to that of Estraderm TTS transdermal patch 50 µg daily. Results show that Aerodiol is as effective as Estraderm in reducing climacteric symptoms (measured using the Kupperman index). Interestingly, Aerodiol is equally effective in reducing night sweats and improving sleep disorders whether given as a morning or evening dose.

Moreover, Aerodiol is as well tolerated as the Estraderm patch system. Regarding gynecological tolerance, moderate or severe mastalgia was reported significantly less frequently with Aerodiol ($p = 0.02$). Locally, Aerodiol's nasal route seems to be at least as well tolerated as the transdermal route. Importantly, however, when asked to indicate their preferred therapy (after having used both systems), 66% of women chose to continue therapy with Aerodiol - principally for its efficacy, discretion, convenience and rapidity of administration.

PULSED ESTROGEN THERAPY

Aerodiol, with its extensive and rapid absorption across the nasal mucosa, introduces a new concept in HRT: pulsed estrogen therapy. This pulsed effect ensures effective estrogenization of the target tissues with an original pharmacokinetic profile, differing from the somewhat flatter, more sustained kinetic profiles of transdermal and oral therapy.

Cellular mode of action

Current evidence suggests that the efficacy of estrogen therapy is directly related to the number of activated receptors, rather than to estradiol plasma levels. At the cell membrane (Figure 6), Aerodiol's pulse creates a high diffusion gradient across which estradiol passes rapidly into the cell. Once inside the cell, the estradiol molecule binds to a specific site on a nuclear receptor. Subsequent activation of this ligand-receptor complex leads to the synthesis of different proteins.

The activated ligand-receptor complex triggers a cascade of DNA synthesis, a prolonged process that helps to explain Aerodiol's sustained efficacy over 24-48 h with a once-daily dosage regimen.

Clinical implications of pulsed estrogen therapy

Clinically, studies show conclusively that Aerodiol's once-a-day pulse of estrogen is as effective as reference oral estradiol 2 mg[21] and transdermal estradiol 50 µg[22] in reducing climacteric symptoms and markers of bone turnover. This confirms that a once-daily 'switching on' of estrogen receptors is sufficient to ensure sustained efficacy (and that constant receptor stimulation may well be unnecessary).

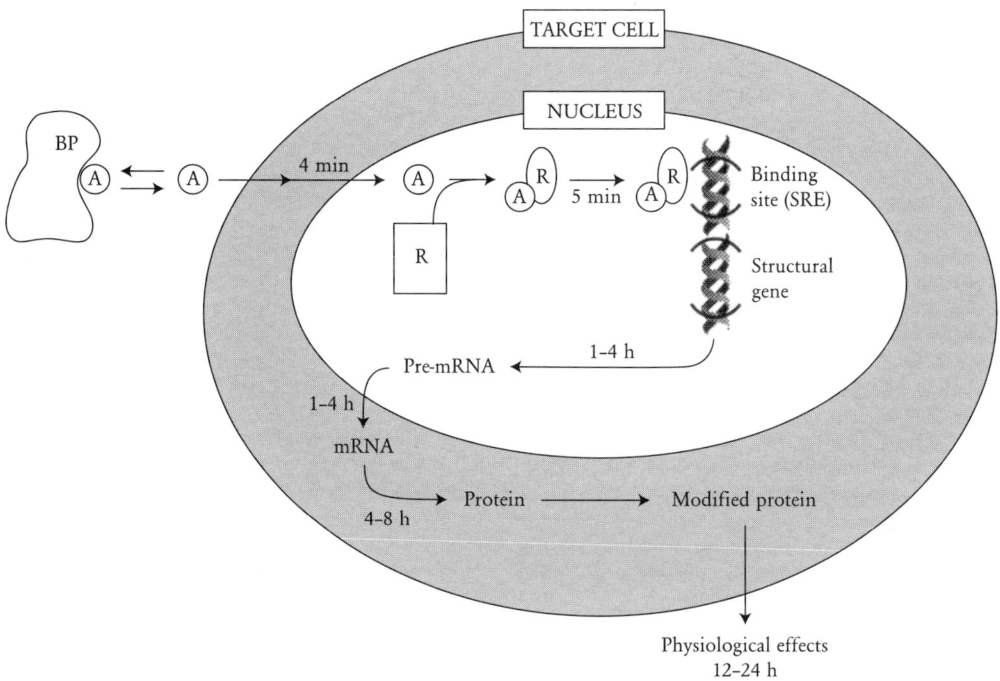

Figure 6 Cellular mode of action of Aerodiol. Adapted from reference 19. A, Aerodiol; R, receptor; BP, binding protein. Copyright © 1997, Lippincott-Raven

Regarding gynecological tolerance, Aerodiol's pulsed profile seems to promote less mastalgia and metrorrhagia than the more sustained estrogen receptor stimulation produced by oral estradiol 2 mg[21]. Whether such a difference in effect on breast and endometrial tissue is due to pharmacokinetic or more tissue-specific differences remains a subject for further investigation.

CONCLUSION

Given the favorable risk-benefit argument for HRT use and the forecast increase in the population of menopausal women, the role of HRT can be expected to increase significantly in the future. In a domain where patient influence is as least as great as physician influence, an increase in choice can only be beneficial, particularly if new choices bring additional clinical and/or practical benefits. Aerodiol presents physicians and women with an appealing new choice, one which is effective, well tolerated, and which offers easy dose adaptation and which, from the woman's perspective in particular, is practical, discrete and easy to use.

ACKNOWLEDGEMENT

This paper has been reproduced with permission from *Medicographia* 1999;21:256-61.

References

1. Kupperman H, Blatt M, Wiesbader H, Filler W. Comparative clinical evaluation of estrogenic preparations by the menopausal and amenorrheal indices. *J Clin Endocrinol* 1953;13:688–703
2. Steingold K, Laufer L, Chetkowski R, *et al.* Treatment of hot flashes with transdermal estradiol administration. *J Clin Endocrinol Metab* 1985;61: 627–32
3. Cauley JA, Seeley DG, Ensrud K, Ettinger B, Black D, Cummings SR. Estrogen replacement therapy and fractures in older women. Study of Osteoporotic Fractures Research Group. *Ann Intern Med* 1995;122:9–16
4. Grodstein F, Stampfer MJ, Colditz GA, *et al.* Postmenopausal hormone therapy and mortality. *N Engl J Med* 1997;336:1769–75
5. Thacker H, Menopause. *Women's Health Primary Care* 1997;24:205–21
6. de Lignieres B, Basdevant A, Thomas G, *et al.* Biological effects of estradiol-17β in postmenopausal women: oral versus percutaneous administration. *J Clin Endocrinol Metab* 1986;62:536–41
7. Stanczyk F, Shoupe D, Numez V, *et al.* A randomized comparison of nonoral estradiol delivery in postmenopausal women. *Am J Obstet Gynecol* 1988; 159:1540–6
8. Frenkel Y, Kopernik G, Lazer S, *et al.* Acceptability and skin reactions to transdermal estrogen replacement therapy in relation to climate. *Maturitas* 1994; 20:31–6
9. Grebe SK, Adams JD, Feek CD. Systemic sensitization to ethanol by transdermal estrogen patches. *Arch Dermatol* 1993;129:379–80
10. Schipper N, Hermens W, Romeijn S, Verhoef J, Merkus F. Nasal absorption of 17-beta-estradiol and progesterone from a dimethyl-β-cyclodextrin inclusion formulation in rats. *Int J Pharm* 1990;64: 61–6
11. Hermens W, Deurloo M, Romeijn S, Verhoef J, Merkus F. Nasal absorption enhancement of 17-β-estradiol by dimethyl-β-cyclodextrin in rabbits and rats. *Pharm Res* 1990;7:500–3
12. Hermens W, Belder C, Merkus J, Hooymans P, Verhoef J, Merkus F. Intranasal estradiol administration to oophorectomized women. *Eur J Obstet Gynecol Reprod Biol* 1991;40:35–41
13. Hermens W, Belder C, Merkus J, Hooymans P, Verhoef J, Merkus F. Intranasal administration of estradiol in combination with progesterone to oophorectomized women: a pilot study. *Eur J Obstet Gynecol Reprod Biol* 1992;43:65–70
14. Studd J, Pornel B, Marton I, *et al.* Efficacy and acceptability of intranasal 17β-oestradiol for menopausal symptoms: randomized dose-response study. *Lancet* 1999;853:1574–8
15. Nogradi M. Dimethyl-β-cyclodextrin. *Drugs Future* 1984;9:577–8
16. Technologie Servier, Orléans, France. The *in vitro* metabolism of [^{14}C]-RAMEB and [^{14}C]-17β-estradiol by nasal epithelium of rat, dog, monkey

and man. *Internal Report, PB-93-21400-028. NP6447*
17. Jones N, Quraishi S, Mason J. The nasal delivery of systemic drugs. *Int J Clin Pract* 1997;51:308–11
18. Lievertz R. Pharmacology and pharmacokinetics of estrogens. *Am J Obstet Gynecol* 1987;156:1289–93
19. Robinson JA, Spelsberg T. Mode of action at the cellular level with specific reference to bone cells. *Estrogens Antiestrogens* 1997;5:43–62
20. Data on file
21. Mattsson L, Christiansen CI, *et al.* Clinical equivalence of intranasal and oral 17β-estradiol for menopausal symptoms. *Am J Obstet Gynecol* Submitted
22. Lopes P, Calaf J, *et al.* Efficacy and tolerability of intranasal and transdermal estradiol in early postmenopausal women. Abstract presented at the *9th International Menopause Society World Congress on the Menopause*, Oct 1999, Yokohama
23. Garnero P, Tsouderos Y, Marton I, Pelissier C, Varin C, Delmas PD. Effects of intranasal 17β-estradiol on bone turnover and serum insulin-like growth factor I in postmenopausal women. *J Clin Endocrinol Metab* 1999;84:2390–7
24. Data on file (Gompel)

Hormones and hemostasis 63

A. Cano

THE HEMOSTATIC SYSTEM

Hemostasis is a physiological mechanism that maintains blood fluidity within the vascular tree. The privation of that function leads to disorders such as acute coronary heart syndrome, which is increasingly recognized as the primary consequence of a local imbalance of the hemostatic mechanism[1-3]. Furthermore, hemostasis prevents the loss of blood through breach disruptions in the normal vasculature. To accomplish this, hemostasis is regulated by a complex mechanism based upon a dynamic equilibrium between procoagulants and anticoagulants, together with pro- and antifibrinolytic activities.

In the normal state, the system works to prevent the local accumulation of activated blood-clotting enzymes and complexes. In the case of a vascular injury, circulating platelets are exposed to the subendothelial layers and, subsequently, attach to the injured surface and become highly adherent. The bound platelets degranulate and provide receptors for the assembly of blood-clotting enzyme complexes[4-6]. Together with the activation of platelets, exposure to non-vascular cell-bound tissue factor in the subendothelial space activates the extrinsic pathway of blood coagulation (Figure 1). The coagulation cascade has the remarkable ability to amplify the signal generated by a small initiating stimulus into a potentially explosive chain reaction. This is accomplished by the well-orchestrated participation of distinct procoagulant factors, which are zymogens providing a reservoir ready to transform into active proteases, then receiving the suffix 'a'.

The limiting factor of this potentially uncontrolled reaction is provided by natural anticoagulant mechanisms. Antithrombin III and protein C, with the concurrent participation of its cofactor, protein S, are the main factors in this system. The activity of antithrombin III is potentiated by the presence of endogenous heparan sulfate, whereas protein C is activated by thrombin in the presence of thrombomodulin, a protein bound to endothelial cells. The antithrombin III pathway inhibits several activated coagulation enzymes by forming complexes, such as thrombin–antithrombin III complexes (TAT), which are rapidly cleared from the circulation by the reticuloendothelial system. The thrombomodulin-activated protein C (APC) inhibits coagulation by proteolytic cleavage of activated factors VIII and V; the R506Q mutation in factor V, also known as factor V Leiden, is therefore a major cause of resistance to APC[7].

Finally, fibrinolysis is a mechanism of the hemostatic system that regulates fibrin formation through a controlled degradation of fibrin by plasmin. Plasmin is a powerful protease which is derived from plasminogen, a zymogen whose activation is regulated by a system of activators and inhibitors. Among them, tissue plasminogen activator (t-PA) is produced in the endothelium and, in the presence of fibrin, activates plasminogen to produce plasmin. Plasminogen activator inhibitor type 1 (PAI-1) is produced in endothelial and hepatic cells and, in balance with t-PA, constitutes the major modulator of fibrinolysis[8]. Other minor regulators of fibrinolysis are the activators factor XIIa and urokinase plasminogen activator, and the inhibitors histidine glycoprotein and α_2-antiplasmin[8].

It is important to note that, together with the self-limitation of the activation of the cascade, as determined by the interplay between prothrombotic and anticoagulant mechanisms, the clot is a focal lesion. This characteristic may be understandable in the context of the local endothelial disruption that generates an imbalance in the system, as described above, but may be puzzling in cases of systemic alterations in the hemostatic

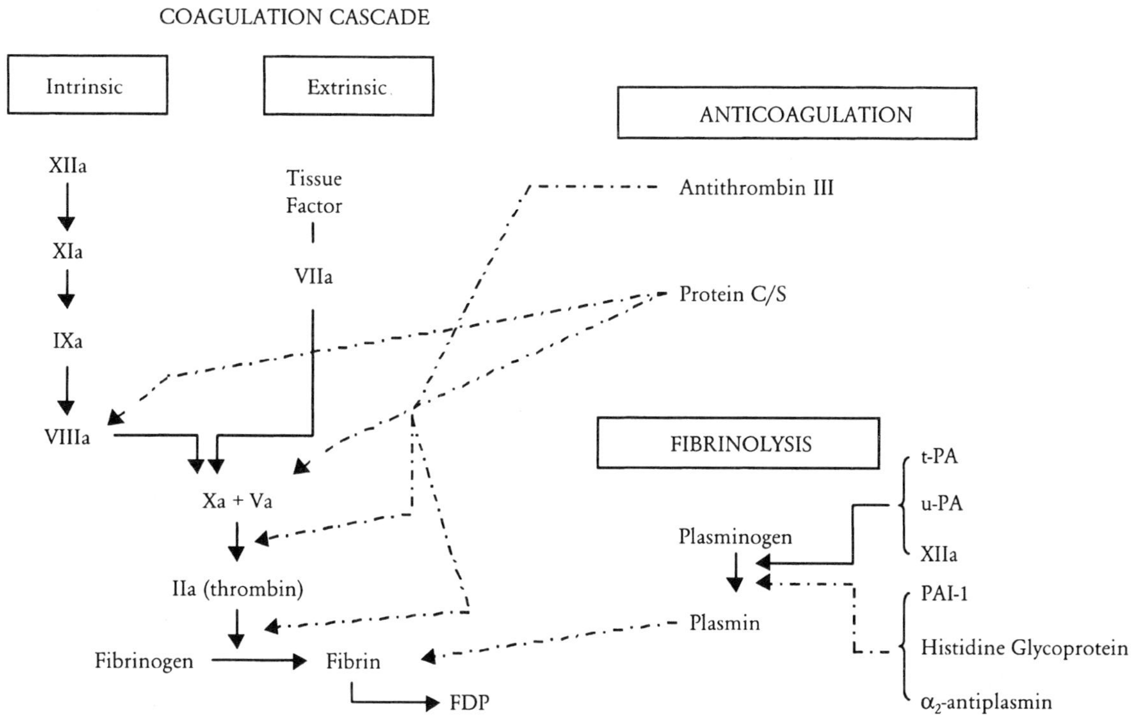

Figure 1 A schematic representation of the coagulation cascade, the anticoagulation system and fibrinolysis, the three mechanisms that regulate the hemostatic system. On the left-hand side, the coagulation cascade is represented by both the intrinsic and the extrinsic arms, described through only the activated forms of the distinct enzymes. Coagulation is initiated by the interaction of tissue factor bound to the cell membrane with factor VIIa. Activation of factor X links the extrinsic and intrinsic pathways, although factor VIIa also activates factor IX (not shown in the Figure). Factor Xa converts prothrombin to thrombin in a reaction activated by factor Va. Anticoagulation is initiated by the antithrombin III and the protein C/S pathways. Antithrombin III neutralizes thrombin instantly and also inhibits other enzymes of the cascade, such as XIa, IXa, and Xa. The protein C/S pathway interacts with thrombomodulin (not shown in the Figure) to inactivate factors Va and VIIIa. The fibrinolytic activity resides in the conversion of plasminogen to plasmin, a protease that degrades fibrin. Plasminogen is activated by tissue plasminogen activator (t-PA), urokinase plasminogen activator (u-PA) and factor XIIa, whereas plasminogen activator inhibitor type 1 (PAI-1) exerts an antifibrinolytic effect, together with histidine glycoprotein and α_2-antiplasmin. Links are represented by solid (when stimulatory) or dashed (when inhibitory) arrows. FDP, fibrin degradation products

system, which also produce thrombotic lesions in discrete areas of the vascular tree. The correct understanding of the factors that determine the focality of the thrombotic lesion is becoming a crucial point in the clarification of the mechanisms of hemostasis.

FACTORS DETERMINING THE FOCALITY OF THROMBOTIC LESIONS

There is actually little doubt that, in keeping with the triad of Virchow, the three mechanisms that affect the thrombotic phenotype are the two already mentioned (local injury to the vessel wall and procoagulant activation of the hemostatic equilibrium) and a decrease in blood flow. The relative involvement of each of these three determinants in the formation of a clot at a certain site of the vascular tree is as yet unknown.

The weight of the vessel wall factor is probably of particular relevance when considering the hemostatic actions of the ovarian steroids, where there seems to be a trend favoring venous thrombosis, whereas the opposite is true for the arterial tree. In addition to this general segregation into either the venous or the arterial vessels, there may also be thrombotic lesions specifically linked to a more concrete vascular site. The frequent location of thrombotic lesions at the portal, hepatic and mesenteric veins in cases of paroxysmal nocturnal hemoglobinuria[9,10] is a clear example.

In some cases, there is also a certain association between the nature of the hemostatic imbalance and the phenotype of the lesion. For example, congenital deficiencies of antithrombin III, protein C and protein S are more often associated with a higher risk of deep-venous, but not arterial, thrombosis[11,12]. However, mutations in the factor V gene (factor V Leiden) and in the prothrombin gene determine a higher risk for deep venous thrombosis of both the legs and brain[13,14], and also arterial thrombosis of the coronary tree in women who smoke[13,15].

To further complicate matters, it seems that distinct combinations of the three Virchow mechanisms may also create specific phenotypes, as is the case with the higher perioperative risk of venous thrombotic episodes resulting from decreased flow, focal disruption of the vessel wall, and deficiencies in the anticoagulant system[16].

Given the complexity of this scenario, the enlightening of the effects of the ovarian steroids is a rather intricate task. A rational approach might be, perhaps, to contrast the clinical observations with the biological data, since this might help to raise hypotheses on the currently unknown actions of hormones. This should be done while keeping in mind that the net effect of hormone replacement therapy (HRT) on clotting and fibrinolysis and its potential clinical implications are still unclear; existing data are derived from population-based studies or small trials assessing the biological intermediates of hemostasis, whose variability and definitive clinical relevance have not been completely confirmed.

CLINICALLY OBSERVABLE EFFECTS OF HORMONES ON THE HEMOSTATIC SYSTEM

One important lesson of the numerous studies on the thrombogenic role of ovarian steroids is that this is a dose-dependent phenomenon mainly linked to estrogens[17]. The coronary heart disease (CHD) events detected in women using the old oral contraceptives were drastically reduced when the estrogenic component was diminished. The more recent data provided by studies in women using the modern preparations with either 30 or 20 μg of ethinylestradiol have shown neutral effects on CHD[18]. The relative risk for venous thrombosis, on the other hand, still seems to be increased, although the absolute risk is as low as 4.6 cases per 10 000 exposed woman years[19].

The distinct formulations employed in HRT almost universally include natural estrogens. Their lower potency is clearly reflected in their markedly diminished effect on hemostasis, the effect on thrombin generation being virtually immeasurable[20]. The perception exists that, within the estrogenic dose range accomplished by HRT, the improvement in fibrinolytic capacity may exceed the activation of baseline coagulation, as suggested by the preservation of a marked reduction in PAI-1 in the presence of undetectable activation of coagulation[21,22]. In fact, there is general agreement on the protective effect of HRT on arterial thrombogenesis. Nonetheless, four distinct retrospective studies[23-26] have presented concordant data on an association between the use of HRT and a mean relative risk of deep venous thrombosis oscillating between 2.1 and 3.6. Together with the variables at work in this different behavior of the arterial and venous trees, the fact that the lower estrogen-progestin dosages used in HRT maintain the venous thrombotic risk of oral contraceptives may possibly result from risk factors other than the induction of a hemostatic imbalance.

The clinical effects of progestins seem to be less important. As for estrogens, part of the information on progestin action has been gathered from studies in the field of contraception, with the use of progestin-only pills. Although the data are scarce and not devoid of controversy, most authors agree that there is no consistent pattern of clinical effects on hemostasis[17,27]. There has been recent controversy, however, on the risk of venous thromboembolism among users of gestodene and desogestrel, two third-generation progestins, versus levonorgestrel-containing combined oral contraceptives. The retrospective nature of the original studies, together with the possible influence of several types of bias[19,28], have deactivated the original safeguards put in place against the use of third-generation oral contraceptives. Moreover, as confirmed in a recent review, an analysis of 17 comparative studies showed no difference between the desogestrel- and gestodene-containing and the levonorgestrel-containing oral contraceptives[29].

In short, the inconsistencies linked to the role of progestins in thrombogenesis leave estrogens as the main factors in this scenario. The following sections, therefore, will review the biological data concerning the action of estrogens on two factors of Virchow's triad, the balance between the procoagulant, anticoagulant and fibrinolytic factors, and the endothelium. There are fewer data concerning the modifications of blood flow in venous territories.

THE BIOLOGICAL EFFECT OF ESTROGENS ON THE HEMOSTATIC BALANCE

As mentioned above, the procoagulant factors are inactive zymogens that require activation to develop their potential functionality. It is important to note that the coagulant factors are present in concentrations far in excess of the physiological need. Accordingly, changes in the plasma levels of inactive zymogens, as occurs after the use of estrogens in HRT, may have little impact. The genes of some procoagulant factors, including factor XII[30], factor VII[31], factors VIII and IX[20] and fibrinogen[31-33], have been found to be regulated by estrogen.

It seems, therefore, and this is an important conclusion when trying to measure clinically any activation of coagulation, that functional measurements should be preferable to the assessment of protein concentrations of zymogens[34]. The TAT complexes, for example, may give a better idea of the amount of thrombin that has been produced. Fibrinopeptide A, a peptide that is released from fibrinogen by the action of thrombin, may be taken to gain information on thrombin activity. However, both the TAT complexes and fibrinopeptide A may be artificially increased by venipuncture and have a short half-life, two factors that make their reliable measurement difficult. The fragment 1+2 (F1+2) constitutes the amino terminus of the prothrombin, which is split during prothrombin activation, and has a long half-life; F1+2 is therefore a reliable marker of the generation of thrombin. The degradation products of fibrin may be taken, for similar reasons, as an indicator of fibrinolytic activity, since the activity of plasmin cannot be measured directly due to the short half-life of the enzyme. The use of estrogens in oral contraception, and at a lower level in replacement therapy after the menopause, has been suggested to increase slightly markers of thrombin generation and activity, such as the prothrombin F1+2, TAT complexes and fibrinopeptide A[35], although this issue remains debatable in the literature.

The activators of the anticoagulant system reside mainly on the endothelium, as is the case with thrombomodulin (protein C) and heparin-like glycoproteins (antithrombin III). Other modulators of the protein C/S pathway are factor V, which acts as a cofactor, and the C4b-binding protein, an inhibitor of the complement pathway that forms a complex with protein S. A decrease in C4b-binding globulin, as induced by estrogens in one study[36], elevates the amount of free protein S, thus increasing its activity. Both protein S and antithrombin III exhibit a very wide range of normality, an important point that invalidates any conclusion obtained from small modifications in their circulating levels, as has been described for estrogens[37] (Figure 2). The level at which antithrombin III would significantly increase the risk of thrombosis is unknown, but studies in families with congenital antithrombin III deficiency suggest that it would have to be reduced to about 50% of its normal activity. The prevalence of congenital deficiencies in any of the three components

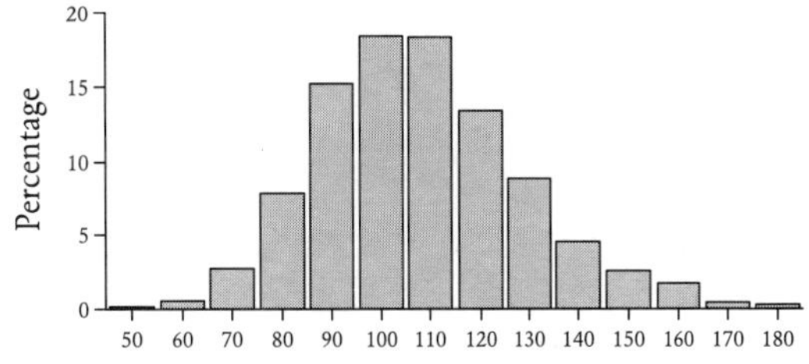

Figure 2 Distribution of plasma antithrombin III levels among 6737 women, aged 45–64 years, who participated in the Atherosclerosis Risk in Communities Study. From reference 37, with permission

of the anticoagulant system is, however, rare. This is at variance with the prevalence of APC resistance due to factor V Leiden, which varies from 2 to 15% in the white population[38].

The increased susceptibility of the population with genetic deficiencies in the anticoagulant system may influence the higher relative risk of venous thromboembolism ascribed to estrogens. This association has been clearly observed for oral contraceptives[39,40]. In fact, the continuous activation of the coagulation cascade *in vivo* seems to be confirmed by the detection of low, but measurable, plasma levels of reaction products of coagulation and fibrinolysis in the normal population. This tonic low-grade activation of coagulation requires the continuous activity of the anticoagulant and fibrinolytic systems. The reduction in the 'safety margin' determined by a genetic deficiency in any of the components of the anticoagulant system may condition a higher thrombotic risk, which is increased by estrogens[36,38-40]. Nonetheless, this effect must be small in HRT users in whom, as mentioned above, the lower estrogenic dose leaves the hemostatic balance very close to neutrality, if not displaced towards the antithrombotic side (see below). Therefore, the extremely low, but still detectable, increased risk of venous thrombosis with HRT may be influenced by alternative variables. The older age of women receiving HRT may possibly exert an influence, since age is a demonstrated risk factor for venous thrombosis[41]. Variables distinct from the activation of procoagulants, such as the reduction in the venous blood flow, the third mechanism of Virchow's triad, may also be operative. This is actually the likely mechanism operating in the prothrombotic effect of immobilization or, more clearly, venous occlusion.

THE RELEVANCE OF PARTICULAR RISK MARKERS

The scant consideration received by the changes induced by estrogens on the levels of circulating procoagulant zymogens or members of the anticoagulant system contrasts with the attention paid to factors whose concentrations have been considered to be clinically relevant. There is general agreement on the value of these factors, despite the awareness of the fact that much of the evidence supporting their relevance comes from retrospective studies and, as a consequence, suffers from methodological insufficiencies. As shown by clinical observations, there may be preferential identification of particular markers with either venous or arterial thrombosis.

Apart from the implication of the other two components of Virchow's triad, there is evidence favoring the concept of hypercoagulability as a main determinant of venous thrombosis. This conclusion is obtained from, first, the observation of a high prevalence of APC resistance or other anticoagulant deficiencies[14,40,42] among patients with venous thrombosis and, second, the association of recognized triggers of venous thrombosis, such as immobilization, trauma or venous occlusion, with increased coagulant activity as indicated by raised F1+2 levels and fibrin degradation products[34].

At the arterial tree, an increase in either the level of fibrinogen or the activity of factor VII has been associated with a higher risk of myocardial infarction, possibly the most severe complication of arterial thrombosis[43-47]. The hypofunctional status of the fibrinolytic system may also be relevant, as suggested by the rise in PAI-1 detected in CHD and the poor prognosis linked to that increase[47-56]. Elevated levels of lipoprotein(a) have been shown to behave as an independent risk factor for cardiovascular disease, an observation that may possibly also be ascribed to hypofunctional fibrinolysis, since several studies have found that lipoprotein(a) interferes with the fibrinolytic system because of its structural similarity to plasminogen[57]. Furthermore, the generation of plasmin has been shown to be inhibited in postmenopausal women with high lipoprotein(a) levels[58]. However, the role of lipoprotein(a) as an independent risk factor is not completely clear[59] and there are no clinical data demonstrating that lowering the lipoprotein(a) level results in a reduced CHD risk. The same criticism may be applied to factor VII and fibrinogen.

THE EFFECT OF HRT

Some reports suggest that HRT increases the concentration of factor VII[22,60-62], although this was not confirmed in other studies, where factor VII remained unchanged[63,64] or even decreased[31,65,66]. An interesting observation supporting the inductive effects of estrogens comes from the observation of a close interrelationship between factor VII and triglyceride[67], since estrogens, particularly through the oral route, are known to increase triglyceride levels. A reduction in the level of circulating fibrinogen during the administration of HRT has been detected in most[31–33,62,66,68,69], but not all, studies[46], with no difference between estrogen and combined HRT.

Fibrinolysis seems to be enhanced by HRT in most studies. A prospective study involving 75 postmenopausal women demonstrated a reduction in PAI-1 and an increase in t-PA in women on HRT, both effects remaining after 1 year of treatment. The reduction in PAI-1 was observed in women receiving oral, but not transdermal, estrogens. In a cohort of 749 women from the Framingham Offspring Study, it was shown that high estrogen status was associated with greater fibrinolytic potential (lower PAI-1 levels)[70]. Similar profibrinolytic changes were observed in other studies with several HRT regimens[22,62,69,71]. A recent study has clarified some molecular aspects of the estrogenic action on the circulating levels of PAI-1[72]. The 4/5 guanosine (4G/5G) polymorphism in the promoter region of the PAI-1 gene has been shown to be associated with higher levels of plasma PAI-1 activity. The 4G allele has a higher activity than the 5G allele, because the 5G allele contains an additional binding site for a DNA-binding protein that could be a transcriptional repressor[73,74]. In a group of postmenopausal women with coronary heart disease, the levels of PAI-1 correlated with the 4G allele dosage (Figure 3)[72]. Furthermore, the HRT-induced decrease in PAI-1 correlated with the 4G allele dosage (Figure 4)[72].

Additional effects on fibrinolysis may be brought about by changes in the circulating concentration of lipoprotein(a). Increases in the concentration of lipoprotein(a) were detected under the hypoestrogenic status of the menopause, either natural[75] or surgical[76]. Accordingly, the administration of estrogens is followed by a reduction in lipoprotein(a) levels[62,75,77,78], an effect that is not downregulated by progestins[75]. Interestingly, the decrease in lipoprotein(a) levels by HRT is particularly evident in women undergoing higher lipoprotein(a) increases with the menopause, and after treatment with oral estrogens, with or without progestins[58]. Also of interest is the fact that the

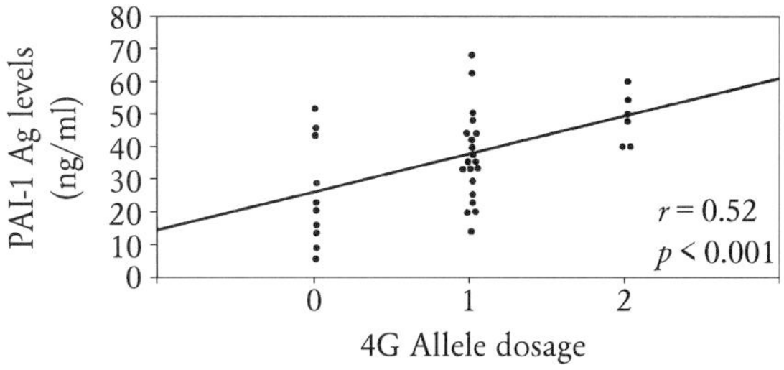

Figure 3 Correlation between plasminogen activator inhibitor type 1 (PAI-1) antigen levels and 4G allele dosage in a group of women with coronary heart disease. The 4G/4G genotype, ascribed to the 2 category at the x axis, is associated with the highest PAI-1 levels. From reference 72, with permission

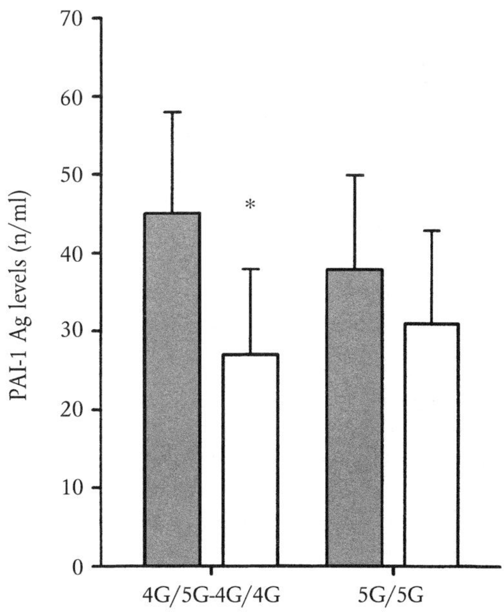

Figure 4 Influence of the plasminogen activator inhibitor type 1 (PAI-1) promoter 4G/5G genotype on the variation in PAI-1 antigen levels under hormone replacement therapy (HRT). The presence of the 4G allele (4G/5G or 4G/4G genotype) determined susceptibility to HRT, as shown by the bars on the left, where the levels of antigenic PAI-1 significantly decreased. In contrast, PAI levels remained unchanged in cases with the 5G/5G genotype, as shown by the bars on the right. Values are mean ± SEM; tinted bars, PAI-1 levels before HRT; open bars, PAI-1 levels after 3–4 months HRT;* $p < 0.05$. From reference 72, with permission

apo(a) component of lipoprotein(a) shows a size polymorphism, with individual isoforms ranging in apparent molecular weight from approximately 250 to 800 kD[79,80]. The low-molecular-weight apo(a) isoforms show higher plasmin inhibition than high-molecular-weight apo(a) isoforms and tend to accumulate in women who suffer higher lipoprotein(a) increases in the menopause, and who are the most estrogen-sensitive population sample[58].

In summary, most of the observed actions of HRT on relevant risk factors affecting the hemostatic balance seem to promote a beneficial effect. The available clinical observations, despite the methodological limitation of the studies, seem unanimous in suggesting a very low, but detectable, risk of venous thrombosis. Therefore, one may speculate on the possible influence of alternative variables, the effect of HRT on either the vessel wall or the blood flow being possible factors.

BIOLOGICAL EFFECTS OF ESTROGENS ON THE VESSEL WALL

Given the lack of a clear prothrombotic effect of HRT when examining the changes induced on relevant hemostatic parameters, attention is being focused on the vascular wall. The endothelium holds a principal position in the control of vascular remodelling and, as mentioned earlier, is the source of crucial antithrombotic substances, such as nitric oxide, prostacyclin, ADPase, thrombomodulin, t-PA and heparan sulfate[81]. In addition, the endothelial membrane is covered by glycoproteins and proteoglycans, which provide a negatively charged environment that impairs the adhesion of platelets and the initiation of the intrinsic pathway of coagulation[82-84]. Endothelial dysfunction, on the other hand, is followed by the release of prothrombotic products, such as von Willebrand factor and platelet activating factor[85-87]. A well-organized system of distinct adhesion molecules[86,88,89], whose expression is potentiated when the endothelial function deteriorates, operates to influence platelet aggregation, a first step in forming a hemostatic plug or a thrombus[4-6]. There is, for example, overexpression of P-selectin, an adhesion molecule also found in activated platelets, which mediates the deceleration of platelets prior to their aggregation.

The development of atherosclerosis, an important difference between the venous and the arterial tree, determines an inflammatory milieu governing endothelial dysfunction[87,90]. Additionally, the initiation and progression of atherosclerosis has been associated with the oxidation of low-density lipoproteins, which may therefore act as an indirect promoter of thrombogenesis[91].

Estrogens are known endothelial protectors, which act through distinct and still incompletely known mechanisms, such as the diminution of the vasomotor tone[92,93], the promotion of vasodilators/antiaggregatory substances such as nitric oxide and prostacyclin[93-95], the decrease of vasoconstrictors/proaggregatory substances such as endothelin-1[96,97], the development of antioxidant effects on low-density lipoproteins[98], the induction of trophic endothelial effects[99-101] and the inhibition of the expression of adhesion molecules[102,103].

In conclusion, there is experimental evidence to suggest that, at the vascular wall, one of the three elements of Virchow's triad, the action of estrogens may be antithrombotic. This action may be conducted through the morphological and functional restoration of the endothelial function and, therefore, may be particularly operative at the arterial level, where atherosclerosis acts as a disturbing endothelial element. This hypothesis may also explain, in part, the contrasting effect on the venous tree, where, in the setting of an already functional endothelium, estrogens seem slightly to increase the thrombotic risk. Most probably, the diminished blood flow, linked with the well-known increased venous distensibility induced by estrogens and progestins[104], may be a component in the paradoxical behavior of the venous tree.

ACKNOWLEDGEMENT

This paper was supported by grant 1FD97-1035-C02-01 from the Spanish Ministry for Education and Culture.

References

1. Fuster V, Badimon L, Badimon JJ, *et al.* The pathogenesis of coronary artery disease and the acute coronary syndromes. *N Engl J Med* 1992;326: 242-50
2. Fuster V, Badimon L, Badimon JJ, *et al.* The pathogenesis of coronary artery disease and the acute coronary syndromes. *N Engl J Med* 1992;326: 310-18
3. Badimon L, Bayés-Genís A. Effects of progestogens on thrombosis and atherosclerosis. *Hum Reprod Update* 1999;5:191-9
4. Kroll MH, Harris TS, Moake JL, *et al.* von Willebrand factor binding to platelet GpIb initiates signals for platelet activation. *J Clin Invest* 1991;88:1568-73
5. Harker LA. Platelets and vascular thrombosis. *N Engl J Med* 1994;330:1006-7
6. Lefkovits J, Plow EF, Topol EJ. Platelet glycoprotein IIb/IIIa receptors in cardiovascular medicine. *N Engl J Med* 1995;332:1553-9
7. Bettina RM, Koeleman BPC, Koster T, *et al.* Mutation in blood coagulation factor V associated with resistance to activated protein C. *Nature (London)* 1994;369:64-7
8. Notelovitz M. Hormone therapy and hemostasis. In Lobo RA, ed. *Treatment of the Postmenopausal Woman. Basic and Clinical Aspects.* New York: Raven Press, 1994:271-81
9. Hillmen P, Lewis SM, Bessler M, *et al.* Natural history of paroxysmal nocturnal hemoglobinuria. *N Engl J Med* 1995;333:1253-8
10. Socie G, Mary JY, de Gramont A, *et al.* Paroxysmal nocturnal haemoglobinuria: long-term follow-up and prognostic factors. *Lancet* 1996;348:573-7
11. De Stefano V, Finazzi G, Mannucci PM. Inherited thrombophilia: pathogenesis, clinical syndromes, and management. *Blood* 1996;87:3531-44
12. Thomas DP, Roberts HR. Hypercoagulability in venous and arterial thrombosis. *Ann Intern Med* 1997;126:638-44
13. Price DT, Ridker PM. Factor V Leiden mutation and the risks for thromboembolic disease: a clinical perspective. *Ann Intern Med* 1997;127:895-903
14. Martinelli I, Sacchi E, Landi G, *et al.* High risk of cerebral-vein thrombosis in carriers of a prothrombin-gene mutation and in users of oral contraceptives. *N Engl J Med* 1998;338:1793-7
15. Rosendaal FR, Siscovick DS, Schwartz SM, *et al.* Factor V Leiden (resistance to activated protein C) increases the risk of myocardial infarction in young women. *Blood* 1997;89:2817-21
16. Pabinger I, Schneider B. Thrombotic risk in hereditary antithrombin III, protein C, or protein S deficiency: a cooperative, retrospective study. *Arterioscler Thromb Vasc Biol* 1996;16:742-8
17. Winkler UH. Effects of progestins on cardiovascular diseases: the haemostatic system. *Hum Reprod Update* 1999;5:200-4
18. Acute myocardial infarction and combined oral contraceptives: results of an international multicentre case-control study. WHO Collaborative Study of Cardiovascular Disease and Steroid Hormone Contraception. *Lancet* 1997;349:1202-9
19. Todd JC, Lawrenson R, Farmer RDT, *et al.* Venous thromboembolism disease and combined oral contraceptives: a re-analysis of the MediPlus database. *Hum Reprod* 1999;14:1500-5
20. Lowe GDO, Rumley A, Woodward M, *et al.* Epidemiology of coagulation factors, inhibitors and activation markers: The Third Glasgow MONICA Survey I. Illustrative reference ranges by age, sex and hormone use. *Br J Haematol* 1997;97:775-84
21. Winkler UH. Menopause, hormone replacement therapy and cardiovascular disease: a review of haemostaseological findings. *Fibrinolysis* 1992;6: 5-10
22. Kroon UB, Silfverstolpe G, Tengborn L. The effects of transdermal estradiol and oral conjugated estrogens on haemostasis variables. *Thromb Haemost* 1994;71:420-3
23. Daly E, Vessey MP, Hawkins MM, *et al.* Risk of venous thromboembolism in users of hormone replacement therapy. *Lancet* 1996;348:977-80
24. Jick H, Derby LE, Myers MW, *et al.* Risk of hospital admission for idiopathic venous thromboembolism among users of postmenopausal oestrogens. *Lancet* 1996;348:981-3
25. Grodstein F, Stampfer MJ, Goldhaber SZ, *et al.* Prospective study of exogenous hormones and risk of pulmonary embolism in women. *Lancet* 1996;348:983-7
26. Gutthan SP, Rodriguez LAG, Castellsague J, *et al.* Hormone replacement therapy and risk of venous thromboembolism: population based case-control study. *Br Med J* 1997;314:796-800
27. Kuhl H. Effects of progestogens on haemostasis. *Maturitas* 1996;24:1-19
28. Balasch J. The 'pill scare II' two years later. *Eur J Contracept Reprod Health Care* 1997;2:149-59
29. Winkler UH. Effects on hemostatic variables of desogestrel- and gestodene-containing oral contraceptives in comparison with levonorgestrel-containing oral contraceptives: a review. *Am J Obstet Gynecol* 1998;179:S51-6
30. Farsetti A, Miniti S, Citarella F, *et al.* Molecular basis of estrogen regulation of Hageman factor XII gene expression. *Endocrinology* 1995;136: 5076-83
31. Kroon UB, Tengborn L, Rita H, *et al.* The effects of transdermal oestradiol and oral progestogens

on haemostasis variables. *Br J Obstet Gynaecol* 1997;104(Suppl 16):32–7
32. Frohlich M, Schunkert H, Hense HW, *et al.* Effects of hormone replacement therapies on fibrinogen and plasma viscosity in postmenopausal women. *Br J Haematol* 1998;100:577–81
33. Conard J, Gompel A, Pelissier C, *et al.* Fibrinogen and plasminogen modifications during oral estradiol replacement therapy. *Fertil Steril* 1997;68: 449–53
34. Winkler UH. Hormone replacement therapy and hemostasis: principles of a complex interaction. *Maturitas* 1996;24:131–45
35. Chae CU, Ridker PM, Manson JE. Postmenopausal hormone replacement therapy and cardiovascular disease. *Thromb Haemost* 1997;77: 770–80
36. Kessler CM, Szymanski LM, Shamsipour Z, *et al.* Estrogen replacement therapy and coagulation: relationship to lipid and lipoprotein changes. *Obstet Gynecol* 1997;89:326–31
37. Conlan MG, Folsom AR, Finch A, *et al.* Antithrombin III: associations with age, race, sex and cardiovascular disease risk factors. *Thromb Haemost* 1994;72:551–6
38. Bertina RM, Rosendaal FR. Venous thrombosis. The interaction of genes and environment. *N Engl J Med* 1998;338:1840–1
39. Vandenbroucke JP, Koster T, Briët E, *et al.* Increased risk of venous thrombosis in oral-contraceptive users who are carriers of factor V Leiden mutation. *Lancet* 1994;344:1453–7
40. Martinelli I, Landi G, Merati G, *et al.* Factor V gene mutation is a risk factor for cerebral venous thrombosis. *Thromb Haemost* 1996;75:393–4
41. Anderson FA, Wheeler HB, Goldberg RJ, *et al.* A population-based perspective of the hospital incidence and case-fatality rates of deep vein thrombosis and pulmonary embolism. The Worcester DVT Study. *Arch Intern Med* 1991;151:933–8
42. Zivelin A, Griffin JH, Xu X, *et al.* A single genetic origin for a common Caucasian risk factor for venous thrombosis. *Blood* 1997;89:397–402
43. Lee AJ, Smith WCS, Lowe GDO, *et al.* Plasma fibrinogen and coronary risk factors: the Scottish Heart Health Study. *J Clin Epidemiol* 1990;43: 913–19
44. Wilhelmsen L, Svärdsudd K, Korsan-Bengtsen K, *et al.* Fibrinogen as a risk factor for stroke and myocardial infarction. *N Engl J Med* 1984;311: 501–5
45. Meade TW, Mellows S, Brozovic M, *et al.* Haemostatic function and ischaemic heart disease: principal results of the Northwick Park Heart Study. *Lancet* 1986;2:533–7
46. Scarabin PY, Alhenc-Gelas M, Plu-Bureau G, *et al.* Effects of oral and transdermal estrogen/progesterone regimens on blood coagulation and fibrinolysis in postmenopausal women. A randomized controlled trial. *Arterioscler Thromb Vasc Biol* 1997;17:3071–8
47. Scarabin PY, Aillaud MF, Amouyel P, *et al.* Associations of fibrinogen, factor VII and PAI-1 with baseline findings among 10,500 male participants in a prospective study of myocardial infarction – the PRIME Study. Prospective Epidemiological Study of Myocardial Infarction. *Thromb Haemost* 1998;80:749–56
48. Aznar J, Estellés A, Tormo G, *et al.* Plasminogen activator inhibitor activity and other fibrinolytic variables in patients with coronary artery disease. *Br Heart J* 1988;59:535–41
49. Páramo JA, Colucci M, Collen D. Plasminogen activator inhibitor in the blood of patients with coronary artery disease. *Br Med J* 1985;291:573–4
50. Hamsten A, Wiman B, De Faire U, *et al.* Increased plasma levels of a rapid inhibitor of tissue plasminogen activator in young survivors of myocardial infarction. *N Engl J Med* 1985;313:1557–63
51. Estellés A, Tormo G, Aznar J, *et al.* Reduced fibrinolytic activity in coronary heart disease in basal conditions and after exercise. *Thromb Res* 1985;40:373–83
52. Hamsten A, De Faire U, Walldius G, *et al.* Plasminogen activator inhibitor in plasma: risk factor for recurrent myocardial infarction. *Lancet* 1987;2:3–9
53. Thogersen AM, Jansson JH, Boman K, *et al.* High plasminogen activator inhibitor and tissue plasminogen activator levels in plasma precede a first acute myocardial infarction in both men and women: evidence for the fibrinolytic system as an independent primary risk factor. *Circulation* 1998;98:2241–7
54. Gottsauner-Wolf M, Sochor H, Hornykewycz S, *et al.* Predictive value of PAI-1 plasma activity and thallium perfusion imaging for restenosis after percutaneous transluminal angioplasty in clinically asymptomatic patients. *Thromb Haemost* 1999;81:522–6
55. Cesari M, Rossi GP. Plasminogen activator inhibitor type 1 in ischemic cardiomyopathy. *Arterioscler Thromb Vasc Biol* 1999;19:1378–86
56. Wiman B. Predictive value of fibrinolytic factors in coronary heart disease. *Scand J Clin Lab Invest Suppl* 1999;230:23–31
57. Edelberg JM, Pizzo SV. Lipoprotein (a): the link between impaired fibrinolysis and atherosclerosis. *Fibrinolysis* 1991;5:135–43
58. Estellés A, Cano A, Falcó C, *et al.* Lipoprotein(a) levels and isoforms and fibrinolytic activity in postmenopause – influence of hormone replacement therapy. *Thromb Haemost* 1999;81:104–10
59. Ridker PM. An epidemiologic reassessment of lipoprotein(a) and atherothrombotic risk. *Trends Cardiovasc Med* 1995;5:225–9
60. Boschetti C, Cortellaro M, Nencioni T, *et al.* Short- and long-term effects of hormone

replacement therapy (transdermal estradiol vs oral conjugated equine estrogens, combined with medroxyprogesterone acetate) on blood coagulation factors in postmenopausal women. *Thromb Res* 1991;62:1-8
61. Habiba M, Andrea A, Philipps B, *et al.* Thrombophilia and lipid profile in postmenopausal women using a new transdermal oestradiol patch. *Eur J Obstet Gynecol Reprod Biol* 1996;66: 165-8
62. Andersen LF, Gram J, Skouby SO, *et al.* Effects of hormone replacement therapy on hemostatic cardiovascular risk factors. *Am J Obstet Gynecol* 1999;180:283-9
63. Saleh AA, Dorey LG, Dombrowski MP, *et al.* Thrombosis and hormone replacement therapy in postmenopausal women. *Am J Obstet Gynecol* 1993;6:1554-7
64. Nabulsi AA, Folsom AR, White A, *et al.* Association of hormone-replacement therapy with various cardiovascular risk factors in postmenopausal women. *N Engl J Med* 1993;328: 1069-75
65. Scarabin PY, Plu-Bureau G, Bara L, *et al.* Haemostatic variables and menopausal status: influence of hormone replacement therapy. *Thromb Haemost* 1993;70:584-7
66. Lindoff C, Peterson F, Lecander I, *et al.* Transdermal estrogen replacement therapy: beneficial effects on hemostatic risk factors for cardiovascular disease. *Maturitas* 1996;24:43-50
67. Skartlien AH, Lyberg-Beckmann S, Holme I, *et al.* Effect of alteration in triglyceride levels on factor VII-phospholipid complexes in plasma. *Arteriosclerosis* 1989;9:798-801
68. PEPI Trial Writing Group. Effects of estrogen/ progestin on heart disease risk factors in postmenopausal women. *J Am Med Assoc* 1995;273: 199-208
69. Meilahn EN, Cauley JA, Tracy RP, *et al.* Association of sex hormones and adiposity with plasma levels of fibrinogen and PAI-1 in postmenopausal women. *Am J Epidemiol* 1996;143:159-66
70. Gebara OCE, Mittleman MA, Sutherland P, *et al.* Association between increased estrogen status and increased fibrinolytic potential in the Framingham Offspring Study. *Circulation* 1995; 91:1952-8
71. Notelovitz M. Progestogens and coagulation. *Int Proc J* 1989;1:229-34
72. Grancha S, Estellés A, Tormo G, *et al.* Plasminogen activator inhibitor-1 (PAI-1) promoter 4G/5G genotype and increased PAI-1 circulating levels in postmenopausal women with coronary artery disease. *Thromb Haemost* 1999;81:516-21
73. Dawson S, Wiman B, Hamsten A, *et al.* The two allele sequences of a common polymorphism in the promoter of the plasminogen activator inhibitor (PAI-1) gene respond differently to interleukin-1 in hepG2 cells. *J Biol Chem* 1993; 268:10739-45
74. Eriksson P, Kallin B, van't Hooft FM, *et al.* Allele-specific increase in basal transcription of the plasminogen-activator inhibitor 1 gene is associated with myocardial infarction. *Proc Natl Acad Sci USA* 1995;92:1851-5
75. Gilabert J, Estellés A, Cano A, *et al.* The effect of estrogen replacement therapy with or without progestogen on the fibrinolytic system and coagulation inhibitors in postmenopausal status. *Am J Obstet Gynecol* 1995;173:1849-54
76. Kim CJ, Ryu WS, Kwak JW, *et al.* Changes in Lp(a) lipoprotein and lipid levels after cessation of female sex hormone production and estrogen replacement therapy. *Arch Intern Med* 1996;156: 500-4
77. Haines CJ, Chung TK, Masarei JR, *et al.* An examination of the effect of combined cyclical hormone replacement therapy on lipoprotein(a) and other lipoproteins. *Atherosclerosis* 1996;119:215-22
78. Honggi W, Lippuner K, Riesen W, *et al.* Long-term influence of the different postmenopausal hormone replacement regimens on serum lipids and lipoprotein(a): a randomised study. *Br J Obstet Gynaecol* 1997;104:708-17
79. Uttermann G, Kraft HG, Menzel HJ, *et al.* Genetics of the quantitative Lp(a) lipoprotein trait. I. Relation of Lp(a) glycoprotein phenotypes to Lp(a) lipoprotein concentrations in plasma. *Hum Genet* 1988;78:41-6
80. Kamboh MI, Ferrel RE, Kottke BA. Expressed hypervariable polymorphism of apolipoprotein(a). *Am J Hum Genet* 1991;49:1063-74
81. Vane JR, Anggard EE, Botting RM. Regularity functions of the vascular endothelium. *N Engl J Med* 1990;323:27-36
82. Marcus AJ, Safier LB, Broekman MJ, *et al.* Thrombosis and inflammation as multicellular processes: significance of cell-cell interactions. *Thromb Haemost* 1995;74:213-17
83. Marcus AJ, Broekman MJ, Drosopoulos JH, *et al.* The endothelial cell ecto-ADPase responsible for inhibition of platelet function is CD39. *J Clin Invest* 1997;99:1351-60
84. Marcum JA, Rosenberg RD. Anticoagulantly active heparin-like molecules from vascular tissue. *Biochemistry* 1984;23:1730-7
85. Ware JA, Heistad DD. Platelet-endothelium interactions. *N Engl J Med* 1993;328:628-35
86. Frenette PS, Wagner DD. Adhesion molecules – part II: blood vessels and blood cells. *N Engl J Med* 1996;335:43-5
87. Cines DB, Pollak ES, Buck CA, *et al.* Endothelial cells in physiology and in the pathophysiology of vascular disorders. *Blood* 1998;91:3527-61
88. Coller BS, Peerschke EI, Scudder LE, *et al.* A murine monoclonal antibody that completely blocks the binding of fibrinogen to platelets

produces a thrombasthenic-like state in normal platelets and binds to glycoprotein IIb and/or IIIa. *J Clin Invest* 1983;72:325-38
89. Phillips DR, Charo IF, Scarborough RM. GPIIb-IIIa: the responsive integrin. *Cell* 1991;65:359-62
90. Ross R. Atherosclerosis - an inflammatory disease. *N Engl J Med* 1999;340:115-26
91. Cox DA, Cohen ML. Effects of oxidized low-density lipoprotein on vascular contraction and relaxation: clinical and pharmacological implications in atherosclerosis. *Pharmacol Rev* 1996;48: 3-19
92. Mendelsohn ME, Karas RH. The protective effects of estrogen on the cardiovascular system. *N Engl J Med* 1999;340:1801-11
93. Sarrel PM. The differential effects of oestrogens and progestins on vascular tone. *Hum Reprod Update* 1999;5:205-9
94. Fogelberg M, Vesterqvist O, Diczfalusy U, *et al.* Experimental atherosclerosis: effects of oestrogen and atherosclerosis on thromboxane and prostacyclin formation. *Eur J Clin Invest* 1990;20:105-10
95. Mikkola T, Turunen P, Avela K, *et al.* 17β-estradiol stimulates prostacyclin, but not endothelin-1, production in human vascular endothelial cells. *J Clin Endocrinol Metab* 1995;80: 1832-6
96. Polderman KH, Stehouwer CDA, van Kamp GJ, *et al.* Influence of sex hormones on plasma endothelin levels. *Ann Intern Med* 1993;118:429-32
97. Chen FP, Lee N, Wang CH, *et al.* Effects of hormone replacement therapy on cardiovascular risk factors in postmenopausal women. *Fertil Steril* 1998;69:267-73
98. Sack MN, Rader DJ, Cannon RO III. Oestrogen and inhibition of oxidation of low-density lipoproteins in postmenopausal women. *Lancet* 1994; 343:269-70
99. Morales DE, McGowan KA, Grant DS, *et al.* Estrogen promotes angiogenic activity in human umbilical vein endothelial cells *in vitro* and in a murine model. *Circulation* 1995;91:755-63
100. Krasinski K, Spyridipoulos I, Asahara T, *et al.* Estradiol accelerates functional endothelial recovery after arterial injury. *Circulation* 1997;95: 1768-72
101. Spyridipoulos I, Sullivan AB, Kearney M, *et al.* Estrogen receptor-mediated inhibition of human endothelial cell apoptosis: estradiol as a survival factor. *Circulation* 1997;95:1505-14
102. Caulin-Glaser T, Watson CA, Pardi R, *et al.* Effects of 17β-estradiol on cytokine-induced endothelial cell adhesion molecule expression. *J Clin Invest* 1996;98:36-42
103. Lip GY, Blann AD, Jones AF, *et al.* Effects of hormone-replacement therapy on hemostatic factors, lipid factors, and endothelial function in women undergoing surgical menopause: implications for prevention of atherosclerosis. *Am Heart J* 1997; 134:764-71
104. Goodrich SM, Wood JE. Peripheral venous distensibility and velocity of venous blood flow during pregnancy or during oral contraceptive therapy. *Am J Obstet Gynecol* 1964;90:740-4

Prescription attitudes of gynecologists towards risk and benefit situations 64

S. Rozenberg, C. Fellemans, J. Barudy Vasquez, J. Vandromme and H. Ham

INTRODUCTION

Hormone replacement therapy (HRT) has been shown to relieve postmenopausal symptoms. There have been a large number of publications suggesting that HRT is also effective in preventing osteoporosis and cardiovascular diseases, although some studies have controverted this[1-6]. Some authors have suggested that the greatest benefit will be obtained by those women who are at high risk for coronary heart disease and those who have pre-existing heart disease; they propose a strategy for identifying patients who would benefit from HRT[3]. Despite the potential health benefit of HRT, the prevalence of its use remains low: less than 10% in some European countries[7-9]. While almost all gynecologists in the UK and in Finland would prescribe HRT to women with climacteric complaints and without contraindications to the treatment, only about 60% of Dutch general practitioners would do so[8,10,11]. Even fewer of the interviewed physicians would prescribe HRT to asymptomatic women. The present studies, conducted among Belgian gynecologists, specifically evaluate the following.

(1) The effect of the patient's age, bone mineral density and individual risk of cardiovascular disease and familial risk of breast cancer on HRT prescription;

(2) Whether other medications are prescribed for osteoporosis instead of HRT;

(3) Whether physicians are willing to prescribe HRT to a patient with a contraindication for HRT (a past history of endometrial cancer) and concurrent indications (climacteric symptoms and osteoporosis).

MATERIALS AND METHODS

Two surveys were used to assess these questions.

Survey 1

Briefly, we summarized the charts of 17 consecutive patients who were postmenopausal and attended a menopause clinic for the first time (original cases)[12]. For each of these charts, we constructed 36 different cases using the following manipulations. Age was modified at two levels: each chart was doubled by either adding or subtracting 10 years according to whether the woman was younger or older than 60 years. The bone mineral density values were also modified. For each case three levels of bone mineral measurements were presented: one with a normal bone mineral density result, one with osteopenia and one with osteoporosis, according to the definitions given by the World Health Organization[13]. Similarly, the cardiovascular risk (three levels) and breast cancer risk (two levels) were also modified. Details of the distribution of the characteristics of the original cases and the constructed cases have been described previously[12].

Thus, starting with 17 original charts we ended up with 612 created cases. Twelve cases were sent out of these 612 files to each of the 1010 practicing Belgian gynecologists. We ensured that these 12 cases corresponded to 12 different original cases. With this constraint, the cases were chosen at random, using a computer program. All the cases that were submitted to the gynecologists were presented as summaries of charts, including a brief personal history, biological results, a normal mammography and the result of bone mineral density measurement at the L2–L4 site using a dual X-ray absorptiometer (Hologic, USA). For each chart, the gynecologists were asked whether they would treat the patient with HRT (closed answer no/yes). They were also asked whether they would prescribe therapies other than HRT (closed answer) and, if so, which ones (open answers). They were assured that their participation would remain anonymous. Two mailings were sent to all Belgian gynecologists within a period of 6 weeks. Statistical analysis was performed using the SPSS software. All decisions regarding prescription were considered as being independent observations without taking into account any physician effect or any effect due to multiplicity of the same cases.

The effect of each of the four factors on prescription rates (univariate analyses) was assessed by χ^2 tests. The significance level was set at $p < 0.01$.

Survey 2

The following case was presented[14]: a 57-year-old woman was treated by total hysterectomy and bilateral salpingo-oophorectomy and lymphadenectomy at the age of 54 years, for a well-differentiated endometrium cancer (stage IA). Since then, cytological smears of the vagina have never shown signs of recurrence. The patient complains of hot flushes, hair loss, skin dryness and loss of libido. Other clinical findings were normal (blood pressure, cholesterol, mammogram), but a bone density result at the L2–L4 site using a dual X-ray absorptiometer revealed osteoporosis (T-score of −3.37).

This case was sent to every practicing Belgian gynecologist ($n = 1363$). The gynecologists were asked whether they would treat this patient with HRT (closed answer no/yes). They could comment on which HRT preparation they would prescribe (open question). A questionnaire including demographic data was included. They were assured that their participation would remain anonymous. Statistical analysis was performed using the SPSS software.

RESULTS

Survey 1

We obtained 388 returns (38.3% response rate) after two mailings (264 on the first mailing and 124 on the second mailing), totalling 4656 cases. A valid response was obtained for 4108 cases.

Overall, the physicians would have prescribed treatment in 67% of the cases. In agreement with the literature, the prescription rates were significantly higher in women who presented climacteric symptoms (87.7% vs. 49%; $p < 0.001$).

A significant association was observed between the increase in prescription rate and the decrease in bone mineral density ($p < 0.001$) (Figure 1). When only women without climacteric symptoms were considered, 32.5% of those with normal bone density, 50.4% with osteopenia and 67.1% with osteoporosis would have been treated ($p < 0.001$) (Figure 2).

The prescription rate was higher ($p < 0.001$) in younger women than in those who were 10 years older. When only women without symptoms were considered, the difference in prescription rate between the younger and the older women was even more pronounced (65.9% vs. 33.4%; $p < 0.001$) (Figure 3). The effect of age and of bone mineral density results on the prescription rate persisted after cases were stratified for both factors. For cases with a mean age of 55 ± 4 years, the

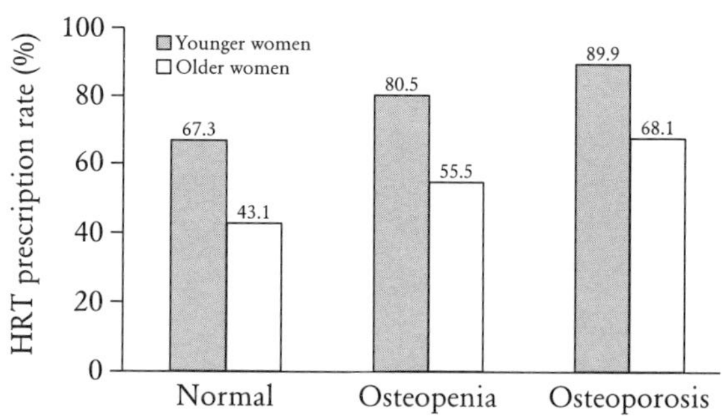

Figure 1 The relationship between hormone replacement therapy (HRT) prescription rates and bone mineral density and age level (differing by 10 years). The prescription rate (%) increased significantly when bone mineral density decreased ($p < 0.001$) and was higher in younger women ($p < 0.001$)

prescription rates were 89.9% for osteoporosis cases, 80.5% for osteopenia cases and 67.3% for cases with a normal bone mineral density result ($p < 0.001$). For the women who were 10 years older, the prescription rates were 68.1% for osteoporosis cases, 55.5% for osteopenia cases and 43.1% for cases with a normal bone mineral density result ($p < 0.001$). The effect of bone mineral density and age persisted in all the subgroups of women having various levels of cardiovascular or breast cancer risk ($p < 0.001$).

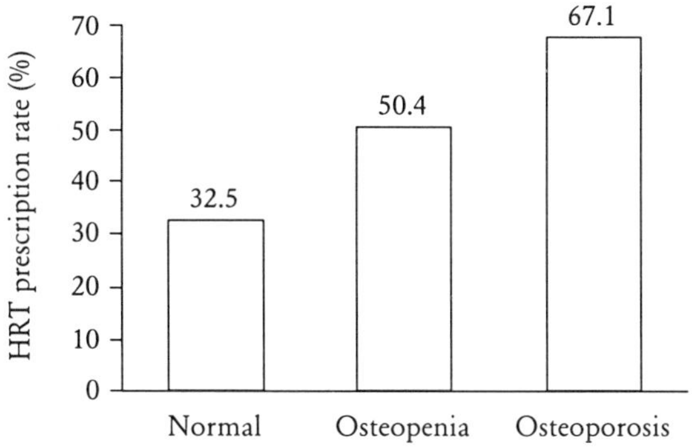

Figure 2 The relationship between hormone replacement therapy (HRT) prescription rates and bone mineral density in women without climacteric symptoms

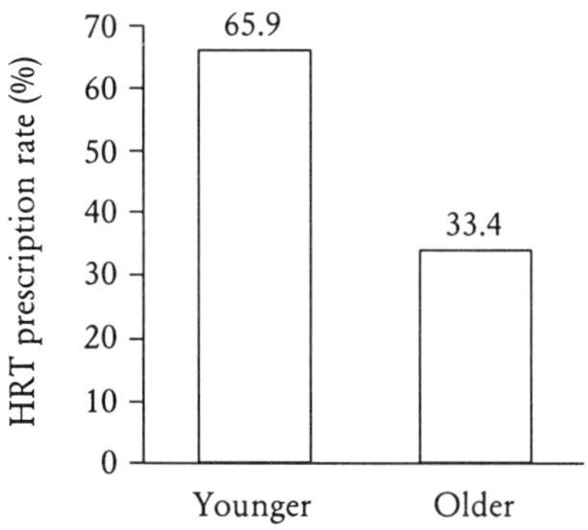

Figure 3 Decrease in prescription rate of hormone replacement therapy (HRT) observed with advancing age and normal bone mineral density ($p < 0.001$)

No significant variation in HRT prescription rate was observed in relation to the cardiovascular risk or to the breast cancer risk.

The prescription rates in relation to bone mineral density for the interventions other than HRT are shown in Table 1. Significantly increased prescription rates were observed for HRT, and for the other regimens calcium, vitamin D, bisphosphonates, calcitonin and fluor in relation to the decrease in bone mineral density ($p < 0.001$). After HRT, calcium was the second most frequently prescribed regimen. It was prescribed 745 times (in 18% of the cases). Other drugs were prescribed less often. Bisphosphonates were prescribed in only 228 cases (6% of the cases).Vitamin D was prescribed 129 times (3% of the cases). Calcitonin ($n = 18$) and fluor ($n = 8$) were very seldom prescribed.

The prescription rates of these regimens in relation to age are presented in Table 2. In cases where HRT had not been prescribed, only slightly higher calcium, bisphosphonates and vitamin D prescription rates were observed in older women than in younger women (not significant).

Survey 2

We obtained 460 returns, of which 18 were considered invalid after one mailing (i.e. a 32% response rate). Overall, the physicians would prescribe treatment in 67% of the cases. Among the physicians who would prescribe HRT, 49% stated that they would prescribe estrogen-only therapy (unopposed

Table 1 Number of cases (with percentages in parentheses) of women with an identical clinical history but three different bone mineral density (BMD) results (normal, osteopenia and osteoporosis) to whom regimens other than hormone replacement therapy were prescribed

Regimens	*Normal BMD*	*Osteopenia*	*Osteoporosis*	*Significance*
Calcium	62 (4.3)	211 (14)	472 (33)	$p < 0.001$
Vitamin D	3 (0.2)	35 (2.3)	91 (6.3)	$p < 0.001$
Bisphosphonates	4 (0.3)	29 (1.9)	195 (13.6)	$p < 0.001$
Calcitonin	0 (0)	0 (0)	18 (1.5)	$p < 0.001$
Fluor	0 (0)	1 (0.1)	7 (0.5)	$p < 0.001$

Table 2 Number of cases (with percentages in parentheses) of women with an identical clinical history but two age levels, differing by 10 years, to whom an osteoporosis regimen was prescribed: younger (mean age ± SD, 55 ± 4 years) and older (mean age ± SD, 65 ± 4 years)

	Younger women	*Older women*	*Significance*
Calcium	397 (19.5)	348 (16.8)	$p < 0.05$
Vitamin D	61 (3)	68 (3.2)	NS
Bisphosphonates	126 (6.1)	102 (4.9)	NS
Calcitonin	10 (0.5)	8 (0.4)	NS
Fluor	3 (0.1)	5 (0.2)	NS

estrogens) and 27% would prescribe a combined estrogen–progestin therapy.

Among those who would prescribe HRT, 75% considered that no other investigations were required to help decide whether HRT was needed for this patient, but 84% of those who would not prescribe HRT answered that they needed more information.

DISCUSSION

A very high prescription rate was observed in these surveys compared to the prevalence of HRT prescription in Belgium[9]. The prescription rates that we encountered here cannot be extrapolated to the general population, since the charts we used are not representative of the general population and many women in survey 1 and the patient in survey 2 had severe climacteric symptoms; it is well known that physicians more often prescribe HRT to such patients. In this study, women with typical climacteric symptoms would also have been treated more often than those without symptoms. Apart from climacteric symptoms, we observed that age and bone mineral density influenced HRT initiation. It is well known that HRT is effective in reducing bone loss[15–18]. Women with the lowest bone mass may have the largest benefit from HRT[18]. Our study shows that Belgian gynecologists are willing to adapt their attitude in relation to the bone mineral density result since they initiate HRT more often in women with a low bone mass. One may wonder why gynecologists would have treated only 80% of women with osteoporosis and 50% of women with normal bone mineral density results. A possible explanation is that some physicians may not be familiar with bone mineral density results or did not recognize low bone mineral density as a risk for osteoporosis. On the other hand, the fact that the bone mineral density result was provided in this study may also have increased the awareness of osteoporosis and increased the prescription rate. It is also possible that some physicians may not have been convinced of the net benefit of HRT in some of these patients; they might consider treating some of the patients with osteoporosis with other medications. This seems not to be the case in this study.

The addition of 10 years of age had a large impact on prescription rates, reducing them by about 30%. Perhaps gynecologists do not consider these women as osteoporotic or are not convinced that HRT will be effective for them. It is also possible that physicians believe that these women will not tolerate HRT. Interestingly, this was then not compensated for by a higher prescription of other regimens. Perhaps gynecologists do not feel familiar with these regimens.

In our study, there was no relationship between prescription habits and cardiovascular risk. Unlike osteoporosis data, the cardiovascular effects of HRT have been controversial[2–6,19,20]. In addition, many HRT formulations still give warnings about cardiovascular risks of HRT. Therefore, some physicians may have seen at least some of the cardiovascular risk factors used in the patient descriptions as a contraindication for HRT prescription, while others may have taken them as an indication. Similar results have been found in the UK and in Finland[10,11].

Clinical data and meta-analyses of HRT use and breast cancer risk have suggested an increased associated risk[21]. In our study, a family history of breast cancer in a first-degree relative did not have a noticeable impact on the prescription rate, even in older women who may have an even higher risk of developing breast cancer. It is possible that much lower prescription rates would have been observed in clinical practice if the women were reluctant to use HRT because of a family history, but this was not tested in this study. Our data suggest that the interviewed gynecologists did not consider a positive family history as a contraindication to HRT.

Barakat[22] recently reviewed the place of estrogen replacement therapy (ERT) in women with a history of endometrial cancer. Since only retrospective data exist, a multicenter randomized trial was designed to resolve the question of whether ERT is safe for these patients[22]. In the meantime, opinion leaders have stated that individual judgement must be used in relation to the risk of recurrence and weighted with other indications for ERT: climacteric symptoms and increased osteoporosis risk[23,24]. Our results report that two out of three gynecologists would accept, at least theoretically, the prescription of HRT to a woman with a history of early stage endometrial cancer, no signs of recurrence and recognized indications for HRT (climacteric symptoms and osteoporosis). These results contradict those of earlier surveys where respectively 63% and 25% of general practitioners and 42% and 44% of gynecologists in the UK had considered a history of endometrial cancer (recurrence free) as either an absolute or a relative contraindication to HRT[10]. This change in attitude may be related to a change due to time, or to a variability in prescription intentions or habits between countries.

References

1. Consensus Development Conference. Diagnosis, prophylaxis, and treatment of osteoporosis. *Am J Med* 1993;94:647-50
2. Lobo RA, Speroff L. International consensus conference on postmenopausal hormone therapy and the cardiovascular system. *Fertil Steril* 1994;62: 176-9S
3. Col NF, Eckman MH, Karas RH, Pauker SG, Goldberg RJ, Ross EM. Patient-specific decisions about hormone replacement therapy in postmenopausal women. *J Am Med Assoc* 1997;277:1140-7
4. Grodstein F, Stampfer MJ, Manson JE, *et al.* Postmenopausal estrogen and progestin use and the risk of cardiovascular disease. *N Engl J Med* 1996;335: 453-61
5. Rozenberg S, Liebens I, Vandromme J, Hotimsky A, Van Rijsselberge M. Cardiovascular protection by estrogen: a hemodynamic mechanism? *Int J Fertil Menopaus Stud* 1994;39:36-42
6. Hulley S, Grady D, Bush T, *et al.*, for the Heart and Estrogen/Progestin Replacement Study (HERS) Research Group. Randomized trial of estrogen plus progestin for secondary prevention of coronary heart disease in postmenopausal women. *J Am Med Assoc* 1998;280:605-13
7. Oddens BJ, Boulet MJ, Lehert P, Visser AP. A study on the use of medication for climacteric complaints in Western Europe - II. *Maturitas* 1994;19: 1-12
8. Stouthamer N, Visser AP, Oddens BJ, *et al.* Dutch general practitioners' attitudes towards the climacteric and its treatment. *Eur J Obstet Gynecol Reprod Biol* 1993;50:147-52
9. Rozenberg S, Fellemans C, Kroll M, Vandromme J. The menopause in Europe. *Int J Fertil Women's Med* 2000; in press
10. Norman SG, Studd JWW. A survey of views on hormone replacement therapy. *Br J Obstet Gynaecol* 1994;101:879-87
11. Hemminki E, Topo P, Malin M, Kangas I. Physicians' views on hormone therapy around and after menopause. *Maturitas* 1993;16:163-73
12. Rozenberg S, Kroll M, Vandromme J, Paesmans M, Lefever A, Ham H. Factors influencing the prescription of hormone replacement therapy. *Obstet Gynecol* 1997;90:387-91
13. Report of a World Health Organization (WHO) Study Group. Assessment of fracture risk and its application to screening for postmenopausal osteoporosis. WHO Technical Report, Series 843. Geneva: WHO, 1994
14. Rozenberg S, Barudy Vasquez J. Estrogen replacement therapy in patients with endometrial cancer: a survey of prescription intention of Belgian gynecologists [letter]. *CA Cancer J Clin* 1999;49:190-1
15. Paganini-Hill A, Ross RK, Gerkins VR, Henderson BE, Arthur M, Mack TM. Menopausal estrogen therapy and hip fractures. *Ann Intern Med* 1981;95: 28-31
16. Lindsay R, Hart DM, Clark DM. The minimum effective dose of estrogen for prevention of postmenopausal bone loss. *Obstet Gynecol* 1984;63: 759-63

17. Ettinger B, Genant HK, Cann CE. Long term estrogen replacement therapy prevents bone loss and fractures. *Ann Intern Med* 1985;102:319–24
18. Rozenberg S, Vandromme J, Kroll M, Pastijn A, Degueldre M. Osteoporosis prevention with sex hormone replacement therapy. *Int J Fertil* 1994;39: 262–71
19. Barrett-Connor E. Postmenopausal oestrogen prevention bias. *Ann Intern Med* 1991;115:455–6
20. Posthuma WDW, Westendorp RGJ, Vandenbroucke JP. Cardioprotective effects of hormone replacement therapy in post-menopausal women: is the evidence biased ? *Br Med J* 1994;308: 1268–9
21. Collaborative Group on Hormonal Factors in Breast Cancer. Breast cancer and hormone replacement therapy: collaborative reanalysis of data from 51 epidemiological studies of 52 705 women with breast cancer and 108 411 women without breast cancer. *Lancet* 1997;350:1047–59
22. Barakat RR. Contemporary issues in the management of endometrial cancer. *CA Cancer J Clin* 1998;48:299–314
23. Shoupe D, Mishell DR. Contraindications to hormone replacement therapy. In Lobo RA, ed. *Treatment of the Postmenopausal Woman*. New York: Raven Press, 1994:415–18
24. Breckwoldt M. Can women with previous oestrogen-dependent cancer receive HRT? In Birkhaüser M, Rozenbaum H, eds. *Menopause: European Consensus Development Conference of the European Menopause Society*. Paris: ESKA, 1996:225–8

Further basic and clinical investigations into Alzheimer's disease 65

H. Honjo, K. Tanaka, N. Kikuchi, Y. Kinoshita, T. Hosoda, T. Tamura and M. Urabe

INTRODUCTION

There have been a large number of papers reporting the preventive and possible therapeutic effects of estrogen on Alzheimer's disease. Yet larger and longer clinical trials involving women with Alzheimer's disease and further basic research are needed. In this paper, we summarize the important published findings, including our own data, and report our further basic and clinical investigations into Alzheimer's disease.

AMELIORATIVE EFFECTS OF ESTROGEN

Below, we will summarize the ameliorative effects of estrogen on Alzheimer's disease in clinics. In 1986, Fillit and colleagues[1] reported on an open trial of estradiol therapy for Alzheimer's disease. Serum estrone is higher than estradiol in postmenopausal woman. Almost all of the estrone in the general circulation is in the form of estrone sulfate. Thus, we gave conjugated estrogen (the main component being estrone sulfate) 1.25 mg/day for 6 weeks to seven patients with probable Alzheimer's disease[2]. Scores of the New Screening Test for Dementia (NSD), developed by the Japanese National Institute of Mental Health, improved in six patients. At the same time, another score, Hasegawa's Dementia Scale (HDS, old type) improved in five patients. As long as estrogen treatment continued, ameliorative effects were observed over six cycles (one cycle consisted of conjugated estrogen 0.625 mg/day for 3 weeks and no drugs for 1 week). Ohkura and co-workers also reported the effects of long-term estrogen replacement therapy in female patients with Alzheimer's disease[3].

In order to confirm the ameliorative effects of estrogen, a double-blind study was conducted in 14 women with Alzheimer's disease who received 1.25 mg/day conjugated estrogen or a placebo for 3 weeks. The revised version of Hasegawa's Dementia Scale (HDS-R), the NSD and the Mini Mental State Examination (MMS) showed significant improvements during the 3rd week of the study.

We have suggested four mechanisms to explain the ameliorative effects of estrogen treatment:

(1) Antidepressive effects or mood changes caused by estrogens make patients more active, and consequently patients could get better scores in the dementia tests;

(2) Vascular dilatation in the central nervous system (CNS) caused by estrogen may make neurons more active;

(3) There may be activation of acetylcholine metabolism by estrogens in the CNS, including the hippocampus and the hypothalamus;

(4) Under the influence of estrogen, glia change their form to the more developed type, and the developed-type glia would help neurons in the CNS[4].

A combination of these mechanisms would work in patients with Alzheimer's disease.

The senile plaques in Alzheimer's disease consist of amyloid. The main component of the amyloid is β-protein. Apolipoprotein E (Apo E) accelerates the precipitation of β-protein. At present, the ε4 allele of Apo E is considered to be an important risk factor for Alzheimer's disease[5]. Furthermore, in our study in Japan, the ratio of carriers of the ε4 allele was significantly higher in women with (7/20; 35%) than in those without (24/200; 12%) Alzheimer's disease. Apolipoproteins were analyzed in 68 women (37-67 years of age). Apo E was higher in the women with a serum estradiol level of less than 20 pg/ml. Apo E was remarkably suppressed with hormone replacement therapy (HRT) in the postmenopausal women[6]. This suppression of senile plaques may be an important factor in preventing and delaying the occurrence of Alzheimer's disease[7,8].

In another study we carried out with 57 postmenopausal women, the serum level of low-density lipoprotein (LDL) cholesterol was decreased with HRT in subtypes ε3ε3 and ε3ε4. The serum level of high-density lipoprotein (HDL) cholesterol was increased in subtype ε3ε3. In subtype ε2ε3, HRT was not effective for lipid metabolism. HRT in subtypes ε3ε3 and ε3ε4 may be more effective to protect against arteriosclerosis and additionally to delay the onset of Alzheimer's disease.

ESTROGEN RECEPTOR (ER)-α mRNA, EXON 4-DELETED ER-α mRNA AND ER-β MRNA

Recently, estrogen receptor (ER)-β, which is highly homologous with classical ER-α, has been cloned[9]. Meanwhile, on an mRNA level, many exon-deleted ER-α mRNAs were reported. As basic studies, we first analyzed ER-α mRNA, exon 4-deleted ER-α (D4-ER-α) mRNA and ER-β mRNA in the rat brain. The expression level of ER-α mRNA was higher than that of D4-ER-α mRNA or ER-β mRNA in the cortex, hippocampus and hypothalamus (Figure 1). ER-α mRNA in the hypothalamus was higher than that in the hippocampus. Estradiol treatment following ovariectomy significantly suppressed the expression level of ER-α mRNA in the hypothalamus. The results suggest an important role of estrogen in the substantia innominata in relation to the hypothalamus.

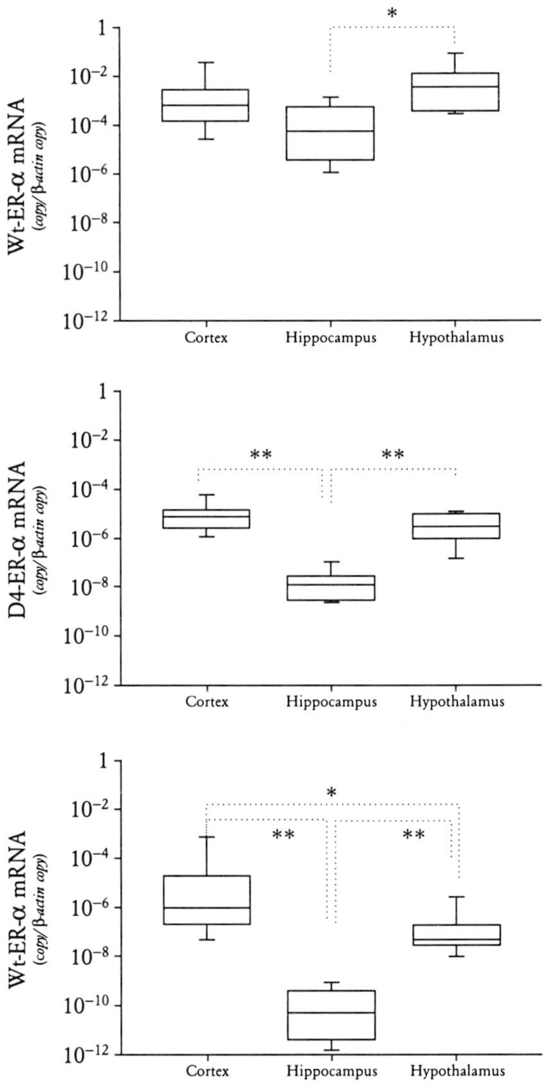

Figure 1 The expression of wild type (Wt) estrogen receptor (ER)-α, exon 4-deleted (D4)-ER-α and Wt-ER-β mRNAs in the cortex, hippocampus and hypothalamus. Wt-ER-α mRNA was present in large amounts in these tissues. The Mann-Whitney test was used for statistical analysis. $^{*}p < 0.05$; $^{**}p < 0.01$. For each set of data, the midline represents the median, the boxes represent the 25th and 75th centiles, and the bars represent the 10th and 90th centiles

EFFECTS ON CHOLINERGIC NEURONS IN THE SUBSTANTIA INNOMINATA

The effects of estrogen on cholinergic neurons in the substantia innominata were investigated with immunocytochemical techniques. Wistar female rats were divided into three groups: control, ovariectomized and estradiol-treated. The rats of the estradiol-treated group were given estradiol for 2 weeks following ovariectomy. The ABC (avidtin-biotin complex) method was used to stain choline acetyltransferase (ChAT). Fluorescence labelling was used to detect fluorogold. The number of positive ChAT-immunoreactive cells decreased in the ovariectomized group and recovered remarkably after estradiol treatment. Fluorogold was injected into the cortex of the forebrain. It was taken up by the projection fibers and transported to cell bodies in the substantia innominata. Fluorogold was localized in cells in the substantia innominata by fluorescence microscopy.

Double staining of ChAT and fluorogold was found in some cells in the substantia innominata. The number of double-labelled cells in the substantia innominata was reduced after ovariectomy and recovered after estradiol treatment (Figure 2). A small number of cells in the substantia innominata showed triple labelling for ChAT, ER-α and fluorogold.

These results indicate the possibility that estrogen had a direct effect on cholinergic neurons projecting from the substantia innominata to the forebrain.

SUPPRESSION OF APOPTOSIS IN ALZHEIMER'S DISEASE WITH ESTROGEN

There are three isotypes of the amyloid protein precursor (APP). β- and α-secretase split off β-amyloid. β-Amyloid consists of 1–42 residues. We used β-amyloid (25–35 residues) for the following study. The rat pheochromocytoma (PC)-12 cell line was used. The PC-12 cell was differentiated morphologically and neurobiologically by nerve growth factor stimulation to produce neuronal cells over a period of 1 week. The differentiated PC-12 dies in a dose-dependent manner with β-amyloid. The survival ratios were elevated (improved) by the addition of estrogen, remarkably so when it was administered in higher concentrations (Figure 3).

The β-amyloid induced DNA fragmentation. DNA fluorescence staining showed nuclear condensation and apoptotic bodies. A flow cytometric analysis showed that apoptotic cells had a tendency to decrease dose-dependently with estradiol treatment.

PROGESTERONE VAGINAL SUPPOSITORIES

Long-term estrogen treatment should be combined with progestogen to suppress the occurrence of uterine endometrial cancer or to prevent uterine bleeding. However, progestogen in the general circulation affects the CNS and sometimes, especially in elderly women, induces a depressive state. When progestogen is administered into the vaginal cavity, a large amount of it essentially concentrates

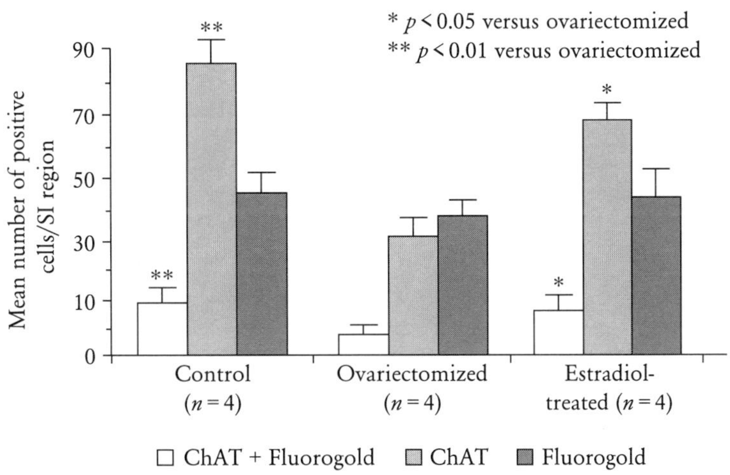

Figure 2 Quantitative analysis of cells double-labelled for choline acetyltransferase (ChAT) and fluorogold. The number of double-labelled cells (mean ± SE) in the substantia innominata (SI) was reduced after ovariectomy, but recovered after estradiol treatment. Student's unpaired t test was used for statistical analysis

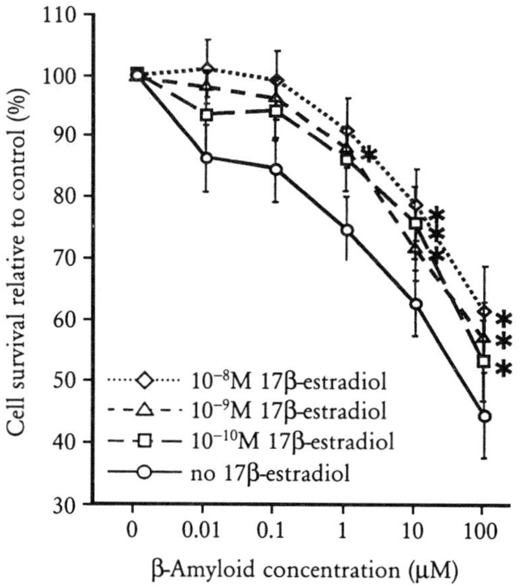

Figure 3 β-Amyloid toxicity and protection by 17β-estradiol. Cell survival was measured by MTT assay in differentiated PC-12 cells 48 h after the addition of β-amyloid. Values are expressed as percentages of cell survival relative to a control culture (not exposed to β-amyloid) for each estradiol concentration (mean ± SEM). Pretreatment with estradiol caused inhibition of MTT reduction dose-dependently (14 separate experiments). Analysis of variance (ANOVA) was used for statistical analysis. $^{*}p < 0.01$ compared with the value of the control culture (untreated with estradiol)

in the uterus and only a small amount of it goes into the general circulation.

In our study, we first mixed progesterone for injection (1 ampule: 50 mg) with the vehicle Witepsol H-15® (1.2 g) and molded the mixture in a container. This type of suppository (H-15) melted too quickly and was difficult to use. Next, the vehicle was changed to Witepsol E-85® (1.32 g; E-85). Some patients claimed vaginal discharge with E-85. The third suppository used (RE) was made with 50 mg progesterone and Witepsol H-15 (1.2 g). This RE was smaller than the other two suppositories and was the easiest to use.

After permission was obtained, a progesterone vaginal suppository was administered to 13 women before they underwent hysterectomy. Serum progesterone was measured before and 2, 4, 8 and 24 h after the administration of the suppository. The serum progesterone level peaked 2 or 4 h after administration. After hysterectomy, endometrial and myometrial progesterone concentrations were measured by radioimmunoassay. The mean endometrial progesterone concentration (ng/g) divided by the maximum serum level of progesterone (ng/ml) was 5.9 ± 6.5 (mean ± SD) (Table 1). Hence, progesterone was concentrated essentially in the endometrium.

Table 1 Endometrial and myometrial progesterone concentrations after a single administration of progesterone

Patient	*Type of suppository*	*Endometrial progesterone concentration* (ng/g)	*Myometrial progesterone concentration* (ng/g)	*Maximum serum progesterone concentration* (ng/ml)	*Endometrial progesterone concentration/maximum serum progesterone concentration*
1	H-15	11.3	7.1	7.9	1.43
2	H-15	2.5	4.6	4.7	0.53
3	E-85	52	54	9.1	5.71
4	E-85	3	2	3.2	0.94
5	E-85	5.9	6.7	9.7	0.61
6	E-85	42	6	2.4	17.50
7	E-85	13	9.3	3.9	3.33
8	E-85		6.4	6	
9	E-85		4.6	3.9	
10	RE	9.6	20	5.1	1.88
11	RE		7.4	11	
12	RE			15	15.33
13	RE	64	5.8	5.3	12.08
Mean		22.6	11.6	6.7	5.9
Standard deviation		23.5	14.2	3.6	6.5

In one case, a progesterone vaginal suppository was administered every day for 5 days before hysterectomy, but no accumulative increase in the progesterone serum level was seen.

HRT AND PROGESTERONE VAGINAL SUPPOSITORIES

Progesterone vaginal suppositories were administered to 17 HRT patients (47–86 years of age). Fifteen patients had experienced HRT regimens containing medroxyprogesterone acetate (MPA) and seven of them claimed some side-effects resulting from MPA, including depressive mood (two patients). One of two patients starting on HRT had complained of depressive status. Progesterone vaginal suppositories were administered to 16 patients cyclically (in most cases, they were administered for 10 days per cycle). To one new patient without depressive status, progesterone vaginal suppositories were administered continuously (E-85 for 8 weeks and RE for 44 weeks), because she wanted to avoid withdrawal bleedings.

Withdrawal and breakthrough bleedings were analyzed in 68 cycles of progesterone vaginal suppository administration. No bleeding occurred in three cycles of RE and withdrawal bleeding occurred in 40 cycles. Breakthrough bleeding occurred in 25 cycles. The amount of bleeding was moderate in most cases.

To examine the effect of treatment on the endometrium, vaginal ultrasonography was performed during progesterone vaginal suppository administration in eight cycles (seven patients). All showed a hyperechoic endometrium, which suggests a progesterone effect. Histological examination was performed during progesterone vaginal suppository treatment in six cycles (five patients). All samples showed a progesterone effect, dating the secretory phase, because of edematous interstitial tissue, etc.

Side-effects included vaginal discharge, which was complained of in a small number of women being treated with RE (i.e. in four of 55 cycles). Genital discomfort was also reported by a small number of women being treated with RE (i.e. in four of 55 cycles). Depressive mood was seen in none of four cycles with H-15, three of 23 cycles with E-85 and six of 55 cycles with RE. The patient to whom progesterone vaginal suppositories were administered continuously did not show any bleeding or depressive mood. In future research, progesterone vaginal suppositories with a lower dose of progestogen should be developed, so that there is sufficient progestogen in the endometrium and no progestogen in the general circulation.

CONCLUSION

With further basic and clinical investigations, the incidence of Alzheimer's disease could be reduced with adequate HRT producing minimal side-effects.

ACKNOWLEDGEMENTS

This study was supported in part by a Grant-in-Aid for General Scientific Research (No. 03454401, No. 07557366 and No. 10671564), the Research Institute for Neurological Disease and Geriatrics, and Works of Scientific Research and Technical Development, Public Health Department of Kyoto Prefectural Government.

References

1. Fillit H, Weinref H, Cholst I, *et al.* Observations in a preliminary open trial of estradiol therapy for senile dementia – Alzheimer's type. *Psychoneuroendocrinology* 1986;11:337–45
2. Honjo H, Ogino Y, Naitoh K, *et al.* *In vivo* effects by estrone sulfate on the central nervous system – senile dementia (Alzheimer's type). *J Steroid Biochem* 1989; 34:521–5

3. Ohkura T, Isse K, Akazawa K, *et al.* Long-term estrogen replacement therapy in female patients with dementia of Alzheimer's type: 7 case reports. *Dementia* 1995;6:99–107
4. Honjo H, Tanaka K, Kashiwagi T, *et al.* Senile dementia - Alzheimer's type and estrogen. *Horm Metab Res* 1995;27:204–7
5. Corder EH, Saunders AM, Strittmatter WJ, *et al.* Gene dose of apolipoprotein E type 4 allele and risk of Alzheimer's disease in late onset families. *Science* 1993;261:921–3
6. Urabe M, Yamamoto T, Kashiwagi K, *et al.* Effect of estrogen replacement therapy on hepatic triglyceride lipase, lipoprotein lipase and lipids including apolipoprotein E in climacteric and elderly women. *Endocr J* 1996;43:737–42
7. Tang M-X, Jacobs D, Stern Y, *et al.* Effect of oestrogen during menopause on risk and age at onset of Alzheimer's disease. *Lancet* 1996;348:429–32
8. Paganini-Hill A, Henderson VW. Estrogen replacement therapy and risk of Alzheimer's disease. *Arch Intern Med* 1996;156:2213–17
9. Kuiper GG, Enmark E, Pelto Huikko M, *et al.* Cloning of a novel estrogen receptor expressed in rat prostate and ovary. *Proc Natl Acad Sci USA* 1996;93: 5925–30

Estrogen therapy and the risk of Alzheimer's disease: an update at the millennium 66

V. W. Henderson

INTRODUCTION: ESTROGEN EFFECTS ON THE CENTRAL NERVOUS SYSTEM

The production of estrogen by the ovaries ceases with the menopause, and levels of circulating estrogens are thereafter greatly reduced[1]. The loss of estrogen affects a variety of reproductive and non-reproductive tissues, including the central nervous system. There are several mechanisms by which estrogen can have an impact on target organs. Most importantly, estrogen interacts with specific receptor proteins located in the cell nucleus to regulate target genes. Both the α-receptor and the recently described β-receptor are found in neurons, and different regions of the nervous system express different levels of these two receptor types[2]. An individual neuron can express either receptor type or none at all; occasionally, both receptor types are present together.

Estrogen actions that occur very rapidly presumably do not involve genomic activation. Many of these rapid effects are thought to be mediated through receptors located within the cell membrane[3]. In addition, it is likely that some biologically important estrogen actions do not require interactions with specific receptors. Finally, estrogens can influence the nervous system indirectly through actions on non-neural tissues, including the cerebral vasculature and the immune system.

ESTROGEN: RELEVANCE TO ALZHEIMER'S DISEASE

In many countries, Alzheimer's disease is the most common cause of dementia, affecting approximately twice as many women as men[4]. The fact that women live longer than men accounts for much of this sex difference in the prevalence of Alzheimer's disease. Apart from longevity, however, the age-specific incidence of Alzheimer's disease may still be somewhat greater for women.

Relatively early in the course of Alzheimer's disease, a striking loss of nerve processes and synapses[5,6] limits communication among neurons. Neuronal death is more prominent later in the disease course. Histopathological features include neurofibrillary tangles within vulnerable neurons and neuritic plaques in the brain substance between neuronal cell bodies. Tangles consist largely of a microtubule protein known as tau. Plaque cores typically include β-amyloid protein proteolytically derived from a larger precursor protein. Also associated with plaques, the presence of reactive astrocytes, activated microglia and complement deposition are taken as evidence for an inflammatory component to the pathology of Alzheimer's disease[7].

Dominantly inherited mutations of genes on chromosome 14 (presenilin-1), chromosome 1 (presenilin-2) and chromosome 21 (amyloid precursor protein) are important determinants of early-onset Alzheimer's disease, in which symptoms first appear before the age of about 60 years. In contrast, autosomal dominant mutations are not believed to play a substantial role in late-onset disease, which is much more common and therefore of much greater importance from a public health perspective. However, it is likely that other genes modify the susceptibility to Alzheimer's disease, particularly the chromosome 19 gene that encodes apolipoprotein E. This lipid transport protein occurs in three common variants (ε2, ε3 and ε4), with increased susceptibility to Alzheimer's disease being associated with the ε4 allele[8]. In Western countries, this allele occurs with a frequency of about 15–20%. Sex modifies the risk conferred by possession of the ε4 allele (greater risk for women than men[9,10]), perhaps explaining reports of an increased incidence of Alzheimer's disease for women.

A number of estrogen actions are relevant to the pathological changes that accompany Alzheimer's disease[11] (Table 1). Estrogen is both neurotrophic and neuroprotective; in addition, estrogen influences specific neurotransmitter systems and proteins associated with Alzheimer's disease. Estrogen modulates nerve growth factor and other neurotrophic factors[12]. Estrogen potentiates the growth of neuronal processes and promotes changes in synaptic plasticity[13]. *In vitro*, estrogen protects against cell death induced by oxidative injury, excitatory amino acids, hypoxia and the β-amyloid protein[14,15]. Effects on the immune system[16], enhancement of cerebral blood flow[17] and augmentation of the transport of glucose across the blood-brain barrier[18] may also be neuroprotective in some circumstances. Estrogen also protects neurons against programmed cell death (apoptosis)[19].

In addition to other neurotransmitters, estrogen influences neurons using acetylcholine[20], noradrenaline[21] or serotonin[22]. The pathology of Alzheimer's disease affects the cell bodies of origin for each of these neurotransmitter systems. The cholinergic system in particular has been linked to memory and attentional deficits in Alzheimer's disease[23]. In animal studies, estrogen is important in maintaining the function and enhancing the effects of cholinergic projections to the hippocampus and cerebral cortex[20]. Preliminary evidence in patients with Alzheimer's disease implies that the beneficial effects of cholinergic therapy are enhanced among women receiving concomitant estrogen therapy[24].

Estrogen has an effect on β-amyloid, tau and apolipoprotein E. The large amyloid precursor protein can be metabolized to different breakdown products. Estrogen inhibits the formation of the β-amyloid fragment[25]. Estrogen promotes neuronal sprouting, a response specifically associated with the induction of tau protein[26]. In some experimental models, sprouting also depends on the availability of apolipoprotein E[27]. Within the brain, apolipoprotein E is involved in neuronal repair processes, and its production by astrocytes and microglia is increased by estrogen[28].

Table 1 Estrogen effects potentially relevant to Alzheimer's disease. Modified from reference 11

Neurotrophic actions
Modulates neurotrophin actions
Potentiates neurite extension
Promotes synaptic plasticity
Neuroprotective actions
Protects against oxidative stress
Protects against excitatory neurotoxicity
Protects against hypoxia
Protects against β-amyloid neurotoxicity
Reduces inflammation
Augments cerebral blood flow
Enhances glucose transport into the brain
Protects against apoptosis
Effects on neurotransmitters
Acetylcholine
Noradrenaline
Serotonin
Others
Effects on proteins involved in Alzheimer's disease
β-Amyloid precursor protein
Tau protein
Apolipoprotein E

ESTROGEN THERAPY AND RISK OF ALZHEIMER'S DISEASE

Several early case-control studies detected no significant association between a history of postmenopausal estrogen therapy (with or without a progestational agent) and a diagnosis of Alzheimer's disease. However, the statistical power in these studies was limited. In the early 1990s, analyses focusing on current estrogen use suggested that estrogen might have a protective effect. For example, within a voluntary cohort in southern California, comparisons between 92 women with Alzheimer's disease and 143 age-equivalent women without dementia suggested that estrogen use was associated with a two-thirds reduction in the risk of Alzheimer's disease (relative risk 0.33, 95% confidence interval 0.15–0.74)[29]. However, estimates of risk based on the current use of hormone therapy are especially liable to bias, as current use may inaccurately reflect prior patterns of hormone use.

Since 1994, seven case-control and cohort studies have assessed the relationship between postmenopausal hormone therapy and the risk of Alzheimer's disease, where the measure of estrogen exposure occurred prior to the onset of dementia symptoms (Table 2). These studies have taken place in the Leisure World retirement community in California[30,31], a large health-maintenance organization in Seattle[32], a community-based urban cohort in New York City[33], a well-characterized longitudinally followed cohort in Baltimore[34], a population-based multicenter Italian cohort[35] and a population-based clinical cohort in Rochester, MN[36]. For most of these studies, information on hormone use had been collected prospectively and in the same way for both cases and controls[30-34,36]. A large proportion of women in several of these studies had used estrogen[30-32,34], a circumstance that increased the statistical power to demonstrate an estrogen effect, if present. Importantly, all but one of these recent epidemiological studies report an association between a woman's use of estrogen after the menopause and protection against Alzheimer's disease, with estimates of risk reduction being about 50% (Table 2).

Surrogate markers of estrogen exposure and risk of Alzheimer's disease

In both Leisure World[31] and the Italian aging study[35], the relationship between estrogen and the risk of Alzheimer's disease was examined indirectly through analyses of three presumptive surrogate markers of increased estrogen exposure: earlier age at menarche, later age at menopause and greater body weight. These analyses provide partial support for a role of estrogen. As predicted, women who experienced menarche at an earlier age had significantly reduced risk estimates for Alzheimer's disease in the Italian study; a trend in the same direction was found in Leisure World. In contrast, neither study found significant associations between age at menopause and risk of Alzheimer's disease. After the menopause, body weight (adiposity) correlates with circulating estrogen levels, since estrogen production occurs primarily through the conversion of androgen precursors in adipose and other peripheral tissues. In Leisure World, lower body weight, as self-reported at the time of cohort enrolment, was a significant predictor of a subsequent diagnosis of Alzheimer's disease. However, retrospective estimates of body weight at age 50 years in the Italian study were unrelated to the risk of Alzheimer's disease.

Amount of estrogen therapy and risk of Alzheimer's disease

Several studies have also considered the relation between the magnitude of a woman's estrogen exposure and the risk of Alzheimer's disease. These analyses, which have assessed exposure in terms of

Table 2 Recent epidemiological studies of Alzheimer's disease and estrogen therapy given prior to the onset of dementia symptoms

Study location	*Source of information on estrogen use*	*Number of Alzheimer's disease cases*	*Number of non-demented control subjects*	*Estrogen use in control subjects (%)*	*Estimate of relative risk**	*95% confidence interval*
Leisure World[31†]	self-report	248	1193	48	0.65	0.49–0.88
Seattle[32]	pharmacy records	107	120	48	1.1	0.6–1.8
New York City[33]	self-report	167	957	15	0.5	0.25–0.9
Baltimore[34]	self-report	34	438	47	0.46	0.21–1.00
Italy[35]	proxy report (cases) self-report (controls)	92	1476	12	0.28	0.08–0.98
Rochester[36]	medical records	222	222	10	0.4	0.2–0.8

*A relative risk estimate of less than 1.0 indicates that estrogen use is associated with a reduced risk of Alzheimer's disease. A relative risk estimate greater than 1.0 indicates that estrogen use is associated with increased risk; †this 1996 study updated an earlier analysis from Leisure World[30], which considered 138 cases and 550 controls; the estimate of risk in the original study was 0.69

the dose of estrogen therapy or the duration of estrogen therapy, tend to support a role for estrogen. In Leisure World, the only study for which dosage information is available, the estimated risk for Alzheimer's disease was significantly lower for increasing doses of the longest-used oral estrogen preparation[31]. With respect to increased duration of estrogen therapy, significant relationships with risk reduction were reported in Leisure World[31], New York City[33] and Rochester, MN[36]. In Leisure World, for example, women who had used estrogen for fewer than 4 years had an estimated relative risk for Alzheimer's disease of 0.83, those who had used estrogen for 4–14 years had a risk of 0.50, and women who had used estrogen for at least 15 years had a risk of 0.44[31] (by definition, women who had never used estrogen therapy had a relative risk of 1.0). This trend for greater risk reduction in association with greater duration of estrogen therapy was highly significant ($p < 0.001$). In the Baltimore cohort, however, there was no link between duration of use and the magnitude of risk reduction[34], although estrogen use *per se* was associated with a reduced risk of Alzheimer's disease.

THE NEW MILLENNIUM

The epidemiological studies reviewed above provide substantial support for the view that estrogen therapy after the menopause may protect against the development of Alzheimer's disease. If confirmed, this association would be of great public health importance. Given the enormous number of women with Alzheimer's disease throughout the world, the burgeoning elderly population, and the huge costs directly and indirectly associated with this illness, any intervention that reduces risk would be invaluable.

Case–control and cohort studies are subject to methodological limitations that are best overcome by carefully conducted, randomized, controlled trials. Two such very large trials are now underway in association with the Women's Health Initiative in the USA and the Women's International Study of Long Duration Oestrogen after Menopause in the UK. Results of these primary prevention trials will not be known until well into the first decade of the new millennium. If findings confirm a protective effect of estrogen, then additional studies will be needed to define optimal timing (e.g. therapy begun immediately after the menopause or delayed to a later age), estrogen preparation (e.g. conjugated estrogens, estradiol or a selective estrogen receptor modulator), estrogen formulation (e.g oral or transdermal), hormone regimen (e.g. intermittent or continuous; estrogen opposed by a progestogen or unopposed estrogen) and hormone dosage. Separate, but closely related, issues of estrogen effects on the brain also require further investigation[37]. These include the possibilities that estrogen priming in women with symptoms of Alzheimer's disease might enhance the effects of other treatment modalities, that estrogen might have a salubrious effect on mood, or that estrogen might augment or preserve cognitive performance in healthy non-demented older women.

References

1. Trévoux R, De Brux J, Castanier M, Nahoul K, Soule J-P, Scholler R. Endometrium and plasma hormone profile in the peri-menopause and post-menopause. *Maturitas* 1986;8:309–26
2. Shughrue PJ, Lane MV, Merchenthaler I. Comparative distribution of estrogen receptor-α and -β mRNA in the rat central nervous system. *J Comp Neurol* 1997;388:507–25
3. Wong M, Thompson TL, Moss RL. Nongenomic actions of estrogen in the brain: physiological significance and cellular mechanisms. *Crit Rev Neurobiol* 1996;10:189–203
4. Jorm AF, Korten AE, Henderson AS. The prevalence of dementia: a quantitative integration of the literature. *Acta Psychiatr Scand* 1987;76:465–79
5. Scheibel ME, Lindsay RD, Tomiyasu U, Scheibel AN. Progressive dendritic changes in aging human cortex. *Exp Neurol* 1975;47:392–403
6. Alford MF, Masliah E, Hansen LA, Terry RD. A simple dot-immunobinding assay for quantification of synaptophysin-like immunoreactivity in human brain. *J Histochem Cytochem* 1994;42:283–7
7. Itagaki S, McGeer PL, Akiyama H, Zhu S, Selkoe D. Relationship of microglia and astrocytes to

amyloid deposits of Alzheimer disease. *J Immunol* 1989;24:173-82
8. Strittmatter WJ, Saunders AM, Schmechel D, *et al.* Apolipoprotein E: high-avidity binding to β-amyloid and increased frequency of type 4 allele in late-onset familial Alzheimer disease. *Proc Natl Acad Sci USA* 1993;90:1977-81
9. Breitner JCS, Wyse BW, Anthony JC, *et al.* APOE-ε4 count predicts age when prevalence of AD increases, then declines: the Cache County study. *Neurology* 1999;53:321-31
10. Bretsky PM, Buckwalter JG, Seeman TE, *et al.* Evidence for an interaction between apolipoprotein E genotype, gender, and Alzheimer's disease. *Alzheimer Dis Assoc Disord* 1999;13:316-21
11. Henderson VW. Estrogen, cognition, and a woman's risk of Alzheimer's disease. *Am J Med* 1997;103(Suppl 3A):11-18
12. Miranda RC, Sohrabji F, Toran-Allerand CD. Presumptive estrogen target neurons express mRNAs for both the neurotrophins and neurotrophin receptors: a basis for potential developmental interactions of estrogen with neurotrophins. *Mol Cell Neurosci* 1993;4:510-25
13. Foy MR, Henderson VW, Berger TW, Thompson RF. Estrogen and neural plasticity. *Curr Direct Psychol Sci* 2000;in press
14. Goodman Y, Bruce AJ, Cheng B, Mattson MP. Estrogens attenuate and corticosterone exacerbates excitotoxicity, oxidative injury, and amyloid β-peptide toxicity in hippocampal neurons. *J Neurochem* 1996;66:1836-44
15. Regan RF, Guo Y. Estrogens attenuate neuronal injury due to hemoglobin, chemical hypoxia, and excitatory amino acids in murine cortical cultures. *Brain Res* 1997;764:133-40
16. Grossman CJ. Interactions between the gonadal steroids and the immune system. *Science* 1985;227:257-61
17. Ohkura T, Teshima Y, Isse K, *et al.* Estrogen increases cerebral and cerebellar blood flows in postmenopausal women. *Menopause* 1995;2:13-18
18. Shi J, Simpkins JW. 17β-Estradiol modulation of glucose transporter 1 expression in blood-brain barrier. *Am J Physiol* 1997;272:E1016-22
19. Pike CJ. Estrogen modulates neuronal Bcl-x_L expression and β-amyloid-induced apoptosis: relevance to Alzheimer's disease. *J Neurochem* 1999;72:1552-63
20. Gibbs RB, Aggarwal P. Estrogen and basal forebrain cholinergic neurons: implications for brain aging and Alzheimer's disease-related cognitive decline. *Horm Behav* 1998;34:98-111
21. Sar M, Stumpf WE. Central noradrenergic neurones concentrate ^{3}H-oestradiol. *Nature (London)* 1981;289:500-2
22. Sumner BEH, Fink G. Estrogen increases the density of 5-hydroxytryptamine$_{2A}$ receptors in cerebral cortex and nucleus accumbens in the female rat. *J Steroid Biochem Mol Biol* 1995;54:15-20
23. Coyle JT, Price DL, DeLong MR. Alzheimer's disease: a disorder of cortical cholinergic innervation. *Science* 1983;219:1184-90
24. Schneider LS, Farlow MR, Henderson VW, Pogoda JM. Effects of estrogen replacement therapy on response to tacrine in patients with Alzheimer's disease. *Neurology* 1996;46:1580-4
25. Xu H, Gouras GK, Greenfield JP, *et al.* Estrogen reduces neuronal generation of Alzheimer β-amyloid peptides. *Nature Med* 1998;4:447-51
26. Ferreira A, Caceres A. Estrogen-enhanced neurite growth: evidence for a selective induction of tau and stable microtubules. *J Neurosci* 1991;11:393-400
27. Stone DJ, Rozovsky I, Morgan TE, Anderson CP, Finch CE. Increased synaptic sprouting in response to estrogen via an apolipoprotein E dependent mechanism: implications for Alzheimer's disease. *J Neurosci* 1998;18:3180-5
28. Stone DJ, Rozovsky I, Morgan TE, Anderson CP, Hajian H, Finch CE. Astrocytes and microglia respond to estrogen with increased apoE mRNA *in vivo* and *in vitro*. *Exp Neurol* 1997;143:313-18
29. Henderson VW, Paganini-Hill A, Emanuel CK, Dunn ME, Buckwalter JG. Estrogen replacement therapy in older women: comparisons between Alzheimer's disease cases and nondemented control subjects. *Arch Neurol* 1994;51:896-900
30. Paganini-Hill A, Henderson VW. Estrogen deficiency and risk of Alzheimer's disease in women. *Am J Epidemiol* 1994;140:256-61
31. Paganini-Hill A, Henderson VW. Estrogen replacement therapy and risk of Alzheimer's disease. *Arch Intern Med* 1996;156:2213-17
32. Brenner DE, Kukull WA, Stergachis A, *et al.* Postmenopausal estrogen replacement therapy and the risk of Alzheimer's disease: a population-based case-control study. *Am J Epidemiol* 1994;140:262-7
33. Tang M-X, Jacobs D, Stern Y, *et al.* Effect of oestrogen during menopause on risk and age at onset of Alzheimer's disease. *Lancet* 1996;348:429-32
34. Kawas C, Resnick S, Morrison A, *et al.* A prospective study of estrogen replacement therapy and the risk of developing Alzheimer's disease: the Baltimore Longitudinal Study of Aging. *Neurology* 1997;48:1517-21
35. Baldereschi M, Di Carlo A, Lepore V, *et al.* Estrogen-replacement therapy and Alzheimer's disease in the Italian Longitudinal Study on Aging. *Neurology* 1998;50:996-1002
36. Waring SC, Rocca WA, Petersen RC, O'Brien PC, Tangalos EG, Kokmen E. Postmenopausal estrogen replacement therapy and risk of AD: a population-based study. *Neurology* 1999;52:965-70
37. Henderson VW. *Hormone Therapy and the Brain: A Clinical Perspective on the Role of Estrogen*. Carnforth, UK: Parthenon Publishing, 2000

Estrogen use and Alzheimer's disease: pharmacogenetic interaction by APOE genotype?

67

A. J. C. Slooter and C. M. van Duijn

INTRODUCTION

Alzheimer's disease, by far the most common type of dementia, is a devastating neurodegenerative disorder. After an extended period of loss of personality and cognition, the disease often results in a state of complete dependency, complicated by psychosis, depression and anxiety[1]. The neuropathological characteristics of Alzheimer's disease include senile plaques, neurofibrillary tangles, amyloid angiopathy and neuronal loss[2]. Senile plaques are extracellular deposits of predominantly β-amyloid. Neurofibrillary tangles are intraneuronal inclusions, which are, in part, composed of abnormally phosphorylated tau proteins.

The prevalence of Alzheimer's disease increases with advancing age. It affects less than 1% of 60–64-year-olds and up to 40% of those over the age of 85 years[3]. Furthermore, the incidence increases with aging, and is estimated to be one per 1000 person-years in 60–64-year-olds and 25 per 1000 person-years in individuals older than 85 years[3].

The etiology of Alzheimer's disease is incompletely understood. Reported risk factors include age, low educational level, smoking, atherosclerosis, exposure to aluminium and previous head injury or depression[3,4]. The use of anti-inflammatory drugs or estrogens seems to decrease the risk of Alzheimer's disease[3,5-16]. Furthermore, multiple genes have been implicated in the etiology of Alzheimer's disease. In the rare early-onset forms, several autosomal dominant mutations have been identified. In addition, a number of susceptibility genes have been studied, though often with inconsistent results. The exception is the apolipoprotein E polymorphism (APOE; protein: apoE), with three common alleles: APOE*2, APOE*3 and APOE*4. The APOE*4 allele is a well-established risk factor for Alzheimer's disease[17,18]. As almost 30% of all individuals carry at least one APOE*4 allele, APOE*4 is the most important genetic risk factor at the population level. However, APOE*4 is neither sufficient, nor necessary, in the etiology of Alzheimer's disease[17,18]. In the majority of cases, Alzheimer's disease most likely results from an interplay of genetic and environmental factors. This article will summarize the putative protective effect of estrogen use on the risk of Alzheimer's disease. In addition, the possible interaction with the APOE genotype is discussed.

ESTROGEN USE AND THE RISK OF ALZHEIMER'S DISEASE

Epidemiological studies on estrogen use and Alzheimer's disease have yielded inconsistent results. Randomized clinical trials are still ongoing and publications are limited to observational studies. At present, 12 investigations on estrogen use and the risk of dementia have been published: four suggested no effect or a slightly increased risk and eight found a decreased risk of dementia[5-16]. A meta-analysis of ten of these investigations reported a 29% decreased risk of developing dementia associated with estrogen use[19]. There were, however, striking differences in methodology across these studies: two used a cohort design and eight a case–control approach. Different diagnostic criteria were used and several studies were subject to recall bias. It should be noted that, in the methodologically superior, prospective follow-up studies, a decreased risk was observed[5,7], which is plausible given the results from neurobiological studies.

POSSIBLE MECHANISM FOR A PROTECTIVE EFFECT OF ESTROGEN ON ALZHEIMER'S DISEASE

Estrogen may have a beneficial effect on the development of Alzheimer's disease through several mechanisms (Figure 1). First, estrogen may be protective for atherosclerosis[20] and may increase cerebral blood flow[21]. As vascular factors seem to be involved in Alzheimer's disease[4], estrogen use may thus have a beneficial effect on the development of Alzheimer's disease. Second, estrogen was found to have neurotrophic effects. Estrogen may promote the activity of growth factors[22], increase neuron viability[22] and maintain neuronal interconnections in brain areas associated with cognition[23]. Estrogen further affects several neurotransmitter systems, in particular the cholinergic system[24]. Third, estrogen may favorably modify the processing of amyloid precursor protein, thereby reducing the accumulation of β-amyloid[22]. In addition, the putative exitotoxic effects of β-amyloid may be diminished by estrogen[25]. Other possible mechanisms include the reversal of glucocorticoid damage, and anti-inflammatory effects[22].

ESTROGEN AND APOE: INVOLVED IN SIMILAR PATHOLOGICAL PROCESSES?

Estrogen may thus act in different ways to prevent or delay the development of Alzheimer's disease. Interestingly, the APOE genotype may also play a role in several of the above-described pathways (Figure 1). As compared to the most common allele, APOE*3, APOE*4 may affect the development of Alzheimer's disease in the opposite way to estrogens. First, atherosclerosis seems to be a risk factor for Alzheimer's disease, particularly in carriers of the APOE*4 allele[4]. Second, the apoE protein may also have neurotrophic effects. It is synthesized after various types of cerebral injury and plays a pivotal role in the supply of lipids to cells under repair[26]. Furthermore, there is some evidence that apoE interacts with growth factors to support neuronal outgrowth and viability[27]. *In vitro*, the addition of apoE4 protein (encoded by the APOE*4 allele) resulted in shorter, stunted neurite extensions as compared to the apoE3 isoform (encoded by the APOE*3 allele)[28]. Third, in the brain of a patient with Alzheimer's disease, the number of plaques and the burden of β-amyloid depends upon the APOE genotype[29]. APOE*4 carriers were found to have an increased density of β-amyloid, while APOE*2 carriers had less β-amyloid depositions[29]. Fourth, like estrogen, apoE may protect against oxidative stress associated with neurodegeneration[30]. The cytotoxic effects of β-amyloid on neuronal cells could be blocked by physiological levels of apoE[31]. The antioxidant activity of apoE appeared to be isoform specific, with apoE2 being most effective, apoE3 moderately effective and apoE4 least effective[31].

However, the above discussion on the role of the apoE protein and estrogens in Alzheimer's disease pathology is rather speculative. Few studies addressed the role of apoE and estrogen at the

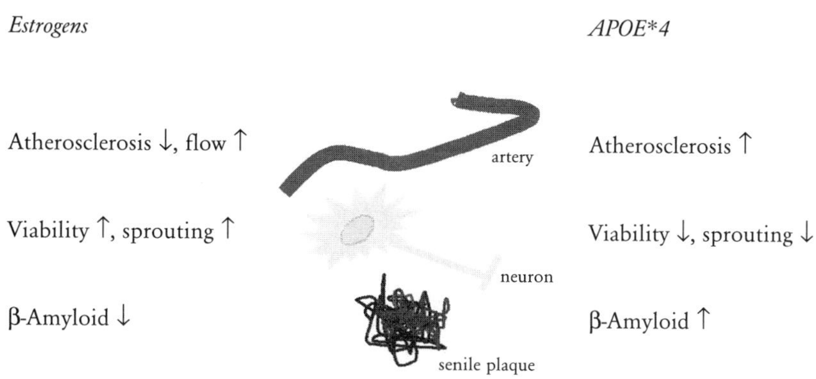

Figure 1 Proposed mechanisms for a beneficial effect of estrogens on Alzheimer's disease and putative mechanism of action of the risk allele APOE*4 relative to the most common allele, APOE*3

same time. It has been reported that estrogen administration inhibits the level of apoE in the plasma[32]. This may reflect antiatherogenic properties of estrogen, as apoE is a component of atherogenic lipoproteins[33]. A reduction in the plasma apoE level by the use of estrogen is not in line with the suggested beneficial effect of estrogen use on Alzheimer's disease, as the level of apoE seems to be reduced in the plasma of patients with Alzheimer's disease[34]. In the brain, the estrogen supply may induce the synthesis of apoE[35]. This may be particularly relevant for carriers of the APOE*4 allele, who were suggested to have a relative deficiency of apoE in the brain as compared to persons without this allele[36]. The beneficial effects of estrogen on the formation of synapses appeared to be dependent upon apoE, as estrogen supply did not enhance synaptic sprouting in apoE knock-out mice[37]. ApoE might therefore be an intermediate factor in the neurotrophic effects of estrogen.

ARE THE EFFECTS OF ESTROGEN USE ON ALZHEIMER'S DISEASE MODIFIED BY APOE?

As estrogens and APOE may be involved in the same processes, the question arises whether the risk of Alzheimer's disease in estrogen-using women differs across the APOE genotypes. Differential effects of estrogen use on the risk of Alzheimer's disease have been discussed in two studies[5,38]. In the first study, 1124 elderly women, who were initially free of Alzheimer's disease, Parkinson's disease and stroke were followed for 1-5 years[5]. A history of estrogen use was obtained from the participants themselves at baseline. The age at onset of Alzheimer's disease was later in women who had used estrogen than in those who had not, and the relative risk was reduced (0.40; 95% confidence interval (CI) 0.22–0.85). This study reported that the strongest effects of estrogen use on the risk of Alzheimer's disease were found in carriers of the APOE*4 allele. In women with one APOE*4 allele, the relative risk of Alzheimer's disease associated with estrogen use was 0.13 (95% CI 0.02–0.95). In women without APOE*4, estrogen use seemed to have a weaker effect, as the relative risk was 0.4 (95% CI 0.2–0.9)[5].

The other report is a population-based, case-control study on early-onset Alzheimer's disease[38]. For each female patient, a female control was matched for age (within 5 years) and place of residence. Information on estrogen use was, for both cases ($n = 109$) and controls ($n = 119$), collected from a relative. Estrogen use was reported less often for patients (10%) than for controls (20%)[38]. This relationship held when adjustments were made for age and education level (odds ratio (OR) 0.34; 95% CI 0.12–0.94)[38]. The inverse association between estrogen use and early-onset Alzheimer's disease seemed to be stronger in APOE*4 (OR 0.37; 95% CI 0.08–1.58) and APOE*2 carriers (OR 0.25; 95% CI 0.02–3.63) than in women with the APOE3E3 genotype (OR 0.60; 95% CI 0.19–1.88), although the difference did not reach statistical significance[38].

DISCUSSION

A recent literature search in PubMed, the internet database of the National Library of Medicine, on 'estrogen' and 'Alzheimer' yielded 261 publications since 1985. The overwhelming majority of these articles are editorials, commentaries, statements, review articles and viewpoints. Not more than 12 publications refer to original data on estrogen use and Alzheimer's disease[5-16]. This discrepancy may reflect the great interest and the desperate need to find treatment for Alzheimer's disease. These 12 publications are all based on observational research and therefore subject to various types of bias. In only two studies is the risk of Alzheimer's disease at follow-up evaluated as a function of estrogen use at baseline[5,7]. Although this design is methodologically better, it cannot be ruled out that women who have used estrogen may have been more healthy and more highly educated and, as a result, less prone to develop Alzheimer's disease. Randomized clinical trials are needed in order to evaluate the risk of Alzheimer's disease at follow-up in women who had a similar risk at baseline.

Assuming that estrogens are, indeed, protective for Alzheimer's disease, it is still unclear whether this effect depends upon the APOE genotype. As discussed above, a modifying effect by APOE was considered in only two studies[5,38]. In the follow-up study by Tang and colleagues, the effects of APOE*4 homozygosity could not be evaluated, as none of these women had taken estrogen[5]. Differences between women with one APOE*4 allele and those without APOE*4 were small and had overlapping confidence intervals[5]. In the case-control study on early-onset Alzheimer's disease, both APOE*2 and APOE*4 were associated with a lower estrogen-related risk of Alzheimer's disease than APOE3E3[38]. This finding is difficult to interpret, as APOE*2 and APOE*4 exert, in many aspects, opposite effects[17,18]. Furthermore, confidence intervals were large and overlapping[38]. An advantage in both studies is the population-based approach that minimizes selection bias[5,38]. Although few neurobiological studies evaluated the effects of *both* estrogens and apoE on the pathophysiology of Alzheimer's disease, the two factors seem to be involved in the same pathways, which supports the above epidemiological observations[5,38]. More research is needed in order to study the possible interaction between estrogens and apoE. In the ongoing trials aimed at finding prevention treatment of Alzheimer's disease in women at risk, stratification by APOE genotype may provide further support for a pharmacogenetic interaction. Hopefully, individuals with a susceptibility to develop Alzheimer's disease may eventually be offered escape from a great tragedy.

References

1. Cummings JL. Dementia: the failing brain. *Lancet* 1995;345:1481-9
2. Mirra SS, Heyman A, McKeel D, *et al.* The Consortium to Establish a Registry for Alzheimer's Disease (CERAD). II. Standardization of the neuropathologic assessment of Alzheimer's disease. *Neurology* 1991;41:479-86
3. Van Duijn CM. Epidemiology of the dementias: recent developments and new approaches. *J Neurol Neurosurg Psychiatry* 1996;60:478-88
4. Hofman A, Ott A, Breteler MMB, *et al.* Atherosclerosis, apolipoprotein E and the prevalence of dementia and Alzheimer's disease in a population-based study: the Rotterdam study. *Lancet* 1997; 349:151-4
5. Tang M-X, Jacobs D, Stern Y, *et al.* Effect of oestrogen during menopause on risk and age at onset of Alzheimer's disease. *Lancet* 1996;348:429-32
6. Waring SC, Rocca WA, Petersen RC, O'Brien PC, Tangalos EG, Kokmen E, Postmenopausal estrogen replacement therapy and the risk of AD: a population-based study. *Neurology* 1999;52:965-70
7. Kawas C, Resnick S, Morrison A, *et al.* A prospective study of estrogen replacement therapy and the risk of developing Alzheimer's disease: the Baltimore Longitudinal Study of Aging. *Neurology* 1997;48:1517-21
8. Mortel KF, Meyer JS. Lack of postmenopausal estrogen replacement therapy and the risk of dementia. *J Neuropsychiatry Clin Neurosci* 1995;7: 334-7
9. Paganini-Hill HA, Henderson VW. Estrogen deficiency and risk of Alzheimer's disease in women. *Am J Epidemiol* 1994;140:256-61
10. Henderson VW, Paganini-Hill HA, Emanuel CK, *et al.* Estrogen replacement therapy in older women: comparisons between Alzheimer's disease cases and nondemented control subjects. *Arch Neurol* 1994; 51:896-900
11. Brenner DE, Kukull WA, Stergachis A, *et al.* Postmenopausal estrogen replacement therapy and the risk of Alzheimer's disease: a population-based case-control study. *Am J Epidemiol* 1994;140:262-7
12. Graves AB, White E, Koepsell TD, *et al.* A case-control study of Alzheimer's disease in Australia. *Ann Neurol* 1990;28:766-74
13. Broe GA, Henderson AS, Creasey H, *et al.* A case-control study of Alzheimer's disease in Australia. *Neurology* 1990;40:1698-707
14. Amaducci LA, Fratiglioni L, Rocca WA, *et al.* Risk factors for clinically diagnosed Alzheimer's disease: a case-control study of an Italian population. *Neurology* 1986;36:922-31
15. Heyman A, Wilkinson WE, Stafford JA, *et al.* Alzheimer's disease: a study of epidemiological aspects. *Ann Neurol* 1984;15:335-41
16. Baldereschi M, Di Carlo A, Lepore V, *et al.* Estrogen-replacement therapy and Alzheimer's disease in the Italian Longitudinal Study on Aging. *Neurology* 1998;50:996-1002
17. Farrer LA, Cupples LA, Haines JL, *et al.* Effects of age, sex, and ethnicity on the association between

apolipoprotein R genotype and Alzheimer disease. A meta-analysis. *J Am Med Assoc* 1997;278:1349–56
18. Slooter AJC, Cruts M, Kalmijn S, *et al.* Apolipoprotein E and dementia. Risk estimates from a population-based incidence study: the Rotterdam Study. *Arch Neurol* 1998;55:964–8
19. Yaffe K, Sawaya G, Lieberburg I, Grady D. Estrogen therapy in postmenopausal women. Effects on cognitive function and dementia. *J Am Med Assoc* 1998;279:688–95
20. Stampfer MJ, Colditz GA, Willett WC, *et al.* Postmenopausal estrogen therapy and cardiovascular disease: ten-year follow-up from the Nurses' Health Study. *N Engl J Med* 1991;325:756–62
21. Ohkura T, Teshima Y, Isse K, *et al.* Estrogen increases cerebral and cerebellar blood flow in postmenopausal women. *Menopause* 1994;2:13–18
22. Henderson VW. The epidemiology of estrogen replacement therapy and Alzheimer's disease. *Neurology* 1997;48(Suppl 7):S27–35
23. Miranda RC, Sohrabji F, Toran-Allerand CD. Interactions of estrogens with the neutrophins and their receptors during neural development. *Horm Behav* 1994;28:367–75
24. Luine VN. Estradiol increases choline acetyltransferase activity in specific basal forebrain nuclei and projection areas of female rats. *Exp Neurol* 1985;89:484–90
25. Goodman Y, Bruce AJ, Cheng B, *et al.* Estrogens attenuate and corticosterone exacerbates excitotoxicity, oxidative injury and amyloid β-peptide toxicity of hippocampal neurons. *J Neurochem* 1996;66:1836–44
26. Poirier J. Apolipoprotein E in animal models of CNS injury and in Alzheimer's disease. *Trends Neurosci* 1994;17:525–30
27. Gutman CR, Strittmatter WJ, Weisgraber KH, *et al.* Apolipoprotein E binds to and potentiates the biological activity of ciliary neurotrophic factor. *J Neurosci* 1997;17:6114–21
28. Nathan BP, Bellosta S, Sanan DA, *et al.* Differential effects of apolipoproteins E3 and E4 on neuronal growth *in vitro*. *Science* 1994;264:850–2
29. Polvikoski T, Sulkava R, Haltia M, *et al.* Apolipoprotein E, dementia, and cortical deposition of β-amyloid protein. *N Engl J Med* 1995;333:1242–7
30. Beal MF. Aging, energy, and oxidative stress in neurodegenerative diseases. *Ann Neurol* 1995;38: 357–66
31. Miyata M, Smith J. Apolipoprotein E allele-specific antioxidant activity and effects on cytotoxicity by oxidative insults and β-amyloid peptides. *Nat Genet* 1996;14:55–61
32. Applebaum-Bowden D, McLean P, Steinmetz A, *et al.* Lipoprotein, apolipoprotein, and lipolytic enzyme changes following estrogen administration in postmenopausal women. *J Lipid Res* 1989;30: 1895–906
33. Mahley RW. Apolipoprotein E: cholesterol transport protein with expanding role in cell biology. *Science* 1988;240:622–30
34. Slooter AJC, De Knijff P, Hofman A, *et al.* Serum apolipoprotein E level is not increased in Alzheimer's disease: the Rotterdam Study. *Neurosci Lett* 1998;248:21–4
35. Stone DJ, Rozovsky I, Morgan TE, *et al.* Astocytes and microglia respond to estrogen with increased apoE mRNA *in vivo* and *in vitro*. *Exp Neurol* 1997;143:313–18
36. Bertrand P, Poirier J, Oda T, *et al.* Association of apolipoprotein E genotype with brain levels of apolipoprotein E and apolipoprotein J (clusterin) in Alzheimer disease. *Mol Brain Res* 1995;33:174–8
37. Stone DJ, Rozovsky I, Morgan TE, *et al.* Increased synaptic sprouting in response to estrogen via an apolipoprotein E-dependent mechanism: implications for Alzheimer's disease. *J Neurosci* 1998;18: 3180–5
38. Slooter AJC, Bronzova J, Witteman JCM, *et al.* Estrogen use and early onset Alzheimer's disease. A population-based study. *J Neurol Neurosurg Psychiatry* 1999;67:779–81

Lipid changes during the peri- and postmenopause and subclinical cardiovascular disease

68

K. A. Matthews, L. H. Kuller, K. Sutton-Tyrrell and D. Edmundowicz

INTRODUCTION

Observational studies of premenopausal women followed through the menopause indicate that the cessation of menses is associated with an increase in total and low-density lipoprotein (LDL) cholesterol, and a small decline in high-density lipoprotein (HDL)-2 cholesterol, relative to premenopausal women[1-3]. No unique changes due to menopausal status are observed for blood pressure, insulin, glucose and weight, although all increase with aging[1-3]. This pattern of findings suggests that the menopause may accelerate atherogenesis in women in part through alterations in lipid metabolism.

Estrogen levels remain at premenopausal levels until immediately prior to the cessation of menses, after which they continue to decline for months to years[4]. Furthermore, considerable variability in postmenopausal women's level of estrogen occurs because of the continued secretion of estradiol from the ovary and the conversion of androstenedione to estrone in fat tissue[5]. In consequence, at least a subset of women may continue to show alterations in estrogen-sensitive risk factors beyond the cessation of menses that are not only due to chronological aging. One purpose of this chapter is to describe changes in lipids and lipoproteins among healthy women from premenopause to 1 year after the cessation of menses, i.e. menopause, and from 1 year to 5 years after the menopause.

Observational studies of the natural menopause have not shown that age at menopause is a risk factor for cardiovascular disease, independent of other cardiovascular risk factors, including age and smoking status[6]. Age and smoking are also predictors of age at menopause[7], as well as cardiovascular disease, so it is difficult to draw firm conclusions about the risk associated with menopause from these findings. It is possible that the natural menopause alters lipid metabolism in a relatively uniform manner, such that absolute risk is higher, even though relative risk among women is not changed, resulting in no apparent effect of the menopause. Recently, we have been evaluating subclinical cardiovascular disease in women using carotid ultrasonography and electron beam computed tomography. The second objective of this chapter is to evaluate the association between subclinical cardiovascular disease, i.e. carotid artery atherosclerosis and coronary calcification, and risk factors measured when women are premenopausal, 1 year after the cessation of menses and 5 years after the cessation of menses. The scientific question is whether or not premenopausal levels of lipids are sufficient to predict postmenopausal subclinical disease or whether menopause-induced changes in lipids add predictive value above and beyond that predicted by premenopausal levels. Depending on the answer, prevention strategies should begin among high-risk women in the pre- or perimenopausal period.

To address these objectives, in the present chapter, we present data from our ongoing epidemiological study, the Healthy Women Study[8]. We began this study in 1983-84, when 541 premenopausal women were enrolled in a study of changes in biological and behavioral characteristics of women as they experienced the menopause. They had been contacted by letter sent to randomly selected women living within certain zip codes in Allegheny County, PA, and subsequently were interviewed by telephone regarding the following eligibility criteria: age range 42–50 years; menstrual bleeding within the last 3 months; no surgical menopause; diastolic blood pressure < 100 mmHg; and no medications known to influence the biological risk factors under study, e.g. estrogens, insulin, and lipid-lowering, thyroid, antihypertensive and psychotropic medications. Sixty per cent of eligible women volunteered. Most of the women were Caucasian because of the sampling procedure and selection criteria, e.g. more African-Americans were excluded based on their blood pressure levels and already being postmenopausal.

All women completed a baseline examination, which included a blood sample being taken for later assays of a number of cardiovascular risk factors, including the focus of the present chapter. Levels of total serum cholesterol[9], total HDL cholesterol[10], HDL subfractions (HDL-2 and HDL-3)[11,12] and triglycerides[13] were measured by a lipid laboratory using the standards of the Centers for Disease Control. LDL cholesterol levels were estimated with the Friedewald equation[14].

After the baseline examination, women reported their menstrual status monthly. When women reported that they had stopped menstruating and/or had taken hormone replacement therapy (HRT) for 12 months, they were considered postmenopausal and their lipids and other risk factors were re-evaluated at that time, and at 2, 5 and 8 years postmenopause. The present report is based on the sample of 372 women who completed examinations approximately 1 and 5 years after the menopause. Of the women, 177 never used HRT, with the remainder using HRT, usually estrogen and progestins, during the follow-up period.

The subclinical disease measures were added to the protocol for women who were evaluated at 5 or 8 years postmenopause. A Toshiba SSA-270A scanner (Tokyo, Japan), equipped with a 5-MHz linear array imaging probe, was used to measure carotid disease in the right and left common carotid arteries, carotid bulb and the first 1.5 cm of the internal and external carotid arteries. Intima media thickness and plaque scores were derived from these recordings. The electron beam computed tomography studies were performed with an Imatron C150 scanner (San Francisco, USA); 30–40 continuous 3-mm-thick transverse images from the level of the aortic root to the apex of the heart were obtained when at maximal breath-holding. During a second pass, 6-mm contiguous images of the aorta were obtained from the aortic arch to the iliac bifurcation. Separate coronary and aortic calcification scores were derived. The reproducibility of both the electron beam computed tomography and carotid ultrasonography measurements was high.

CHANGES IN LIPIDS AND LIPOPROTEINS

At the premenopausal examination, the risk factor levels were relatively low in this sample of women because of the study selection criteria[8]. The changes in total cholesterol, LDL cholesterol and triglycerides were substantial between the premenopausal and 5-year postmenopausal examinations. The changes in total cholesterol and triglycerides did not vary according to HRT use. However, the changes in LDL and total HDL cholesterol between the premenopausal and 5-year postmenopausal evaluations were affected by HRT use: never users of HRT showed a decline in HDL, whereas the HRT users showed an increase; never users showed a larger increase in LDL cholesterol than the other groups.

Changes in total cholesterol, LDL cholesterol and triglycerides between the premenopausal and 1-year postmenopausal examinations were larger than those between the 1-year and 5-year postmenopausal examinations, adjusted for duration of follow-up. Women who used HRT at both postmenopausal examinations experienced a more modest increase in LDL during both periods and a modest increase in HDL during the first period, compared to never users of HRT. These findings are consistent with the notion that changes in estrogen exposure affect lipid metabolism.

Despite the substantial changes in total cholesterol, LDL cholesterol and triglycerides between the premenopausal and 5-year menopausal examinations, and the changes in HDL and LDL cholesterol varying according to HRT use, the correlations between lipid levels measured at the premenopausal and 5-year postmenopausal examinations were moderate to large for the entire group, as well as the HRT groups taken separately. The one exception was triglycerides, where the correlation was significantly larger for never users of HRT than users of HRT. These findings suggest that the rank order of the women's risk factors was fairly stable over the study period of nearly 13 years.

PREMENOPAUSAL LIPID LEVELS AND SUBCLINICAL CARDIOVASCULAR DISEASE

The higher the intima media thickness scores, the greater the premenopausal levels of total cholesterol, LDL cholesterol and triglycerides, and the lower the premenopausal levels of HDL and HDL-2 cholesterol[15]. Similarly, women who had a plaque score of 2 had greater premenopausal levels of total cholesterol, LDL cholesterol and triglycerides, and lower levels of HDL and HDL-2.

Similarly, coronary and aortic calcification scores were linearly and strongly related to the premenopausal levels of LDL and HDL cholesterol, triglycerides and apolipoprotein B[16]. The combination of HDL < 60 mg/dl, triglycerides > 100 mg/dl and LDL cholesterol > 100 mg/dl at the premenopausal examination was particularly likely to be associated with high coronary calcification. For example, among those with premenopausal levels of HDL < 60 mg/dl, 44% of those with high LDL cholesterol and triglyceride levels had coronary calcification scores greater than 100, compared to 11% of those with low LDL cholesterol and triglyceride levels. Relative to non-users of HRT, HRT users had lower coronary calcification scores if they had elevated LDL cholesterol or lowered HDL cholesterol levels when premenopausal.

Women who had high scores regarding both measures of carotid disease and calcification were particularly likely to have an adverse lipid profile. For example, women who had a carotid plaque score of 2 or greater and a coronary calcification score of 11 or greater had premenopausal levels of triglycerides of 116 mg/dl, compared to 73 mg/dl for those with neither.

MENOPAUSE-INDUCED CHANGES IN LIPIDS AND SUBCLINICAL DISEASE

Changes in lipids and lipoproteins between the premenopausal and 1-year postmenopausal examinations were unrelated to intima media thickness when statistical adjustments were made for premenopausal levels. Women who had a plaque score of 0 or 1 had a small increase in HDL cholesterol between the premenopausal and 1-year postmenopausal examinations, adjusted for premenopausal level and age, relative to those with a plaque score of ≥ 2, whose HDL cholesterol levels declined slightly.

Women in the top quartile of the distribution of coronary calcification tended to have no change in HDL cholesterol levels, but a substantial increase in triglyceride levels between the premenopausal and 1-year postmenopausal examinations, whereas those with less or no calcification had a small increase in HDL and triglyceride levels. Women in the top quartile of the distribution of aortic calcification experienced a greater increase in total and LDL cholesterol levels between the premenopausal and 1-year postmenopausal examinations than those with less aortic calcification. These analyses were adjusted statistically for premenopausal levels of risk factors, as well as for age and HRT use.

Taken together, it appears that the menopause-induced changes in lipids and lipoproteins do not strongly influence the natural history of carotid disease, but may influence somewhat the natural history of coronary and aortic calcification. Elevated premenopausal levels of lipids and lipoproteins do strongly influence the natural history of both carotid disease and calcification.

CONCLUDING COMMENTS

In middle-aged healthy women, there are striking and large changes in the levels of lipids and lipoproteins across nearly 9 years. The changes are more substantial during the period prior to the complete cessation of menses than during the 4 years after the menopause, supporting the hypothesis that the perimenopause affects lipid metabolism. Premenopausal levels of lipids are excellent predictors of postmenopausal carotid intima media thickness, plaque, coronary calcification and aortic calcification, especially in combination. This may be due to the fact that the relative rank of women's lipid and lipoprotein levels is fairly stable across the peri- and postmenopausal years, except for increasing triglyceride levels among HRT users. Menopause-induced changes in lipids predict calcification somewhat. It may be that those changes will be better predictors with a longer exposure to the postmenopausal levels, allowing for acceleration of atherosclerosis associated with the menopause.

ACKNOWLEDGEMENT

This research was supported by National Institutes of Health grant HL28266.

References

1. Matthews KA, Meilahn E, Kuller LH, *et al.* Menopause and risk factors for coronary heart disease. *N Engl J Med* 1989;321:641–6
2. Lindquist O. Intraindividual changes of blood pressure, serum lipids, and body weight in relation to menstrual status: results from a prospective population study of women in Goteborg, Sweden. *Prev Med* 1982;11:162–72
3. Hjortland MC, McNamara PM, Kannel WB. Some atherogenic concomitants of menopause: the Framingham Study. *Am J Epidemiol* 1976;103: 304–11
4. Longcope C, Franz C, Morello C, *et al.* Steroid and gonadotropin levels in women during the peri-menopausal years. *Maturitas* 1986;8:189–96
5. Matthews KA, Cauley J. Menopause and mid-life changes. In Hazzard WR, Blass JP, Ettinger WH Jr, Halter JB, Ouslander JG, eds. *Principles of Geriatric Medicine and Gerontology*, 4th edn. New York: McGraw-Hill, 1999:179–90
6. Colditz GA, Willett WC, Stampfer MJ, *et al.* Menopause and the risk of coronary heart disease in women. *N Engl J Med* 1987;316:1105–10
7. Willett W, Stampfer MJ, Bain C, *et al.* Cigarette smoking, relative weight, and menopause. *Am J Epidemiol* 1983;117:651–8
8. Matthews KA, Kelsey SF, Meilahn EN, *et al.* Educational attainment and behavioral and biologic risk factors for coronary heart disease in middle-aged women. *Am J Epidemiol* 1989;129:1132–44
9. Allain CC, Poon LS, Chan CS, *et al.* Enzymatic determination of total serum cholesterol. *Clin Chem* 1974;20:470–5
10. Warnick GR, Albers JJ. A comprehensive evaluation of the heparin-manganese precipitation procedure for estimating high density lipoprotein cholesterol. *J Lipid Res* 1978;19:65–76
11. Gidez LI, Miller GJ, Burstein M, *et al.* Analyses of plasma high density lipoprotein subclasses by a precipitation procedure: correlations with preparative and analytical centrifugation. In Lippel K, ed. *Report of the High Density Lipoprotein Methodology Workshop*, San Francisco, California, 12–14 March 1979. (NIH publication no. 79-1661.) Bethesda, MD: Department of Health, Education and Welfare, Public Health Service, National Institutes of Health, 1979:328–42
12. Gidez LI, Miller GJ, Burstein M, *et al.* Separation and quantitation of subclasses of human plasma high density lipoproteins by a simple precipitation procedure. *J Lipid Res* 1982;23:1206–23
13. Bucolo G, David H. Quantitative determination of serum triglycerides by the use of enzymes. *Clin Chem* 1983;19:476–82
14. Friedewald WT, Levy RI, Fredrickson DS. Estimation of the concentration of low-density lipoprotein cholesterol in plasma, without use of the preparative ultracentrifuge. *Clin Chem* 1982;18: 499–502
15. Sutton-Tyrrell K, Lassila HC, Meilahn E, *et al.* Carotid atherosclerosis in premenopausal and postmenopausal women and its association with risk factors measured after menopause. *Stroke* 1998; 29:1116–21
16. Kuller LH, Matthews KA, Sutton-Tyrrell K, *et al.* Coronary and aortic calcification among women 8 years after menopause and their premenopausal risk factors. *Arterioscler Thromb Vasc Biol* 1999;19: 2189–98

Effects of continuous combined HRT on lipid profile

J. Y. Lee, Y. M. Choi and S. Y. Ku

INTRODUCTION

It is well known that estrogen replacement therapy in postmenopausal women lowers the risk of cardiovascular disease[1]. The cardioprotective effect of estrogen is multifactorial, including estrogen-induced changes in lipid metabolism, blood pressure, coagulation and endothelial functions. The most widely acknowledged mechanism is the favorable effect of oral estrogens on lipoproteins, i.e. an increase in high-density lipoprotein cholesterol and a decrease in low-density lipoprotein cholesterol[2,3].

Most data concerning the risk of cardiovascular disease are for estrogen alone, and information associated with combined therapy is limited. Recent data suggest that estrogen plus progestin combinations would have virtually the same cardioprotective effect as estrogen alone[4,5]. This seems to be true for levonorgestrel[6], norethisterone[7] and medroxyprogesterone acetate[5].

Added progestins may have a negative impact on beneficial estrogen-induced changes in lipoproteins. The impact of added progestins on the lipid profile is variable, depending on the preparation, dose, timing of administration and duration of treatment. Data from many studies in which progestin was added cyclically suggest that synthetic progestins, especially C19 compounds which have androgenic activity, mitigate the advantageous influence of estrogen and have a dose-response effect[8], while C21 compounds, such as medroxyprogesterone acetate, are considered to be less detrimental than C19 compounds[9].

In an effort to increase the compliance and patient acceptance of hormone replacement therapy (HRT), a regimen of continuous combined estrogen-progestin replacement has been proposed[10]. At present, a continuous combined estrogen-progestin replacement regimen has become one of the most widely used regimens of HRT. The importance in assessing the lipoprotein changes caused by continuous combined estrogen-progestin regimens is evident. We evaluated the impact of continuous combined estrogen-progestin replacement therapy on the lipid profiles of Korean postmenopausal women.

MATERIALS AND METHODS

Serum lipid profiles were examined in 145 postmenopausal women every 3 months during 12 months of treatment with conjugated equine estrogen at 0.625 mg and medroxyprogesterone acetate at 2.5 mg daily (continuous combined estrogen-progestin regimen). For comparison, data from 96 women receiving 0.625 mg of conjugated equine estrogen daily (estrogen-only regimen) and 104 women taking conjugated equine estrogen plus 10 mg of medroxyprogesterone acetate on days 1-12 (sequential regimen) were analyzed.

Women were scheduled to be seen at 3, 6, 9 and 12 months. At every visit, fasting morning blood was obtained for the measurement of lipids and lipoproteins.

Cholesterol levels were determined from fasting plasma using the cholesterol oxidase/peroxidase method, and triglyceride levels were determined from fasting plasma using the glycerol phosphate oxidase method. High-density lipoprotein (HDL) cholesterol was separated from the plasma by the precipitation of other lipoproteins with dextran sulfate manganese, and the supernatants were assayed for cholesterol content. Low-density lipoprotein (LDL) cholesterol was calculated using the following standard formula:

$$\text{LDL cholesterol} = \text{total cholesterol} - \text{HDL cholesterol} - \left(\frac{\text{triglyceride}}{5}\right)$$

The changes in LDL cholesterol, HDL cholesterol and triglyceride levels were calculated as percentages of the corresponding baseline values.

RESULTS

There were 145 women receiving the continuous combined estrogen-progestin regimen, 96 on the estrogen-only regimen and 104 receiving the sequential regimen. There were no significant differences in patient characteristics among the three groups (Table 1).

With the continuous combined estrogen-progestin regimen, HDL cholesterol levels increased 11.9% from the baseline at 3 months, 11.1% at 6 months, 13.4% at 9 months and 14.3% at 12 months ($p < 0.05$). When the sequential regimen was given, HDL cholesterol levels increased by 9.6%, 9.2%, 8.9% and 8.4% at 3, 6, 9 and 12 months, respectively ($p < 0.05$). The estrogen-only regimen showed a 15.7% increase in HDL at 3 months, 15.5% at 6 months, 14.4% at 9 months and an 18.4% increase at 12 months ($p < 0.05$). Women on the continuous combined estrogen-progestin regimen showed a lower increase in HDL levels than those who were receiving estrogen-only treatment, while the continuous combined estrogen-progestin regimen induced a higher

Table 1 Patient characteristics by treatment group. Values are mean ± SD

	CCEP regimen ($n = 145$)	*Estrogen-only regimen* ($n = 96$)	*Sequential regimen* ($n = 104$)
Age (years)	54.5 ± 5.3	51.4 ± 3.5	52.1 ± 6.7
Duration of menopause (years)	4.1 ± 1.9	4.4 ± 1.2	3.1 ± 1.3
Weight (kg)	58.3 ± 2.9	61.0 ± 2.9	60.2 ± 3.8
HDL cholesterol (mg/dl)	52 ± 9	54 ± 10	53 ± 11
LDL cholesterol (mg/dl)	127 ± 22	132 ± 28	127 ± 27
Triglycerides (mg/dl)	112 ± 30	129 ± 52	102 ± 52
Total cholesterol (mg/dl)	201 ± 22	212 ± 30	201 ± 29

CCEP, continuous combined estrogen-progestin; HDL, high-density lipoprotein; LDL, low-density lipoprotein

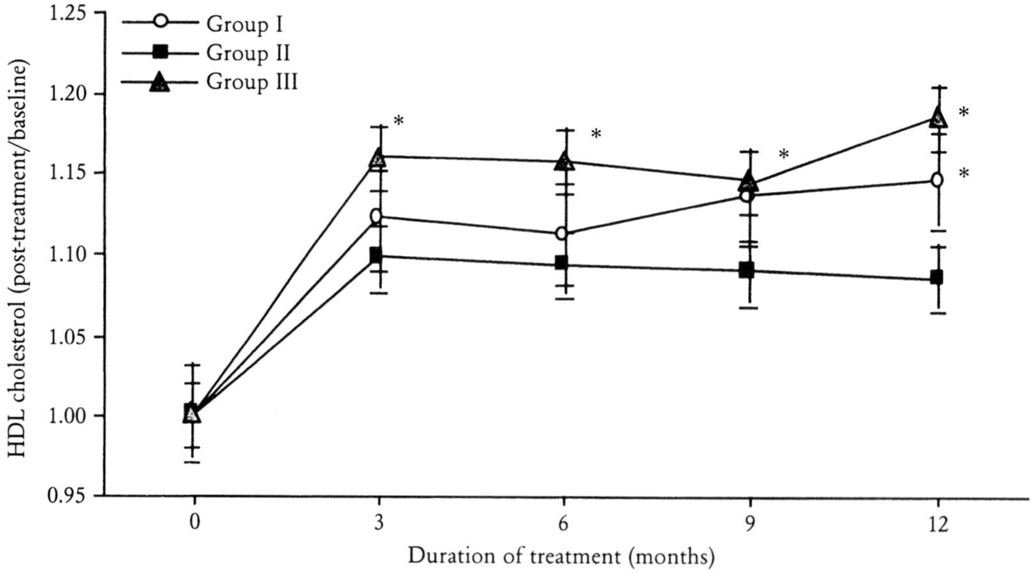

Figure 1 Serum high-density lipoprotein (HDL) cholesterol levels during estrogen replacement therapy. Group I received continuous combined estrogen-progestin therapy, group II received cyclic estrogen-progestin therapy and group III received estrogen-only therapy. Values are given as mean ± SE and expressed as ratios

Table 2 Mean change in high-density lipoprotein (HDL) cholesterol during hormone replacement therapy (HRT), expressed as percentage change ± SE

	Change in HDL cholesterol during HRT			
Regimen	*After 3 months*	*After 6 months*	*After 9 months*	*After 12 months*
CCEP	11.9 ± 2.4*	11.1 ± 2.9*	13.4 ± 2.9*	14.3 ± 3.4*
Estrogen-only	15.7 ± 2.1*	15.5 ± 2.5*	14.4 ± 2.3*	18.4 ± 2.7*
Sequential	9.6 ± 2.0*	9.2 ± 2.7*	8.9 ± 2.8*	8.4 ± 2.2*

*$p < 0.05$; CCEP, continuous combined estrogen-progestin

Table 3 Mean change in low-density lipoprotein (LDL) cholesterol during hormone replacement therapy (HRT), expressed as percentage change ± SE

	Change in LDL cholesterol during HRT			
Regimen	*After 3 months*	*After 6 months*	*After 9 months*	*After 12 months*
CCEP	−13.0 ± 1.7*	−10.1 ± 2.5*	−10.4 ± 3.0*	−7.2 ± 2.8*
Estrogen-only	−7.5 ± 1.9*	−10.8 ± 2.2*	−8.2 ± 2.1*	−2.1 ± 2.6
Sequential	−8.8 ± 1.8*	−6.5 ± 1.7*	−9.8 ± 2.2*	−8.7 ± 2.4*

*$p < 0.05$; CCEP, continuous combined estrogen-progestin

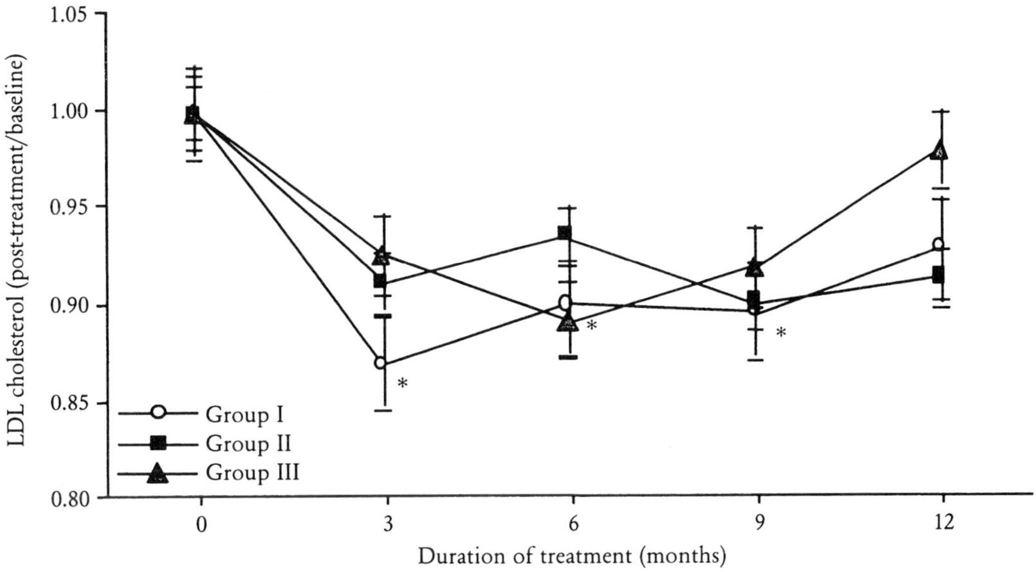

Figure 2 Serum low-density lipoprotein (LDL) cholesterol levels during estrogen replacement therapy. Group I received continuous combined estrogen-progestin therapy, group II received cyclic estrogen-progestin therapy and group III received estrogen-only therapy. Values are given as mean ± SE and expressed as ratios

increase in HDL levels than the cyclic estrogen-progestin therapy (Table 2 and Figure 1). However, these differences were not statistically significant.

On the other hand, the continuous combined estrogen-progestin regimen decreased serum LDL cholesterol levels significantly, in comparison with the baseline, at 3, 6, 9 and 12 months (13.0%, 10.1%, 10.4% and 7.2%, respectively) ($p < 0.05$). With sequential treatment, LDL cholesterol levels decreased 8.8% from the baseline at 3 months,

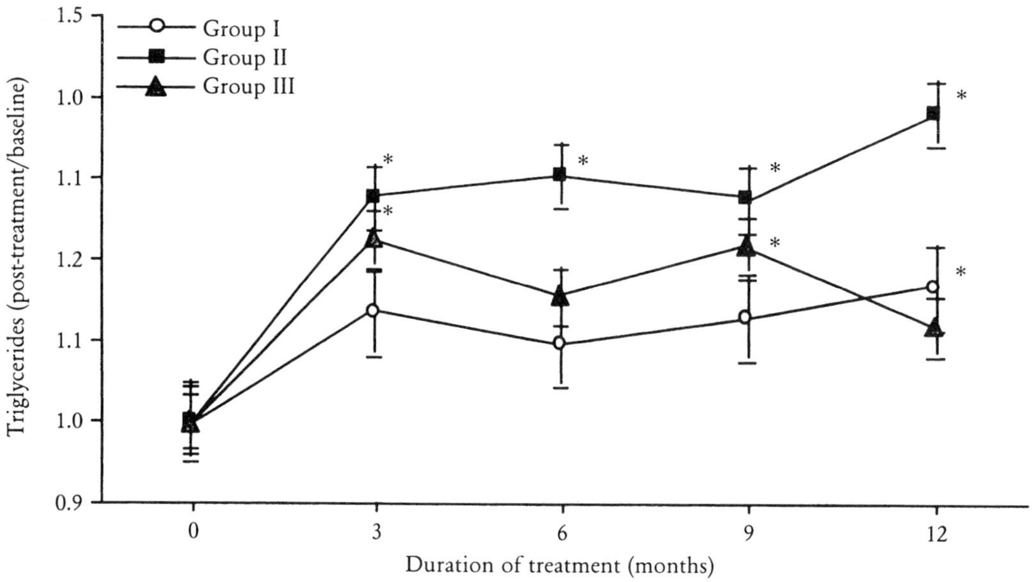

Figure 3 Serum triglyceride levels during estrogen replacement therapy. Group I received continuous combined estrogen–progestin therapy, group II received cyclic estrogen–progestin therapy and group III received estrogen-only therapy. Values are given as mean ± SE and expressed as ratios

Table 4 Mean changes in triglyceride levels during hormone replacement therapy (HRT), expressed as percentage change ± SE

	Change in triglyceride levels during HRT			
Regimen	*After 3 months*	*After 6 months*	*After 9 months*	*After 12 months*
CCEP	13.1 ± 3.9*	9.3 ± 4.4*	12.3 ± 4.6*	16.2 ± 5.8*
Estrogen-only	22.2 ± 3.7*	15.0 ± 4.2*	21.5 ± 4.3*	11.6 ± 4.0*
Sequential	27.2 ± 4.4*	29.9 ± 5.3*	27.1 ± 6.1*	37.5 ± 8.2*

*$p < 0.05$; CCEP, continuous combined estrogen–progestin

6.5% at 6 months, 9.8% at 9 months and 8.7% at 12 months ($p < 0.05$). When unopposed estrogen was used, LDL cholesterol levels decreased by 7.5% at 3 months, 10.8% at 6 months, 8.2% at 9 months and 2.1% at 12 months ($p < 0.05$). There were no significant differences in the decreases in LDL levels between the three HRT regimens (Table 3 and Figure 2).

The continuous combined estrogen–progestin regimen increased triglyceride levels by 13.1% at 3 months, 9.3% at 6 months, 12.3% at 9 months and 16.2% at 12 months ($p < 0.05$). Women on the cyclic regimen also showed significantly increased triglyceride levels compared to the baseline value, ranging from 27.1–37.5% ($p < 0.05$). Patients on the estrogen-only regimen showed an 11.6–22.2% increase in triglyceride levels ($p < 0.05$). The continuous combined estrogen–progestin regimen caused a smaller change in triglyceride levels than unopposed estrogen therapy after 9 months (Table 4 and Figure 3).

None of the three HRT regimens produced any significant change in total cholesterol level, even after 12 months of therapy. The continuous combined estrogen–progestin regimen resulted in a 0.9–6.5% decrease, sequential estrogen–progestin therapy resulted in a 1.7–3.5% decrease and unopposed estrogen resulted in a −1.8–4.6% decrease ($p < 0.05$) (Table 5 and Figure 4).

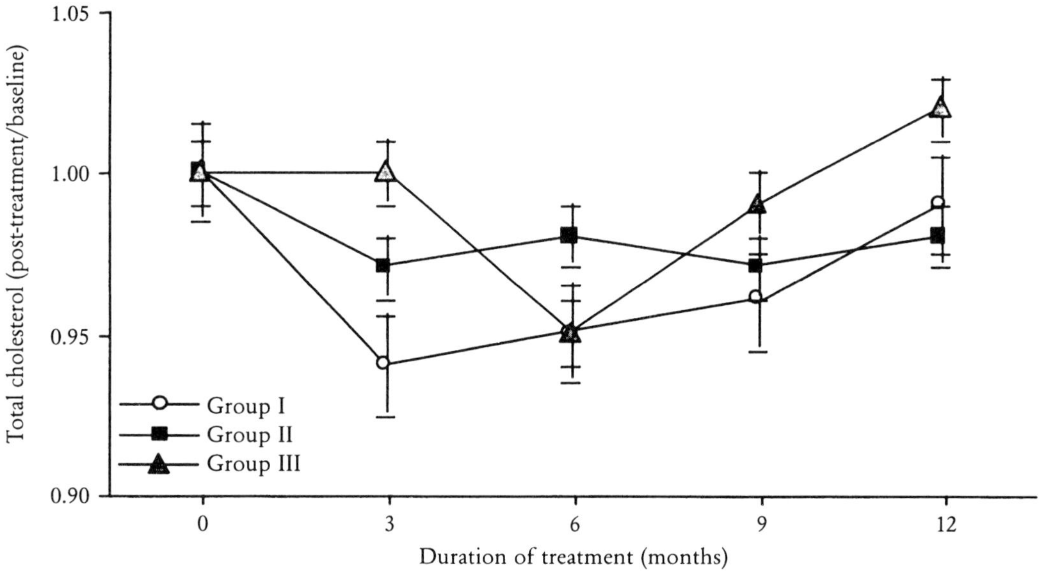

Figure 4 Serum total cholesterol levels during estrogen replacement therapy. Group I received continuous combined estrogen-progestin therapy, group II received cyclic estrogen-progestin therapy and group III received estrogen-only therapy. Values are given as mean ± SE and expressed as ratios

Table 5 Mean change in total cholesterol during hormone replacement therapy (HRT), expressed as percentage change ± SE

	Change in total cholesterol during HRT			
Regimen	*After 3 months*	*After 6 months*	*After 9 months*	*After 12 months*
CCEP	−6.5 ± 1.1	−4.9 ± 1.3	−4.4 ± 1.3	−0.9 ± 1.9
Estrogen-only	−0.2 ± 1.1	−4.6 ± 1.3	−1.5 ± 1.3	1.8 ± 1.4
Sequential	−3.5 ± 1.2	−1.7 ± 1.3	−3.4 ± 1.3	−2.5 ± 1.4

CCEP, continuous combined estrogen-progestin

DISCUSSION

In our study, beneficial changes in lipoprotein levels were observed in women who received the continuous combined regimen, as well as those who were on unopposed estrogen therapy. These data were derived from the use of Premarin® 0.625 mg and Provera® 2.5 mg, as were most of the previous other studies about the effects of continuous combined estrogen-progestin therapy on lipid profiles.

Most studies, including ours, have shown an increase in HDL cholesterol[11-13]. However, some studies showed no change[14,15], and some showed a decrease in HDL cholesterol[16].

It is noteworthy that the increase in HDL was more pronounced in Korean menopausal women (14.3% at 1 year) than in women studied in the Postmenopausal Estrogen/Progestin Interventions (PEPI) trial[13], which found that HDL levels had only increased by approximately 2% at 1 year. The investigation by Lobo and colleagues[12], as well as the PEPI trial[13], showed a smaller increase in HDL cholesterol in women receiving the continuous combined estrogen-progestin regimen than in those receiving unopposed estrogen treatment. These data are in agreement with ours.

Many studies have indicated that estrogen with or without progestins decreases the serum level of

LDL[12,13,15,16]. There seems to be a general agreement that there is no difference in LDL levels whether women are treated with unopposed estrogen, cyclic estrogen-progestin or continuous estrogen-progestin[12,13].

High serum concentrations of triglycerides are another risk factor for cardiovascular disease. Most studies, including ours, have shown an increase in triglyceride levels[12-14,17], while other studies have shown no change or a decrease in triglyceride levels[11,15]. In our study, the continuous combined estrogen-progestin regimen showed a smaller increase in triglyceride levels compared to unopposed estrogen at up to 9 months of treatment. However, the difference was not observed at 12 months of treatment. In contrast, the PEPI trial showed no difference in triglyceride levels between women assigned to estrogen alone (approximately 25% of the baseline at 1 year) and those being treated with continuous estrogen-progestin (approximately 20% of the baseline at 1 year).

The results of this investigation generally agree with those of most previous studies, indicating that postmenopausal women treated with the continuous combined estrogen-progestin regimen show an increase in HDL cholesterol and triglyceride, and a decrease in LDL cholesterol.

To summarize the results of this investigation, a continuous combined estrogen-progestin regimen consisting of conjugated equine estrogen 0.625 mg and medroxyprogesterone acetate 2.5 mg is beneficial to lipid metabolism in that it increases HDL cholesterol and decreases LDL cholesterol. However, continuous combined estrogen-progestin therapy may cause a lower increase in HDL cholesterol when compared to unopposed estrogen. The direct effects of the continuous combined estrogen-progestin regimen on blood vessels should be further studied in order to understand the long-term effects of this therapy on the incidence of coronary heart disease.

References

1. Grady D, Rubin SM, Pettiti DB, *et al.* Hormone therapy to prevent disease and prolong life in postmenopausal women. *Ann Intern Med* 1992;117:1016–37
2. Walsh BW, Schiff I, Rosner B, Greenberg L, Ravnikar V, Sacks FM. Effects of postmenopausal estrogen replacement on the concentrations and metabolism of plasma lipoproteins. *N Engl J Med* 1991;325:1196–204
3. Lobo RA. Effects of hormonal replacement on lipids and lipoproteins in postmenopausal women. *J Clin Endocrinol Metab* 1991;73:925–30
4. Psaty BM, Heckbert SR, Atkins D, *et al.* The risk of myocardial infarction associated with the combined use of estrogens and progestins in postmenopausal women. *Arch Intern Med* 1994;154:1333–9
5. Grodstein F, Stampfer MJ, Manson JE, *et al.* Postmenopausal estrogen and progestin use and the risk of cardiovascular disease. *N Engl J Med* 1996;335:453–61
6. Falkeborn M, Persson I, Adami HO, *et al.* The risk of acute myocardial infarction after oestrogen and oestrogen-progestogen replacement. *Br J Obstet Gynaecol* 1992;99:821–8
7. Hunt K, Vessey M, MePherson K, Coleman M. Mortality in a cohort of long-term users of hormone replacement therapy: an updated analysis. *Br J Obstet Gynaecol* 1990;97:1080–6
8. Christiansen C, Riis BJ. Five years with continuous combined oestrogen/progestogen therapy. Effects on calcium metabolism, lipoproteins, and bleeding pattern. *Br J Obstet Gynaecol* 1990;97:1087–92
9. Vejtorp M, Christensen MS, Vejtorp L, Larsen JF. Serum lipoprotein changes in climacteric women induced by sequential therapy with natural estrogens and medroxyprogesterone acetate or norgestrel. *Acta Obstet Gynecol Scand* 1986;65:391–5
10. Weinstein L, Bewtra C, Gallagher JC. Evaluation of a continuous combined low-dose regimen of estrogen-progestin for treatment of the menopausal patient. *Am J Obstet Gynecol* 1990;162:133–42
11. Kable WT, Gallagher JC, Nachtigall L, Goldgar D. Lipid changes after hormone replacement therapy for menopause. *J Reprod Med* 1990;35:512–18
12. Lobo RA, Pickar JH, Wild RA, Walsh B, Hirvonon E, for the Menopause Study Group. Metabolic impact of adding medroxyprogesterone acetate to

conjugated estrogen therapy in postmenopausal women. *Obstet Gynecol* 1994;84:987–95

13. The Writing Group for the Postmenopausal Estrogen/Progestin Interventions (PEPI) Trial. Effects of estrogen or estrogen/progestin regimens on heart disease risk factors in postmenopausal women. *J Am Med Assoc* 1995;273:199–208
14. Weinstein L. Efficacy of a continuous estrogen-progestin regimen in the menopausal patient. *Obstet Gynecol* 1987;69:929–32
15. AinMelk Y. Comparison of two continuous combined estrogen progestogen regimens in postmenopausal women: a randomized trial. *Fertil Steril* 1996; 66:962–8
16. Al-Azzawi F, Wahab M, Habiba M, Akkad A, Mason T. Continuous combined hormone replacement therapy compared with tibolone. *Obstet Gynecol* 1999;93:258–64
17. Gibbons WE, Judd HL, Luciano BA. Comparison of sequential versus continuous estrogen/progestin replacement therapy on serum lipid patterns. Presented at the *Society of Gynecological Investigation Annual Meeting*, 1991:abstr 491

Managing postmenopausal women with hypercholesterolemia: HRT, statins or both?

70

S. R. Davis

INTRODUCTION

Cardiovascular disease is a major cause of morbidity and the leading cause of mortality in women[1]. Women generally develop coronary heart disease later in life than men, and at nearly all ages the risk of dying acutely following myocardial infarction is several-fold greater in women than men[2]. This has been attributed to a more delayed diagnosis in women, the presence of small vessels, the fact that women are diagnosed when they are older and are more likely to have concurrent disease and the possibility that women may have more untreated risk factors. There is a dramatic increase in coronary heart disease in women in the middle years; however, this is not correlated with natural menopause[3]. Despite this blatant sexual dimorphism, studies involving men dominate the field of cardiovascular disease prevention. Women account for only 14–19% of the subjects included in the large studies of the effects of 3-hydroxy-3-methylglutaryl coenzyme A (HMG Co-A) reductase inhibitors, known as 'statins', as secondary prevention therapy[4-6]. In general, these studies do not have sufficient statistical power to determine fully the effects of statin therapy in women. In women, these studies have not demonstrated a reduction in death from coronary heart disease with statin therapy versus placebo; however, risk reductions in non-fatal myocardial infarction and major coronary heart disease events have been seen in the Scandinavian Simvastatin Survival Study[6] and the Cholesterol and Recurrent Events Trial[7]. This is despite the fact that most prospective studies have shown a positive association between total cholesterol and coronary heart disease in women.

Following the menopause, the lipoprotein profile becomes more atherogenic, with increases in total cholesterol, low-density lipoprotein (LDL) cholesterol and triglycerides. Observational epidemiological studies indicate that postmenopausal estrogen therapy reduces the risk of coronary heart disease in women, with the greatest benefit apparent for those at greatest risk[8]. This is consistent with the observation that postmenopausal estrogen therapy improves lipids in normolipemic women, with a 5–10% reduction in total cholesterol, a 10–15% reduction in LDL cholesterol and a 5–10% increase in high-density lipoprotein (HDL) cholesterol[9,10].

DOES HRT REDUCE CORONARY HEART DISEASE EVENTS OR MORTALITY IN WOMEN?

The Heart and Estrogen/Progestin Replacement Study (HERS) is the only double-blind placebo-controlled trial of hormone therapy as secondary prevention for heart disease in women to have been conducted[11]. This study, which has been widely publicized, involved 2763 postmenopausal women with coronary heart disease who were randomized to receive either conjugated equine estrogens (CEE) 0.625 mg plus medroxyprogesterone acetate (MPA) 2.5 mg or placebo, with a follow-up of 4.1 years.

Mean changes in lipoprotein lipids in the first year of HERS were consistent with intervention studies such as the Postmenopausal Estrogen/Progestin Interventions (PEPI) Trial[12]. There was a mean decrease in LDL cholesterol of 14%, with a concomitant increase in HDL cholesterol of 8%[11]. Nevertheless, no significant differences in myocardial infarction or coronary heart disease death between active and placebo groups were observed. Furthermore, there were no differences in fracture rates, cancer occurrence or total mortality. Unexpectedly, in the first year following randomization, there was an increase in coronary heart disease events and non-fatal myocardial infarctions in the treated group versus controls and, in all follow-up years, there was a significant increase in venous thrombotic events in the women who received hormone replacement therapy (HRT). The interpretation of this study is difficult and extrapolation to other subpopulations of women at risk or other forms of HRT is significantly limited. HERS was complicated by a 25% drop-out rate in the HRT group by 3 years. Forty-five per cent of the subjects were on lipid-lowering drugs at enrolment and, during the course of the study, 22% of patients who received placebo versus 18% of the HRT users commenced statins. Eight per cent of the placebo subjects reported additional HRT use, whereas 18% of the HRT users switched to placebo during the study. Despite this, analysis was performed on the basis of intention to treat. Taken together, the high rate of use of lipid-lowering therapy, the decline in HRT use by users enrolled on this randomized therapy, and the high rate of increase of use by placebo patients makes the interpretation of the outcomes confusing.

With respect to the increased venous thrombotic events in HRT users, 13% of subjects were current smokers, 19% were diabetic, 67% would be classified as obese and 10% had clinical congestive cardiac failure, each of these in itself being an adequate contraindication for oral estrogen therapy because of enhanced thrombotic risk. Hence, it is not surprising that such a high rate of venous thrombotic events was observed.

In summary, there are insufficient data from secondary coronary heart disease intervention studies in women employing either HRT or statin therapy to guide us as to how heart disease can be best prevented in women. Studies in this category published to date appear either to lack statistical power or to be confounded by the skew of the population's clinical characteristics.

The proposed mechanisms by which estrogen protects against cardiovascular disease include favorable lipoprotein lipid effects, antioxidant effects, enhanced vascular endothelial cell function, modulation of vascular smooth muscle reactivity, possible antithrombotic effects in the arterial system, facilitation of collateral vessel growth, effects on the extracellular matrix and plaque stabilization, and favorable effects on body fat distribution[13]. We have specifically addressed the favorable lipoprotein lipid effects and evaluated the clinical effects of estrogen and progestin continuous combined therapy versus simvastatin in hypercholesterolemic postmenopausal women[14]. This study of 58 postmenopausal women with a mean fasting total cholesterol of 8 mmol/l compared the effects of simvastatin 10 mg versus continuous combined CEE 1.25 mg and MPA 5 mg (therapy H), with a randomized cross-over design[14].

We observed and reported for LDL cholesterol mean decreases of 24% (95% confidence interval (CI) 23–29%) and 36% (95% CI 32–40%) with H and simvastatin, respectively, while HDL cholesterol was increased by 7% by both simvastatin and H. Therapy H, but not simvastatin, caused a significant increase in triglycerides, while H significantly lowered lipoprotein(a) (mean decrease 27%, 95% CI 20–34%); however, simvastatin had no effect.

We then went on to compare the effects of continuous CEE/MPA versus simvastatin versus combined H and statin therapy in hypercholesterolemic postmenopausal women[15]. The combination therapy (H plus simvastatin) was more effective than either therapy alone in lowering total cholesterol ($p = 0.01$) and LDL cholesterol ($p < 0.0001$). No further beneficial effect on HDL cholesterol was observed, whereas the combination prevented the increase in triglycerides evident with H alone. Lipoprotein(a) fell with H plus simvastatin, but the effect was not different from that observed with H alone.

In a similar study, but without employing MPA, Koh and colleagues[16] measured post-ischemia flow-mediated dilatation (FMD) of the brachial artery in women receiving either CEE alone, simvastatin alone or CEE plus simvastatin. They observed a significant increase in percentage FMD with each therapy alone, and no further increase by combining the two therapies. Williams and co-workers[17] investigated the effects of adding MPA to CEE on vascular reactivity in a primate model. They observed a diminution of the beneficial effect on vascular reactivity of estrogen replacement with the addition of MPA. Williams and co-workers also reported unfavorable effects with the addition of MPA to estrogen therapy on plaque size in the coronary arteries of cynomolgus female monkeys[18]. In contrast, other animal studies indicate that the accumulation of cholesterol in the proximal aorta is not adversely affected by the addition of norethisterone acetate[19].

We have also looked at the effects of parenteral estrogen in the form of estradiol implants[20] and transdermal estradiol patches[21] on lipoprotein lipids, and observed less profound effects on LDL cholesterol and total cholesterol, with little change in both HDL and triglycerides, in normolipemic women than those seen with oral estrogen therapy.

Thus, the effects of HRT on lipoproteins and vascular reactivity appear to depend significantly upon the mode of administration, the concurrent use of a progestin and, if so, the type of progestin used and the amount of estrogen dose administered. In addition, the percentage change in lipoprotein lipids with HRT administration is significantly greater in those with a more adverse profile at baseline[14].

TRANSLATION INTO CLINICAL PRACTICE

Prospective observational epidemiological studies support the cardioprotective effect of postmenopausal HRT. *In vitro* and *in vivo* mechanistic and animal studies provide plausible biological explanations supportive of these cardioprotective effects. Yet, despite these findings and the evidence that a reduction in LDL cholesterol prevents cardiovascular disease, secondary intervention studies of both HRT and statins in women are inconclusive. Although in our and other studies statin therapy is more potent in normalizing an adverse lipoprotein profile, the combination of statin and HRT may maximize the desired therapeutic effect on lipids in hypercholesterolemic postmenopausal women. However, different progestins appear to have differing cardiovascular effects, some of which may be adverse.

In view of the conflicting research outcomes and the necessity to rely on surrogate end-points, the decision to recommend HRT at present should not be based solely on cardiovascular disease risk, but on a comprehensive assessment of all the benefits and risks for each individual woman.

References

1. Rich-Edwards JW, Manson JE, Hennekens CH, Buring JE. The primary prevention of coronary heart disease in women. *N Engl J Med* 1995;332: 1757–66
2. Vaccarino V, Parsons L, Every NR, Barron HV, Krumholtz HM. Sex-based differences in early mortality after myocardial infarction. *N Engl J Med* 1999;341:217–25
3. Colditz GA, Willett WC, Stampfer MJ, Rosner B, Speizer FE, Hennekens C. Menopause and the risk of coronary heart disease in women. *N Engl J Med* 1987;316:1105–10
4. The LIPID Study Group. Prevention of cardiovascular events and death with pravastatin in patients with coronary heart disease and a broad range of initial cholesterol levels. *N Engl J Med* 1998;339:1349–57
5. Schram JHN, Boerrigter PJ, The YT. Influence of two hormone replacement therapy regimens, oral oestradiol valerate and cyproterone acetate versus transdermal oestradiol and oral dydrogesterone, on lipid metabolism. *Maturitas* 1995;22:121–30
6. Scandinavian Simvastatin Survival Study Group. Randomised trial of cholesterol lowering in 4444 patients with coronary heart disease: the Scandinavian Simvastatin Survival Study (4S). *Lancet* 1994;344:1383–9
7. Sacks FM, Pfeiffer MA, Lemuel AM. The effect of pravastatin on coronary events after myocardial infarction in patients with average cholesterol levels. *N Engl J Med* 1996;335:1001–9
8. Grodstein F, Martinez ME, Platz EA, *et al.* Postmenopausal hormone use and risk for colorectal cancer and adenoma. *Ann Intern Med* 1998;128: 705–12

9. Lobo RA. Clinical review 27: effects of hormonal replacement on lipids and lipoproteins in postmenopausal women. *J Clin Endocrinol Metab* 1991; 73:925-30
10. Walsh BW, Schiff I, Rosner B, Greenberg L, Ravnikar V, Sachs FM. Effects of postmenopausal estrogen replacement on the concentrations and metabolism of plasma lipoproteins. *N Engl J Med* 1991;325:1196-204
11. Hulley S, Grady D, Bush T, *et al.*, HERS Research Group. Randomized trial of estrogen plus progestin for secondary prevention of coronary heart disease in postmenopausal women. *J Am Med Assoc* 1996;280:605-12
12. The Writing Group for the PEPI Trial. Effects of estrogen or estrogen/progestin regimens on heart disease risk factors in postmenopausal women. *J Am Med Assoc* 1995;273:199-208
13. Gerhard M, Ganz P. How do we explain the clinical benefits of estrogen? *Circulation* 1995;92:5-8
14. Darling GM, Johns JA, McCloud PI, Davis SR. Estrogen and progestin compared with simvastatin for hypercholesterolemic postmenopausal women. *N Engl J Med* 1997;337:595-601
15. Darling GM, Johns JA, McCloud PI, Davis SR. Concurrent use of simvastatin and estrogen/progestin therapy compared with each therapy used alone for the treatment of hypercholesterolemia in postmenopausal women *Climacteric* 1999;2:181-8
16. Koh KK, Cardillo C, Bui MN, *et al.* Vascular effects of estrogen and cholesterol-lowering therapies in hypercholesterolemic postmenopausal women. *Circulation* 1999;99:354-60
17. Williams JK, Honore EK, Washburn SA, Clarkson TB. Effects of hormone replacement therapy on reactivity of atherosclerotic coronary arteries in cynomolgus monkeys. *J Am Coll Cardiol* 1994;24: 1757-61
18. Williams JK, Delansorne R, Paris J. Estrogens, progestins, and coronary artery reactivity in atherosclerotic monkeys. *J Steroid Biochem Mol Biol* 1998; 65:219-24
19. Haarbo J, Leth-Espensen P, Stender S, Christiansen C. Estrogen monotherapy and combined estrogen-progestogen replacement therapy attenuate aortic accumulation of cholesterol in ovariectomized cholesterol-fed rabbits. *J Clin Invest* 1991;87:1274-9
20. Davis SR, McCloud PI, Strauss BJG, Burger HG. Testosterone enhances estradiol's effects on postmenopausal bone density and sexuality. *Maturitas* 1995;21:227-36
21. Davis SR, Newman A. A pilot study of the effects of continuous combined transdermal oestrogen-oral progesterone theapy on lipoprotein lipids in hypercholesterolemic postmenopausal women. *Clin Endocrinol* 1999;50:405

Female sexual interest, response and attractiveness in relation to age, the menopause and hormone replacement therapy 71

N. L. McCoy

INTRODUCTION

In any consideration of female sexuality, it is important to orient our thinking around the three components of female sexuality proposed by Beach[1]. He named two components that also characterize male sexuality: proceptivity or sexual desire, and responsivity, or the ability to respond sexually. In the case of men, these components have often been referred to as libido and potency. Beach named a third component of female sexuality, that of attractivity. When applied to the human female, this component refers to a woman's sexiness or her value as a sexual stimulus and her ability to attract men. Although sexual interest and the ability to respond sexually in relation to aging and the menopause have been studied repeatedly by sex researchers, this third component of female sexuality has been notably absent from such studies. Its potential importance as a factor in the sexual lives of women after the menopause and as they age make it imperative that we begin to include it in our research.

RESEARCH ON MENOPAUSE AND SEXUALITY

Despite the paucity and methodological problems of studies concerning the effects of the menopause on sexuality, the results of such research paint a fairly consistent picture. There are at least 16 studies[2–18], conducted in nine different countries, that have examined at least one aspect of sexuality at two or more points during the menopausal transition period[19]. Sexual interest has been the most frequently studied and ten of 11 of these studies[2–5,8,11–13,17,18] have found a decline in sexual interest with progression through the menopausal transition. Eight of eight studies[3–5,8,14,16–18] have found a decline in frequency of sexual intercourse, and six of six[3,6,9,10,13,17] have found an increase in vaginal dryness. Four of these studies[4,8,17,18] have examined capacity for orgasm and three[4,8,18] of them found a decline. Three studies[4,13,17] have examined a woman's satisfaction with her sex partner or her relationship, with two[4,17] reporting a decline. Three studies have examined painful sexual intercourse[5,6,17] and two[5,6] of them reported an increase.

It is important to remember that changes in sexuality reported by these studies are relative to earlier phases in the menopausal transition and do not indicate an absence of sexual activity, response, pleasure or satisfaction. Moreover, social variables, such as socioeconomic status[8] and cultural views of sexuality[18], also play a role in the sexual changes associated with the menopausal transition.

MENOPAUSE AND HORMONES

If the menopause marks a relative decline in sexuality, then it is likely that cessation of cycling and the decreases in hormone production are implicated in this decline. Of course, it is possible that just the knowledge that she is at the end of her reproductive life depresses a woman's sexuality, but, for the majority of women, this seems unlikely. One estimate[20] of the changes in hormone production after the menopause indicates a drop in estradiol production of 85%, a reduction in estrone of 58%, a decline in androstenedione of 67% and a reduction in testosterone of 29%. Thus, the biggest postmenopausal change is in estradiol production and the smallest change is in testosterone production. Not surprisingly, we now have considerable evidence that the postmenopausal ovary produces significant amounts of androstenedione and testosterone[21-24]. Both Judd and colleagues[21] and Longcope and co-workers[22] have found significant amounts of androstenedione and testosterone in ovarian arterial and venous blood of postmenopausal women. Andreyko and colleagues[23] gave a gonadotropin-releasing hormone (GnRH) agonist to postmenopausal women and found a significant decline in testosterone and no change in dehydroepiandrosterone sulfate, suggesting decreased androgen secretion of ovarian but not adrenal origin. Finally, Sluijmer and associates[24] found that the amount of ovarian stromal hyperplasia in postmenopausal women was positively correlated with ovarian vein levels of testosterone and androstenedione. Such work suggests that at least half of postmenopausal women, and probably more, have significant amounts of androgens produced by their postmenopausal ovaries.

The obvious conclusion from this work is that naturally postmenopausal women will not typically be androgen deficient. However, women who have had their ovaries surgically removed do not have the possibility of androgen secretion by their postmenopausal ovaries. Furthermore, Cumming and colleagues[25] have shown that such ovariectomized women had a significantly lower production of adrenal androgens, particularly dehydroepiandrosterone sulfate. Thus, postmenopausal women without their ovaries are likely to be androgen deficient, as well as hormone deficient, compared to naturally menopausal women.

RESEARCH ON AGING AND SEXUALITY

The more recent research focus on menopause as a major variable affecting sexuality was preceded by a number of relatively large studies that focused mainly on age[14,26-39]. Because of their size, findings from these studies offer additional information, adding to the picture of the effects of aging on women's sexuality. A major finding in all of the studies that have examined both men and women[14,26,28-32,34-38] was that of a sex difference, with men reporting more sexual activity than women at all ages studied. If we examine the findings for women, age was the major variable associated with declines in sexual interest and activity. However, it is important to recognize that age as a variable is naturally confounded with menopause. This is because age in older populations reflects years since the menopause[39] and years with decreased hormone levels for the majority of women.

The most interesting finding from this body of research is that marital status is a major determinant of continued sexuality in aging women. For all studies examined in which marital status was a variable[26,27,29-31,35,37-39], it was a significant predictor of female sexual activity. In a related finding, a large magazine survey[40] recently conducted by the American Association of Retired Persons found that, beginning with the age grouping of 50–54 years, there were more men with partners than women, and the gap progressively increased over successive age groupings. Thus, it appears that, with menopause, advancing age and the death of husbands or male partners, women are unlikely to find a new partner. Given that women who are married are apt to be sexually active, this suggests that it may not be sexual motivation that is lacking, but sexual attractiveness and the ability to attract a new partner.

Recent research published by Wildt and Sir-Petermann[41] has taken a first step in examining the issue of sexual attractiveness. In that study, two researchers each estimated the age of 100 perimenopausal women ranging in age from 35 to 55 years. Plasma estradiol levels were obtained, and the authors reported a significant correlation between estimated age and plasma estradiol level; age was overestimated when estradiol was low and underestimated when estradiol was high. Thus, we might hypothesize that, for naturally postmenopausal women, hormone replacement therapy (HRT) that uses transdermal modes of delivery and/or specifically raises plasma free estradiol levels may increase sexual attractiveness and consequently the chance of finding a new partner for those who do not have one.

Besides marital status, the other important variable reported by many of these studies[26,27,31,33,34,38] is past sexuality. Not surprisingly, a woman who was highly sexual in her youth is more apt to maintain her sexuality with aging. Religiosity played a negative role in the oldest studies[14,27,33] and in one study of women of advanced age[38], but most studies have apparently not asked about religion. Health is obviously important, but individuals with health problems often do not participate in studies of aging and sexuality. However, one older study[26] and the recent magazine survey[40] discussed above reported that health played a significant role.

HORMONE REPLACEMENT THERAPY AND SEXUALITY

Given what the research tells us about declines in various aspects of female sexuality after the menopause and with years since the menopause, an examination of placebo-controlled research on the effects of HRT on sexuality is of interest[42]. Because surgically menopausal women are likely to have significantly lower androgen levels than naturally menopausal women, careful attention must be paid to who the subjects are in these studies.

Placebo-controlled studies of HRT and sexuality

To date, there are three placebo-controlled studies[43-45] examining the effects of testosterone on sexual interest: in one[44], all subjects had surgical removal of ovaries; in a second[43], one-third of the subjects had surgical removal of ovaries; and in the third[45], all women but one who received testosterone were naturally menopausal. In both studies involving surgically menopausal women, sexual interest increased with testosterone. In the study of naturally menopausal women, there was no change in sexual interest and it was apparent, as a result of the radioimmunoassay used, that the endogenous production of testosterone in these women had been lowered by replacement with oral methyltestosterone. Moreover, two studies giving 17β-estradiol - one orally[46] and one transdermally[47] - to naturally menopausal women reported an increase in sexual interest.

Three old studies[48-50] gave high-dose oral contraceptive hormones to hysterectomized and to ovariectomized, hysterectomized women; two of them found an increase in sexual interest, one[48] with mestranol combined with norethynodrel and the other[49] with ethinylestradiol. The third study[50] using a combination of mestranol and norethisterone, found no change. The estrogens in these studies are no longer used in HRT.

There are five placebo-controlled trials with conjugated equine estrogens, two[51,52] with surgically menopausal women and three[45,53,54] with naturally menopausal women. None of these studies found an increase in sexual interest. This is not surprising, given that the oral first-pass effect of conjugated equine estrogens results in a significant increase in sex hormone-binding globulin[55-59] and significantly lower bioavailable testosterone[56,59] levels.

Nine placebo-controlled studies[43,45,47,49-54] have examined the effects of hormones on the vaginal health of both surgically and naturally menopausal women. Regardless of the type of estrogen used or what was measured (vaginal cytology or lubrication or vaginitis), all but one of these studies[45] reported significant improvement. However, only one study[47] of six[45,47,50,52-54] that examined the effects of HRT on painful sexual intercourse found significant improvement. This may simply reflect that it takes longer for improvement in painful sexual intercourse to occur than the time frame provided by these studies.

One study[49] of five placebo-controlled studies[44,47,49,53,54] has reported a change in frequency of orgasm with HRT. This 1980 study[49] found an increase in orgasm using a high dose of ethinylestradiol with a group of younger, surgically menopausal subjects. Finally, no placebo-controlled study examining the frequency of sexual intercourse[44,45,49,53,54] has reported a significant increase in frequency associated with the use of either estrogens or androgens[44,45].

Conclusions

The following conclusions can be drawn from the research carried out to date:

(1) Vaginal dryness shows improvement with all types of estrogens and modes of delivery tested.

(2) Testosterone increases sexual interest in surgically menopausal women and in mixed groups of naturally and surgically menopausal women.

(3) No good evidence exists to indicate that physiological levels of testosterone increase sexual interest in naturally menopausal women. Moreover, evidence suggests that, in naturally menopausal women, exogenous testosterone decreases the endogenous production of testosterone.

(4) No evidence exists to suggest that conjugated equine estrogens increase sexual interest in either surgically or naturally postmenopausal women. Because oral structurally non-human estrogens increase sex hormone-binding globulin and decrease bioavailable testosterone, in some cases they may actually decrease sexual interest[52].

(5) Two studies suggest that structurally human estradiol can increase sexual interest in naturally menopausal women. This may be because estradiol acts to increase sexual attractiveness or sexual interest or both.

(6) No hormone replacement regimen has as yet significantly increased the frequency of sexual intercourse in placebo-controlled research. One hypothesis is that, unless sexual attractiveness is significantly affected, no increase is likely. To date, no research has attempted to examine the effects of HRT on sexual attractiveness.

FUTURE RESEARCH

We clearly need more research concerning the menopause and its effect on sexuality. Specifically, we need research on the effects of continuous versus cyclic hormone replacement regimens and of different hormone products and types of delivery systems on sexuality. We need to follow women longitudinally to see the effects of HRT on sexuality over time and to compare such women with those not using HRT over the same time period.

We need research on the relationship of sexual attractiveness to the frequency of sexual intercourse experienced by postmenopausal women; do hormones and/or pheromones increase the sexual attractiveness of postmenopausal women and their sexual activity? Is this particularly the case for unmarried or unpartnered women?

These topics for research are not important simply because they may suggest ways to improve the sexual lives of postmenopausal women. Their greatest importance lies in their ability to reveal what types of HRT - drugs, regimens, and modes of delivery - may actually be impairing women's sexuality. We should not be creating sexual problems with HRT that then lead to further treatment with additional drugs.

References

1. Beach FA. Sexual attractivity, proceptivity, and receptivity in female mammals. *Horm Behav* 1976;7:105-38
2. Bachmann GA, Leiblum SR. Sexuality in sexagenarian women. *Maturitas* 1991;13:43-50
3. Bachmann GA, Leiblum SR, Sandler B, *et al.* Correlates of sexual desire in post-menopausal women. *Maturitas* 1985;7:211-16
4. Bottiglioni F, De Aloysio D. Female sexual activity as a function of climacteric conditions and age. *Maturitas* 1982;4:27-32
5. Dennerstein L, Smith AMA, Morse CA, *et al.* Sexuality and the menopause. *Psychosom Obstet Gynecol* 1994;15:59-66
6. Hagstad A. Gynecology and sexuality in middle-aged women. *Women Health* 1988;13:57-80

7. Hallstrom T. *Mental Disorder and Sexuality in the Climacterium*. Stockholm: Scandinavian University Books, 1973
8. Hallstrom T. Sexuality of women in middle age: the Goteborg study. *J Biosoc Sci* 1979;6(Suppl):165–75
9. Holte A. Prevalence of climacteric complaints in a representative sample of middle-aged women in Oslo, Norway. *J Psychosom Obstet Gynaecol* 1991;12: 303–15
10. Holte A. Influences of natural menopause on health complaints: a prospective study of healthy Norwegian women. *Maturitas* 1992;14:127–41
11. Huerta R, Mena A, Malacara JM, *et al.* Symptoms at the perimenopausal period: its association with attitudes toward sexuality, life-style, family function and FSH levels. *Psychoneuroendocrinology* 1995; 20:135–67
12. Huerta R, Mena A, Malacara JM, *et al.* Symptoms at the menopausal and premenopausal years: their relationship with insulin, glucose, cortisol, FSH, prolactin, obesity and attitudes towards sexuality. *Psychoneuroendocrinology* 1995;20:851–64
13. Hunter M, Battersby R, Whitehead M. Relationships between psychological symptoms, somatic complaints and menopausal status. *Maturitas* 1986; 8:217–28
14. Kinsey AC, Pomeroy WB, Martin CE, *et al. Sexual Behavior in the Human Female*. Philadelphia: WB Saunders, 1953
15. Koster A, Garde K. Sexual desire and menopausal development: a prospective study of Danish women born in 1936. *Maturitas* 1993;16:49–60
16. McCoy N, Cutler W, Davidson JM. Relationships among sexual behavior, hot flashes, and hormone levels in perimenopausal women. *Arch Sex Behav* 1985;14:381–90
17. McCoy NL, Davidson JM. A longitudinal study of the effects of menopause on sexuality. *Maturitas* 1985;7:203–10
18. Tungphaisal S, Chandeying V, Sutthijumroon S, *et al.* Postmenopausal sexuality in Thai women. *Asia-Oceania J Obstet Gynecol* 1991;17:143–6
19. McCoy NL. Methodological problems in the study of sexuality and the menopause. *Maturitas* 1998;29:51–60
20. Longcope C, Jaffee W, Griffing G. Production rates of androgens and oestrogens in post-menopausal women. *Maturitas* 1981;3:215–23
21. Judd HL, Judd GE, Lucas WE, *et al.* Endocrine function of the post-menopausal ovary: concentration of androgens and estrogens in ovarian and peripheral vein blood. *J Clin Endocrinol Metab* 1974;39:1020–4
22. Longcope C, Hunter R, Franz C. Steroid secretion by the postmenopausal ovary. *Am J Obstet Gynecol* 1980;138:564–8
23. Andreyko JB, Monroe SE, Marshall LA, *et al.* Concordant suppression of serum immunoreactive luteinizing hormone (LH), α-subunit bioactive LH, and testosterone in postmenopausal women by a potent gonadotropin-releasing hormone antagonist (Detirelix). *J Clin Endocrinol Metab* 1992;74: 399–405
24. Sluijmer AV, Heineman MJ, Koudstaal J, *et al.* Relationship between ovarian production of estrone, estradiol, testosterone, and androstenedione and the ovarian degree of stromal hyperplasia in postmenopausal women. *Menopause* 1998; 5:207–10
25. Cumming DC, Rebar RW, Hopper BR, *et al.* Evidence for an influence of the ovary on circulating dehydroepiandrosterone sulfate levels. *J Clin Endocrinol Metab* 1982;54:1069–71
26. Newman G, Nichols CR. Sexual activities and attitudes in older persons. *J Am Med Assoc* 1960;173: 33–5
27. Christenson CV, Gagnon JH. Sexual behavior in a group of older women. *J Gerontol* 1965;20:351–6
28. Pfeiffer E, Vervoerdt A, Wang H-S. Sexual behavior in aged men and women. I. Observations on 254 community volunteers. *Arch Gen Psychiatry* 1968; 19:753–8
29. Verwoerdt A, Pfeiffer E, Wang H-S. Sexual behavior in senescence: changes in sexual activity and interest of aging men and women. *J Geriatr Psychiatry* 1969;2:163–80
30. Verwoerdt A, Pfeiffer E, Wang H-S. Sexual behavior in senescence. II. Patterns of sexual activity and interest. *Geriatrics* 1969;24:137–54
31. Pfeiffer E, Davis GC. Determinants of sexual behavior in middle and old age. *J Am Geriatr Soc* 1972;20:151–8
32. Pfeiffer E, Vervoerdt A, Davis GC. Sexual behavior in middle life. *Am J Psychiatry* 1972;128:1262–7
33. Christenson CV, Johnson AB. Sexual patterns in a group of older never-married women. *J Geriatr Psychiatry* 1973;6:80–98
34. De Nicola P, Peruzza M. Sex in the aged. *J Am Geriatr Soc* 1974;22:380–2
35. Persson G. Sexuality in a 70 year old urban population. *J Psychosom Res* 1980;24:335–42
36. George LK, Weiler SJ. Sexuality in middle and late life: the effects of age, cohort, and gender. *Arch Gen Psychiatry* 1981;38:919–23
37. Todarello O, Boscia FM. Sexuality in aging: a study of a group of 300 elderly men and women. *J Endocrinol Invest* 1985;8(Suppl 2):123–30
38. Bretschneider JG, McCoy NL. Sexual interest and behavior in healthy 80- to 102-year-olds. *Arch Sex Behav* 1988;17:109–29
39. Lindgren R, Berg G, Hammar M, *et al.* Hormonal replacement therapy and sexuality in a population of Swedish postmenopausal women. *Acta Obstet Gynecol Scand* 1993;72:292–7
40. Jacoby S. Great sex: what's age got to do with it? The AARP/Modern Maturity survey on sexual attitudes and behavior. *Mod Maturity* 1999; Sept-Oct:41–5, 91

41. Wildt L, Sir-Petermann T. Oestrogen and age estimations of perimenopausal women. *Lancet* 1999; 354:224
42. McCoy NL. Sexualité, hormonothérapie substitutive et qualité de vie après la ménopause [Sexuality, hormone replacement therapy, and quality of life after menopause]. In *Stéroïdes, Ménopause et Qualité de Vie*. Paris: Elsevier Scientific Editions, 1995:81-100
43. Greenblatt RB, Barfield WE, Garner JF, *et al.* Evaluation of an oestrogen, androgen, oestrogen-androgen combination, and a placebo in the treatment of the menopause. *J Clin Endocrinol Metab* 1950;10:1547-58
44. Sherwin BB, Gelfand MM, Brender W. Androgen enhances motivation in females: a prospective, crossover study of sex steroid administration in the surgical menopause. *Psychosom Med* 1985;47:339-51
45. Myers LS, Dixen J, Morrissette D, *et al.* Effects of estrogen, androgen, and progestin on sexual psychophysiology and behavior in postmenopausal women. *J Clin Endocrinol Metab* 1990;70: 1124-31
46. Fedor-Freybergh P. The influence of oestrogens on the wellbeing and mental performance in climacteric and postmenopausal women. *Acta Obstet Gynecol Scand* 1977;64(Suppl):1-91
47. Nathorst-Böös J, Wiklund I, Mattsson L-A, *et al.* Is sexual life influenced by transdermal estrogen therapy? A double blind placebo-controlled study in postmenopausal women. *Acta Obstet Gynecol Scand* 1993;72:656-60
48. Bakke JL. A double-blind study of a progestin-estrogen combination in the management of the menopause. *Pacific Med Surg* 1965;73:200-5
49. Dennerstein L, Burrows GD, Wood C, *et al.* Hormones and sexuality: effect of estrogen and progestogen. *Obstet Gynecol* 1980;56:316-22
50. Paterson MEL. A randomised, double-blind, cross-over study into the effect of sequential mestranol and northisterone on climacteric symptoms and biochemical parameters. *Maturitas* 1982;4: 83-94
51. Utian WH. The true clinical features of postmenopause and oophorectomy, and their response to oestrogen therapy. *S Afr Med J* 1972;46:732-7
52. Coope J, Thomson JM, Poller L. Effects of 'natural estrogens' replacement therapy on menopausal symptoms and blood clotting. *Br Med J* 1975;4: 139-43
53. Campbell S. Double blind psychometric studies on the effects of natural estrogens on post-menopausal women. In Campbell S, ed. *The Management of the Menopause and the Post-Menopausal Years*. Lancaster: MTP Press, 1976;149-58
54. Campbell S, Whitehead M. Oestrogen therapy and the menopausal syndrome. *Clin Obstet Gynaecol* 1977;4:31-47
55. Geola FL, Frumar AM, Tataryn IV, *et al.* Biological effects of various doses of conjugated equine estrogens in postmenopausal women. *J Clin Endocrinol Metab* 1980;51:620-5
56. Mathur RS, Landgrebe SC, Moody LO, *et al.* The effect of estrogen treatment on plasma concentrations of steroid hormones, gonadotropins, prolactin and sex hormone-binding globulin in postmenopausal women. *Maturitas* 1985;7: 129-33
57. L'Hermite M. Risks of estrogens and progestogens. *Maturitas* 1990;12:215-46
58. Lorrain J, Lalumiere G, Filion A, *et al.* Use of transdermal estrogen gel in postmenopausal women. *Menopause Management* 1999;8:11-15
59. Simon J, Klaiber E, Wiita B, *et al.* Differential effects of estrogen-androgen and estrogen-only therapy on vasomotor symptoms, gonadotropin secretion, and endogenous androgen bioavailability in postmenopausal women. *Menopause* 1999;6:138-46

Psychosomatic aspects of sexuality among married middle-aged women

72

F. Horiguchi, H. Ohta and S. Nozawa

INTRODUCTION

Although Japanese teenagers and men speak freely about sex, middle-aged women are reluctant to talk about their own sexuality. Because the traditional role of women within the family system was to bear and raise children, and this role ended after reaching midlife, it was considered shameful for women older than 40 years to have a sex life or to become pregnant. Consequently, it has been difficult to collect data, and little information is available on the sexuality of Japanese menopausal women in general. Even women who present at menopause clinics because of menopausal symptoms seldom discuss matters related to their own sexuality. Although menopausal women may sense various changes, such as reduced sexual response, loss of interest in sex or frigidity[1], the most direct expressions of sexual life are usually coital pain and sexual abstinence.

We studied how family relationships affect sexual attitudes and behavior among women presenting with menopausal symptoms at the Menopause Clinic of Keio University Hospital. Historical changes in the concept of sexuality among Japanese women have also been discussed.

SUBJECTS AND METHODS

All subjects were legally married women who presented to our menopause clinic because of physical and mental symptoms related to the menopause. Unmarried women, divorcees and widows were excluded. A total of 52 women aged 45–55 years (mean 51.2 years) were enrolled. All subjects were leading normal lives and had no evidence of serious disease. Before enrolment, gynecological and breast examinations were performed. Other tests related to the general health of menopausal women, including examinations for osteoporosis and cardiovascular disease, were also performed.

All subjects were interviewed by means of a questionnaire on menopausal symptoms. They then filled in the Cornell Medical Index health checklist[2] and underwent the Yatabe-Guilford character test and sentence completion test[3]. To rule out severe depression, some patients were tested according to the self-rating depression scale of Zung[4].

RESULTS AND DISCUSSION

Baseline characteristics of the subjects

Among the 52 patients enrolled, eight (15.4%) were premenopausal and still had regular menstrual cycles, 15 (28.8%) were perimenopausal and had irregular cycles, 11 (21.2%) were postmenopausal and 18 cases (34.6%) had undergone hysterectomy. The ovaries remained in only one of the patients who had undergone hysterectomy; the other 17 patients had undergone concurrent bilateral oophorectomy. There was no evidence of functional ovaries in 28 women (53.8%); 24 women (46.2%) had functional ovaries. However, even premenopausal women with functional ovaries complained of symptoms similar to those experienced by postmenopausal women. In such patients, pharmacological treatment, such as hormone replacement therapy (HRT), may be of limited benefit, and psychosomatic treatment may be indicated[5].

Pharmacological therapy of menopausal symptoms

Among the treatments used to manage menopausal symptoms, including unidentified complaints, the most commonly prescribed was hormone preparations, given to 18 of the 52 patients (34.6%). Minor tranquillizers were given to nine patients (17.3%) and antidepressants to six (11.5%). Other types of treatment included herbal medicine, autonomic nervous system regulators and vitamins. No patient had a marked improvement in symptoms in response to any of these treatments.

Sexual activity in menopausal women

Seven of the eight premenopausal women (87.5%), 13 of the 15 perimenopausal women (86.7%) and all 11 of the postmenopausal women (100.0%) were sexually active. The proportion of sexually active subjects was lowest among women who had undergone hysterectomy; 15 of the 18 women (83.3%), who had normal follicle stimulating hormone (FSH) levels, were sexually active. Overall, 46 of the 52 women (88.5%) were sexually active despite concerns about physical and psychological symptoms related to the menopause. This proportion is consistent with statistics on induced abortion[6] and birth rate[7] among women 45 years of age or older.

Frequency of coital pain among menopausal women (Table 1)

Among the 46 sexually active women (88.5%), 20 had coital pain (43.5%). The incidence of coital pain was highest in women who had natural menopause (54.5%) or surgically induced menopause (57.1%), in whom FSH levels were high and estradiol levels were low. These findings suggested a relationship between coital pain and the menopause. Some premenopausal women also had coital pain.

Hormone treatment and coital pain (Table 2)

The 17 women received three types of therapy for menopausal symptoms: HRT with estrogen and progesterone; depot injections of testosterone (49 mg) with estrogen (1 mg); and HRT plus estradiol and testosterone. Although coital pain persisted in seven of the 17 treated patients (41.2%), it resolved in the other ten (58.8%), indicating that hormone therapy seemed to be effective. However, when the response was analyzed according to the type of medication given, we found that pain resolved in the patients (six of nine; 66.7%) who received estrogen plus testosterone. This rate was higher than the response rate with the other two treatments (50%). The addition of testosterone to HRT, which includes progesterone, was therefore not very effective. Coital pain is attributed to insufficient lubrication and a gradual loss of sexual drive[8]. Although the reasons remain speculative, it seems that these problems are improved by estrogen plus testosterone. Studd and

Table 1 Frequency of coital pain in menopausal patients ($n = 46$)

Menstrual status	*No. of patients*	*Patients with coital pain*	
		n	*%*
Premenopause	7	2	28.6
Perimenopause	13	4	30.8
Postmenopause	11	6	54.5
Hysterectomy			
FSH normal	1	0	0
FSH elevated	14	8	57.1
Total	46	20	43.5

FSH, follicle stimulating hormone

Table 2 Coital pain in patients receiving hormone medication ($n = 17$)

Hormone preparations	*No. of users*	*Patients with coital pain*	
		n	*%*
HRT	6	3	50.0
Estradiol (1 mg) + testosterone (49 mg)	9	3	33.3
HRT + estradiol (1 mg) + testosterone (49 mg)	2	1	50.0
Total	17	7	41.2

HRT, hormone replacement therapy

Thom[9] reported that a testosterone-induced increase in sexual drive might influence coital pain.

A relationship between coital pain and the menopause was suggested, but all women did not respond to hormone treatment. We therefore concentrated on vaginal findings and psychological factors as reasons for the lack of response to hormone treatment.

Vaginal scores in women with coital pain (Table 3)

In the 20 women with coital pain, vaginal scores were calculated on the basis of symptoms such as the degree of flow, dryness and itchiness. Vaginal symptoms were assessed according to a three-grade scale and were scored from 0 to 9 points. The average vaginal score was 6 points in premenopausal women, substantially higher than the score of 1 or 2 points in perimenopausal and postmenopausal women. Despite no evidence of infection or inflammation, two women complained of flow, vaginal dryness and vulval itchiness for prolonged periods.

These findings are consistent with the symptoms associated with decreasing estrogen levels. However, in some patients, vaginal symptoms and coital pain were probably not directly related to the menopause. Furthermore, among the four perimenopausal women, the three who received hormone therapy had lower vaginal symptom scores. Most postmenopausal women and women undergoing hysterectomy who received no hormone treatment also had low vaginal scores. Utian[10] and Leiblum and colleagues[11] emphasized the relationship between vaginal symptoms and the menopause. Although coital pain appeared to be related to the menopause, there was no relationship between ovarian hormones and vaginal score in some women. Psychological factors may therefore influence pain.

Coital pain in women receiving antidepressants and hormones

The six women with coital pain who had depression received antidepressants. Three of these patients continued to experience coital pain. The response to HRT was unclear because one patient responded and one did not.

Coital pain in women receiving minor tranquillizers and hormones

The proportion of patients who took mild tranquillizers for mental health problems and had coital pain was not particularly high: only three out of nine women. Although patient 8 was receiving HRT and experienced coital pain, no pain was reported by patients 4 and 5, who were given testosterone. Menopausal patients who were treated with minor tranquillizers did not often complain of coital pain.

Psychological tests (Figure 1)

The Cornell Medical Index was assessed in 45 women with menopausal symptoms. Six women (13.3%) and 11 women (24.4%), i.e. a total of 17

Table 3 Vaginal score in patients with coital pain ($n = 20$)

		Patients treated with hormones		*Vaginal score**	
Menstrual status	*No. of patients*	*n*	*%*	*Mean*	*Range*
Premenopause	2	0	0	6	2.5–9
Perimenopause	4	3	75.0	2	0–5
Postmenopause	6	1	16.7	2	0–4
Hysterectomy					
FSH normal	1	0	0	1	1
FSH elevated	7	2	28.6	1	0–1.5
Total	20	6	30.0	2.4	0–9

*Vaginal symptoms were scored from 0 to 9 points; FSH, follicle stimulating hormone

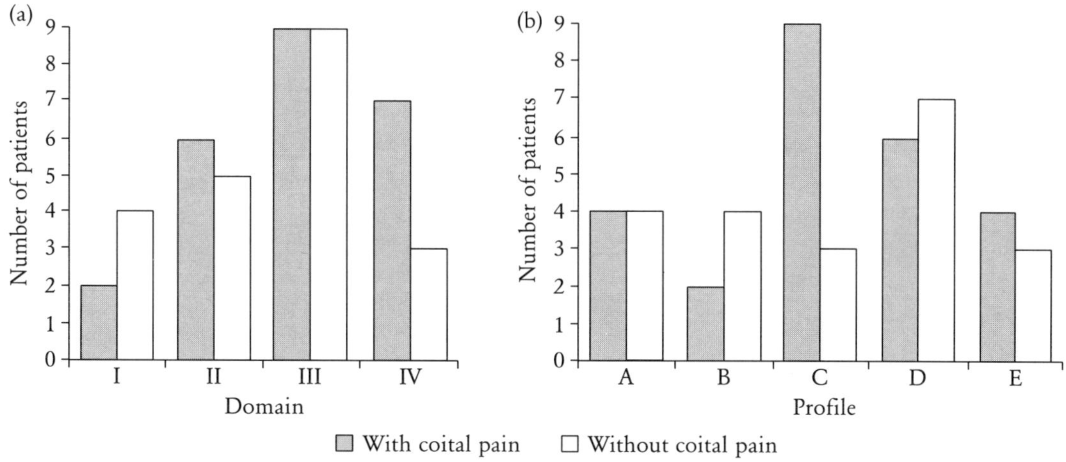

Figure 1 Results of psychological tests (Cornell Medical Index ($n = 45$) (a) and Yatabe–Guilford character test ($n = 46$) (b)), in menopausal patients with or without coital pain

patients (37.8%), were classified as domains I and II, respectively, which are normal. Eighteen women (40.0%) and ten women (22.2%), i.e. a total of 28 patients (62.2%), belonged to domains III and IV, respectively, which indicate neurotic tendencies. The majority of women thus had neurotic tendencies. Seven of the ten women with coital pain (70.0%) were classified as domain IV. The Yatabe- Guilford test was performed on 46 women. The highest frequency of coital pain was found in calm-type women (nine of 12; 75.0%), who are usually socially and emotionally stable, followed by eccentric-type women (four of seven; 57.1%), who are very emotionally unstable.

These results suggest that mild-mannered women tend to suffer pain without taking positive action to resolve the problem. Both psychological tests indicate that coital pain is experienced mainly by calm-type women, who tend to have neurotic symptoms; coital pain is apparently related to personality type.

Table 4 Image of husband among patients with coital pain ($n = 20$)

	Patients	
Image of husband	*n*	%
Negative image of husband		
dissatisfaction	10	50.0
violence	2	10.0
delusion	1	5.0
illness	1	5.0
total	14	70.0
Positive image of husband	6	30.0
Total	20	100.0

Family relationships among women with coital pain (Table 4)

Fourteen of 20 women (70.0%) had a negative assessment of their husbands. The most common reason (ten women) was dissatisfaction with their husband. Other reasons included their husband's violence, wild fantasies of jealousy towards their husband and illness. Only six women (30.0%) were on good terms with their husbands and gave their husbands a positive assessment.

One woman had a negative self-evaluation and doubted her attitude towards her role as a wife. Although some anxiety was caused by factors such as her daughter's divorce or illness, she expressed no opinion about her sons. Through counselling, some women realized that their husband's attitude was related to, and influenced by, their own reproductive function crisis, caused by factors such as menopausal symptoms and surgery (hysterectomy and other procedures). These women endeavored to be cheerful and to get closer to their husbands. Such realization helped the wives achieve satisfaction and a sense of security, even if they could not obtain a complete sexual response or the same kind of response as previously. On the other hand, sexual intercourse may no longer be enjoyed because of instability caused by psychological factors. The interpersonal relationship between such women and their husbands must be improved, because pharmacological therapy provided little or no benefit.

Abstinence (Table 5)

Sexual abstinence was reported by one premenopausal woman, two perimenopausal women, two women who underwent simple hysterectomy and one woman who underwent a radical operation for early cervical cancer. The duration of abstinence ranged from 1 to 17 years. Hormone replacement therapy was given to only patient 4, who demonstrated no symptomatic improvement. Even when a self-administered questionnaire was used, only the two women who underwent total hysterectomy with bilateral oophorectomy reported having vaginal symptoms. On vaginal examination, however, there were no clear-cut signs of inflammation. The other four women had no flow, vaginal dryness or itchiness. Psychological tests showed that many women were classified as domain III or IV according to the Cornell Medical Index, indicating a neurotic tendency. On the Yatabe-Guilford test, two women were classified as emotionally unstable eccentric type and two as calm type.

The motive for abstinence in patient 1 (premenopausal) was gestational toxicosis; her second child was delivered by Cesarean section. The patient, who was very sensitive to pain, fell into a panic because of postsurgical pain. Subsequently, she has been afraid of becoming pregnant again and has abstained from sexual intercourse. We suppose that she has had some reason to refuse her husband and has not even attempted to use contraception. Since she delivered her first child vaginally, we believe that she might have tolerated the birth of a second child. The patient should have been given adequate support when she underwent Cesarean section.

Patient 2 had a timid disposition and was easily worried. The patient had a calm-type personality according to the Yatabe-Guilford test. She was being observed for polymenorrhea and uterine myoma, suspected because of uterine hemorrhage and an abnormal Papanicolaou smear. She experienced increasing insomnia and anxiety and has subsequently abstained from sexual intercourse. In addition, she has been taking analgesics, hormones, mild tranquillizers, sleeping pills and herbal medicines for indefinite complaints and premenstrual tension for a prolonged period.

Patient 3 experienced domestic tension and palpitations at mealtimes and ceased sexual activity 4 years ago, after her husband had undergone surgery for gastric cancer. At this time she was already becoming less involved with her husband.

Patient 4 had had a total hysterectomy with bilateral oophorectomy. She got divorced 4 years later and remarried. Although she currently shares the same outlook on life as her husband and is satisfied with married life, she has abstained from sexual intercourse ever since surgery. Although she previously received HRT, it recently became ineffective against indefinite complaints. Treatment was switched to drugs such as testosterone and herbal medicine, but she has not responded. The patient now finds life not worth living.

Table 5 Psychological factors in women abstaining from sexual intercourse ($n = 6$)

Patient no.	*Cornell Medical Index (domain)*	*Yatabe-Guilford test (type of profile)*	*Motivation for abstinence*
1	III	director	panic caused by pain after Cesarean section
2	II	calm	uterine hemorrhage and abnormal Papanicolaou smear
3	IV	average	husband's illness
4	IV	eccentric	loss of motherhood caused by hysterectomy
5	IV	eccentric	husband refused to talk over sexual intercourse with her after hysterectomy
6	II	calm	anxiety of recovery from hysterectomy

Patient 5 had a total hysterectomy because of uterine myoma 10 years ago. After surgery, her husband refused to talk to her about their sexual intercourse, so she rejected him and has abstained ever since.

Patient 6 had pelvic cavity inflammation after undergoing hysterectomy, making her very anxious. Although she still had pain after recovery, she continued to have sexual intercourse, but had symptoms such as vaginal itchiness and dryness. She finally had to abstain because of anxiety about recovering from the effects of hysterectomy.

CONCLUSION

Although coital pain and abstinence are often attributed to the menopause in middle-aged women, we found that coital pain and abstinence from sexual intercourse were frequently unrelated to vaginal score, menopause and hormone treatment, suggesting the involvement of psychological causes. Factors such as marital relationships, personality, and history of childbirth and total hysterectomy played an important role in coital pain and sexual abstinence. Middle-aged women with these problems are likely to benefit substantially from early psychological intervention.

References

1. Dennerstein L. Well-being, symptoms and the menopausal transition. *Maturitas* 1996;23:147–57
2. Brodman K, Erdmann AJ Jr, Lorge I, *et al.* The Cornell Medical Index – Health Questionnaire III. The evaluation of emotional disturbance. *J Clin Psychol* 1952;8:119–24
3. Indow T, Sano K, Namiki H, *et al.* A mathematical model for interpretation in projective tests: an application to SEIKEN SCT. *Jpn Psychol Res* 1962; 4:163–72
4. Zung WWK. A self-rating depression scale. *Arch Gen Psychiatry* 1965;12:63–70
5. Lean E, van Lunsen RH. Hormones and sexuality in postmenopausal women: a psychological study. *J Psychosom Obstet Gynecol* 1997;18:126–33
6. Ministry of Health and Welfare, Japan. Live birth by age of mother and total birth order, 1951–1996. *Maternal and Child Health Statistics of Japan*. Tokyo: Mothers' and Childrens' Health and Welfare Associations, 1998:50
7. Ministry of Health and Welfare, Japan. Induced abortion by age of woman 1960–1996. *Maternal and Child Health Statistics of Japan*. Tokyo: Mothers' and Childrens' Health and Welfare Associations, 1998:64
8. Dennerstein L, Smith AM, Morse CA, *et al.* Sexuality and menopause. *J Psychosom Obstet Gynecol* 1994; 15:59–66
9. Studd JWW, Thom MH. Ovarian failure and aging. *Clin Endocrinol Metab* 1981;10:89–113
10. Utian WH. Definitive symptoms of postmenopause – incorporating use of vaginal parabasal cell index. *Front Horm Res* 1975;3:74–93
11. Leiblum S, Backmann G, Kemmann E, *et al.* Vaginal atrophy in the postmenopausal woman. *J Am Med Assoc* 1983;249:2195–8

Dyspareunia: differential diagnosis and treatment guidelines

73

A. Graziottin and E. Castoldi

INTRODUCTION

Dyspareunia is described as a persistent or recurrent pain experienced primarily during sexual intercourse, which causes personal distress[1]. The traditional focusing on activity - coital sex - instead of on the location -'where does it hurt?'- and the characteristics of pain, has kept dyspareunia in a psychosexual domain. This has led to a substantial dismissal of its biological basis and a consequent diagnostic omission of its medical characteristics that are deeply rooted in the gynecologist's specialist domain. Meana and colleagues[2] found that the location of the pain and its onset during an episode of intercourse were the strongest predictors of the presence and type of organicity. Psychosocial variables, such as situational factors, relationship adjustment and history of sexual abuse, had no predictive value and women with dyspareunia did not differ significantly from controls on these measures[2].

Dyspareunia affects an estimated 10-15% of sexually active women[3,4], with increasing prevalence after the menopause, when it affects on average 3-15%[5,6] of women still sexually active in the general population and 12-33%[4,7] of women attending medical offices, the wide range of prevalence being due to selection biases and methodological problems[8]. Vaginal changes may be problematic for about 40-60% of menopausal women.

A different diagnostic - and cultural - approach, namely to consider dyspareunia as a pain disorder and not 'simply' as a sexual disorder, is necessary to address correctly the many different issues it implies, as an indicator both of physical damage and a negative emotional experience[1,2,9].

The aim of this paper is to analyse the leading medical causes of dyspareunia in the postmenopause. Psychogenic or relational cofactors will be only briefly mentioned.

Leading causes of introital and mid-vaginal dyspareunia in the postmenopause may be summarized as follows:

(1) Hormonal (loss of estrogen and androgen) with subsequent vulvovaginal dystrophy;

(2) Sexual (vaginismus, loss of libido, arousal disorders);

(3) Inflammatory (vaginitis, vestibulitis, postcoital cystitis, usually secondary to the mechanical trauma);

(4) Iatrogenic (outcomes of perimenopausal physical therapies - namely laser and diathermocoagulation - and surgery, episiotomy, repair for rhagas and hemorrhoids, plus postmenopausal colporrhaphy and perineorrhaphy);

(5) Muscular (levator ani tender and trigger points; tension myalgia of the pelvic floor);

(6) Neurological (systemic and local, i.e. pudendal neuralgia);

(7) Immunological (Sjögren syndrome) and dismetabolic (diabetes);

(8) Vascular causes (have only recently been reported).

Multifactorial causes appear to interact in the individual patient and careful diagnosis should recognize potential overlapping of different medical etiologies, i.e. muscle hypertonicity, either lifelong (as in primary vaginismus)[10] or acquired (following vestibulitis[11-14]), persisting arousal disorders and vaginal dryness (as a defense mechanism to prevent further coitus and pain) and/or reactive posture[15,16]. All of the above more frequently cause superficial or introital and mid-vaginal dyspareunia.

Deep causes of dyspareunia, although less frequently found during the postmenopausal years than in the fertile age, include:

(1) Endometriosis;

(2) Pelvic inflammatory disease;

(3) Pelvic varicocele;

(4) Referred pain;

(5) Outcome of radiotherapy;

(6) Abdominal cutaneous nerve entrapment syndrome.

ETIOLOGY OF INTROITAL AND MID-VAGINAL DYSPAREUNIA

It is worth noting that textbooks usually report only 'superficial' or 'deep' dyspareunia. If women are asked 'where the pain is' and objective examination of painful points is carried out, mid-vaginal pain is reported on average in more than half of the patients.

Hormonal loss and urogenital dystrophy

Symptoms of urogenital dystrophy, secondary to estrogen deprivation after the menopause, occur 10 or more years after the last menstrual period[17]. Clinical experience has correlated postmenopausal vaginal dystrophy with mucosal thinning, reduced vaginal length and elasticity, reduced introital caliber and poor lubrication, the leading causes of vaginal dryness and dyspareunia, which are increasingly complained of in the absence of hormonal replacement therapy (HRT)[18]. Conversely, HRT, even local treatment, was shown to improve all these parameters in a significant number of patients[19], leading to the reduction or disappearance of dyspareunia. However, Laan and Lunsen[20] found that vaginal dryness correlated more with premenopausal pre-existing arousal disorders than with postmenopausal loss of estrogen *per se*. It is possible that women with pre-existing arousal disorders might be at higher risk for postmenopausal vaginal dryness, owing to the concurrence of premenopausal sexual problems (arousal disorders include the often associated loss of libido[21,22]) and biological factors, such as the reduced effect of estrogen on vasoactive intestinal polypeptide[23]. Vascular factors could concur with premenopausal sexual problems, but this has only recently been given clinical attention in women, in contrast to the study of vascular factors in the etiology of male arousal disorders[24].

Vulvar involution, secondary to loss of hormones, may concur with sexual pain through two mechanisms: introital pain, owing to scarring and skin retraction; and clitoral pain and dysfunction, because of the parallel anatomic involution. The clitoral cavernosal erectile tissue consists of smooth muscle and connective tissue and is reduced by half between infancy and the postmenopausal years. Tarcan and co-workers[25] showed that the percentage of clitoral cavernosal smooth muscle in the age group 6 months–15 years was $65 \pm 1.5\%$, in 44–54-year-old women it was $50 \pm 1.2\%$ and in 55–90-year-old women it was $37 \pm 1.3\%$ (ANOVA, $p = 0.0001$). This study revealed a strong link between increase in age and decrease in clitoral cavernosal smooth muscle fibers. It could be the anatomic basis of the complaint: 'My clitoris is dead', reported by 20% of postmenopausal women in the study of Sarrel and Whitehead[26], where the loss of clitoral response correlated well with arousal disorders with basic biological roots, involving all the cavernosal tissue of the genital area and leading to a more complex form of 'sexual pain-related disorder'. Clinicians should pay more clinical attention to the semiology of the external genitalia and vagina when dyspareunia is complained of. Testosterone 2% cream seems to reduce the anatomic and functional involution of the clitoris and vulvar area in the postmenopause, but controlled studies are still lacking.

Iatrogenic

Perineal surgery may cause acquired dyspareunia, because of retracting scars and a long-lasting reflex hypertonicity of the pelvic floor, leading to secondary vaginismus[10,27–32].

Postmenopausal surgery, namely posterior colporrhaphy and perineorrhaphy have been considered to cause dyspareunia because of vaginal stenosis[33-35]. Francis and Jeffcoate[33] reported apareunia and dyspareunia in 70 of 140 women after prolapse repair; in 43 of these women, introital narrowing to one finger breadth or less had occurred. They recommended that posterior colpoperineorrhaphy be omitted whenever possible.

However, some authors present opposite findings[36,37]. According to the cross-sectional study of Weber and co-workers[36], vaginal anatomy, measured by introital caliber, length and vulvovaginal atrophy, does not correlate well with sexual function, particularly symptoms of dyspareunia and vaginal dryness. Specifically, a lack of estrogen replacement therapy (ERT) in postmenopausal women was not associated with dyspareunia and vaginal dryness. Patient selection biases may partly account for these controversial findings on the role of anatomy and sex hormones. Being conscious of the potential sexual side-effects of pelvic surgery and active prevention are essential to maintain a functional sexual response when surgery is complete. After surgery, a clinical history should look for these complications and a physical examination should pay attention to the quality of local scars (retraction, pain, mucocutaneous and myofascial trigger points, and signs of nerve entrapment syndrome), vaginal anatomic outcome (introital caliber, vaginal length and post-repair elasticity), the tone of pelvic floor muscles and their role as causes or cofactors in introital and mid-vaginal dyspareunia.

Rehabilitation of the pelvic floor muscles, stretching and relaxation of contracted muscles, massage of painful scars, improved trophism with at least local ERT, and, after muscle relaxation has been obtained, active dilatation of the introitus with fingers and dilators seem to be clinically useful in reducing dyspareunia until a normal coital function is restored (provided that libido is present and arousal adequate), although no controlled study has been performed so far in the author's knowledge.

Sexual and relational

Different aspects of the sexual response are closely interdependent. Arousal disorders[21,23], leading to vaginal dryness, may be secondary to vascular[24], hormonal or involutional causes[5,19,25,38-40], or secondary to loss of libido, difficulty in reaching orgasm, dissatisfaction or frank dyspareunia of whatever cause. Relational factors, including the real desirability of the partner, may further modulate the sexual response from a psychodynamic point of view, concerning the experience of pain during intercourse, and should be properly investigated and treated, if present.

Inflammatory

Vulvitis, vaginitis and vestibulitis are the most familiar causes of dyspareunia to gynecologists[11,14,41-43] during the fertile age. They may also be important in the postmenopause, particularly in sexually active women when sexually transmitted diseases are in play, leading to pelvic inflammatory disease, which also emerges in the postmenopausal years. Vaginitis resulting from common pathogens (e.g. *Escherichia coli*) is a more frequent complication of postmenopausal hypoestrogenic dystrophy. Systemic and/or local ERT (or HRT) is the treatment of choice when colonic saprophytes are in play; the major effect occurs between 1 and 3 months after the start of treatment, with changes in pH and cytological findings[19]. An estimated 10–25% of women receiving systemic hormone replacement therapy still experience the symptoms of urogenital atrophy[44]. For these women it is likely that low-dose local preparations in addition to systemic therapy will have a beneficial effect[19]. Because of the high frequency of mistakes when diagnosis is limited to a clinical evaluation, a sample should be obtained with a swab every time that inflammation is considered to be the cause of dyspareunia, to avoid useless and potentially damaging 'generic' antibiotic treatments. Lifestyle should be properly addressed[11,42,45,46], particularly when recurrences are frequent.

Postcoital cystitis[19,22] may frequently be a symptom related to dyspareunia, mainly in the postmenopause when dystrophic vaginal dryness is associated with dystrophy of the trigonal and urethral areas and with a secondary spasm of the perivaginal muscles, leading to a complex vulnerability to a coital mechanical trauma[47].

Active and passive relaxation of the pelvic floor should integrate the HRT.

Muscular

Muscular causes of dyspareunia are the least familiar to gynecologists, who are trained to recognize the hypotonic conditions of the pelvic floor, but are usually totally deprived of any training in diagnosing the hypertonic conditions, including tender and trigger points, levator ani myalgia and so on[13-16,47-52].

Secondary 'defensive' contraction of the perivaginal pelvic floor until frank vaginismus (when the condition is worsened by a phobic attitude and active coital avoidance) is a common outcome when long-lasting dyspareunia is experienced, particularly in nulliparous women or when coitus is resumed after years of postmenopausal estrogen loss.

Routine evaluation of the pelvic floor in a relaxed and contracted condition, and an active search for levator ani tender and/or trigger points, should be part of all gynecological examinations and are mandatory when dyspareunia is complained of.

Neurological

Neurological causes are also usually undiagnosed causes of chronic dyspareunia[14,48,53,54]. They may be systemic, for example, when neurological damage associated with multiple sclerosis, diabetes mellitus and collagen disease is involved. More frequently, peripheral and especially local neurological causes, secondary to the involvement of the pudendal nerve, are the hidden causes of a persisting dyspareunia, which is often associated with other 'cloudy' symptoms (clitoralgia, cystalgia, urgency and pain mimicking sciatica) that all have pudendal dysfunction in common secondary to compression and/or trauma - the so-called 'nerve entrapment syndrome'[53,55,56].

The pudendal nerve, composed of three roots derived from S2, S3 and S4 (with its sensory, motor and autonomic components) supplies the vast majority of the perineum. It may be compressed in the pudendal canal (Alcock canal), which is formed between the ischial bone and a fascial sheath from the internal obturator muscle, or between the sacrospinous and the sacrotuberous ligament, where the nerve turns around the falciform process before entering the pudendal canal[55].

Pudendal neuralgia has been reported after surgical and non-surgical trauma (perineal and/or vertebral trauma)[53,55]. The diagnostic tests for evaluation are radiographic studies of the lumbosacral spine and evoked potentials. The approach for proven pudendal entrapment syndrome is surgical, with pudendal nerve decompression[57-59].

Systemic and local autoimmune and metabolic diseases

Altered vaginal epithelium, chronic inflammatory changes in the vaginal wall or chronic cervicitis and systemic vasculitis could be responsible for reduced vaginal secretion and lubrication in autoimmune disease (Sjögren's disease)[40,60].

Other pathologies, such as systemic lupus erythematosus, may predispose to vaginal candidiasis, which is more frequent after immunosuppressive therapy, and neuropathies[41].

Diabetes mellitus may lead to dyspareunia due to a number of factors: *Candida* vaginal infections are frequent because of local glucose increases; local infections - vaginitis and vulvitis - may be enhanced secondary to the reduced diabetes-dependent immune response; vascular dysfunction secondary to diabetic microangiopathy may complicate the loss of the vascular response secondary to the menopause; and pain may be finally triggered by a peripheral neuropathy, leading to dysesthesia[41].

Finally, dismetabolic disorders, such as celiac disease, may cause atrophia of the vulvovaginal epithelium, leading to dyspareunia[61].

All of the above most frequently cause superficial and mid-vaginal dyspareunia.

ETIOLOGY OF DEEP DYSPAREUNIA

Deep causes of dyspareunia, although less frequently found during the postmenopausal years than in the fertile age, include endometriosis[62], pelvic inflammatory disease (PID)[63], adhesions[64], pelvic varicocele[65], referred pain[49], outcome of radiotherapy[66], and abdominal cutaneous nerve entrapment syndrome[67]. Endometriosis requires continuous combined treatments to avoid the worsening of menstrual pain. The possibility of PID, particularly subclinical, should be kept in mind, as an increasing number of postmenopausal women are sexually active and may engage in unprotected sex with new partners. Pelvic varicocele is a rare cause of dyspareunia, increasingly recognized thanks to intravaginal echography. Referred pain, from muscular, connective and mucocutaneous trigger points, is increasingly recognized as an important cause of chronic pelvic pain and dyspareunia. Pelvic radiotherapy is an issue in cancer survivors still engaging in sex. Abdominal cutaneous nerve entrapment syndrome may be another overlooked cause of chronic pelvic pain and deep dyspareunia.

CONCLUSION

Pain, including dyspareunia, has a solid biological basis that may cause and/or be associated with emotional and relational symptoms. Gynecologists should enrich their clinical competence with a more active knowledge of the biological basis of the female sexual disorders that are rooted in their specialist domain, and strive to increase their 'physician impact factor', i.e. their ability to cure and care with diagnostic skill and empathy.

An interdisciplinary sex pain clinic, where different specialists discuss individual cases, may increase the diagnostic accuracy for those patients presenting with more difficult clinical pictures. However, the majority of postmenopausal women complaining of dyspareunia may be actively helped by a listening gynecologist who is willing to make a good semiological evaluation of the pelvic floor and of the most frequent medical causes of painful sex, and who is able to address them in a competent and well-tailored treatment design.

References

1. Meana M, Binik YM, Khalife S, *et al.* Dyspareunia: more than bad sex [Editorial]. *Pain* 1997;71:211-2
2. Meana M, Binik YM, Khalife S, *et al.* Dyspareunia: sexual dysfunction or pain syndrome? *J Nerv Ment Dis* 1997;185:561-9
3. Lauman EO, Gagnon JH, Michaci RT, *et al. The Social Organization of Sexuality.* Chicago: University of Chicago Press, 1994
4. Lauman EO, Gagnon JH, Michaci RT, *et al.* Sexual dysfunction in the United States: prevalence and predictors. *J Am Med Assoc* 1999;10:537-42
5. Osborn M, Hawton K, Gath D. Sexual dysfunction among middle aged women in the community. *Br Med J* 1988;296:959-62
6. Di Benedetto P, Graziottin A. *Piacere e Dolore.* Trieste: Libreria Goliardica Editrice, 1997
7. Dow MGT, Hart DM. Hormonal treatments of sexual unresponsiveness in postmenopausal women: a comparative study. *Br J Obstet Gynaecol* 1983;90:361-6
8. Myers LS. Methodological review and meta-analysis of sexuality and menopause research. *Neurosci Biobehav Rev* 1995;19:331-41
9. Russo CM, Brose WG. Chronic pain. *Annu Rev Med* 1998;49:123-33
10. Butcher J. ABC of sexual health. Female sexual problems. II. Sexual pain and sexual fears [Clinical review]. *Br Med J* 1999;318:110-12
11. Bergeron S, Binik YM, Khalife S, *et al.* Vulvar vestibulitis syndrome: a critical review. *Clin J Pain* 1997;13:27-42
12. Goetsch MF. Vulvar vestibulitis: prevalence and historic features in a general gynecologic practice population. *Am J Obstet Gynecol* 1991;164:1609-16
13. Gilliland R, Heymen JS, Altomare DF, *et al.* Biofeedback for intractable rectal pain: outcome and predictors of success. *Dis Colon Rectum* 1997;40: 190-6
14. Reid R. The management of genital condylomas, intraepithelial neoplasia and vulvodynia. *Obstet Gynecol Clin North Am* 1996;23:917-91
15. Paavonen J. Diagnosis and treatment of vulvodynia. *Ann Med* 1995;27:175-81
16. Sinaki M, Merritt JL, Stillwell GK. Tension myalgia of the pelvic floor. *Mayo Clin Proc* 1977;52:717-22

17. Iosif CS. Effects of protracted administration of estriol on the lower genitourinary tract in postmenopausal women. *Acta Obstet Gynecol Scand* 1992;251:115–20
18. Greendale GA, Judd JL. The menopause: health implications and clinical management. *J Am Geriatr Soc* 1993;41:426–36
19. Cardozo L, Bachmann G, McClish D, *et al.* Meta-analysis of estrogen therapy in the management of urogenital atrophy in postmenopausal women: second report of the Hormones and Urogenital Therapy Committee. *Obstet Gynecol* 1998;92:722–7
20. Laan E, Lunsen RHW. Hormones and sexuality in postmenopausal women: a psychophysiological study. *J Psychosom Obstet Gynecol* 1997;18:126–33
21. Graziottin A. The biological basis of female sexuality. *Int Clin Psychopharmacol* 1998;13(Suppl 6):S15–22
22. Masters WH, Johnson VE, Kolodny RC. *Heterosexuality*. Glasgow: Harper Collins Publishing, 1994
23. Levin RJ. The mechanism of human female sexual arousal. *Ann Rev Sex Res* 1992;3:1–48
24. Goldstein I, Berman JR. Vasculogenic female sexual dysfunction: vaginal engorgement and clitoral erectile insufficiency syndromes. *Int J Impotence Res* 1998;10:S84–90
25. Tarcan T, Park K, Goldstein I, *et al.* Histomorphometric analysis of age-related structural changes in human clitoral cavernosal tissue. *J Urol* 1999;161: 940–4
26. Sarrel PM, Whitehead MI. Sex and menopause: defining the issues. *Maturitas* 1985;7:217–24
27. Weber AM, Walters MD, Schover LR, *et al.* Vaginal anatomy and sexual function. *Obstet Gynecol* 1995; 86:946–9
28. Jeffcoate TNA. Posterior colpoperineorrhaphy. *Am J Obstet Gynecol* 1959;77:490
29. Korlof B, Nylen K, Tillenger G, *et al.* Different methods of reconstruction after vulvectomies for cancer of the vulva. *Acta Obstet Gynecol Scand* 1975;54:41
30. Woodruff JD, Genadry R, Poliakoff S. Treatment of dyspareunia and vaginal outlet distortions by perineoplasty. *Obstet Gynecol* 1981;57:750–4
31. Reid R. Flash lamp excited dye laser. *Contemp Obstet Gynecol* 1995;40:78–90
32. Reid R, Omoto KH, Precop SL, *et al.* Flashlamp-excited dye laser therapy of idiopathic vulvodynia is safe and efficacious. *Am J Obstet Gynecol* 1995;172: 1684–96, discussion 1696–701
33. Francis WJA, Jeffcoate TNA. Dyspareunia following vaginal operations. *J Obstet Gynaecol Br Commonw* 1961;68:1–10
34. Haase P, Skibsted L. Influence of operations for stress incontinence and/or genital descensus on sexual life. *Acta Obstet Gynecol Scand* 1988;67: 659–61
35. Holley RL, Varner RE, Gleason BP, *et al.* Sexual function after sacrospinous ligament fixation for vaginal vault prolapse. *J Reprod Med* 1996;41:355–8
36. Weber AM, Walters MD, Schover LR, *et al.* Vaginal anatomy and sexual function. *Obstet Gynecol* 1995; 86:946–9
37. Given FT, Muhlendorf IK, Browning GM. Vaginal length and sexual function after colpopexy for complete uterovaginal eversion. *Am J Obstet Gynecol* 1993;169:284–8
38. Barlow DH, Cardozo L, Francis RM, *et al.* Urogenital ageing and its effect on sexual health in older British women. *Br J Obstet Gynaecol* 1997;104: 87–91
39. Sarrel PM. Sexuality and menopause. *Obstet Gynecol* 1990;75(Suppl):26S–30S
40. Mulherin DM, Sheeran TP, Kumararatne DS, *et al.* Sjögren's syndrome in women presenting with chronic dyspareunia. *Br J Obstet Gynaecol* 1997;104: 1019–23
41. Faro S. Vaginitis: diagnosis and management. *Int J Fertil Menopausal Stud* 1996;41:115–23
42. Heller DS, Randolph P, Young A, *et al.* The cutaneous vulvar clinic revisited: 5 years experience of the Columbia Presbyterian Medical Center Cutaneous Vulvar Service. *Dermatology* 1997;195:26–9
43. Friedrich EG Jr. Vulvar vestibulitis syndrome. *J Reprod Med* 1987;32:110–14
44. Smith RJN, Studd JWW. Recent advances in hormone replacement therapy. *Br J Hosp Med* 1993;49:799–809
45. Ashman RB, Ott AK. Autoimmunity as a factor in recurrent vaginal candidosis and the minor vestibular gland syndrome. *J Reprod Med* 1989;34:264–6
46. Horowitz BJ. Mycotic vulvovaginitis: a broad overview. *Am J Obstet Gynecol* 1991;165:1188–92
47. Travell J, Simons D. *Myofascial Pain and Dysfunction. The Trigger Points Manual*, Vol 1. Baltimore, MD: Williams and Wilkins, 1983
48. Wesselmann U, Burnett AL, Heinberg LJ. The urogenital and rectal pain syndromes. *Pain* 1997;73: 269–94
49. Slocumb JC. Neurological factors in chronic pelvic pain: trigger points and the abdominal pelvic pain syndrome. *Am J Obstet Gynecol* 1984;149:536–43
50. De Lancey JO, Sampselle CM, Punch MR. Kegel dyspareunia: levator ani myalgia caused by overexertion. *Obstet Gynecol* 1993;82:658–9
51. Heah SM, Ho YH, Tan M, *et al.* Biofeedback is effective treatment for levator ani syndrome. *Dis Colon Rectum* 1997;40:187–9
52. Thiele GH. Coccygodynia: cause and treatment. *Dis Colon Rectum* 1963;6:422–36
53. Turner MLC, Marinoff SC. Pudendal neuralgia. *Am J Obstet Gynecol* 1991;165:1233–6
54. McKay M. Subsets of vulvodynia. *J Reprod Med* 1988;33:695–8

55. Andersen KV, Bovim G. Impotence and nerve entrapment in long distance amateur cyclists. *Acta Neurol Scand* 1997;95:233–40
56. Gillespie L, Bray R, Levin N, *et al.* Lumbar nerve root compression and interstitial cystitis - response to decompressive surgery. *Br J Urol* 1991;68:361–4
57. Robert R, Prat Pradal D, Labat JJ, *et al.* Anatomic basis of chronic perineal pain: role of the pudendal nerve. *Surg Radiol Anat* 1998;20:93–8
58. Shafik A, el Sherif M, Youssef A, *et al.* Surgical anatomy of the pudendal nerve and its clinical implications. *Clin Anat* 1995;8:110–15
59. Shafik A. Pudendal canal syndrome as a cause of vulvodynia and its treatment by pudendal nerve decompression. *Eur J Obstet Gynecol Reprod Biol* 1998; 80:215–20
60. Tayal SC, Watson PG. Dyspareunia in undiagnosed Sjögren's syndrome. *Br J Clin Pract* 1996;50:57–8
61. Costello C, Smith JR. Vulvodynia associated with coeliac disease. *Br J Obstet Gynaecol* 1996;103:1162–3
62. Fukaya T, Hoshiai H, Yajima A. Is pelvic endometriosis always associated with chronic pain? A retrospective study of 618 cases diagnosed by laparoscopy. *Am J Obstet Gynecol* 1993;169:719–22
63. Sweet RL, Gibbs RS. Pelvic inflammatory disease. In Sweet R, Gibbs RS, eds. *Infectious Disease of the Female Genital Tract (Part 1).* Baltimore, MD: Williams and Wilkins, 1985:53–77
64. Rapkin AJ. Adhesions and pelvic pain: a retrospective study. *Obstet Gynecol* 1986;68:13–15
65. Beard RW, Highman JH, Pearce S, *et al.* Diagnosis of pelvic varicosities in women with chronic pelvic pain. *Lancet* 1984;2:946–9
66. Andersen BL. Sexual functioning complications in women with gynecologic cancer. Outcomes and directions for prevention [Review]. *Cancer* 1987;60 (Suppl 8):2123–8
67. Bonica JJ. Pelvic and perineal pain caused by other disorders. In Bonica JJ, ed. *The Management of Pain II.* Philadelphia: Lea and Febiger, 1990;69:1383–94

The role of selective estrogen receptor modulators in the prevention of cardiovascular disease

74

N. K. Wenger

INTRODUCTION

Interest in postmenopausal hormone therapy for cardioprotection derives from evidence that coronary heart disease (CHD) predominates in postmenopausal women, that CHD has an earlier onset and an increased relative risk of coronary death in women with bilateral oophorectomy or premature ovarian failure, and that CHD is the leading cause of mortality in American women. Furthermore, women have less favorable outcomes following myocardial infarction and myocardial revascularization procedures than do their male counterparts[1-3]. Selective estrogen receptor modulators (SERMs), non-hormonal agents that bind with high affinity to estrogen receptors, exhibit both estrogen agonist-like effects and estrogen antagonist-like effects, depending on the target tissue. Thus, these compounds offer the estrogen-like potential for cardioprotection, without some of the risks of estrogen therapy.

POSTMENOPAUSAL ESTROGEN THERAPY: INFORMATION REGARDING CARDIOPROTECTION

A sizeable literature[4,5] describes favorable and consistent observational data for the cardioprotective effect of estrogen in postmenopausal women, with a 35–50% coronary survival benefit seen in hormone users compared with non-users. This relates both to unopposed estrogen therapy and to combined estrogen–progestin use. Whether this reflects a true protective effect of hormone therapy or the selection of low-risk women for such therapy remains uncertain. More pronounced benefit is described for women with documented CHD and with severe as compared with mild to moderate CHD. A few contradictory reports have appeared in recent years[6], with data suggesting a lack of cardiac protection. Inherent weaknesses of observational studies include the selection bias just cited, compliance bias and healthy survivor bias, all of which may spuriously inflate the cardioprotection attributed to hormone use. Therefore, randomized trial data with clinical outcomes are necessary for definitive evaluation. Several such trials are currently under way[7,8].

Biologically plausible mechanisms of estrogen benefit augment the interest in its use[4,9]. Estrogen favorably affects lipid levels, increasing high-density lipoprotein (HDL) cholesterol and decreasing low-density lipoprotein (LDL) cholesterol concentrations by 10–15% each, with a decrease also reported in lipoprotein (a) (Lp(a)). An undesired effect is that estrogen uniformly elevates triglyceride levels. Other favorable metabolic and coagulation features include a decrease in fibrinogen, a decrease in plasminogen activator inhibitor-1 (PAI-1) and an increase in fibrinolysis. These improvements in lipid profiles and other intermediate markers for CHD have been documented in a randomized, placebo-controlled intermediate outcomes trial, the Postmenopausal Estrogen/Progestin Intervention (PEPI) trial[10]. Although a decrease in homocysteine levels has been reported, an unfavorable estrogen effect is an increase in levels of C-reactive protein, a marker of inflammation[11]. Major recent attention has been focused on the vascular effects of estrogen, both receptor and non-receptor mediated. Estrogen has antioxidant effects, limiting oxidation of LDL and thereby increasing nitric oxide availability; nitric oxide is a potent vasodilator. Estrogen use is associated with decreased levels of endothelin and with enhanced prostacyclin production, which also favor vasodilatation. There is also modulation of ion channels with calcium antagonist effects and opening of potassium channels with resultant vasodilatation. There is decreased proliferation and migration of smooth muscle cells, an early step in atherosclerotic lesion formation. A number of studies suggest that estrogen may decrease plaque formation or rupture, with resultant reduction in the risk of coronary occlusion.

Although a number of the non-cardiovascular effects of estrogen also provide benefit, including the prevention of bone loss and osteoporotic fractures, and reduction of menopausal and urogenital symptoms of estrogen deficiency, its attendant risks are of concern. Unopposed estrogen use is associated with atypical or adenomatous endometrial hyperplasia, a precursor of endometrial cancer, such that concurrent administration of a progestin is indicated for women with an intact uterus. The major problem for women regarding hormone use is the risk of breast cancer. Breast cancer risk appears to be most prominent in women with more than 5 years of hormone use and for women older than 60 years of age, with both long-term use and older age characteristic of women who use hormones for cardioprotection[12,13]. Furthermore, there is a two- to three-fold increased risk of venous thromboembolism and an increased risk of gallbladder disease. Women often discontinue estrogen use owing to undesirable side-effects, predominantly vaginal bleeding and breast pain or tenderness.

The only randomized controlled clinical trial data for postmenopausal hormone therapy available to date derive from the Heart and Estrogen/progestin Replacement Study (HERS)[14], a trial of estrogen plus progestin in postmenopausal women younger than 80 years of age with established CHD and an intact uterus. In the 2763 women followed for an average duration of 4.1 years, treatment with 6.25 mg of conjugated equine estrogen plus 2.5 mg of medroxyprogesterone acetate daily did not reduce the primary outcome measure, i.e. non-fatal myocardial infarction or coronary death. Despite the 11% decrease in LDL cholesterol and 10% increase in HDL cholesterol in the hormone group compared with the placebo group, there was also no difference in other cardiovascular outcomes, including coronary revascularization procedures, hospitalization for unstable angina or heart failure, peripheral arterial disease and stroke or transient ischemic attack. There was a three-fold increased relative risk of venous thromboembolism, and a 40% increased risk of gallbladder disease. Of major concern was the statistically significant time trend in coronary events, such that hormone-treated women had an excess of coronary events in year 1 (relative risk 1.52) with fewer events in years 4 and 5 (relative risk 0.67). The mechanism(s) responsible for these early and late effects remain poorly understood, but may be clarified with longer-term follow-up of the HERS cohort. Therefore, current recommendations are that postmenopausal women with established CHD do not initiate this hormone regimen for cardioprotection. Nonetheless, given the favorable pattern of coronary events after several years of therapy, it might be appropriate for currently treated women with CHD to continue such hormone therapy.

These adverse outcomes of hormone use further stimulated interest in the role of selective estrogen receptor modulators (SERMs) to reduce CHD risk in postmenopausal women.

CURRENTLY AVAILABLE SERMs

The two SERMs for which clinical data are available are tamoxifen, a non-steroidal triphenylethylene derivative used for the prevention and treatment of breast cancer; and raloxifene, a benzothiophene derivative, approved for the prevention and treatment of osteoporosis. Raloxifene, in addition to its role in the prevention of osteoporosis, is currently under investigation for the prevention of breast cancer.

Tamoxifen, however, is an incomplete SERM, in that, unlike raloxifene, it induces endometrial proliferation and increases the risk for endometrial cancer. Therefore, it is unlikely to be evaluated for cardioprotection, particularly given its currently recommended duration of use limited to 5 years (tamoxifen prescribing information: Zeneca Inc., Wilmington, DE; 1998). Nonetheless, in clinical trials involving women with breast cancer, tamoxifen had a favorable effect on lipid

Table 1 Effects of hormone replacement therapy (HRT) and selective estrogen receptor modulators on surrogate markers of coronary disease. From reference 15, with permission

	HRT	*Tamoxifen*	*Raloxifene*
Lipoproteins			
HDL-C	improved	no effect	no effect
LDL-C	improved	improved	improved
Triglycerides	worsened	worsened or no effect	no effect
Lp(a)	improved	–	improved
Coagulation factors			
Fibrinogen	improved	improved	improved
PAI-1	improved	–	no effect
Inflammatory markers			
Homocysteine	improved	–	no effect or improved
CRP	worsened	–	no effect

HDL, high-density lipoprotein; C, cholesterol; LDL, low-density lipoprotein; Lp(a), lipoprotein(a); PAI-1, plasminogen activator inhibitor-1; CRP, C-reactive protein

profiles, reduced fibrinogen levels and levels of Lp(a), but did not increase HDL cholesterol (Table 1)[15]. Tamoxifen also has favorable antioxidant effects. Although reduction in the incidence of fatal and non-fatal myocardial infarction was reported from the randomized controlled clinical trials conducted by the National Surgical Adjuvant and Breast and Bowel Project (NSABP), the Scottish Cancer Trial's Breast Group and the Stockholm Breast Cancer Study Group, a recent meta-analysis did not identify a significant reduction in cardiovascular mortality in tamoxifen-treated women[16].

PRECLINICAL STUDIES OF RALOXIFENE SUGGESTING THE POTENTIAL FOR CARDIOPROTECTION

A spectrum of preclinical studies has suggested that the SERM raloxifene shares many of the favorable effects of estrogen on lipid metabolism and on the blood vessel wall. Raloxifene decreased the concentration of serum cholesterol in ovariectomized rats and limited the accumulation of cholesterol in the aorta of ovariectomized, cholesterol-fed rabbits[17]. In the latter model, this benefit was independent of changes in serum cholesterol levels. Raloxifene blocked the oxidation of human HDL and enhanced the release or availability of nitric oxide from vascular endothelium[18,19]. Inhibition of vascular smooth muscle cell migration was also shown to be related to raloxifene use. Although raloxifene inhibited cholesterol accumulation in the aorta of ovariectomized, cholesterol-fed rabbits[17], there was no effect on coronary atherosclerosis in ovariectomized monkeys compared with the effect of estrogen therapy[20].

INTERMEDIATE-OUTCOMES: CLINICAL TRIAL DATA FOR RALOXIFENE

Raloxifene, given to 390 healthy postmenopausal women, was examined for its effect on intermediate outcomes, i.e. cardiovascular risk factors and other metabolic parameters (Tables 1 and 2)[21–24]. In this randomized clinical trial[21], raloxifene significantly decreased the levels of both total and LDL cholesterol, without an increase in total HDL cholesterol or in serum triglyceride levels. Despite the lack of increase in total HDL cholesterol, there was a substantial increase in HDL_2, the subfraction considered to provide cardioprotection. Raloxifene also lowered levels of Lp(a) and fibrinogen. Whether these favorable effects on coronary risk factors will translate into reductions in coronary events must be determined by a randomized clinical trial.

In two osteoporosis trials[22,23], raloxifene also reduced total cholesterol and LDL cholesterol levels, did not alter total HDL but increased HDL_2, increased lipoprotein(a) 1 and lowered apolipoprotein B; serum triglyceride levels were not increased significantly (Table 2). These effects of raloxifene on markers of cardiovascular risk

Table 2 Effects of raloxifene on markers of risk of coronary heart disease, in three studies. From reference 24, with permission

	Change (%)					
Treatment	*LDL-C*	*HDL-C*	*TC*	*Triglycerides*	*Lp(a)*	*Fibrinogen*
Draper *et al.*, 1996[22] (mean change)						
Placebo	−4.0	+4.4	−1.4	–	–	–
Raloxifene:						
200 mg/day	−9.5	+5.7*	−5.3	–	–	–
600 mg/day	−12.6	+1.5*	−9.7*	–	–	–
Postmenopausal estrogen therapy	−11.2	+20.9	−1.4	–	–	–
Delmas *et al.*, 1997[23] (median change)						
Placebo	−1.0	−4.7	−1.2	0	–	–
Raloxifene						
30 mg/day	−6.2†	−3.1	−5.2†	0	–	–
60 mg/day	−10.1†	−3.7	−6.4†	+3.2	–	–
150 mg/day	−14.1†	−4.5	−9.7†	+0.5	–	–
Walsh *et al.*, 1998[21] (median change)						
Placebo	+1	+1	–	0	+3	−2
Raloxifene						
60 mg/day	−11‡	+1**	–	−4**	−4†,**	−12††,‡
120 mg/day	−11‡	+4††	–	0**	−4†,**	−14††,‡
HRT	−13‡	+11‡	–	+20‡	−16‡	−3

LDL-C, low-density lipoprotein cholesterol; HDL-C, high-density lipoprotein cholesterol; TC, total cholesterol; Lp(a), lipoprotein (a); HRT, hormone replacement therapy; *$p < 0.05$ compared with postmenopausal estrogen therapy; †$p < 0.05$ compared with placebo; ‡$p < 0.001$ compared with placebo; **$p < 0.001$ compared with HRT; ††$p < 0.05$ compared with HRT

resemble those of tamoxifen. Indeed, these are the attributes that may underlie the apparent cardioprotective effect of tamoxifen seen in some but not all reports of clinical trials of tamoxifen in women with breast cancer.

The safety profile of raloxifene in approximately 8000 postmenopausal women enrolled in osteoporosis studies is important. There was no evidence of endometrial proliferation or bleeding. The occurrence of breast pain or tenderness did not differ from that in women receiving placebo. There was no increase in the risk of endometrial cancer, and a significantly reduced risk of breast cancer was evident[21,23].

The symptomatic side-effects of raloxifene include hot flushes and leg cramps, but these were not of a severity to cause greater discontinuation of the drug than of placebo in these clinical trials. The serious adverse effect of raloxifene is a two- to three-fold increase in the risk of venous thromboembolism, comparable to that associated with postmenopausal hormone therapy.

THE RALOXIFENE USE FOR THE HEART (RUTH) TRIAL

Because both preclinical and clinical trial data suggest that raloxifene may decrease cardiovascular risk in postmenopausal women, a cardiovascular outcomes trial of raloxifene is currently under way. The Raloxifene Use for The Heart (RUTH) trial plans to enroll 10 000 postmenopausal women older than 55 years of age in 26 countries, with a scheduled follow-up of approximately 5 years. The primary clinical outcome is a combination of coronary death and non-fatal myocardial infarction. Secondary outcomes include all-cause mortality, all-cause hospitalizations, coronary revascularization procedures, stroke, breast cancer and fractures. Women eligible for participation in the RUTH trial include those with prior myocardial infarction, coronary artery bypass graft surgery, percutaneous transluminal coronary angioplasty and women with angina pectoris and angiographically documented CHD. Women at increased risk for CHD, i.e. those with multiple risk factors (diabetes mellitus, peripheral arterial disease, smoking, hypertension, hyperlipidemia), will also be included. Criteria for exclusion are a history of venous thromboembolism, breast or other cancer, class III-IV heart failure, severe hepatic or renal disease, and anticipated survival of under 5 years. Participating women cannot take estrogen, estrogen/progestin, tibolone, or other selective estrogen receptor modulator drugs. They also cannot take cholestyramine or any other investigational drug.

SUMMARY

Because raloxifene has beneficial estrogen-like effects in preventing bone loss and decreasing vertebral fractures, without estrogen agonist effects on the endometrium or breast, use of this category of drugs suggests the ability to segregate the beneficial and adverse effects of estrogen. Clinical trial data are requisite to determine whether the SERM raloxifene offers cardioprotection for postmenopausal women. Nonetheless, as with estrogen, raloxifene increases the risk of venous thromboembolism.

References

1. Wenger NK. Coronary heart disease: an older woman's major health risk. *Br Med J* 1997;315: 1085-90
2. Chandra NC, Ziegelstein RC, Rogers WJ, *et al.* Observations of the treatment of women in the United States with myocardial infarction: a report from the National Registry of Myocardial Infarction-I. *Arch Intern Med* 1998;158:981-8
3. Edwards FH, Carey JS, Grover FL, *et al.* Impact of gender on coronary bypass operative mortality. *Ann Thorac Surg* 1998;66:125-31
4. Wenger NK. Postmenopausal hormone therapy: is it useful for coronary prevention? *Cardiol Clin* 1998;16:17-25
5. Barett-Connor E, Grady D. Hormone replacement therapy, heart disease and other considerations. *Annu Rev Publ Health* 1998;19:55-72
6. Sidney S, Petitti DB, Quesenberry CP Jr. Myocardial infarction and the use of estrogen and estrogen-progestogen in postmenopausal women. *Ann Intern Med* 1997;127:501-8
7. The Women's Health Initiative Study Group. Design of the Women's Health Initiative clinical trial and observational study. *Control Clin Trials* 1998;19:61-109
8. Vickers MR, Mead TW, Wilkes HC. Hormone replacement therapy and cardiovascular disease: the case for a randomized controlled trial. *Ciba Found Symp* 1995;191:150-64
9. Gerhard M, Ganz P. How do we explain the clinical benefits of estrogen? From bedside to bench. *Circulation* 1995;92:5-8
10. Writing Group for the PEPI Trial. Effects of estrogen or estrogen/progestin regimens on heart disease risk factors in postmenopausal women: the Postmenopausal Estrogen/Progestin Interventions (PEPI) trial. *J Am Med Assoc* 1995;273:199-208
11. Cushman M, Meilahn EN, Kuller LH, *et al.* Hormone replacement therapy (HRT) and markers of hemostasis and inflammation in elderly women [abstr]. *Circulation* 1998;97:84
12. Grodstein F, Stampfer MJ, Colditz GA, *et al.* Postmenopausal hormone therapy and mortality. *N Engl J Med* 1997;336:1769-75
13. Collaborative Group on Hormonal Factors in Breast Cancer. Breast cancer and hormone replacement therapy: collaborative reanalysis of data from 51 epidemiological studies of 52,075 women with breast cancer and 108,411 women without breast cancer. *Lancet* 1997;350:1047-59
14. Hulley S, Grady D, Bush T, *et al.*, for the Heart and Estrogen/progestin Replacement Study (HERS) Research Group. Randomized trial of estrogen plus progestin for secondary prevention of coronary heart disease in postmenopausal women. *J Am Med Assoc* 1998;280:605-13
15. Wenger NK, Grady D. Postmenopausal hormone therapy, selective estrogen receptor modulators, and coronary heart disease in women. *J Endocrinol Invest* 1999;22:616-24
16. Early Breast Cancer Trialists' Collaborative Group. Tamoxifen for early breast cancer: an overview of the randomised trials. *Lancet* 1998;351:1451-67
17. Bjarnason NH, Haarbo J, Byrjalsen I, *et al.* Raloxifene inhibits aortic accumulation of cholesterol in

ovariectomized, cholesterol-fed rabbits. *Circulation* 1997;96:1964–9

18. Zuckerman SH, Bryan N. Inhibition of LDL oxidation and myeloperoxidase-dependent tyrosyl radical formation by the selective estrogen receptor modulator raloxifene (LY139481 HCL). *Atherosclerosis* 1996;126:65–75
19. Rahimian R, Laher I, Dube G, *et al.* Estrogen and selective estrogen receptor modulator LY117018 enhance release of nitric oxide in rat aorta. *J Pharmacol Exp Ther* 1997;283:116–22
20. Clarkson TB, Anthony MS, Jerome CP. Lack of effect of raloxifene on coronary artery atherosclerosis of postmenopausal monkeys. *J Clin Endocrinol Metab* 1998;83:721-6
21. Walsh BW, Kuller LH, Wild RA, *et al.* Effect of raloxifene on serum lipids and coagulation factors in healthy, postmenopausal women. *J Am Med Assoc* 1998;279:1445–51
22. Draper MW, Flowers DE, Huster WJ, *et al.* A controlled trial of raloxifene (LY139481) HCL: impact on bone turnover and serum lipid profile in healthy postmenopausal women. *J Bone Miner Res* 1996;11:835–42
23. Delmas PD, Bjarnason NH, Mitlak BH, *et al.* Effects of raloxifene on bone mineral density, serum cholesterol concentrations, and uterine endometrium in postmenopausal women. *N Engl J Med* 1997;337:1641–7
24. Wenger NK. Effects of selective estrogen receptor modulators on coronary disease risk factors. *Contemp Obstet Gynecol* 1999;44(suppl):17–31

The potential effects of SERMs on breast cancer prevention

75

C. A. Stuenkel

INTRODUCTION

Women are increasingly aware of the potential risks and sequelae of osteoporosis and coronary heart disease, but breast cancer remains their greatest fear. Globally, the risk of breast cancer varies significantly between nations. Differences in risk may be due to diet, environmental factors or differences in reproductive patterns. Measures to reduce estrogen stimulation of the breast from either exogenous or endogenous sources might reduce breast cancer incidence. The evolution of selective estrogen receptor modulators (SERMs), pharmacological agents with estrogen agonist action in some tissues (ideally, the bone and cardiovascular system) and estrogen antagonist effects in other tissues (ideally, the breast and uterus), could provide alternative preventive strategies for postmenopausal women. In two large clinical trials, the SERMs tamoxifen and raloxifene reduced the risk of breast cancer. Questions remain, however, about efficacy, safety and candidates for the chemoprevention of breast cancer.

BREAST CANCER: THE SCOPE OF THE PROBLEM

Breast cancer is the most common malignancy in women[1]. In 1990, 796 000 cases were reported, representing 21% of all new cases of cancer in women. By 2010, over 1.35 million new cases are anticipated. In 1990, breast cancer claimed 314 000 lives, 14.1% of all cancer deaths in females. Worldwide, breast cancer is the leading cause of cancer mortality in women.

ESTROGEN EXPOSURE AND RISK OF BREAST CANCER

Increased exposure to exogenous or endogenous estrogen might increase the risk of breast cancer. Early menarche, late menopause and prolonged hormone replacement therapy (HRT) have all been identified as possible contributing factors. The Collaborative Group on Hormonal Factors in Breast Cancer collected and re-analyzed data from 51 epidemiological studies in 21 countries, representing 90% of the world-wide evidence[2]. Of the 52 705 women with breast cancer and 108 411 women without breast cancer who were included, approximately one-third were postmenopausal, one-third had used HRT at some time and one-third of HRT users had used hormones for more than 5 years. Increasing duration of HRT was associated with a 2.3% per year increased relative risk of breast cancer. After 5 years, the risk increased by 35%. The higher risk, however, declined to the normal range 5 years after therapy was discontinued.

The uncertain risk of breast cancer with prolonged HRT remains a concern. Fear of breast cancer has often been cited as a reason why postmenopausal women do not continue taking HRT for longer than a few years. More definitive data about HRT and breast cancer risk should be forthcoming from two large randomized clinical trials: the Women's Health Initiative (WHI) in the USA and the Women's International Study of long Duration Oestrogen after Menopause (WISDOM) trial in the UK.

The risk of HRT is important to establish, but the contribution of endogenous estrogen may be more significant for a greater number of women. In the Collaborative Group re-analysis, women with a late menopause had an increased risk of breast cancer of 2.8% per year for every year that menopause was delayed[2]. More recently, in the Study of Osteoporotic Fractures, a prospective observational study of 9704 women at least 65 years of age followed for 3.2 years, the risk of breast cancer was correlated with a single measure of serum bioavailable estradiol in 97 cases of breast cancer and 244 controls[3]. For women with bioavailable estradiol in the highest quartile (≥ 6.83 pmol/l), the relative risk of breast cancer was found to be 3.6 times that of women with the lowest concentration. The authors proposed using a single measurement of bioavailable estradiol to identify women at highest risk of breast cancer who might benefit from chemopreventive therapy.

TAMOXIFEN FOR BREAST CANCER PREVENTION

The idea to use a SERM with antiestrogen actions in the breast for cancer prevention stems from tamoxifen trials in women with early breast cancer. The recent analysis by the Early Breast Cancer Trialists' Collaborative Group included randomized clinical trials initiated before 1990 comparing adjuvant tamoxifen therapy to placebo in women to whom tamoxifen was given before the recurrence of breast cancer[4]. Data were collected and analyzed centrally on 37 000 women from 55 trials, representing 87% of the world-wide evidence. In women with estrogen-receptor-positive breast cancer, 5 years of tamoxifen therapy significantly reduced breast cancer recurrence by 47% and reduced overall mortality by 26%. Regardless of estrogen receptor status, 5 years of tamoxifen therapy reduced contralateral breast cancer by 47%, with the benefit persisting for an additional 5 years after tamoxifen therapy was stopped.

THE BREAST CANCER PREVENTION TRIAL

To investigate whether the preventive benefits of tamoxifen might extend to healthy women at high risk for breast cancer, the National Surgical Adjuvant Breast and Bowel Project established the P-1 Breast Cancer Prevention Trial (BCPT)[5]. This study was initiated in 1992, enrolled 13 388 women from the USA and Canada at increased risk for breast cancer, and randomly assigned participants to placebo or tamoxifen 20 mg orally per day (Table 1). Five years of follow-up was planned. Eligibility was based on breast cancer risk: women ≥ 60 years of age, women with a history of lobular carcinoma *in situ* and women between 35 and 59 years of age with a 5-year predicted breast cancer risk of ≥ 1.66% based on the Gail model. The Gail model for risk assessment is a computer algorithm based on a multivariate logistic regression model provided by the National Cancer Institute that takes into account age, number of first-degree relatives with breast cancer, number of previous breast biopsies, presence of atypical hyperplasia on biopsy, age at first live birth and age at menarche.

After 55 months of follow-up, an independent Data and Safety Monitoring Board terminated the

Table 1 Summary of randomized breast cancer prevention trials

	BCPT[5]	*Royal Marsden Hospital trial*[6]	*Italian study*[7]	*MORE*[8]
SERM	tamoxifen	tamoxifen	tamoxifen	raloxifene
Dosage (mg/day)	20	20	20	60 or 120
No. of women	13 175	2471	5408	7705
Breast cancer risk	high (Gail model)	family history	hysterectomy/oophorectomy	osteoporosis
Median age (years)	39% < 50	47	51	67
Estrogen use (%)	< 10	26	14	< 10
Median follow-up period (months)	55	70	46	40

BCPT, Breast Cancer Prevention Trial; MORE, Multiple Outcomes of Raloxifene Experience; SERM, selective estrogen receptor modulator study because of the significant 50% reduction in both invasive and non-invasive breast cancer incidence with tamoxifen therapy versus placebo (Table 2). The beneficial effect of tamoxifen was evident only in women with estrogen-receptor-positive cancer. Based upon the BCPT findings, the Food and Drug Administration in the USA approved the use of tamoxifen, 20 mg per day for 5 years, for the prevention of breast cancer in women with a 5-year risk of at least ≥ 1.66%.

Enthusiasm following the publication of the results of the BCPT has been tempered by safety concerns regarding tamoxifen. Endometrial cancer (Table 3) and venous thromboembolic events (Table 4) increased significantly, as did a trend toward an increase in stroke, particularly for women over 50 years of age. All endometrial cancers, however, were Stage I; no endometrial cancer deaths occurred. There was no overall risk or benefit when rates of ischemic heart disease were compared between tamoxifen and placebo groups. The rates for myocardial infarction, severe angina or acute ischemic syndromes were not significantly different. A non-significant reduction in fractures of the hip, spine and wrist was observed, with 137 total fractures in the placebo group and 111 fractures in the tamoxifen group (relative risk 0.81, 95% confidence interval 0.63–1.05).

Table 2 Breast cancer incidence and estrogen receptor status

	Cancer incidence				*Receptor status*					
	Total cancers		*Invasive cancers*		*ER-positive*		*ER-negative*		*Unknown*	
	Placebo	*Treated*	*Placebo*	*Treated*	*Placebo*	*Treated*	*Placebo*	*Treated*	*Placebo*	*Treated*
BCPT[5]	244	124*	175	89	130	41	31	38	14	10
RR			0.51		0.31					
95% CI			0.39–0.66		0.22–0.45					
Royal Marsden Hospital trial[6]	36	34	32	30	–	–	–	–	–	–
RR	1.1									
95% CI	0.7–1.7									
Italian study[7]	22	19	–	–	8	10	–	–	–	–
MORE[8†]	32	22	27	13	20	4	4	7	3	2
RR	0.35		0.24		0.10					
95% CI	0.21–0.58		0.13–0.44		0.04–0.24					

*Non-invasive cancers were significantly reduced (RR 0.50, 95% CI 0.33–0.77); †twice as many women received treatment with raloxifene as with placebo; BCPT, Breast Cancer Prevention Trial; MORE, Multiple Outcomes of Raloxifene Experience; RR, relative risk; CI, confidence interval

Table 3 Endometrial cancer in breast cancer prevention trials

	BCPT[5]	*Royal Marsden Hospital trial*[6]	*Italian study*[7]	*MORE*[8]
Cases				
placebo	15	1	–	4
treatment	36	4	–	6
Risk ratio	2.53			0.8
95% confidence interval	1.35–4.97			0.2–2.7

BCPT, Breast Cancer Prevention Trial; MORE, Multiple Outcomes of Raloxifene Experience

Table 4 Venous thromboembolic events in breast cancer prevention trials

	Pulmonary embolus	*DVT*	*Combined thromboembolic events (pulmonary embolus + DVT)*		
	BCPT[5]	*BCPT*[5]	*Royal Marsden Hospital trial*[6]	*Italian study*[7]	*MORE*[8]
Cases					
placebo	6	22	4	4	8
treatment	18	35	7	7	49*
Risk ratio	3.01	1.60	–	–	3.1
95% confidence interval	1.15–9.27	0.91–2.86			1.5–6.2

*Twice as many women received treatment with raloxifene as with placebo; DVT, deep vein thrombosis; BCPT, Breast Cancer Prevention Trial; MORE, Multiple Outcomes of Raloxifene Experience

OTHER TAMOXIFEN PREVENTION TRIALS

Concurrent with the Breast Cancer Prevention Trial in North America, two other tamoxifen prevention trials were under way in the UK and Europe (Table 1). Contrary to the findings of the BCPT, an interim analysis of both the Royal Marsden Hospital Tamoxifen Chemoprevention Trial[6] and the Italian Tamoxifen Prevention Study[7] failed to reveal a reduction of breast cancer incidence with tamoxifen therapy (Table 2).

An interim analysis of the Royal Marsden Hospital Tamoxifen Chemoprevention Trial[6], published after 70 months of follow-up of 2494 women in the 8-year trial, showed no difference in breast cancer rates between placebo and tamoxifen therapy (Table 2), although the rate of breast cancer was relatively high in the placebo group (Figure 1). The authors postulated that genetically transmitted breast cancers, characterized by a strong family history, might predominate in their population, which might explain the lack of tamoxifen effect. Genetic testing of the cohort who developed breast cancer and re-evaluation after the completion of the trial may shed further light on the differences in outcome from the BCPT.

The second negative trial, the Italian Tamoxifen Prevention Study[7], required hysterectomy for study eligibility (Table 1). Of the 5408 enrollees, 48% had undergone bilateral oophorectomy in addition to hysterectomy. These authors postulated that the low incidence of breast cancer in their placebo group was due to the high rate of oophorectomy, and the lack of effect of tamoxifen (Table 2) might be due to a lower anticipated benefit in women at low risk of breast cancer (Figure 1). Final analysis of this trial is also pending.

RALOXIFENE AND BREAST CANCER PREVENTION

In addition to tamoxifen, other SERMs with different risk/benefit profiles are under investigation. Raloxifene has been approved in the USA for osteoporosis prevention and treatment. Interest in raloxifene for breast cancer prevention originates from the recent findings of decreased breast cancer incidence in women taking raloxifene compared to women on placebo in the Multiple Outcomes of Raloxifene Experience (MORE) trial[8]. Breast cancers were reduced equally by 65% with both the 60 mg and 120 mg doses of raloxifene (Figure 1). Similar to the tamoxifen experience, estrogen-receptor-positive cancers were preferentially reduced (Table 2).

Raloxifene, in contrast to tamoxifen, did not increase endometrial cancer (Table 3). However, the risk of venous thromboembolic events is similar for the two agents (Table 4) and comparable to the increased risk reported with HRT in the Heart and Estrogen/progestin Replacement Study[9]. Raloxifene has already been reported to reduce bone loss and osteoporotic fractures[10]. Ongoing trials will establish whether or not raloxifene therapy will reduce coronary events.

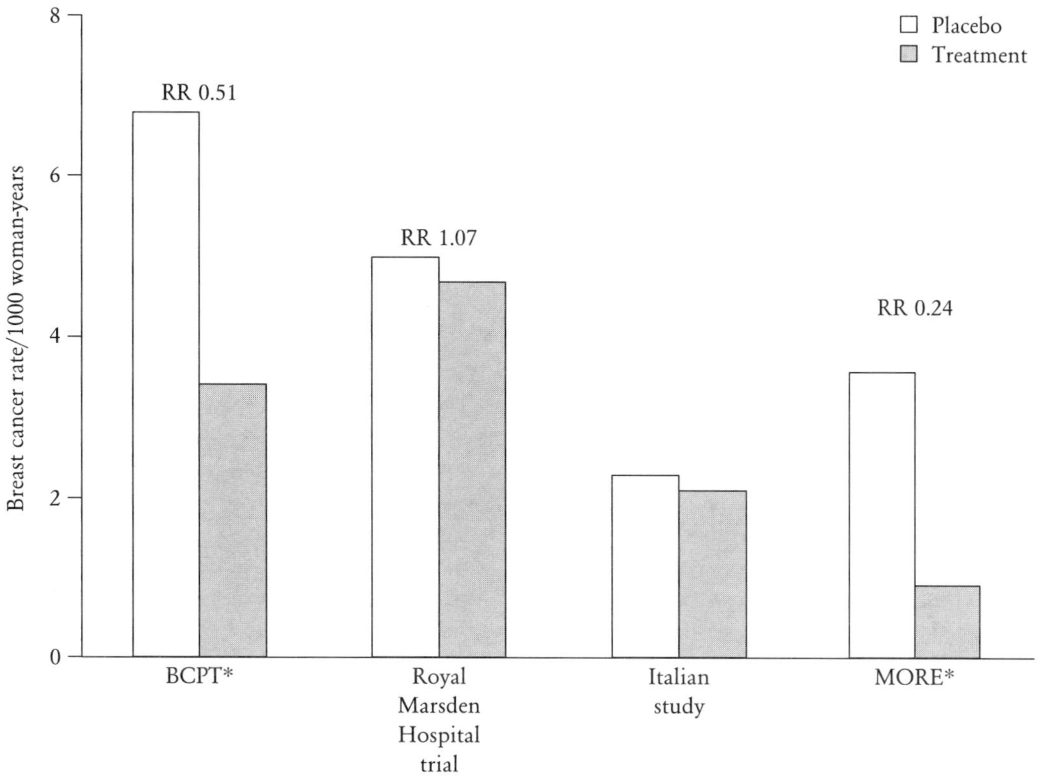

Figure 1 Breast cancer rates in chemoprevention trials. Women in the Breast Cancer Prevention Trial (BCPT) had the highest rate of breast cancer. Placebo rates in the Royal Marsden Hospital trial were twice that of the Italian group, which had the lowest placebo rate. Women in the Multiple Outcomes of Raloxifene Experience (MORE) trial had rates intermediate between the Italian and the Marsden trials. The majority of women in the MORE trial would have qualified for the BCPT based on age criteria. *Rates are for invasive cancers. RR, relative risk

RECOMMENDATIONS FOR BREAST CANCER REDUCTION

The American Society of Clinical Oncology (ASCO) reviewed the breast cancer prevention trials and developed clinical recommendations[11]. They concluded that tamoxifen, 20 mg/day for up to 5 years, may be offered to women with a defined 5-year projected risk of breast cancer of ≥ 1.66%. Women should be carefully counselled regarding the risks and benefits of tamoxifen. At this time, there is no evidence that co-morbidity or -mortality is reduced with tamoxifen therapy.

The ASCO review also stated that it is premature to recommend raloxifene to lower the risk of developing breast cancer outside of a clinical trial setting. Several ongoing clinical trials will further assess the effect of raloxifene on breast cancer. The CORE trial (Continuous Outcomes Relevant to Evista) will enrol 5000 of the MORE participants for an additional 4 years of follow-up, extending the raloxifene experience to 8 years. The RUTH trial (Raloxifene Use for the Heart) is enrolling 10 000 women with documented coronary heart disease or risk factors for heart disease. In addition to coronary events and deaths, breast cancer is an outcome measurement.

To evaluate specifically women at high risk for breast cancer, the National Cancer Institute initiated the STAR trial (Study of Tamoxifen and Raloxifene)[12]. The STAR trial will determine whether raloxifene is more or less effective than tamoxifen at reducing the incidence of invasive breast cancer in postmenopausal women who are at increased risk for the disease and whether raloxifene reduces the rate of endometrial cancer compared to tamoxifen. The STAR trial is currently enrolling 22 000 women who have a 5-year risk of breast cancer ≥ 1.66% according to the Gail model used in the BCPT. Women will be randomized to tamoxifen 20 mg/day or raloxifene 60 mg/day. The study will be event driven; follow-up is anticipated for 5 years.

BREAST CANCER PREVENTION: REMAINING QUESTIONS

Though the breast cancer prevention trials have provided important new information, new questions are also raised. As elaborated in the ASCO assessment, additional studies are needed to determine the safety and efficacy of chemopreventive agents. Issues related to patient selection still remain: is the minimum criterion for the Gail model really the most appropriate group, or should preventive therapy be reserved for women at higher risk (as enrolled in the BCPT)? While 5 years of tamoxifen therapy have been shown to be optimal in women with a history of breast cancer, is 5 years the optimum duration for the prevention of breast cancer? Would longer therapy be more effective? Will more cancers be prevented or might more cancers ultimately be promoted (as with > 5 years of tamoxifen therapy)? What happens when tamoxifen or raloxifene is combined with HRT? Is there any role for the use of tamoxifen and raloxifene in combination or sequentially? Is it safe to start raloxifene after a course of tamoxifen in women with a history of breast cancer?

CONCLUSION

In spite of the unanswered questions, two agents have now been shown in randomized clinical trials to reduce the incidence of breast cancer in women. We are on the threshold of a new era in which breast cancer prevention is a reality. Further elucidation of the risks and benefits of raloxifene and tamoxifen, and the development of other SERMs under investigation, will hopefully lead to agents that prevent breast cancer and provide additional health benefits while minimizing the endometrial and thromboembolic risks.

References

1. Parkin DM, Pisani P, Ferlay J. Global cancer statistics. *CA Cancer J Clin* 1999;49:33–64
2. Collaborative Group on Hormonal Factors in Breast Cancer. Breast cancer and hormone replacement therapy: collaborative reanalysis of data from 51 epidemiological studies of 52 705 women with breast cancer and 108 411 women without breast cancer. *Lancet* 1997;350:1047–59
3. Cauley JA, Lucas FL, Kuller LH, *et al.* Elevated serum estradiol and testosterone concentrations are associated with a high risk for breast cancer. *Ann Intern Med* 1999;130:270–7
4. Early Breast Cancer Trialists' Collaborative Group. Tamoxifen for early breast cancer; an overview of the randomized trials. *Lancet* 1998;351:1451–67
5. Fisher B, Costanino JP, Wickerham L, *et al.* Tamoxifen for prevention of breast cancer: report of the National Surgical Adjuvant Breast and Bowel Project P-1 Study. *J Natl Cancer Inst* 1998;90: 1371–88
6. Powles T, Eeles R, Ashley S, *et al.* Interim analysis of the incidence of breast cancer in the Royal Marsden Hospital tamoxifen randomized chemoprevention trial. *Lancet* 1998;352:98–101
7. Veronisi U, Maisonneuve P, Costa A, *et al.* Prevention of breast cancer with tamoxifen: preliminary findings from the Italian randomized trial among hysterectomised women. *Lancet* 1998;352:93–7
8. Cummings SR, Eckert S, Krueger KA, *et al.* The effect of raloxifene on risk of breast cancer in postmenopausal women. *J Am Med Assoc* 1999;281: 2189–97
9. Hulley S, Grady D, Bush T, *et al.* Randomized trial of estrogen plus progestin for secondary prevention of coronary heart disease in postmenopausal women. *J Am Med Assoc.* 1999;280:605–13
10. Ettinger B, Black DM, Mitlak BH, *et al.* Reduction of vertebral fracture risk in postmenopausal women with osteoporosis treated with raloxifene. *J Am Med Assoc* 1999;282:637–45

11. Chlebowski RT, Collyar DE, Somerfield RM, *et al.* American Society of Clinical Oncology technology assessment on breast cancer risk reduction strategies: tamoxifen and raloxifene. *J Clin Oncol* 1999;17: 1939-55

12. Jordan VC, Morrow M. Tamoxifen, raloxifene, and the prevention of breast cancer. *Endocr Rev* 1999;20: 253-78

Raloxifene: safety considerations and side-effects

76

D. W. Purdie

Raloxifene as a selective estrogen receptor modulator is, by definition, an agent that will selectively agonistically engage estrogen receptors in bone and the cardiovascular system while selectively antagonistically engaging estrogen receptors in the endometrium and breast tissue. An absolute minimum of adverse events is to be anticipated in these areas. Since raloxifene will often be prescribed to patients who cannot, will not or should not take conventional hormone replacement therapy (HRT) formulations, it is essential that, overall, it has a safety and side-effect profile which confers significant advantages over its parent regimen. Raloxifene has been subjected to the most meticulous safety examinations since it emerged from its phase II trials; volunteer exposure to the drug now amounts to some 33 000 woman-years.

Overall, raloxifene is safe, with no reports of excess all-cause mortality in treated patients. There have been no reports of significant blood dyscrasias and no reports of neoplasia. Vital signs and general hematological and biochemical parameters appear to be unaffected by the drug.

The engagement of breast and uterine receptors by conventional HRT regimes is a major factor in the rejection of such treatments by patients and in the high rate of discontinuation observed in many studies. Our own and other studies have shown that a return to cyclic bleeding and the fear of breast cancer are, respectively, the first and second reasons most commonly advanced by patients who fail to continue with treatment[1]. It is to address these problems, among others, that the selective estrogen receptor modulators (SERMs) were developed.

With regard to the uterus, both animal studies and human trials have shown convincingly that raloxifene, in contrast to estrone or estradiol, is not associated with profileration of the endometrium[2]. Histologically, it is not associated either with eosinophilia or stromal histological changes and there is no evidence of an increase in uterine blood flow - again as seen with estradiol. The endometrial depth as measured by ultrasound over 24 months is no greater than the depth observed in placebo-treated controls and clinically this is attested by the fact that there has been no excess of reports of vaginal bleeding among raloxifene-treated patients, again compared to controls[3]. Therefore, raloxifene does not appear to share the partial endometrial agonism of tamoxifen which has been reported to cause endometrial proliferation, hyperplasia and neoplasia in a number of reports. A recent report[4] from the Multiple Outcomes Raloxifene Evaluation (MORE) trial showed no increase in the risk of endometrial cancer in treated women who displayed a relative risk of 0.8 (95% CI 0.2–2.7).

The effects of raloxifene on breast tissue have been covered elsewhere in this symposium and, in summary, raloxifene may be said to cause no excess of mastalgia over that observed in controls and its effect upon the incidence of breast cancer is most encouraging, with a significant reduction in estrogen receptor-positive breast cancers observed in raloxifene-treated osteoporotic women.

With regard to adverse events in general, careful observation was made throughout the phase III clinical trials for the occurrence of side-effects. In the MORE study, which randomized 7700 women to raloxifene or placebo, three significant side-effects were observed, which were more common in the raloxifene 60 mg group than in controls. These side-effects were hot flushes, leg cramps and peripheral edema. However, the incidence of clinically severe hot flushes and leg cramps was extremely low, as is attested by the fact that only about 1 in 11 of patients entered in the MORE study withdrew, citing such side-effects as the reason for withdrawal. Overall, three-quarters of all patients randomized to raloxifene reported no hot flushes and, in those who did, the duration and severity were usually transient and mild, respectively.

The most significant side-effect noted with raloxifene was venous thromboembolic phenomena. In summary, the excess of such events was comparable to the excess observed in previous studies involving conventional HRT and often occurred within the first 6 months of therapy. A recent report on the outcomes from the MORE trial showed an overall relative risk of venous thromboembolic events of 3.1 (95% CI 1.5-6.2). Thus the same caveat should apply to the use of raloxifene as applies to the use of conventional HRT. It should be used with caution in any patient displaying a personal or family history of deep venous thrombosis (DVT) and should be regarded as contraindicated where such a history is backed up by radiological confirmation of the event. As is well known, there is a major mismatch between suspicion of DVT and actuality, and therefore in practical terms if the patient's history shows that she had been anticoagulated at the time of the suspected venous thromboembolic event then this should probably be taken as equivalent to confirmation.

In summary, raloxifene, given in its standard dose of 60 mg/day, is well tolerated and should prove a valuable adjunct to the range of treatments available to the physician charged with the prevention and treatment of postmenopausal osteoporosis, specially where the patient is personally or clinically disbarred from the use of conventional estrogen.

References

1. Purdie DW, Steel SA, Howey S, *et al.* The technical and logical feasibility of population examination using DEXA and directed HRT intervention: with two year follow up. *Osteoporosis Int* 1996;3:S31-6
2. Boss SM, Huster WJ, Neild JA, *et al.* Effects of Raloxifene on the endometrium of postmenopausal women. *Am J Obstet Gynecol* 1997;177:1458-64
3. Delmas PD, Bjarnason NH, Mitlak BH, *et al.* Effects of raloxifene on bone mineral density, serum cholesterol and endometrium in postmenopausal women. *N Engl J Med* 1997;337:1641-7
4. Cummings SR, Eckert S, Krueger KA, *et al.* The effect of raloxifene on risk of breast cancer in postmenopausal women. Results from the MORE randomized trial. *J Am Med Assoc* 1999;281:2189-97

Aging of the hypothalamic–pituitary–gonadal axis in men

77

J. M. Kaufman

In men, androgen production as well as fertility can be largely preserved until very old age. Indeed, aging in healthy men is normally not accompanied by abrupt or drastic alterations of gonadal function. Aging of the reproductive system in males thus differentiates itself from that in women, in whom the menopause, the ineluctable consequence of ovarian depletion of oocytes, signals the rather abrupt end of reproductive function and near total cessation of gonadal hormone production. Therefore, an 'andropause', defined as the male equivalent of the menopause, does not exist. Nevertheless, gonadal function in healthy men does not remain unaffected by the aging process. Aging in healthy men is accompanied by a substantial, albeit variable, progressive decline of Leydig cell function and more subtle changes in Sertoli cell function and spermatogenesis.

DECLINING LEYDIG CELL FUNCTION IN AGING MEN

Testosterone production and serum levels

Several early reports have shown decreased testosterone production rates in elderly men, but aging is also accompanied by a reduction of the metabolic clearance rate of testosterone[1-3]. In any case, it is now well established from the findings of a series of cross-sectional studies (see references 4 and 5 for review), more recently confirmed by longitudinal studies[6,7] involving large groups of healthy men, that serum testosterone levels decrease with age. The mean total serum testosterone level in the male population decreases by about 30% between the ages of 25 and 75 years[4,5]. Most of the testosterone in the circulation is bound to serum proteins, i.e. tightly bound to sex hormone binding globulin (SHBG) or rather weakly bound to albumin; only the free and part of the albumin-bound testosterone is readily available for biological action at the tissue level. Looking at the biologically active fractions of testosterone, the effect of aging on the androgen status is even more pronounced, with an approximately 50% decrease between the ages of 25 and 75. The steeper decline of the free (or bioavailable) serum testosterone levels as compared to the total serum testosterone levels is explained by an age-associated increase in SHBG binding capacity[8]. There is a circadian variation of serum testosterone in men, with the highest levels in the early morning and the lowest levels in the late afternoon, which is markedly blunted in elderly men[9]. Therefore, the age-related decline in serum (free) testosterone is most clearly demonstrated when blood sampling is performed in the morning before 10.00.

Whereas the mean serum testosterone levels in the adult male population decrease with age, there is a remarkable interindividual variability of serum total and free testosterone levels, with some men having frankly low serum testosterone levels while many others have preserved testosterone secretion and serum levels well within the normal range for young adults. However, with advancing age, the distribution of serum testosterone levels in the population shifts towards lower values with a progressively larger proportion of men having subnormal values relative to those in young adults. More than one out of five men over the age of 60 years present with subnormal serum testosterone levels, this proportion increasing to over one out of three of the men older than 80 years[4,8]. The age-related decrease of free (bioavailable) serum testosterone levels is paralleled by a decrease of similar magnitude of the testosterone concentrations in most, but not all, tissues[10]. As to testosterone metabolites, there is a significant age-related decrease of serum levels of 5α-androstane-3α-17βdiol-glucuronide[11]. There is no apparent decrease of dihydrotestosterone, but serum levels are not a reliable parameter of tissular dihydrotestosterone formation. The effectiveness of testosterone aromatization increases with age, probably owing to increased fat mass, resulting in maintained total serum estradiol levels in the elderly; there is, however, a significant age-related decrease of bioavailable estrogen levels[12].

Factors affecting serum testosterone levels in elderly men

The mechanisms underlying the striking inter-individual variability of serum testosterone levels in the elderly (as well as in younger men) are still not fully explained. However, several factors contributing to this variability have been identified and include genetic, physiological and lifestyle-related factors (see references 5 and 13 for review).

Twin studies have shown that total serum testosterone levels as well as SHBG levels and free testosterone levels are partly determined by genetic factors, but the nature of the underlying genetic mechanisms has not yet been elucidated. As to the physiological factors, the circadian rhythm of serum testosterone should not play a major role if serum testosterone levels are consistently measured in the morning (but in daily clinical practice serum testosterone levels are often measured later during the day). There is an ultradian rhythm of serum testosterone, this hormone being secreted episodically. Nevertheless, when looking at serum testosterone levels in two blood samples obtained at 1-year intervals in a large group of elderly men, we observed a rather good correlation ($r = 0.8$). The occurrence of seasonal variations of serum testosterone with an amplitude of about 25% have also been reported.

Several metabolic and hormonal factors influence SHBG serum levels and thus also serum total testosterone levels. In clinical studies, the body mass index (BMI) emerges as an important determinant of SHBG levels with, for the whole range of clinically encountered BMI values, a highly significant negative correlation between SHBG and testosterone serum levels, an effect probably mediated in part by insulin. In elderly men, this inverse relationship between BMI and SHBG levels can be clearly demonstrated, notwithstanding the background of an age-related rise of SHBG levels. Whereas moderate obesity affects only total serum testosterone by lowering SHBG binding capacity, in morbid obesity (BMI > 35–40) free testosterone levels are also decreased, as a result of neuroendocrine disturbances.

As to factors related to lifestyle, reports on the effects of diet on serum testosterone levels have not been concordant, but the available data indicate that fiber-rich vegetarian diets are associated with higher SHBG and testosterone levels in comparison with Western-type diets with high fat content.

Prolonged fasting transiently suppresses testosterone production through reduced gonadotropic testicular stimulation. Smoking has been associated with higher testosterone levels than in non-smokers, this effect being observed both in young and in elderly men, with the difference amounting to 5–15% of the levels in non-smokers[5]. Both physical and psychological stress, as well as strenuous physical activity, have been shown to suppress serum testosterone levels transiently. Alcohol abuse, also in the absence of cirrhosis of the liver, may accentuate the age-associated decrease of serum testosterone.

The 30% decrease in serum total testosterone and 50% decrease in serum free testosterone observed between the ages of 25 and 75 years in ambulatory, healthy men can be further accentuated by a series of intercurrent diseases with higher prevalence in the elderly population (see references 5, 13 and 14 for review). Acute critical illness, acute myocardial infarction and surgical injury have been shown to cause profound, but generally transient, decreases of free testosterone levels. Several chronic diseases can induce more long-standing decreases in testosterone levels. The latter include, non-exhaustively, diabetes mellitus, coronary atherosclerosis (low testosterone cause or consequence?), chronic renal failure, rheumatoid arthritis (mainly during acute flares) and peri-arteritis nodosa. Sleep apnea syndrome is accompanied by relative hypogonadism, with massive obesity often being a contributing factor. Finally, one should also consider a possible role of medications, among which a special mention should be made of glucocorticoids, resulting in a high prevalence of subnormal serum testosterone levels during chronic use.

Physiopathology of declining Leydig cell function in senescence

The decrease of serum free testosterone levels in healthy aging men is the result of the combined effects of primary testicular changes, of altered neuroendocrine regulation of Leydig cell function and of an independent increase of serum SHBG levels (see references 5 and 15–18 for review).

Changes at the testicular level are revealed by a diminished response of testicular testosterone upon stimulation with human chorionic gonadotropin (hCG) (as a substitute for luteinizing hormone (LH)), the anatomical substrate for this observation being an age-related reduction of the number of Leydig cells in the testes. However, although the response to hCG is reduced in the elderly as compared to the young, a substantial response is still seen in most elderly men.

In accordance with the existence of a primary testicular defect in the elderly is the observation of a modest increase of basal serum (LH) levels. However, this increase is not always clearly present, and it is in any case of rather modest amplitude. As the reserve secretory capacity of the testes of elderly men, although diminished, is still sufficient, one might expect that the decreased testicular activity would be compensated for by increased production of pituitary LH such as to normalize serum testosterone levels. The fact that this is generally not observed indicates that aging is also accompanied by alterations in the neuroendocrine regulation of Leydig cell function, LH secretion being inadequate in the face of a prevalent relative hypoandrogenism. Several observations have confirmed the existence of age-related changes in the central compartment of the gonadal axis. First of all, the marked blunting of the circadian rhythm for testosterone, which is centrally regulated, has already been mentioned. Second, there are changes in the pulsatile pattern of LH secretion in the elderly, with an unchanged LH pulse frequency, but a reduced number of large-amplitude LH pulses and a reduced mean LH pulse amplitude. In fact, an unchanged LH pulse frequency should also be regarded as inappropriate. Indeed, in young men hypoandrogenism results in a compensatory increase of LH pulse frequency, which is not observed in the elderly.

The pituitary response to small physiological doses of exogenous gonadotropin releasing hormone (GnRH) is perfectly well maintained in the elderly. This indicates that the deficient LH secretion in the elderly results from hypothalamic rather than primary pituitary changes, with inadequate secretion of GnRH, the hypothalamic hormone that governs gonadotropin secretion. Further findings pointing towards changes at the hypothalamic level are the blunting of the circadian rhythm and a decreased response of LH secretion upon opiate receptor blockade. An important observation is that elderly men are more sensitive to the negative feedback effects of circulating testosterone on LH secretion. Also, this increased sensitivity to the negative feedback effects of testosterone points towards a hypothalamic component, since testosterone exerts its main feedback activity by acting on the so-called 'hypothalamic GnRH pulse generator'.

The mechanisms underlying the age-associated increase of serum SHBG levels are yet to be elucidated. A plausible working hypothesis is that this increase is the consequence of the reduced activity of the somatotropic axis, with reduced circulating levels of insulin-like growth factor-I (IGF-I). Several studies have shown an inverse correlation between IGF-I and SHBG serum levels; the increased circulating SHBG levels in young, growth-hormone-deficient men can be normalized by substitution with growth hormone. Increased plasma binding capacity results in a reduction of the biologically active free testosterone fraction, which in elderly men is not adequately compensated for by an increase of LH and testosterone secretion.

Clinical significance of age-related hypoandrogenism

Many of the clinical changes observed in healthy aging men are reminiscent of the clinical picture of hypogonadism in young men. Indeed, aging in men is generally accompanied by a decrease in general well-being, in virility, in sexual pilosity, in skin thickness, in energy and in muscular mass and strength, by an increase in upper and central body fat, by osteopenia, by decreases in libido and sexual drive and by a greatly increased frequency of impotence (see references 5, 13, 17 and 19–21 for review).

It therefore seems plausible that these clinical changes may be at least in part the consequence of (or accentuated by) the relative hypoandrogenism of the elderly. However, a causal link between hypoandrogenism and clinical changes in elderly men is still rather poorly documented by cross-sectional studies. Indeed, correlations between prevalent androgen levels and clinical variables such as fat mass, muscle mass and bone mineral content have been documented, but these associations are usually rather weak. An association between decreased androgen levels and decreased libido has been shown in some but not in all studies. Decreased androgen levels have also been associated with a more atherogenic serum lipid profile, but again these associations are rather weak. There are many possible reasons for the failure to show a stronger relationship between prevalent androgen levels and clinical indexes. First, these clinical changes are certainly multifactorially determined. Furthermore, the effects of hypoandrogenism may be confounded by the high prevalence of intercurrent diseases in the elderly male population. Also, long-term changes in serum androgens are imperfectly assessed by a single point testosterone measurement. Another explanation may be the existence of threshold effects for the action of androgens at the tissue levels. For instance, it has been shown that, in young men with artificially induced hypogonadism, normal sexual function can be restored with subnormal testosterone levels[22].

In any case, cross-sectional studies can never give proof of a causal relationship between hormonal changes and clinical changes. Therefore, it is important to perform longitudinal studies assessing prospectively the clinical changes in men with normal and in men with subnormal serum testosterone. Another approach is to assess the effects of testosterone replacement therapy in elderly men with subnormal testosterone levels. Recently, the results of the first well-controlled prospective clinical trials became available[23-25]. These preliminary findings showed a beneficial effect of testosterone treatment on body composition, with a decrease of fat mass and an increase of muscle mass, the findings for muscle strength being less consistent. There have also been reports of a modest beneficial effect of testosterone treatment on the bone mineral content in elderly men with borderline serum testosterone levels.

Whereas it is likely that hypoandrogenism in elderly men contributes to the clinical changes, it is clear that hypoandrogenism can be responsible for only some of these clinical changes. In this context, it is noteworthy that the relative hypoandrogenism of the elderly does not appear to play an important role in the high prevalence of erectile dysfunction. Indeed, in this regard other factors and in particular co-morbidity (e.g. diabetes, atherosclerosis, neurological pathology) play a more determinant role.

In the present state of the art it would not be reasonable to propose large-scale substitution therapy in the elderly. First, many outstanding questions have to be answered. At present, we do not know what are normal testosterone levels for the elderly. We need more information on possible changes in the sensitivity to androgen actions in older men; this sensitivity may differ according to the tissue being considered. On the other hand, there is also no reason to withhold androgen substitution treatment to elderly men who are clearly hypogonadal (i.e. with symptoms of hypogonadism and clearly low serum testosterone levels) after careful evaluation for possible contraindications such as active prostatic disease, elevated blood hematocrit or sleep apnea.

SERTOLI CELL FUNCTION AND SPERMATOGENESIS IN ELDERLY MEN

Aging in healthy men is accompanied by a progressive increase of mean follicle stimulating hormone (FSH) serum levels. This has generally been interpreted as indicating an age-related decrease of Sertoli cell function and spermatogenesis. However, most studies concerning the influence of age on the quality of the ejaculate have observed only minor changes, with a somewhat reduced ejaculate volume and somewhat decreased motility of the spermatozoa, with normal or even increased sperm concentration[26,27]. Moreover, a decreased ejaculatory frequency, as observed in elderly men[27], might account for at least part of these age-related changes, but may also mask more subtle changes in spermatogenic activity[28]. Further limitations of the few available studies on the quality of the ejaculate are the facts that they included only small numbers of men over the age of 60 years and that they may not have been representative of the overall elderly male population, as they often consisted of men attending a fertility clinic.

Recently, serum inhibin B has been shown to be the physiologically important form of inhibin in men, produced by the Sertoli cells and exerting negative feedback regulation of pituitary FSH secretion[29]. Serum inhibin B has been validated as a valuable marker of Sertoli cell function and spermatogenesis. In a recent study involving a large group of community-dwelling healthy men, we observed that the serum inhibin levels were somewhat lower in men after age 35 years compared to younger men, but were little affected by the aging process thereafter[30]. This finding supports the view that Sertoli cell function and spermatogenesis are fairly well maintained in aging men. Nevertheless, we observed the previously described progressive increase of serum FSH levels, with a progressive and marked age-related decrease of the ratio of serum inhibin B over serum FSH. The latter observation indicates that, whereas Sertoli cell function is well preserved in the elderly, this necessitates an increased drive by pituitary FSH.

SUMMARY

Aging in healthy men is accompanied by a progressive, albeit variable, decline of Leydig cell function, resulting in a progressive decrease of mean serum total testosterone with a more marked decrease of mean serum free testosterone in the population. After the age of 60 years, more than 20% of men present with subnormal levels as compared to those in young men. The decline in bioavailable androgen levels results from primary testicular changes, inadequate neuroendocrine compensatory mechanisms and an independent increase of serum SHBG levels.

Sertoli cell function and spermatogenesis in elderly men appear to be generally better preserved than androgen production. It appears that, in the case of Sertoli cell function and spermatogenesis, the age-related testicular changes are more adequately compensated for by an appropriate increase of pituitary FSH secretion.

ACKNOWLEDGEMENT

Part of this work has been supported by grant G0058.97 of the Fonds von Wetenschappellijk Onderzoek Vlaanderen.

References

1. Vermeulen A, Rubens R, Verdonck L. Testosterone secretion and metabolism in male senescence. *J Clin Endocrinol Metab* 1972;34:730-5
2. Giusti G, Gonneli P, Borreli D, *et al.* Age related secretion of androstenedione, testosterone and dihydrotestosterone by the human testes. *Exp Gerontol* 1975;10:241-5
3. Baker HWG, Burger HG, de Kretser DM, *et al.* Endocrinology of aging: pituitary testicular axis. In James VHT, ed. *Proceedings of the 5th International Congress of Endocrinology.* Amsterdam: Excerpta Medica Foundation, 1977:179-83
4. Vermeulen A. Androgens in the aging male - Clinical review 24. *J Clin Endocrinol Metab* 1991;73: 221-4
5. Kaufman JM, Vermeulen A. Declining gonadal function in elderly men. *Baillière's Endocrinol Metab* 1997;11:289-309
6. Pearson UJD, Blackman MR, Metter EJ, *et al.* Effect of age and cigarette smoking on longitudinal changes in androgens and SHBG in healthy males [abstr P2-129]. *Abstracts of the 77th Annual Meeting of the Endocrine Society.* Bethesda, MD: The Endocrine Society, 1995:322

7. Morley JE, Kaiser FE, Perry HM, *et al.* Longitudinal changes in testosterone, SHBG, LH, and FSH in healthy older males [abstr P1-158]. *Abstracts of the 10th International Congress of Endocrinology.* Bethesda, MD: The Endocrine Society, 1996:174
8. Vermeulen A, Kaufman JM, Giagulli VA. Influence of some biological indices on sex hormone binding globulin and androgen levels in aging and obese males. *J Clin Endocrinol Metab* 1996;81:1821-7
9. Bremner WJ, Vitiello MV, Prinz PN. Loss of circadian rhythmicity in blood testosterone levels with aging in normal men. *J Clin Endocrinol Metab* 1983;56:1278-81
10. Deslypere JP, Vermeulen A. Aging and tissue androgens. *J Clin Endocrinol Metab* 1981;53:430-4
11. Deslypere JP, Sayed A, Punjabi U, *et al.* Plasma 5α-androstane-3α, 17-diol and urinary 5α-androstane-3α, 17-diol glucuronide, parameters of peripheral androgen action: a comparative study. *J Clin Endocrinol Metab* 1982;54:386-91
12. Ferrini RL, Barrett-Connor E. Sex hormones and age: a cross-sectional study of testosterone and estradiol and their bioavailable fractions in community-dwelling men. *Am J Epidemiol* 1998; 147:750-4
13. Kaufman JM, Vermeulen A. Androgens in male senescence. In Nieschlag E, Behre HM, eds. *Testosterone - Action Deficiency Substitution.* Berlin: Springer, 1998:437-73
14. Handelsman DJ. Testicular dysfunction in systemic disease. *Endocrinol Metab Clin* 1994;23:839-52
15. Kaufman JM, Deslypere JP, Giri M, *et al.* Neuroendocrine regulation of pulsatile luteinizing hormone secretion in elderly men. *J Steroid Biochem* 1990;37:421-30
16. Vermeulen A, Kaufman JM. Role of the hypothalamo-pituitary function in the hypoandrogenism of healthy aging. *J Clin Endocrinol Metab* 1992;74:1226A-1226C
17. Tsitouras PD, Bulat T. The aging male reproductive system. *Endocrinol Metab Clin* 1995;24:297-315
18. Tenover JS, Matsumoto AM, Plymate SR, *et al.* The effects of aging in normal men on bioavailable testosterone and luteinizing hormone secretion: response to clomiphene citrate. *J Clin Endocrinol Metab* 1987;65:1118-26
19. Kaufman JM. Androgens, bone metabolism and osteoporosis. In Oddens B, Vermeulen A, eds. *Androgens and the Aging Male.* Carnforth, UK: Parthenon Publishing, 1996:39-60
20. Schiavi RC, Schreiner-Engel P, Mandeli J, *et al.* Healthy aging and male sexual function. *Am J Psychiatry* 1990;147:767-71
21. Tenover JS. Androgen administration to aging men. *Endocrinol Metab Clin* 1994;23:877-89
22. Gooren LJG. Androgen levels and sex functions in testosterone treated hypogonadal men. *Arch Sex Behav* 1987;16:463-76
23. Sih R, Morley JE, Kaiser FE, *et al.* Testosterone replacement in older hypogonadal men: a 12 month randomized controlled trial. *J Clin Endocrinol Metab* 1997;82:1661-7
24. Snyder PJ, Peachey H, Hannoush P, *et al.* Effect of testosterone treatment on bone mineral density in men over 65 years of age. *J Clin Endocrinol Metab* 1999;84:2647-53
25. Snyder PJ, Peachey J, Hannoush P, *et al.* Effect of testosterone treatment on body composition and muscle strength in men over 65 years of age. *J Clin Endocrinol Metab* 1999;84:2647-53
26. Nieschlag E, Lammers U, Freischem CW, *et al.* Reproductive functions in young fathers and grandfathers. *J Clin Endocrinol Metab* 1982;55: 676-81
27. Rolf C, Behre M, Nieschlag E. Reproductive parameters of older compared to younger men of infertile couples. *Int J Androl* 1996;19:135-42
28. Cooper TG, Keck C, Oberdieck U. Effects of multiple ejaculations after extended periods of sexual abstinence on total motile and normal sperm numbers as well as on accessory gland secretions from healthy normal and oligospermic men. *Hum Reprod* 1993;8:1251-8
29. Illingworth PJ, Groome NP, Byrd W, *et al.* Inhibin B: a likely candidate for the physiologically important inhibin form in men. *J Clin Endocrinol Metab* 1996;81:1321-5
30. Mahmoud AM, Goemaere S, Comhaire FH, *et al.* Serum inhibin B in healthy aging men. *Abstracts Endo '99. 81st Annual Meeting of the Endocrine Society,* San Diego, California, 1999:abstr P3-320

Fertility and fertility-related problems in the aging male

78

E. Nieschlag, M. Brinkworth, C. Rolf and A. Lerchl

The end of the millennium has seen great changes in health and lifestyle among most populations in the world. The expectations for length and quality of life, at least in developed countries such as Germany and Japan, are much greater now than ever before. One consequence of this is that individuals are not only now able to become parents at an older age, but many now choose to do so. Associations between risks for fertility and for the health of the offspring with advancing maternal age are well-documented, but the issue has not been adequately researched regarding the male. The purpose of this paper is to present evidence concerning any age-related impairment of male reproductive function and to consider the implications of advanced paternal age for the health of the offspring.

Although controversial for many years, it is now known that serum levels of testosterone show a slight age-related decline in healthy men, which might imply an impairment of reproductive function[1]. However, the decline is only small and probably partly due to a concomitant increase in the concentration of sex hormone binding globulin[2]. Only slight rises in gonadotropin levels occur up to a relatively advanced age (> 70 years), after which they may increase more[3], but what this implies for the efficacy of spermatogenesis is not known.

Data on semen parameters and testicular histology are very limited because of the scarcity of samples from healthy men. However, we have been able to show that elderly men attending our clinic as volunteers with proven prior fertility had comparable semen values (sperm concentration, morphology and motility, and hamster oocyte penetration test results) to those of younger patients or volunteers[3]. We were recently able to confirm these findings for infertility patients[4], which argues against an age-related decline in reproductive function.

Direct evidence of changes in fertility with age is hard to come by; however, birth statistics demonstrate that men are still able to father children to a much more advanced age than women. Data on the age of parents of children born in 1997 show that five men aged 71 years became fathers in Japan, while in Germany 27 71-year-olds became fathers (Figure 1). These men were about 20 years older than the oldest women to give birth in either country in that year (Figure 1). This is despite the fact that population age-distribution data from the Statistisches Bundesamt (Germany) and the Statistics Bureau (Japan) show that there is little difference in the proportion of males and females in either country and that, above the age of 60 years, there are indeed more women than men. Although there could be other (for example, social) reasons for this difference in the oldest reproductive ages, it is likely that the fertility of men is maintained for much longer than that of females.

The incidence of genetic disorders among the offspring of older mothers and fathers has been investigated in a number of studies. It is widely accepted that non-disjunction during meiosis in developing oocytes leads to an increased occurrence of syndromes associated with trisomy of various chromosomes. That this does not happen in the male presumably reflects a particular feature of this process in females rather than a general age-related deterioration in the fidelity of gametic division. However, there is evidence of an increased rate of spontaneous abortions with increasing age of the father (mirrored by an increase in pre-implantation losses in litters sired by old rats[5]), which suggests a decrease in the genetic quality of sperm produced by older men.

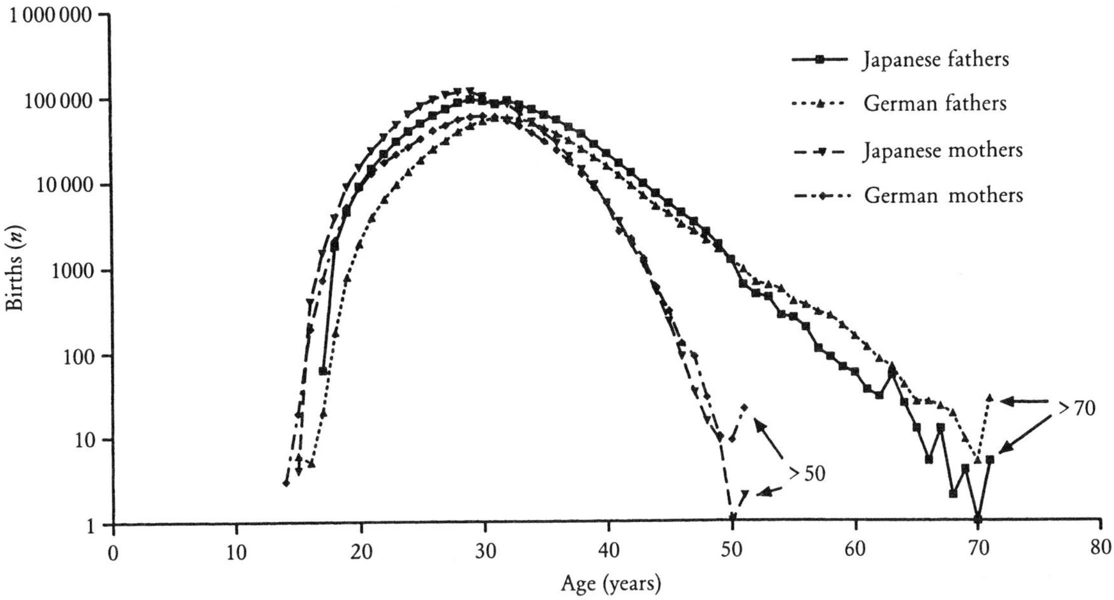

Figure 1 The age distribution of parents in Germany and Japan in 1997 (total: 66 340 (Germany) and 1 175 006 (Japan)). The points indicate the total number of children born to parents of a given age by sex (male or female) and nationality (German or Japanese). Data provided by the Statistisches Bundesamt (Germany) and the Statistics Bureau, Management and Co-ordination Agency (Japan)

This could have a number of causes, among which age-related increases in germ-line mutations and impairment of DNA repair and/or apoptotic processes are perhaps the most likely.

The mutation rate in the male germ line may partly be influenced by the higher number of cell divisions undertaken by male germ cells, but has a separate, age-dependent component[6]. The mutation rate in germ cells can be estimated directly by polymerase chain reaction-based methods if it is very high (~ 1%)[7]. Coding sequences never have spontaneous mutation rates as high as that, but mini- or microsatellites are often mutated at a detectable frequency.

The analysis of genetic diseases yields an indirect approach to the detection of germ-line mutations. In a study of fathers of children with genetic diseases (achondroplasia, polyposis coli, neurofibromatosis and Duchenne muscular dystrophy), their mean age was 6 years older than that of the controls[8], demonstrating an increased risk of genetic abnormality in the germ line with increasing age[9]. One explanation could be increasingly defective repair processes, which could also imply an increased sensitivity to genotoxins.

A number of genetic diseases have been associated specifically with paternal transmission, including: lipoprotein lipase deficiency caused by complete paternal isodisomy for chromosome 8[10]; type III spinal muscular atrophy (probably) caused by paternal isodisomy for chromosome 5[11]; and pyknodysostosis caused by paternal disomy for chromosome 1[12]. Such defects are potentially inducible by genotoxins, since smoking has been associated with increased disomy in sperm, even in young men[13]. Thus, if the risk of genetic aberrations arising in the germ line increases with age, older men may also have a higher chance of passing on genetic disease as a result of longer genotoxin exposure.

Little is known about whether the DNA repair capacity in developing spermatogenic cells declines with age, but recent studies have indicated a role for reduced paternal germ-cell apoptosis in the transmission of mutations leading to genetic defects in the offspring. Conflicting results have been obtained in rodents, since aged male rats show an increase in germ-cell apoptosis[14], but old mice do not[15]. However, oxidative stress in old male mice has been shown to decrease germ-cell apoptosis[15]. This could be significant, because work from our Institute has demonstrated an association between reduced paternal germ-cell apoptosis and the appearance of abnormalities among the offspring following long-term, low-dose cyclophosphamide exposure[16]. Furthermore, aging *per se* in male rats has been found to lead to lowered birth weight among the offspring[5]. Since apoptosis is known to occur (spontaneously) in the testes of both old[17] and young men[18], if the aged rodent models prove to be suitable for humans, genotoxins could be particularly hazardous for the male germ line in older, compared with younger, men.

References

1. Belanger A, Candas B, Dupont A, *et al.* Changes in serum concentrations of conjugated and unconjugated steroids in 40- to 80-year-old men. *J Clin Endocrinol Metab* 1994;79:1086–90
2. Gray A, Feldman HA, McKinlay JB, *et al.* Age, disease, and changing sex hormone levels in middle-aged men: results of the Massachusetts Male Aging Study. *J Clin Endocrinol Metab* 1991;73: 1016–25
3. Nieschlag E, Lammers U, Freischem CW, *et al.* Reproductive functions in young fathers and grandfathers. *J Clin Endocrinol Metab* 1982;55:676–81
4. Rolf C, Behre HM, Nieschlag E. Reproductive parameters of older compared to younger men of infertile couples. *Int J Androl* 1996;19:135–42
5. Serre V, Robaire B. Paternal age affects fertility and progeny outcome in the Brown Norway rat. *Fertil Steril* 1998;70:625–31
6. Crow JF. The high spontaneous mutation rate: is it a health risk? *Proc Natl Acad Sci USA* 1997;94: 8380–6
7. May CA, Jeffreys AJ, Armour JA. Mutation rate heterogeneity and the generation of allele diversity at the human minisatellite MS205 (D16S309). *Hum Mol Genet* 1996;5:1823–33
8. Risch N, Reich EW, Wishnick MM, *et al.* Spontaneous mutation and parental age in humans. *Am J Hum Genet* 1987;41:218–48
9. Bazhenova MD, Kozlova SI, Al'tshuler BA, *et al.* Analysis of the relation of the frequency of new gene mutations for Mendelian diseases to parental age. *Genetika* 1984;20:1726–32
10. Benlian P, Foubert L, Gagne V, *et al.* Complete paternal isodisomy for chromosome 8 unmasked by lipoprotein lipase deficiency. *Am J Hum Genet* 1996;59:431–6
11. Brzustowicz LM, Allitto BA, Matseoane D, *et al.* Paternal isodisomy for chromosome 5 in a child with spinal muscular atrophy. *Am J Hum Genet* 1994;54:482–8
12. Gelb BD, Willner JP, Dunn TM, *et al.* Paternal uniparental disomy for chromosome 1 revealed by molecular analysis of a patient with pycnodysostosis. *Am J Hum Genet* 1998;62:848–54
13. Rubes J, Lowe X, Moore D 2nd, *et al.* Smoking cigarettes is associated with increased sperm disomy in teenage men. *Fertil Steril* 1998;70:715–23
14. Barnes CJ, Covington BWt, Lee M. Effect of aging and dietary restriction on rat testicular germ cell apoptosis. *J Gerontol A Biol Sci Med Sci* 1999;54: B199–204
15. Barnes CJ, Covington BWt, Cameron IL, *et al.* Effect of aging on spontaneous and induced mouse testicular germ cell apoptosis. *Aging* 1998;10: 497–501
16. Brinkworth MH, Nieschlag E. Association of cyclophosphamide-induced male-mediated, foetal abnormalities with reduced paternal germ-cell apoptosis. *Mutation Res* 1999;in press
17. Brinkworth MH, Weinbauer GF, Bergmann M, *et al.* Apoptosis as a mechanism of germ cell loss in elderly men. *Int J Androl* 1997;20:222–8
18. Hikim AP, Wang C, Lue Y, *et al.* Spontaneous germ cell apoptosis in humans: evidence for ethnic differences in the susceptibility of germ cells to programmed cell death. *J Clin Endocrinol Metab* 1998;83:152–6

Epidemiological correlates of erectile dysfunction (impotence) and its biomedical significance

79

J. B. McKinlay

INTRODUCTION

There was very little reliable information on erectile dysfunction available until the very end of the 20th century[1]. Pioneering contributions made during the 1950s were not extended into later decades and half-century-old findings had little relevance to very different subsequent cohorts. That situation has changed dramatically - more has been learned about erectile dysfunction (a medical condition formerly termed 'impotence') during the past decade than was known during the rest of the 20th century combined. Prior to about 1985, most information on erectile dysfunction was based on clinical impressions and studies of convenience samples of atypical patients. Many considered erectile dysfunction to be a psychological problem, or a medical condition with, primarily, psychogenic origins. Erectile dysfunction is now receiving deserved attention for various reasons:

(1) There is increased understanding of the basic pathophysiology of erectile dysfunction;

(2) The recent, rapid, world-wide aging of the population is focussing attention on the health concerns of older people;

(3) Changes in urological practice (especially a decline in surgical procedures) are refocussing attention on erectile dysfunction;

(4) The recent availability of user-friendly oral medications (compared to surgery, penile injections and vacuum devices) has increased public interest in erectile dysfunction - the publicity surrounding oral sildenafil (Viagra®) may have increased public awareness and health education;

(5) Issues concerning the quality of life associated with major medial conditions (e.g. diabetes, coronary heart disease, cancer and depression) are receiving increased attention;

(6) Erectile dysfunction received 'official' recognition as a medical and public health problem at a 1992 National Institutes of Health Consensus Development Conference[2].

FROM OBSERVATION TO EXPERIMENTATION

Figure 1 summarizes the recent development of scientific knowledge concerning erectile dysfunction. Moves to the right-hand side of the figure (indicated with the bold arrow) represent improvement in the knowledge base, from uncontrolled observations to experimental evidence from field trials. Prior to about 1980, and with the notable exceptions of Kinsey[3] and Masters and Johnson[4], little was known about erectile dysfunction - clinical opinion prevailed. As the saying goes, everyone has a right to an opinion, but not every opinion is right! Real progress was made after the 1992 National Institutes of Health Consensus Conference on erectile dysfunction. Once a working definition was agreed upon ('the persistent inability to attain and maintain a penile erection adequate for sexual performance') investigators could begin to measure erectile dysfunction.

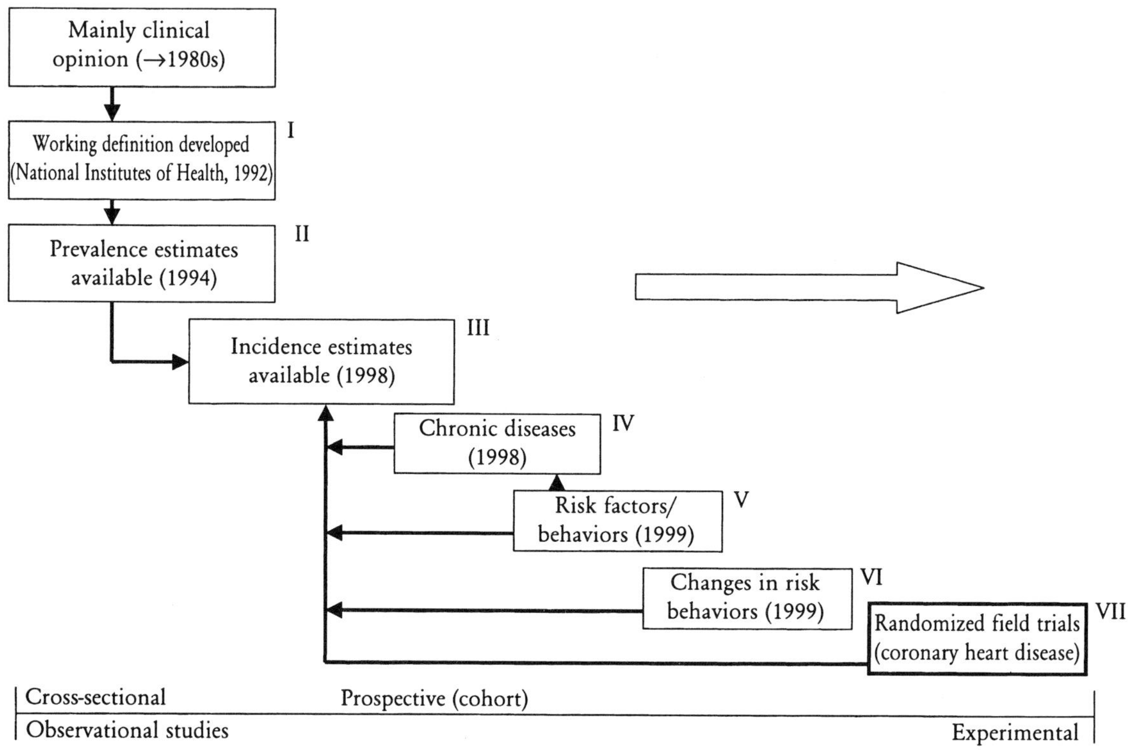

Figure 1 From observation to experimentation: history of the development of scientific knowledge concerning erectile dysfunction

THE MASSACHUSETTS MALE AGING STUDY (MMAS)

The Massachusetts Male Aging Study (MMAS) is the first major epidemiological investigation of erectile dysfunction[5,6]. It is unique in its scope, research design and field methods. The MMAS is a random-sample prospective study of health and aging in middle-aged men, addressing specific conditions of importance to older men (prostate cancer, hormone status and erectile function) in the context of comprehensive information on physiology, behavior, illness, medication, anthropometrics, sexual activity, psychology and life-style[7]. The MMAS baseline study (1987–89) established a cohort of 1709 men aged 40–70 years, of whom 1156 were re-interviewed in 1995–97. Figure 2 summarizes the overall research design of the MMAS, which had certain methodological advantages over earlier work:

(1) The cohort was a large, population-based random sample (not a selected clinic sample);

(2) The design was truly prospective (thus providing unbiased baseline data);

(3) Interviews were conducted in subjects' homes (including an inventory of current medications as well as body measurements, blood sampling and questionnaire data collection);

(4) A private, self-administered sexual activity instrument represented the state-of-the science in subjective assessment of erectile function;

(5) Blood drawing and handling were timed and controlled for diurnal variation and pulsatile emission to ensure accurate determination of 12 serum androgen and other hormone levels in a Centers for Disease Control-certified laboratory;

(6) Supplemental medical information was gathered from hospital records and state and national death registries.

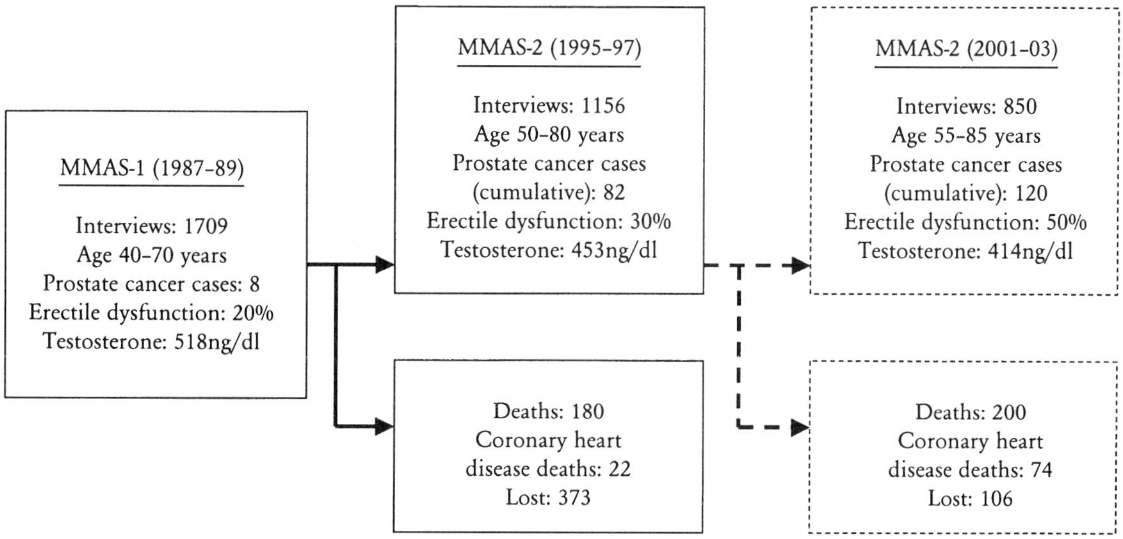

Figure 2 Description of the Massachusetts Male Aging Study (MMAS) cohort: MMAS-1 (1987–89), MMAS-2 (1995–97) and a proposed MMAS-3 (2001–03)

The MMAS is the largest population-based study to date with information on the prevalence, incidence and etiology of erectile dysfunction. It is the only large random sample study to provide longitudinal data regarding the epidemiology of erectile dysfunction and other aspects of sexual function in men over the age of 60 years. The study has provided important new cross-sectional and longitudinal information regarding changes in hormone status and sexual function with respect to aging, the relation of these changes to erectile dysfunction and prostate cancer, and preliminary evidence for a relationship between erectile dysfunction and cardiovascular disease.

PREVALENCE AND WORLD-WIDE BURDEN

Figure 3 summarizes the prevalence of minimal, moderate and complete erectile dysfunction from the baseline MMAS (1987–89). It should be noted that these estimates improve upon and refine our earlier published estimates[5], mainly as a result of a better method (a new discriminant function) for estimating erectile dysfunction in a population-based epidemiological study[8]. Our new approach is less susceptible to selection bias, results in less missing data and has greater construct validity than our earlier widely accepted method[5]. The prevalence and degree of erectile dysfunction (minimal, moderate and complete) clearly increases with age: while 8% of men in their 40s report either moderate or complete erectile dysfunction, this approaches 40% in men aged 60–69 years. In short, men between the ages of 60 and 69 years experience more than four times the level of moderate or complete erectile dysfunction compared to their 40–49-year-old counterparts.

Using recent MMAS estimates, Figure 4 shows the likely world-wide (age-adjusted) prevalence of erectile dysfunction between 1995 and 2025 (employing the most conservative (or lowest) United Nations population projections). The world-wide prevalence of erectile dysfunction will probably increase from 152 million men in 1995 to 322 million men in 2025 – an increase of 170 million[9]. Much of this increase is associated with the aging of the world's population. Other related factors (secular increases in weight, dietary changes, smoking behavior and an emerging diabetes pandemic) are also contributing to the increase.

The MMAS has provided the first incidence rates for erectile dysfunction. Incidence rates (which comprise new cases of a condition, or a transition from a non-diseased to a diseased state) obviously require prospective data for their calculation. Prior to the MMAS, the only published

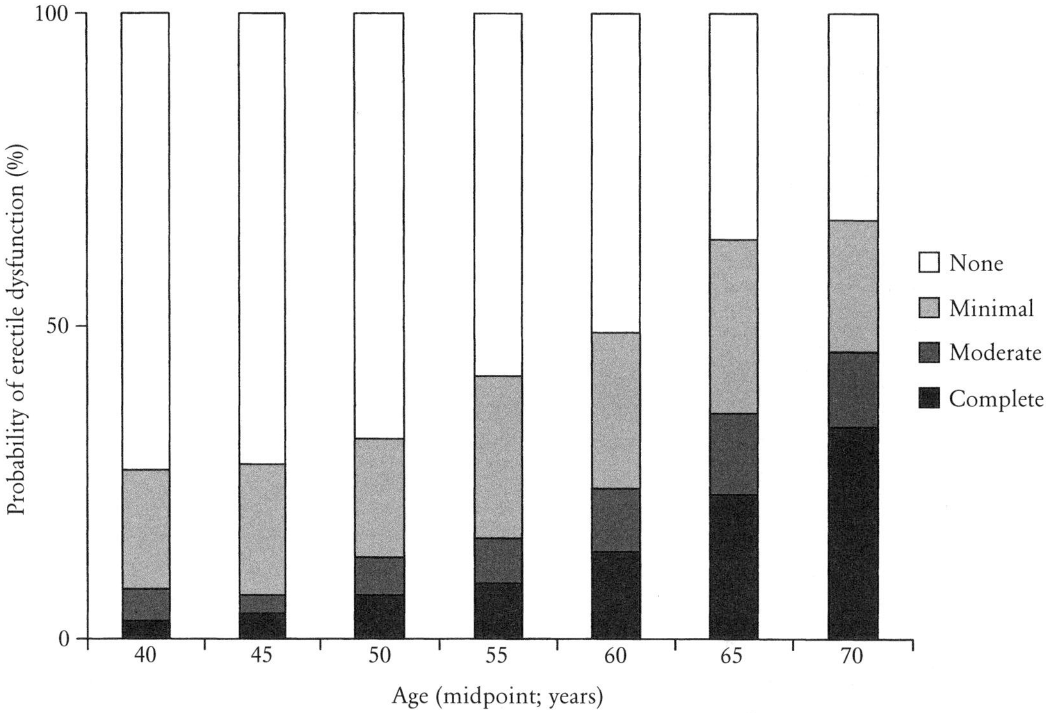

Figure 3 Prevalence of erectile dysfunction in the Massachusetts Male Aging Study, 1987–89 ($n = 1626$). From reference 8

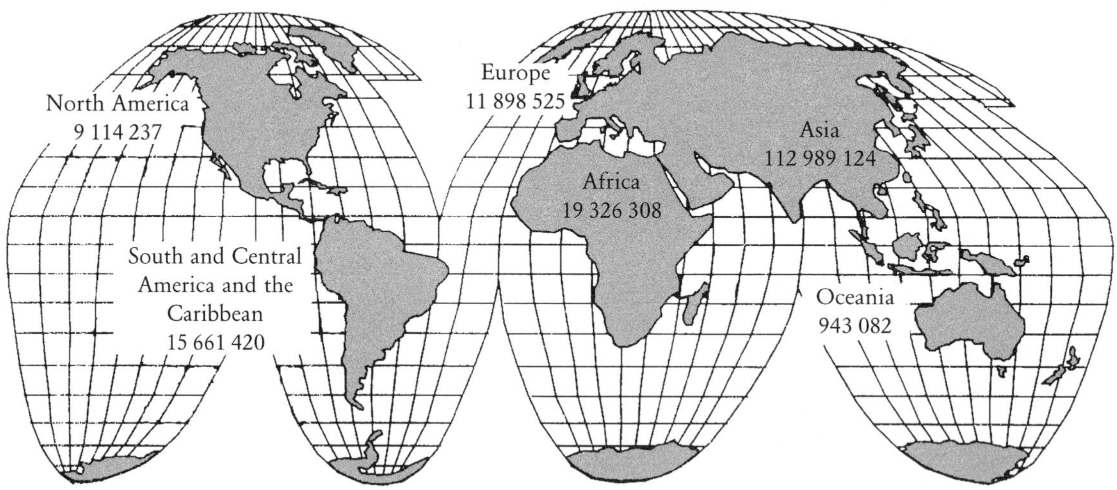

Figure 4 The likely world-wide increase in the (age-adjusted) prevalence of erectile dysfunction between 1995 and 2025: world total increase = 169 932 786. From reference 16. The most conservative (lowest) projection was employed. Prevalence estimates of erectile dysfunction were employed from the Massachusetts Male Aging Study (MMAS) 1987–89 for ages 40–69 years and the MMAS 1995–97 for ages 70–79 years

estimate of the incidence of erectile dysfunction was from a convenience sample of 3250 men aged 26–83 years visiting a preventive medicine clinic in Texas between 1987 and 1991[10]. Johannes and colleagues[11] have reported age-category-specific incidence rates for erectile dysfunction and show

Table 1 Estimated number of new cases of erectile dysfunction (ED) annually in the USA (men aged 40–69 years). Data is from the Massachusetts Male Aging Study and 1990 US Census data

Age	*Number of men at risk*	*Age-specific incidence rate for ED/1000*	*Expected number of new ED cases*
40–49	11 928 664	12.4	147 915
50–59	7 540 415	29.8	224 704
60–69	5 282 236	46.4	245 096
Total	24 751 315		617 715

how they differ by sociodemographic status (education, income) and also health status.

Once reliable incidence rates were established (Table 1), it was possible to relate the presence of various chronic disease conditions (e.g. heart disease, diabetes, hypertension and depression) to the development of new cases of erectile dysfunction. Various risk factors and lifestyles have been linked to the development of chronic diseases (e.g. cholesterol, smoking, lack of physical activity and hypertension are thought to be precursors of coronary heart disease). It was possible with the MMAS to determine whether these risk behaviors (which are related to major diseases) are also linked to the development of erectile dysfunction, independent of the chronic diseases for which they are precursors. This linkage marked a distinct step to the right in Figure 1. Elsewhere, we have looked at how both active and passive smoking are related to the development of erectile dysfunction. The adjusted rate of incident erectile dysfunction was significantly higher in cigarette smokers (24%) than in non-smokers (14%), with an adjusted odds ratio (OR) of 1.97 and a 95% confidence interval (CI) of 1.07–3.63. Passive exposure to cigarette smoke (if present both at home and at work) doubled the odds of incident erectile dysfunction (adjusted OR 2.07, 95% CI 1.04–4.13). Cigar smoking was also strongly predictive of incident erectile dysfunction, with an adjusted OR of 2.45 and a 95% CI of 1.9–5.50. Former smokers were no more likely than non-smokers to incur erectile dysfunction. Passive exposure to cigarette smoke at home and work increased the odds of incident erectile dysfunction (OR 2.07). In other words, this exposure to passive smoking had the same effect on erectile dysfunction as active smoking. Among smokers, each increment of passive exposure increased the likelihood of incident erectile dysfunction. Cigar smokers had an equivalent increase in the incidence of erectile dysfunction (OR 2.45). It is noteworthy that all three forms of smoking (cigarettes, cigars and passive exposure) had equivalent independent effects on erectile dysfunction.

Weight is a strong independent behavioral predictor of erectile dysfunction. The adjusted rate of incident erectile dysfunction in men who were overweight (body mass index > 30.0 kg/m^2) at baseline was 22%, significantly higher than in those who were not overweight (12%), with an adjusted OR of 1.96 and a 95% CI of 1.17–3.28.

While these new results represent a desirable move from cross-sectional to prospective analyses of cohort data, they still remain observational. The next step – representing a type of 'quasi-experiment' – was to see if changes in the risk factors that are known to be associated with erectile dysfunction result in changes in incident erectile dysfunction. Using MMAS data, Derby and colleagues[12] recently examined the extent to which changes in smoking, heavy drinking, sedentary lifestyle and obesity are associated with incident erectile dysfunction. Physical activity (an increase from baseline to T_2) (the 1995–97 follow-up) seemed to be beneficial: those becoming more active seemed to have less erectile dysfunction than those who did not change their activity level.

MEASURING ERECTILE DYSFUNCTION IN EPIDEMIOLOGICAL FIELD STUDIES

As noted above, the 1992 National Institutes of Health Consensus Development Conference developed a working definition of erectile dysfunction: 'the persistent inability to attain and maintain a penile erection adequate for sexual performance'[2]. That landmark conference also called for 'major research efforts to improve diagnostic classification for epidemiologic purposes'. It was a milestone event because it underscored key features of erectile dysfunction:

(1) That it is a subjectively identified state for each man (the means for its 'objective'

measurement with technology still require improvement and validation).

(2) That it focuses on behavior (penile erections) and not underlying aspects of libido (sexual drive or interest).

(3) That erectile dysfunction, like most medical conditions, is not an either/or condition.

Degrees of erectile dysfunction are recognized in the MMAS, where important distinctions are made between complete erectile dysfunction, moderate erectile dysfunction, minimal erectile dysfunction and no erectile dysfunction[5,6,8]. The MMAS often combines 'complete erectile dysfunction' and 'moderate erectile dysfunction' into a single category. 'Minimal erectile dysfunction' is often considered a transitional state (influenced perhaps by mood or episodic depression) and usefully grouped together with 'no erectile dysfunction'.

Several well-known questionnaires are available for the measurement of erectile dysfunction[13,14]. These instruments were developed in clinical settings, mainly for self-selected atypical populations seeking treatment for erectile dysfunction; they have limited use in field studies with population-based samples (not patients). Major limitations of these questionnaires are:

(1) They are lengthy and increase respondent burden (with multiple detailed queries on sensitive topics);

(2) If items are omitted or skipped (common in self-administered questionnaires), it is often difficult to calculate an overall score (resulting in missing data);

(3) Wordy questionnaires present difficulties for poorly educated respondents and increase translational misunderstandings when used in cross-cultural studies.

There is a need for a simple appropriate method for validly measuring degrees of erectile dysfunction in population-based epidemiologic studies. Just one question has been shown to provide useful information in many other areas of health care. We developed such a question for erectile dysfunction (Table 2) and have carefully assessed its metric properties against the two established indices

Table 2 A single question to assess the degree of erectile dysfunction

Impotence means not being able to get and keep an erection that is rigid enough for satisfactory sexual activity. How do you describe yourself?

Not impotent:	always able to get and keep an erection good enough for sexual intercourse.
Minimally impotent:	usually able to get and keep an erection good enough for sexual intercourse.
Moderately impotent:	sometimes able to get and keep an erection good enough for sexual intercourse.
Completely impotent:	never able to get and keep an erection good enough for sexual intercourse.

previously developed and validated in clinical settings[15]. It should be noted that the MMAS single question approach may be inappropriate for clinical studies, which require instruments that are sensitive enough to detect changes with medical and surgical treatments, or which must optimize case finding (specificity) where screening is followed by clinical evaluations.

The MMAS-2 follow-up provided a unique opportunity to rigorously compare a single question approach to measuring erectile dysfunction, with the two major existing questionnaires: the International Index of Erectile Function (IIEF)[13] and the Brief Male Sexual Function Inventory (BMSFI)[14] (Table 3). We embedded an experiment within the MMAS study: of the 1156 respondents to the 1995–97 follow-up, 505 were randomly selected to complete either the IIEF ($n = 254$) or the BMSFI ($n = 251$), in addition to our brief MMAS single question self-assessment. The results were reassuring. The proportions not classified because of missing data were as follows: MMAS = 11%; MMAS single question = 9%; IIEF = 18%; IIEF-5 = 18% and BMSFI = 8%. The overall prevalence of moderate to severe erectile dysfunction as determined by the MMAS single question was 25% (95% CI 20–29%). This was the same as the 25% prevalence (95% CI 19–32%) of moderate or severe erectile dysfunction using the IIEF. The MMAS single question correlated well with the other measures of erectile dysfunction (for example, with the IIEF, $r = 0.71$–0.78, $p < 0.001$); however,

Table 3 Comparison of the Massachusetts Male Aging Study (MMAS) single question with other major questionnaires

	MMAS	*MMAS single question*	*IIEF*[13]	*IIEF-5*[13]	*BMSFI*[14]
Features					
Number of respondents	505	505	254	254	251
Length (number of questions)	– (13)	✓✓ (1)	– (6)	– (5)	✓ (3)
Percentage of questions not classified	– (11)	✓ (9)	– (18)	– (18)	✓ (8)
Cost (US$)					
Translational difficulty	–	✓✓	–	✓	✓
Usability (e.g. NHANES)	–	✓✓	–	✓	✓
	–	✓✓	–	✓	✓✓
Estimates					
Prevalence of erectile dysfunction (%)	26.7	24.9	25.5	54.3	35.8
(95% CI)	(23-31)	(20-29)	(19-32)	(48-61)	(30-42)

Correlation of MMAS single question with IIEF = 0.71. IIEF, International Index of Erectile Function; BMSFI, Brief Male Sexual Function Inventory; NHANES, National Health and Nutrition Examination Survey; –, inappropriate; ✓, appropriate; ✓✓, most appropriate

the estimated prevalence of moderate to severe erectile dysfunction differed (59.5%, 25.5%, 54.3% and 24.9% using the BMSFI, IIEF, IIEF-5 and MMAS single question, respectively). A single, direct question appears to provide a practical means of assessing erectile dysfunction in population-based studies. With further development, it should be possible to include a single question concerning erectile dysfunction in large national health studies (e.g. NHANES) to provide estimates of erectile dysfunction for selected population groups and geographic regions.

HEALTH SERVICES RESEARCH AND ERECTILE DYSFUNCTION

Very little health services research has focussed specifically on erectile dysfunction. There were obviously limits to what the MMAS could study. In a future MMAS (planned for 2001-03), we plan to follow subjects into later years and add important questions concerning health-care utilization for erectile dysfunction. The willingness of older men to, first, actually seek medical care and, second, receive appropriate effective treatment once the health system has been accessed, are now important public health issues, especially with the availability of apparently effective, well-tolerated user-friendly oral preparations. We have recently considered some of the health services research and policy implications for many countries of the availability of new treatments for erectile dysfunction[9].

While the MMAS could not include questions concerning health-care utilization for erectile dysfunction, some new data are available for the USA from a national survey sample recently (1999) conducted for the American Association of Retired Persons[16]. Figure 5 summarizes the results, which show that only about 10% of men report seeking or receiving treatment for 'sexual problems' and only half of these (5% of all US males > 45 years of age) have ever tried or are using sildenafil (Viagra).

In summary:

(1) Erectile dysfunction is a prevalent medical condition;

(2) It has behavioral precursors that are amenable to change;

(3) It has serious implications for quality of life;

(4) Despite the availability of new pharmacological interventions, the vast majority of aging men (even those reporting complete or moderate erectile dysfunction) do not seek medical care for the condition.

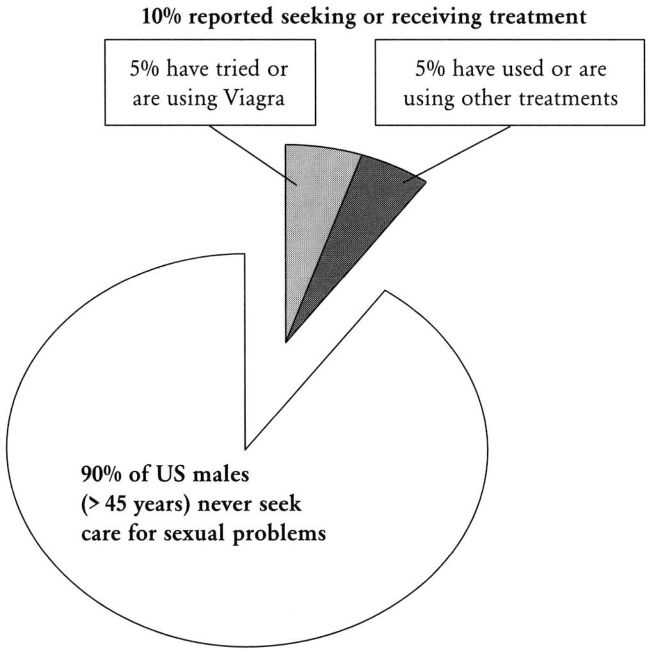

Figure 5 Only a tiny proportion of US males seek treatment for erectile dysfunction: results from a national survey ($n = 1384$, men: $n = 639$). From reference 17

ACKNOWLEDGEMENTS

The Massachusetts Male Aging Study (MMAS) is supported by grants from the National Institutes of Health, NIDDK (DK 44995) and NIA (AG 04673). All members of the MMAS Team made important contributions to this paper: Andre Araujo, Isik Aytack, Carol Derby, Henry Feldman, Irwin Goldstein, Katherine Johannes, Kenneth Kleinman, Robert Krane, Christopher Longcope and Beth Mohr. Lisa Marceau and Agnes Migliaccio assisted with the development of the final manuscript.

References

1. Krane RJ, Goldstein I, de Tejada IS. Impotence. *N Engl J Med* 1989;321:1648–59
2. National Institutes of Health Consensus Development Panel on Impotence. Impotence. *J Am Med Assoc* 1993;270:83–90
3. Kinsey AC, Pomeroy WB, Martin CE. *Sexual Behavior in the Human Male*. Philadelphia: WB Saunders, 1948
4. Masters WH, Johnson VE. Human sexual response. Boston, MA: Little, Brown and Co., 1966
5. Feldman HA, Goldstein I, Hutzichristov D, *et al.* Impotence and its medical and psycholosocial correlates: results from the Massachusetts Male Aging Study. *J Urol* 1994;151:54–61
6. McKinlay JB. Medical and psychological influences on erectile dysfunction – results from a community study. Presented at the *9th Scientific Congress of the Kuwait Medical Association, October, Kuwait. Sociology, Epidemiology and Biostatistics.* 1994:353–8
7. McKinlay JB, Longcope C, Gray A. The questionable physiologic and epidemiologic basis for a male climacteric syndrome: preliminary results from the Massachusetts Male Aging Study. *Maturitas* 1989; 11:103–5

8. Kleinman KP, Feldman HA, Johannes CB, McKinlay JB. A new surrogate variable for erectile dysfunction status in the Massachusetts Male Aging Study. *J Clin Epidemiol* 2000;in press
9. Aytac IA, McKinlay JB, Krane RJ. The likely worldwide increase in erectile dysfunction between 1995 and 2025 and some possible policy consequences. Br J Urol Int 1999;84:450–6
10. Wei M, Macera CA, Davis DR, Hornung CA, Nankin HR, Blair SN. Total cholesterol and high density lipoprotein cholesterol as important predictors of erectile dysfunction. *Am J Epidemiol* 1994;140:930–7
11. Johannes CB, Araujo AB, Feldman HA, Derby CA, Kleinman, KP, McKinlay JB. Incidence of erectile dysfunction in men ages 40–69: longitudinal results from the Massachusetts Male Aging Study. *J Urol* 2000;in press
12. Derby CA, Mohr B, Goldstein I, Feldman HA, Johannes CB, McKinlay JB. Modifiable risk factors and incidence of erectile dysfunction: implications for prevention. Submitted, 1999
13. Rosen RC, *et al.* The International Index of Erectile Function (IIEF): a multidimensional scale for assessment of erectile dysfunction. *Urology* 1997;49: 822–30
14. O'Leary MP, *et al.* A brief male sexual function inventory for urology. *Urology* 1995;46:694–706
15. Derby CA, Araujo AB, Johannes CB, Feldman HA, McKinlay JB. Measurement of erectile dysfunction in propulation-based studies: the use of a single question self-assessment in the Massachusetts Male Aging Study. Submitted, 1999
16. United Nations. *World Population Prospects: the 1996 Revision.* New York: United Nations, 1997
17. American Association of Retired Persons (AARP). Washington, DC: AARP, *Modern Maturity*, September 1999

Impact of urogenital aging on the quality of life

80

D. Hudita

Many of the anatomical and functional disturbances experienced by women after the menopause are associated with a decline in sex hormones.

Embryological data show that the female genital and urinary systems develop from the primitive urogenital sinus. Different studies have shown that organs of the urogenital trigone have estrogen receptors. There are data that show that decreases in estrogen levels negatively influence the lower urinary tract and genital area.

Some epidemiological studies have shown an increase of urogenital disturbances in the menopause, implicating estrogen deficiency. All these urogenital complaints appear after 2 or 3 years and become stronger with age. Although these disturbances are not life-threatening, they affect women's quality of life.

Estrogen deficiency modifies the urogenital area in three respects: atrophy, urinary micturition complaints and recurrent urinary tract infections. Atrophy induces genital and sexual disturbances. The genital complaints are connected with atrophy, and these are summarized in Table 1.

Urinary complaints also depend on atrophy and estrogen deprivation (Table 2). The prevalence of urogenital complaints is not known exactly. Many women do not ask for treatment because of the belief that this is an inevitable part of normal aging, or because they are embarrassed.

In 1996 in Sydney, at the *8th World Congress of Menopause*, Nachtigall[1] reported that postmenopausal women have a variety of troubles in their organs, but that urogenital atrophy occurs in practically 100%. Nobody will die from it, but they will live a miserable life.

One of the first studies on urogenital comfort, and certainly the best known, is that by Iosif and Bekassy[2], in 1984. In their study on 902 randomly selected women aged 61, urinary incontinence had a prevalence of 29.2% (stress incontinence 40.1%, mixed incontinence 32.7%, urge incontinence 27.2%). The onset of troubles after the menopause

Table 1 Genital complaints secondary to atrophy

Symptoms	*Signs*	*Laboratory findings*	*Diagnosis*
Soreness, itching, burning, vaginal dryness	scant vaginal fluid, vaginal hyperemia, reduction of vaginal folds, petechiae, bleeding on light contact	parabasal cells Döderlein's bacillus ↓ pH ↑ cornified cells ↓	vaginal atrophy
Abnormal vaginal discharge	scant vaginal fluid, vaginal hyperemia, reduction of vaginal folds, petechiae, bleeding on light contact	parabasal cells Döderlein's bacillus ↓ pH ↑ cornified cells ↓ fecal flora	atrophic vaginitis
Dyspareunia, decline of libido	scant vaginal fluid, vaginal hyperemia, reduction of vaginal folds, petechiae, bleeding on light contact, reduction of vaginal width	parabasal cells Döderlein's bacillus ↓ pH ↑ cornified cells ↓	sexual disturbances

Table 2 Urinary complaints secondary to atrophy

Micturition disorders	*Urinary incontinence*	*Urodynamic investigations*	*Diagnosis*
Frequent micturition, urgency	yes	bladder excitability	urge incontinence
Frequent micturition, leakage with effort	yes	low ureteral pressure	stress incontinence
Frequent micturition, urgency, leakage with effort	yes	bladder excitability, low ureteral pressure	mixed incontinence
Frequent micturition, urgency, leakage with effort, dysuria fever	yes	positive urine microbiology	urinary tract infection (recurrent)

occurred in 30% of women. Infection of the lower urinary tract was found in 13% of cases, sometimes associated with urinary incontinence, but recurrent infection was found in only 5.4%. Although these data are impressive, only 4% of women reported current oral estrogen treatment, probably more having topical treatment.

A study in Western European women on their experience of urogenital aging problems and their management was carried out by Barlow, Samsioe and van Geelen in 1994 in six European countries. They examined a cohort of 3000 women aged 55–75 years[3]. Urogenital aging symptoms were recognized in 29.3% of the postmenopausal women. The intensity of symptoms was considered to be moderate by 48% of the women and as severe by only 11.2%. Dysuria (8.3%), urinary incontinence (7.4%), urinary frequency (12.7%) and recurrent urinary tract infections (7.4%) were the urogenital symptoms reported. The clinical intensity of the symptoms was different for each woman.

The increase of awareness among the general population in 1984–94 and an increase of available information could explain the difference in the prevalence of symptoms in these two studies. Statistical data in the USA show that the number of women suffering urogenital symptoms is 20 million. The most prevalent symptom, and a large handicap, is urinary incontinence. This is recognized by 11 million women according to the National Institute of Diabetes and Digestive and Kidney Disease (NIDDK). Palmer's study in 1994 reported the estimated prevalence of urinary incontinence in social residents as 40–60%.

All these urogenital symptoms are an important influence on the quality of life of women. For many years, studies were conducted on menopausal symptoms only, and the results of treatment were analyzed only for medical reasons. Quality of life, according to the World Health Organization, is 'Not only the absence of illness but complete well-being from the physical, mental and social point of view of the individual person'.

Problems experienced by these women are urine leakage, an unpleasant odor, urinary infections, perineal rash and skin infections. Women also have sleep disturbances, restricted social interactions, reduced sexual activity, loss of self-esteem and depression. Employment becomes a problem, and social and private life is changed.

The symptoms before and after treatment have to be quantified in an objective manner. There are questionnaires adapted for the menopause: the Women's Health Questionnaire, the Self-Rating of Climacteric Symptoms, the French questionnaire 'Qualifemme', and so on[4–8]. The main aim of these questionnaires is to transform women's subjective data into objective, quantifiable data.

For more than 10 years the medical community has been concerned about the role of menopausal urinary incontinence in decreasing quality of life. Urinary incontinence is considered a new health-related quality of life measure[9]. The question 'Do you consider this accidental loss of urine a problem that interferes with your day-to-day activities or bothers you in other ways?' is the best predictor of a subject's response to quality of life measures. Symptoms that are best correlated with quality of life measures are frequency of episodes of incontinence, amount of urine loss and frequency of micturition.

There are two specific questionnaires for urinary incontinence: the Incontinence Impact Questionnaire (IIQ) and the Urinary Distress Inventory (UDI). They have long versions, with 30 items on the IIQ and 19 items on the UDI, and short forms, with seven and six items, respectively. The short-form versions may be more useful in many clinical trials and for general clinical practice[10] (Table 3). This is exemplified by the study of Robinson and colleagues in 1998, on 384 community-dwelling incontinent women[10]. This questionnaire consists of a series of questions with the following available responses (scores): Not at all, 0; Slightly, 1; Moderately, 2; Greatly, 3. Each of the instruments is further subdivided into subclasses, which address specific aspects of life quality: social, emotional and physical.

Table 3 Items in the short forms of the Incontinence Questionnaire and the Urogenital Distress Inventory[10]

Has urine leakage or prolapse affected the following:
Household chores
Physical recreation
Entertainment activities
Travel > 30 min away from home
Social activities
Emotional health (nervousness, depression, etc.)
Feeling frustrated
Do you experience, and if so, how much are you bothered by the following:
Frequent urination
Leakage related to feeling of urgency
Leakage related to activity, coughing, or sneezing
Small amounts of leakage (drops)
Difficulty emptying the bladder
Pain or discomfort in lower abdominal or genital area

Associations between demographic characteristics, incontinence symptoms, quality of life measures, and the questions on inconvenience were statistically evaluated using Pearson correlations and the Goodman–Kruskal rank correlation for ordinal data. A logistic regression analysis using the proportional odds logistic model was used to determine which of the patient's characteristics and incontinence symptoms were predictive for the scores for quality of life measurement and the global questions on inconvenience (Table 4).

To account for the preponderance of '0' responses, the mean scores were converted to ordinal data as follows: an average score of 0.0 was evaluated as 0, those of 0.01–0.50 as 1, those of 0.51–1.50 as 2 and all mean scores of 1.51–3.00 as 3 (Table 5).

A higher Incontinence Impact Questionnaire score reflects lower quality of life. In addition, younger women were more likely to have a poorer quality of life score than the elderly.

For a long period of time and for many people, especially men, sexual life after the menopause is less attractive. In 1845, Colombat de l'Isere stated that the female was compelled to yield to the power of time and that postmenopausal women cease to contribute to the survival of the species and henceforward live only for themselves. Their features are stamped with the impress of age and their genital

Table 4 Associations of patient-reported incontinence symptoms with Incontinence Impact Questionnaire, the Urogenital Distress Inventory and the question on how much the patient was bothered[10]

Self-reported measure	*Impact questionnaire*	*Distress questionnaire*	*'Bothered' question*
Leakage in past 3 months	0.40	0.48	0.58
Number of accidents/week	0.32	0.44	0.50
Number of leaks/day	0.25	0.26	0.37
Number of leaks/night	0.09	0.16	0.53
Urine lost (drops–gushes)	0.28	0.27	0.52
Urine lost (moisture–wet floor)	0.34	0.26	0.54
Status in past year	0.14	0.22	0.37
Number of voids/day	0.24	0.34	0.41
Number of times awakened	0.18	0.20	0.40
Ever asked about urinary incontinence	0.18	0.11	0.14
Ever made a clinician aware	0.22	0.28	0.20

organs are sealed with the signet of sterility ... It is prudent to avoid all circumstances as might tend to awaken any erotic thoughts in the mind, and everything calculated to cause regret for charms lost and enjoyments that are ended forever. This is an erroneous position. Exact information about sexual life in postmenopausal women is difficult to obtain in a society where sexuality is thought to be a prerogative only of youth. The genital symptom that usually comes first in the menopause is a feeling of dryness in the vagina. This symptom could appear in the peri- and even the premenopausal period. It is very important, for later consequences, to be aware that vaginal disturbances are in connection with estrogen deprivation.

Vaginal dryness is accompanied by some other symptoms: itching, smarting pain, burning, soreness. The entire genital area undergoes an atrophic change: reduction of pubic fat, atrophic minor lips, thin atrophic vaginal mucus with reduction of vaginal folds, petechiae, bleeding at light contact. These indicate vaginal atrophy and, later, atrophic vaginitis[11-13]. All these complaints contribute to discomfort, even pain, caused by atrophy and vaginal infection, but the most important complaint is dyspareunia - painful intercourse that diminishes sexual satisfaction (Table 6). In connection with estrogen deprivation there is a decrease of neurosteroids that causes a loss of sexual interest, which contributes to the lack of satisfaction or depression in menopausal women[12-15].

The prevalence of different genital symptoms described by Iosif and Bekassy[2] shows vaginal dryness at 38.8%, followed by loss of interest in sexual relations (32.7%) and vaginal pain or discharge (15%). It is important to make the association of genital disturbances with urinary tract disorders. Urinary incontinence, rash of the perineum,

Table 5 Regression analysis of patient characteristics and incontinence symptoms with Incontinence Impact Questionnaire, Urogenital Distress Inventory and question on how much the patient was bothered

Variable	*Impact questionnaire (ordinal)*	*Distress questionnaire (ordinal)*	*'Bothered' question (number)*
Leakage in past 3 months	1.30 (1.18-1.44)	1.34 (1.20-1.50)	1.50 (1.30-1.74)
Urine lost (drops-gushes)	2.64 (1.65-4.24)	1.57 (0.99-2.47)	1.98 (1.30-1.74)
Number of voids/day	1.14 (1.06-1.23)	1.18 (1.10-1.27)	1.08 (0.99-1.19)
Number of times awakened	1.15 (1.06-1.24)	1.15 (0.99-1.33)	1.24 (1.10-1.41)
Ever asked about incontinence	1.89 (1.19-3.00)	1.67 (1.02-2.74)	1.25 (0.65-2.40)
Age (reference: 60-65 years)			
66-70 years	0.61 (0.32-1.14)	0.92 (0.52-1.61)	0.50 (0.22-1.14)
71-75 years	0.51 (0.27-0.97)	0.53 (0.32-0.89)	0.43 (0.23-0.81)
76-80 years	0.25 (0.13-0.48)	0.56 (0.27-1.15)	0.31 (0.13-0.75)
> 80 years	0.30 (0.14-0.66)	0.52 (0.27-1.00)	0.49 (0.20-1.19)
Education (reference: less than high school)			
high school	1.15 (0.68-1.94)	1.14 (0.65-2.01)	1.78 (0.87-3.61)
some college	1.54 (0.74-3.22)	1.83 (0.95-3.53)	1.90 (0.66-5.44)
college degree	1.91 (0.75-4.83)	1.34 (0.72-2.48)	1.41 (0.44-4.48)

Table 6 Menopausal status and sexual health problems

	Premenopausal		*Perimenopausal*		*Postmenopausal*		
Sexual health problem	*Sometimes*	*Often*	*Sometimes*	*Often*	*Sometimes*	*Often*	*p Value*
Post-coital bleeding/irritation	8.70	5.98	12.28	7.02	12.90	9.68	NS
Lack of lubrication	22.28	14.13	24.56	19.30	12.63	44.21	0.0001
Dyspareunia	15.76	8.70	14.04	10.53	17.89	16.84	NS
Difficulty reaching orgasm	32.61	25.00	28.07	36.84	21.05	34.74	NS
Vaginismus	16.85	9.78	19.30	7.02	13.86	20.00	NS
Vaginal infection	10.33	4.35	24.56	7.02	8.42	2.11	0.01

urinary leakage and odor are mostly responsible for the decline in sexual interest and for unpleasant intercourse. In the study of Barlow and colleagues in 1994 on 3000 women from six countries in Europe[3], 49.1% were sexually active, with 20.7% for women over 65. Vaginal itching and burning after the menopause was reported by 10.6% of the women; 16.5% thought it was severe and 40.7% moderate. Dyspareunia was reported in 6.7%, but was thought of as a severe problem by 12.7% and moderate by 48%. Vaginal signs of atrophy accompanied it in 39.4%. The frequency of intercourse was reported by 23.2% as once per week or more, and by 23.2% as less than once per month. It is illustrative that sexually active women have a more healthy vaginal status than abstinent women. An American study[16] reported in 1995 that postmenopausal women anticipate menopausal troubles and adapt to the new status with a relatively rich sexual life - 54% being sexually active, but 55% showing a loss of sexual interest (Table 7). Sexual health problems at the menopause show that lack of lubrication and vaginal infection have a large influence on decreasing quality of life[14,17].

Bachmann[18] elaborated a vaginal health index able to assess genital atrophy and thus give women objective data for a reason for treatment and a prediction of recovery after treatment (Table 8)[16]. There are five parameters: overall elasticity, fluid secretion, pH, epithelial mucosa and moisture, with five degrees of impairment. A lower score corresponded to greater vaginal atrophy.

This is a good example of the woman taking decisions, so we will be sure of her awareness and compliance with treatment[19,20].

Normal genital health for postmenopausal women can be realized by estrogen therapy. This leads to cessation of genital complaints and accordingly to a normal sexual life. In turn, this will improve self-esteem and social and family interactions.

CONCLUSIONS

(1) Urogenital aging - an old problem is newly recognized.

Table 7 Age and frequency of sexual activity[16]

	35–49 years (%)			*> 50 years (%)*			
Sexual activity	*Never*	*Sometimes*	*Often*	*Never*	*Sometimes*	*Often*	*p Value*
Sexual fantasy	20.59	47.06	32.35	44.86	45.79	9.35	0.0001
Kissing	22.06	19.12	58.82	21.50	19.63	58.88	NS
Masturbation	42.54	47.76	9.70	55.56	41.67	2.78	NS
Foreplay	24.44	42.22	33.33	32.71	43.93	23.36	0.01
Oral sex	42.96	42.22	14.81	67.59	27.78	4.63	0.0001
Vaginal intercourse	25.19	45.93	28.89	34.26	45.37	20.37	0.002
Anal intercourse	93.33	5.19	1.48	99.07	0.93	0.00	NS

Table 8 Vaginal health index[16]

*Overall elasticity**		*Fluid secretion type and consistency*	*pH*	*Epithelial mucosa*	*Moisture*
1	None	none	6.1	petechiae noted before contact	none, mucosa inflamed
2	Poor	scant, thin yellow	5.6–6.0	bleeds with light contact	none, mucosa not inflamed
3	Fair	superficial, thin white	5.1–5.5	bleeds with scraping	minimal
4	Good	moderate, thin white	4.7–5.0	not friable, thin mucosa	moderate
5	Excellent	normal (white flocculent)	< 4.6	not friable, normal mucosa	normal

*Lower score corresponds to greater urogenital atrophy

(2) Urogenital aging is not life threatening but has a major impact on quality of life in postmenopausal women.

(3) Urinary incontinence is the most debilitating for postmenopausal women; urge incontinence is a new health-related measure for quality of life. It is a cause for institutionalization, with heavy physiological and economic burdens.

(4) Lower genital tract disorders and sexual dysfunction increase with age, according to atrophic changes.

(5) Estrogen therapy is the most widely available regimen for alleviation of the negative impact of urogenital aging on quality of life.

References

1. Nachtigall L. Towards better recognition of urogenital aging. *Am J Obstet Gynecol* 1998;178:S243-4
2. Iosif CS, Bekassy Z. Prevalence of genito-urinary symptoms in the late menopause. *Acta Obstet Gynecol Scand* 1984;63,S257-60
3. Barlow DH, Samsioe G, van Geelen JM. A study of women's experience of the problems of urogenital ageing and its management. *Maturitas* 1997;27: S239-47
4. Comet D. Qualifemme®, echelle francaise de qualite de la vie en menopause: utilisation en routine. *Reprod Hum Horm* 1997;X:29-32
5. Le Floch J-P. Validation d'un questionnaire d'evaluation de la qualitee de la vie en menopause. *Reprod Hum Horm* 1997;X:11-21
6. Rozenbaum H. Editorial. *Reprod Hum Horm* 1997;X:2
7. Wiklund I. Modalites d'evaluation de la qualite de la vie de la femme menopause. *Reprod Hum Horm* 1997;X:S3-10
8. Zartanian M. Evaluation de la qualite de vie chez la femme menopausee en France. Resultats d'une etude multicentrique. *Reprod Hum Horm* 1997; X:S23-8
9. Doren M. Urogenital aging - creation of improved awareness. *Am J Obstet Gynecol* 1998;178:S254-6
10. Robinson D, Pearce K, Preisser J, Dugan E, Suggs P, Cohen S. Relationship between patient reports of urinary incontinence symptoms and quality of life measures. *Obstet Gynecol* 1998;91:224-8
11. Molander U, Milsom I, Ekelund P, Mellstrom D. An epidemiological study of urinary incontinence and related urogenital symptoms in elderly women. *Maturitas* 1990;12:51-60
12. Samsioe G. Urogenital aging - a hidden problem. *Am J Obstet Gynecol* 1998;178:S245-9
13. Samsioe G, Jansson I, Mellstrom D, Svanborg A. Occurrence, nature and treatment of urinary incontinence in a 70-year-old female population. *Maturitas* 1985;7:335-42
14. Foidart JM, Vervliet J, Buytaert P. Efficacy of sustained-release vaginal oestriol in alleviating urogenital and systemic climacteric complaints. *Maturitas* 1991;13:99-107
15. Wright HJ. The female perspective: women's attitudes toward urogenital aging. *Am J Obstet Gynecol* 1998;178:S250-3
16. Bachmann G. Urogenital ageing: an old problem newly recognized. *Maturitas* 1995;22(Suppl):S1-5
17. Griebling TL, Nygaard E. The role of estrogen replacement therapy in the management of urinary incontinence and urinary tract infection in postmenopausal women. *Endocrinol Metab Clin North Am* 1997;26:347-60
18. Bachmann GA. The clinical platform for the 17beta-estradiol vaginal releasing ring. *Am J Obstet Gynecol* 1998;178:S257-60
19. Fantl JA, Cardozo L, McClish DK. The Hormones and Urogenital Therapy Committee. Estrogen therapy in the management of urinary incontinence in postmenopausal women: a meta-analysis. First report of the Hormones and Urogenital Therapy Committee. *Obstet Gynecol* 1994;83:12-18
20. Fantl JA, Bump RC, Robinson D, McClish DK, Wyman JF. The Continence Program for Women Research Group. Efficacy of estrogen supplementation in the treatment of urinary incontinence. *Obstet Gynecol* 1996;88:745-9

Vaginal microecology and local immune system in postmenopausal women

81

V. Smetnik, V. Balan, A. Ankirskaja and G. Suchich

INTRODUCTION

The postmenopause is characterized by universal hormonal changes and aging processes and, as a result, urogenital atrophy develops[1,2]. According to epidemiological data, the frequency of urogenital atrophy varies from 30–70%[3,4]. However, only 4–14% of postmenopausal women develop recurrent urinary tract infection (RUTI)[5–7]. There is a big difference between the data obtained by different authors. This may be due to different methodological approaches or the absence of a conventional definition of RUTI in postmenopausal women. In one paper, RUTI is defined as the 'occurrence of more than two episodes of infection of the previous year'[7]. Another paper defined RUTI by the occurrence of proven episodes of infection within a 6-month period[8].

Thus, all postmenopausal women have a similar hormonal status, aging process and urogenital atrophy, but only a small number of them develop true vaginitis and RUTI. The following question arises: 'What is the protective mechanism against infection?' We investigated this question in two ways: studying the vaginal microecology and estimating the local immunity in vaginal tissue.

METHODS

Postmenopausal women, all non-smokers aged 49–69 years with vaginal symptoms (dryness, dispareunia, vulvar itching and burning) and a body mass index less than 26, were enrolled in the study. None of the patients had used hormone replacement therapy (HRT) for a period of at least 1 year and antibiotics for at least 3 months before the beginning of the study. Exclusion criteria were sexually transmitted diseases and diabetes. In total, we enrolled 100 women in the study, after they had given informed consent. All patients had been married, but 24% were widowed and 20% were divorced at the beginning of the study. Women were divided into three groups: in group I ($n = 37$) the women had a menopausal duration of 3–5 years; in group II ($n = 36$) they had a menopausal duration of 6–10 years; and in group III ($n = 27$) the women had a menopausal duration of more than 10 years. A complex microbiological investigation, including microscopy of Gram-stained vaginal smears, was undertaken to evaluate vaginal microcenosis. Cultures were used to study facultative obligate anaerobic and microaerophilic micro-organisms, using quantitative methods. Using immunohistochemical methods, we studied the organization of CD8, CD14, CD56 T-cells and CD72 B-cells in vaginal tissue from patients with vaginal atrophy using CD-line monoclonal antibodies (Immunotech, Marseille, France).

RESULTS

According to our data, four variants of vaginal microcenosis in the postmenopause can be found: subnormocenosis, vaginal atrophy, bacterial vaginosis and bacterial non-specific vaginitis (Table 1).

Subnormocenosis differs from normocenosis by a slightly decreased, but still dominant number of lactobacilli, a moderate pH increase and the appearance of intermediate cells without an inflammatory reaction. Subnormocenosis is a variant of vaginal microcenosis that can be distinguished from vaginal atrophy, because in vaginal atrophy we observed lack or absence of lactobacilli, the appearance of parabasal cells and a bigger pH increase, still without an inflammatory reaction. We assumed that subnormocenosis was a physiological variant of vaginal microcenosis in

Table 1 Variants of vaginal microcenosis in postmenopausal women

Characteristic	*Normocenosis*	*Subnormocenosis*	*Vaginal atrophy*
Lactobacilli (colony-forming units/ml)	dominant; 10^7–10^8	dominant; 10^5–10^7	10^3–10^5, or absent
Opportunistic micro-organisms (colony-forming units/ml)	$< 10^3$–10^5	$< 10^3$–10^6	10^2–10^4, or absent
Cytology	superficial cells	intermediate and superficial cells	parabasal and intermediate cells
Leukocytes	≤ 10 cells in vaginal fluid	≤ 10 cells in vaginal fluid	< 10 cells in vaginal fluid, or absent
pH	3.8–4.5	4.0–4.5	≥ 5.0

postmenopausal women. Therefore, the term 'subnormocenosis' was introduced. The distribution of the variants of vaginal microcenosis, which depend on the duration of the postmenopause, is shown in Table 2.

Thus, postmenopausal estrogen deficiency in patients with vaginal atrophy resulted in a decrease or elimination of lactobacilli from the vaginal microflora. However, we could not find opportunistic micro-organisms. This suggests that there are other mechanisms of protection against pathogens in the female urogenital tract, for example immune protection.

We investigated some indicators of the local immune system in vaginal tissue obtained from 11 postmenopausal women with vaginal atrophy. The distribution of cells labelled with monoclonal antibodies in vaginal tissue is presented in Table 3. The organization of the immune cells in different histological structures of the vaginal wall in patients with vaginal atrophy was distinct. The supressor cytotoxic (CD8) and natural killer (CD56) cells, which are not usually present in healthy women of childbearing age, were highly increased and distributed throughout the lamina propria and stroma in the same manner, but there were only a few of them in the epithelium. We suggest that both types of these cells play an important role in protection against pathogens. After 6 months of HRT, we observed the disappearance of these cells. This is not only additional evidence for an important role of the local immune system in postmenopausal women, but also proof that the process can be reversed.

Table 2 Frequency of microcenosis variants depending on the duration of the postmenopause

	Duration of postmenopause		
Variant of microcenosis	*1–5 years* ($n = 37$)	*6–10 years* ($n = 36$)	*11–19 years* ($n = 27$)
Subnormocenosis *n* (%)	23 (62.2)	13 (36.1)	7 (25.9)
Vaginal atrophy *n* (%)	3 (8.1)	18 (50.0)	20 (74.1)
Bacterial vaginosis *n* (%)	10 (27.0)	5 (13.9)	0 (0)
Non-specific vaginitis *n* (%)	1 (2.7)	0 (0)	0 (0)

Table 3 Distribution of cells labelled with monoclonal antibodies in vaginal tissue in patients with vaginal atrophy. Values are mean ± SE

Cell marker	*Epithelium*	*Lamina propria*	*Stroma*
CD4	absent	absent	absent
CD8	9.8 ± 4.2	89.5 ± 15.25	28.65 ± 4.1
CD14	0.23 ± 0.11	9.45 ± 2.7	5.5 ± 2.35
CD56	4.05 ± 1.9	90.75 ± 8.9	26.45 ± 2.25
CD72	absent	absent	absent

DISCUSSION

The vagina, with its unique microflora, forms a balanced ecosystem. This ecosystem changes with variations in the levels of hormones. Lactobacilli play an important role in the maintenance of homeostasis within the dynamic vaginal ecosystem by preventing colonization and infection by pathogenic organisms[9]. Lactobacilli dominate in the vaginal microflora at 10^7–10^8 colony-forming units/ml of vaginal fluid in healthy premenopausal women[10]. Lactobacilli are believed to interfere with pathogens by different mechanisms. Lactobacilli may protect the vaginal epithelium through a series of barrier (self-aggregation, adherence) and interference (receptor-binding interference, coaggregation with potential pathogens) mechanisms[11]. Lactobacilli produce antimicrobial compounds such as lactic acid, hydrogen peroxidase[12,13] and possible biosurfactants[14], which may result in the inhibition of the growth of pathogens. Thus, we can suggest that vaginal subnormocenosis in postmenopausal women protects the vagina against pathogens by different mechanisms. As the incidence of subnormocenosis in postmenopausal women with vaginal atrophy without an inflammatory reaction decreases, other mechanisms of protection begin to work. The regulation of mucosal immunity in the female reproductive tract through the reproductive cycle is well established[15]. In an experimental study on ovariectomized rats, estradiol was shown to have an inhibitory effect on vaginal antigen presentation by macrophage/dendritic cells[16]. This effect was reversible. The local immune defence system (secretory component and IgA cells) has been studied in female cervical and endometrial specimens in the proliferative and secretory phases, and was found to be hormone-dependent[17]. In our study, we used immunohistochemistry to evaluate the organization of CD4, CD8, CD14, CD56 and CD72 cells in the vaginal tissue of postmenopausal women. A significant increase in the numbers of CD8 and CD56 (natural killer) cells was found to depend on the increase in duration of the postmenopause[18]. Recently, an increased activity of natural killer cells was demonstrated in blood samples obtained from postmenopausal women[19]. According to our data, an efferent arm of local immune system activation (supressor and cytotoxic CD8 cells and natural killer (CD56) cells) may be due to a lack of estradiol inhibitory action in the postmenopause. The phenotype of CD8 cells characterizes two lymphocyte groups: supressor and cytotoxic lymphocytes and they may act like immunoregulators and influence T-helper activity[20]. It has been proposed that the biological effect of these cells may contribute to virus replication and be involved in antimicrobial protection[21]. Natural killer cells play a very important role in non-specific or 'non-adaptive' immune responses. We suggest that subnormocenosis and the activation of local vaginal immune protection in the post-menopause in part provide biological protection against aging in the female.

CONCLUSION

Urogenital aging during the menopause is associated with a special type of vaginal microcenosis – so-called 'subnormocenosis' – which is a condition different, but similar to, normocenosis and which provides physiological protection against infection in postmenopausal women. In the absence of protective vaginal microflora, the local immune system is the real protective mechanism in the female genital tract.

References

1. Samsioe G. Urogenital aging – a hidden problem. *Am J Obstet Gynecol* 1998;178:245–9
2. Ulmsten U. On urogenital aging. *Maturitas* 1995; 21:163–9
3. Barlow DH, Samsioe G, Van Green JM. A study of European women's experience of the problems of urogenital ageing and its management. *Maturitas* 1997;27:239–47
4. Palasious S. Postmenopausal vaginal atrophy and HRT. In Birkhäuser M, Rosenbaum H, eds. *IV European Congress on Menopause, Vienna.* Paris: ESKA, 1998:305–14

5. Iosif C, Bekassy Z. Prevalence of genito-urinary symptoms in the late menopause. *Acta Obstet Gynecol Scand* 1984;63:257–60
6. Malander U, Milson I, Ekelund P, *et al.* An epidemiological study in urinary incontinence and regulated urogenital symptoms in elderly women. *Maturitas* 1990;13:51–60
7. Stenberg Å, Heimer G, Ulmsten U, *et al.* Prevalence of genitourinary and other climacteric symptoms in 61 year old women. *Maturitas* 1996;24:31–6
8. Stevenson JC, Gaspard V, Avonac B, *et al.* Points to consider for the development of new indications for hormone replacement therapies and estrogen-like molecules. *Climacteric* 1998;1:12–17
9. McGroarty JA. Probiotic use of lactobacilli in the human female urogenital tract. *FEMS Immunol Med Microbiol* 1993;6:251–64
10. Sobel JD. Vaginitis and vaginal flora: controversies abound. *Curr Opin Infect Dis* 1996;9:42–7
11. Boris S, Suarez JE, Vazquez F, *et al.* Adherence of human vaginal lactobacilli to vaginal epithelial cells and interaction with uropathogens. *Infect Immunol* 1998;66:1985–9
12. Reid G, McGroarty JA, Angotti R, *et al.* Lactobacillus inhibitor production against *Escherichia coli* and coaggregation ability with uropathogens. *Can J Microbiol* 1998;34:345–51
13. Hiller SL, Lan RJ. Vaginal microflora in postmenopausal women who have not received estrogen replacement therapy. *Clin Infect Dis* 1997;25(Suppl 2):5123–6
14. Velraeds MCM, Van der Mei HC, Reid G, *et al.* Inhibition of initial adhesion of uropathogenic *Enterococcus feacalis* by biosurfactants from *Lactobacillus* isolates. *Appl Environ Microbiol* 1996;62: 1958–63
15. Wira CR, Stern J. Endocrine regulation of the mucosal immune system in the female reproductive tract: control of IgA, IgG and secretory component during the reproductive cycle at implantation and throughout pregnancy. In Pasqualini JR, Scholler RS, eds. *Hormones and Fetal Pathophysiology* New York: Marcel Decker, Inc., 1992:343
16. Wira CR, Rossol RM. Antigen-presenting cells in the female reproductive tract: influence of sex hormones on antigen presentation in the vagina. *Immunology* 1995;84:505–8
17. Kondi-Paphitis A, Carvounis H, Kairi E, *et al.* Expression of local immune defence system in the female genital tract. *Eur J Gynecol Oncol* 1999;20: 141–3
18. Balan VE. *Urogenital Disturbances in the Climacterium (Clinic, Diagnosis, HRT).* Moscow: Delight Printing and Publishing, 1998:287
19. Albrecht AE, Hartman BX, Scholten C, *et al.* Effect of estrogen replacement therapy on natural killer cell activity in postmenopausal women. *Maturitas* 1996;25:217–22
20. Hastin J, Van der Eynde JP. Cytologic evaluation of the effects of ovarian estrogens given in postmenopause. *Acta Gynecol* 1977;21:225–8
21. Brondz BD. *T-Lymphocytes and their Receptors in Immunological Recognition.* Moscow: Nauka, 1987: 470

Update in assessment of the patient with postmenopausal urethrovesical dysfunction

82

H. E. O'Connell

INTRODUCTION

The major forms of urethral and bladder dysfunction in postmenopausal women include incontinence, voiding dysfunction, recurrent urinary tract infection and interstitial cystitis. This paper will provide an update on the evaluation of each of these problems. A thorough history and examination, a residual volume measurement, cystometrogram and abdominal leak-point pressure determination permit the characterization of most incontinence and voiding disorders. Bladder discomfort and recurrent urine infection in the absence of incontinence require a different diagnostic path.

INCONTINENCE AND VOIDING DYSFUNCTION: CLINICAL EVALUATION

Urinary incontinence occurs regularly in about 31% of middle-aged Western women[1]. The incidence of incontinence also increases with age, though it is a common problem in all age groups. The bladder, urethra or both may be responsible for either incontinence or voiding dysfunction. Determination of the cause of either problem requires a systematic approach. Stress incontinence in a surgically fit patient is a condition which is curable in most cases. It is often associated, however, with other conditions such as detrusor instability and voiding dysfunction. The latter conditions are not as reliably cured. When leakage is the presenting problem, it is important to determine its severity. A conservative strategy without an accurate diagnosis is sometimes acceptable, especially if the patient is not particularly bothered by the problem. If the problem has an effect on the patient's quality of life, restricts her activities, results in the need for regular pad wearing, is associated with recurrent urinary infection, or if conservative treatment is not resolving a problem that bothers the patient, accurate characterization of the problem is appropriate.

Urge incontinence – detrusor instability/poor compliance

Urge incontinence is a symptom which may be defined as urinary leakage preceded by an uncontrollable desire to void. Usually the patient has the symptom of urgency as well, i.e. after sensing the urge to pass urine, the patient hurries to the toilet, reaching it before leakage occurs. The patient knows that, if they defer voiding, they are at risk of leaking. Frequency, nocturia and enuresis are related symptoms. If elevated bladder storage pressures are the cause of these symptoms, recurrent urinary tract infections may also occur. In this setting, the infection is likely to be secondary to elevated bladder pressure rather than being the cause of the incontinence *per se*.

Urge incontinence may be due to either poor bladder compliance or detrusor instability, reflex activity that is difficult or impossible to inhibit. When the latter occurs, the term 'overactive' detrusor is also used. A cystometrogram is useful, as it reliably diagnoses poor bladder compliance. Detrusor instability is not reliably diagnosed with a cystometrogram, as many as 50% of cases having a normal study. The bladder may be poorly compliant as a result of a disturbance of the neurological control mechanism responsible for bladder relaxation. Fibrosis also causes poor bladder compliance. This secondary process may occur in neurogenic states, particularly in the presence of an indwelling catheter. Other chronic bladder conditions, such as interstitial cystitis, cyclophosphamide or tiaprofenic acid (Surgam®) cystitis and Bacillus Calmette Guerrin (BCG) cystitis, may also develop sufficient fibrosis to cause poor compliance. When urge incontinence, detrusor instability or poor compliance occur, a neurological cause should be considered.

The fact that the bladder is 'overactive' does not mean that bladder emptying function is satisfactory. The bladder reflex activity responsible for the incontinence may be poorly sustained or lack voluntary control, and inadequate emptying may occur in a patient who has severe leakage. With this combined problem, an underlying neurological lesion is sometimes causative, but often, especially in the elderly, diabetic patients and those with a history of bladder overdistention injury, a neurological condition may not be found. Patients who have urge incontinence must have an evaluation of their emptying function. This requires a residual bladder volume estimate, which is easily achieved with ultrasound. In the context of previous stress incontinence surgery, urethral hypersuspension should be excluded by palpation of the urethra during a valsalva maneuver and cough. This condition can cause slow flow, high residual volumes and detrusor instability. A pressure flow study with fluoroscopy may also be helpful.

Urge incontinence may be idiopathic. However, an underlying and treatable cause should be sought. Possible causes that may be cured include stress incontinence, urethral obstruction and genital prolapse. These conditions should be sought, as any reversible factor may be useful to minimize a condition that is often difficult to cure.

When the sensation of urgency occurs, but there are no accompanying episodes of incontinence, the patient's symptoms are likely to be due to bladder hypersensitivity or interstitial cystitis, rather than a problem with detrusor overactivity. In this situation, bladder filling is associated with discomfort, and leakage does not occur with deferral of voiding. Hypersensitivity states of the bladder, with or without observable inflammation, often cause the sensation of a need to void. The patient is desperate to void in order to relieve their discomfort, rather than because they fear that leakage will occur. In such patients, leakage is unusual unless a secondary problem has arisen with bladder compliance, or a co-existing condition such as detrusor instability or stress incontinence is present.

Stress or exertion-related leakage

When leakage occurs during physical exertion, it is usually due to urethral dysfunction. The proximal urethra should be located intra-abdominally and when the abdominal pressure rises during exertion, that pressure should be transferred to the urethra to maintain it passively closed[5]. When the urethra moves excessively due to changes in its support, leakage occurs via this mechanism. Such a urethral condition is referred to as urethral hypermobility. This condition may be cured by an operation which stops movement of the proximal urethra during exertion.

A second mechanism by which the urethra may leak in response to abdominal pressure is referred to as intrinsic sphincter deficiency. In this latter condition, the urethra may be immobile and therefore always subject to the passive closure force of the abdomen. Despite its correct position, however, when intrinsic sphincter deficiency exists, the urethra leaks easily even with minimal exertion, often resulting in severe leakage. This condition occurs if the proximal urethral integrity is disturbed by direct destruction or neurological or vascular injury to the urethral wall components. Damage to the urethral wall may result from prior surgery such as repeated surgery for stress incontinence, urethral diverticulectomy, bladder neck incision, prolonged catheter drainage and pelvic irradiation. Other risk factors for intrinsic sphincter deficiency, probably mediated neurologically, include myelodysplasia, Shy–Drager syndrome, abdominoperineal resection, radical hysterectomy and spinal cord injury or infarction. A recent study[6] indicated that simple hysterectomy may also be a significant risk factor for intrinsic sphincter deficiency. Correction of such a disorder has to be aimed at improving mucosal coaptation or urethral wall integrity. This may be achieved with a pubovaginal sling and, in many cases, a submucosal injectable agent may be used.

Typically high impact activity, such as vigorous coughing and sport, are associated with urethral hypermobility in the absence of intrinsic sphincter deficiency. Intrinsic sphincter deficiency, however, is associated with minimal exertion such as rising to an upright position, bending, blowing the nose and walking. It may be difficult to discern the difference clinically between intrinsic sphincter deficiency and poor compliance, and therefore a urodynamic study, preferably guided by fluoroscopy, is required. In the elderly, the amount of physical exertion performed may be negligible and these patients may not have the classical symptoms of stress incontinence. Again, accurate characterization of urethral dysfunction is important, as stress incontinence is readily treatable and often curable, and the clinical picture may suggest an alternative diagnosis.

Combinations of urethral and bladder disorders

Intrinsic sphincter deficiency and urethral hypermobility are not mutually exclusive conditions. Furthermore, any bladder disorder does not preclude a urethral disorder. Thus, a patient with spina bifida typically has poor bladder compliance, poor bladder sensation, intrinsic sphincter deficiency and poor bladder emptying function due to detrusor areflexia[7].

Genital prolapse

Genital prolapse may also occur with any urethral or detrusor disorder. A patient may have a large cystocele, detrusor instability, intrinsic sphincter deficiency and urethral hypermobility. In the management of large cystoceles, it is important to evaluate the urethra after reduction of the cystocele, as large cystoceles may mask urethral dysfunction. Prospective identification of urethral dysfunction facilitates correction of the combined problem and may be associated with a better outcome than having a standard treatment for all cystoceles[8].

PHYSICAL EXAMINATION

A pelvic examination should include evaluation of urethral hypermobility, genital prolapse and the pelvic floor. A neurological examination is also indicated, especially where incontinence is severe and associated with voiding dysfunction. A urine microscopy and culture should be obtained. A residual volume estimate is also appropriate in all cases.

URODYNAMIC EVALUATION

Urodynamic testing and imaging of the urinary tract is a continuation of the history and physical examination. The history and physical examination guides the clinician to determine which questions will be answered by a urodynamic examination and imaging studies. It is advantageous for the patient if evaluation is discrete, quick, accurate, reliable and makes a difference to the treatment choice.

Is urge incontinence or severe leakage due to poor bladder compliance?

A cystometrogram permits evaluation of bladder compliance. This is an easy test to perform and fulfils the characteristics noted above. Poor compliance may predispose a patient to upper urinary tract deterioration or recurrent significant urinary tract infection[7]. With the aid of fluoroscopy, morphological concomitants of poor compliance, such as trabeculation, diverticulum formation and vesicoureteric reflux, may be identified.

Is stress incontinence present and, if so, what type?

After bladder compliance has been shown to be normal, sphincteric function may be meaningfully evaluated. Stress incontinence occurs when maneuvers to increase abdominal pressure result in leakage in the absence of a rise in pressure due to the detrusor. Normally, the urethra prevents leakage driven by abdominal pressure. With fluoroscopy, urethral movement during exertion may be accurately demonstrated. The urethra may be open even before exertion occurs. Intrinsic sphincter deficiency may be quantified by the determination of abdominal leak-point pressure. Intrinsic sphincter deficiency is associated with a low abdominal leak-point pressure. Where the cause of stress incontinence is urethral hypermobility in the absence of intrinsic sphincter deficiency, the abdominal leak-point pressure is high (> 80 cmH_2O). The urethra may be hypermobile and close poorly in which case fluoroscopy or physical examination will reveal the urethral descent (> 2 cm) and the abdominal leak-point pressure will be low (< 60 cmH_2O).

Abdominal leak-point pressure determination permits broad stratification of urethral pathophysiology[9]. An algorithm is presented in Figure 1, which may be used to guide therapy. Topical or oral estrogens may be used in any of these categories to assist in urethral closure, urethral support and improve detrusor control. Pelvic floor exercises may be useful in all diagnostic groups.

Recurrent urinary tract infection and interstitial cystitis

An overview of these topics for the non-urologist may be found in reference 2. A complete description of the evaluation of recurrent urinary tract infections and interstitial cystitis is beyond the scope of this text. Useful references include 3 and 4.

CONCLUSIONS

Evaluation of incontinence and voiding dysfunction does not have to be torture. A thorough clinical evaluation supported by the discriminant use of urodynamic and imaging studies provides a useful framework for the treatment of urethral and vesical dysfunction in postmenopausal women.

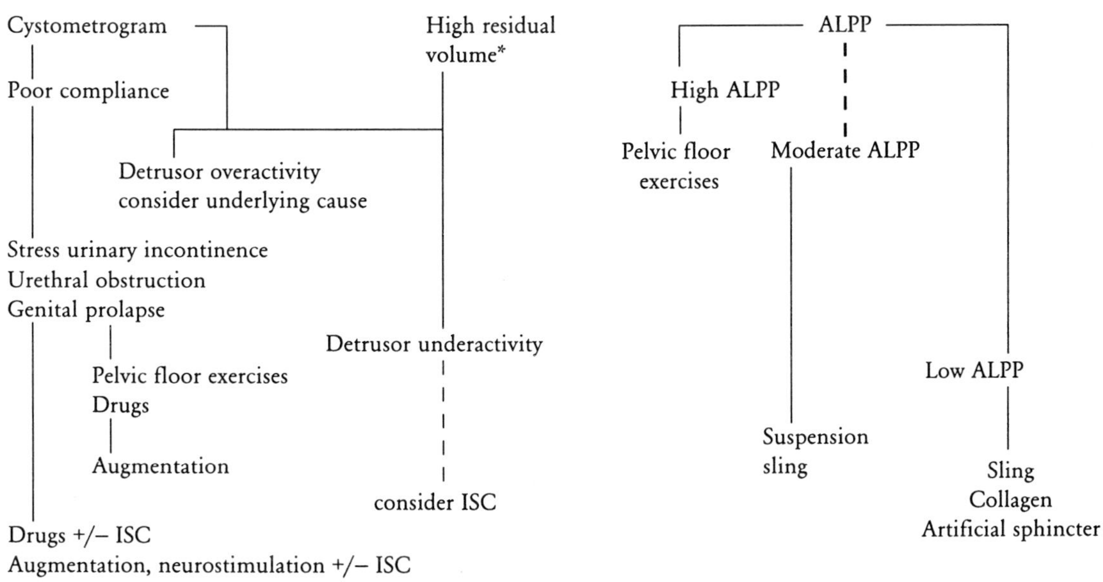

Figure 1 Determination of abdominal leak-point (ALPP): use of findings to determine treatment *Consider urethral obstruction; ISC, intermittent self-catheterization

References

1. Burgio KL, Matthews KA, Engel BT. Prevalence, incidence and correlates of urinary incontinence in healthy, middle aged women. *J Urol* 1991;146: 1255–9
2. O'Connell HE, McKertich K. Common urological problems in women. *Aust Fam Phys* 1998;12: 1098–2004
3. Wein AJ, Hanno PM, eds. Interstitial cystitis: an update of current information. *Urology* 1997;49:5
4. Kunin CM. *Urinary Tract Infections - Detection, Prevention and Management.* Baltimore: Williams and Wilkins, 1997
5. McGuire EJ, Herlihy E. The influence of urethral position on urinary continence. *Invest Urol* 1997; 15:205–7
6. Morgan JL, O'Connell HE, McGuire EJ. Is intrinsic sphincter deficiency a complication of simple hysterectomy. *J Urol* 1999; submitted
7. McGuire EJ, Woodside JR, Borden TA, *et al.* Prognostic value of urodynamic testing in myelodysplastic patients. *J Urol* 1981;126:205–9
8. Ghoniem GM, Walters F, Lewis V. The value of the vaginal pack test in large cystoceles. *J Urol* 1994;152: 931–4
9. McGuire EJ, Fitzpatrick CC, Wan J, *et al.* Clinical assessment of urethral sphincter function. *J Urol* 1993;150:1452–4

Behavioral intervention for incontinence in clinical practice

83

C. M. Sampselle

INTRODUCTION

Urinary incontinence, the involuntary leakage of urine, affects between 25% and 34% of community-dwelling women[1]. It imposes heavy costs related to treatment or management of the condition as well as costs resulting in decreased quality of life. Women are at greater risk for urinary incontinence subsequent to pregnancy and childbirth[2], to hysterectomy[3] and to aging[4,5].

Recognizing the widespread impact of urinary incontinence on the health and well-being of women, the Association of Women's Health, Obstetric and Neonatal Nurses (AWHONN) designed a research project to focus on this condition[6]. The project was entitled 'Continence for Women: AWHONN's Third Research Utilization Project'. That 3-year project, begun in 1995, consisted of three phases. Phase I, for planning, included the development of an evidence-based protocol that has been presented in detail in a previous publication[7], as well as the development of data management forms and the plan for implementation of the project. Phase II, for implementation, entailed site recruitment, resulting in the inclusion of 21 ambulatory women's health-care sites that participated throughout the project, the training of nurses to use the evidence-based protocol, and data collection. Phase III, for evaluation, involved assessment of the success of the process that enabled clinicians to use the protocol. The aim of the study reported here was to test the effectiveness of an evidence-based protocol for urinary incontinence in increasing identification of women with the condition and improving patient outcomes.

HYPOTHESES

The project investigated two broad research questions:

(1) Would change occur in clinical practice after clinicians were trained to identify urinary incontinence and to intervene using an evidence-based protocol?

(2) Would patient outcomes be positively affected after the protocol was instituted in the clinical setting?

The following hypothesis was related to practice change. Hypothesis 1: More women will screen positive for urinary incontinence when routine screening is implemented, compared to the proportion who disclose the condition, as reported in the literature.

The hypotheses related to patient outcomes were as follows. Hypothesis 2: Urinary incontinence episodes will decrease in frequency. Hypothesis 3: Urine loss per episode will decrease in volume. Hypothesis 4: The cost of self-management of urinary incontinence will decrease. Hypothesis 5: The amount of bother associated with incontinence will decrease. Hypothesis 6: The number of activities avoided because of incontinence will decrease.

METHODS

The initial sample consisted of 1474 women screened for incontinence as a part of the routine history collected in their respective ambulatory settings. Four screening questions were asked of all women (Figure 1).

1. Do you ever leak urine/water when you don't want to?
2. Do you ever leak urine/water when you cough, laugh, or exercise?
3. Do you ever leak urine/water on the way to use the bathroom?
4. Do you ever use pads, tissue, or cloth in your underwear to catch urine?

Figure 1 Screening questions

Of the total sample screened, 57% (842) responded 'always' or 'sometimes' on at least one of the four screening items. The specific measures identified for each variable of interest and the analyses selected to test each hypothesis are detailed below.

Hypothesis 1

The proportion of women who responded positively to one or more of the four screening questions was compared to the percentages (38–41%) of women identified by the survey[8,9] who indicated that they had incontinence and had discussed the problem with a health-care provider. Using the aggregate number of women reported by participating sites who answered any of the first four screening questions positively as the denominator, the proportion who completed the basic evaluation was calculated.

Hypothesis 2

Data for variables used for testing of hypotheses 2–6 were collected on the Basic Evaluation Form (Figure 2) at baseline prior to treatment and at 4 months after treatment. Respondents indicated the volume of urine lost per episode of incontinence by selecting one of five categories (less than once a week, once a week, more than once a week, once a day, more than once a day). Differences in the usual frequency of urine leakage were determined by comparing the response on this item at baseline with that on the same item on the ongoing evaluation administered 4 months later.

Hypothesis 3

Differences in amount of urine loss per episode were assessed by comparison of baseline indications of a selected category that estimated the volume of urine lost, on average, per episode of incontinence (damp, wet, cupful, flood) with the same item in the ongoing evaluation.

Hypothesis 4

A cost estimate was calculated by obtaining retail prices of all levels of protection, from panty liners to absorbent pants/super pads in two regional areas (Washington, DC and Arizona). The mean cost of each type of protection was multiplied by the number of reported changes per day and then multiplied by 7 to derive an estimated cost per week. These estimates were compared between the baseline and the ongoing evaluations.

Hypothesis 5

A difference in the level of bother (ranging from 1 which signified no bother to 5, a great deal of bother) was compared between the baseline and the ongoing evaluation.

Hypothesis 6

Women were asked to indicate specific activities they avoided such as shopping, exercising or travelling. The percentage of women who reported avoiding particular activities at baseline was compared to the percentage who reported avoiding those activities at the time the ongoing evaluation was administered.

Analysis

The statistical analyses were performed using the Statistical Package for the Social Sciences[10]. The χ^2 test, the *t* test and repeated measures analysis of variance were used for assessment of group differences in demographic characteristics and for hypothesis testing. Descriptive statistics were generated from the 1474 cases initially screened across the 21 participating sites. To conduct hypothesis testing of the effects on continence status, we analyzed

Date: [ ][ ] / [ ][ ] / [ ][ ]   Site: [ ][ ][ ]   Participant: [ ][ ][ ]

FIGURE 2   14

Continence for Women Project: Basic Evaluation

1. How long have you had the problem of leaking when you don't want to? — [ ][ ] months [ ][ ] years

2. On average, how often do you lose urine/water during a typical week? —
   - ○ Less than once a week
   - ○ Once a week
   - ○ More than once a week
   - ○ Once a day
   - ○ More than once a day

3. How would you describe the amount of urine you usually leak? —
   - ○ Damp/ a few drops
   - ○ Wet/enough to wet underpants
   - ○ Quite wet/a cupful (soaks pads/other protection)
   - ○ Very wet/floods/soaks through outer clothes

4. How much does this leakage bother you? Not at all ○ 1 ○ 2 ○ 3 ○ 4 ○ 5 Very Much

5. Are you currently using pads for protection against urine leakage?
   - ○ No — Skip to #6
   - ○ Yes — What type? ○ Panty liner ○ Sanitary pad ○ Larger pad ○ Absorbent pant — How many times **per day** do you need to change pads? ○ 1 or fewer ○ 2 ○ 3 ○ 4 ○ 5 ○ 6 or more

6. How many days **last week** did you leak urine? — ○ 0 ○ 1 ○ 2 ○ 3 ○ 4 ○ 5 ○ 6 ○ 7

7. Are you avoiding certain activities because of a urine/water loss problem?
   - ○ No — Skip to #8
   - ○ Yes — ○ Shopping ○ Exercising ○ Traveling ○ Visiting friends/family ○ Dating ○ Having sex ○ Dancing ○ Playing sports

8. On average, how many times do you urinate/pass water during the day? [ ][ ] night? [ ][ ]

9. Are you having burning or discomfort when you urinate/pass water? — ○ Yes ○ No

10. Do you have a history of: *(check as many as apply)*
    - ○ Diabetes
    - ○ Stroke
    - ○ Multiple Sclerosis
    - ○ Spinal cord injury or surgery
    - ○ Constipation
    - ○ Problems walking
    - ○ Previous treatment for urine loss

11. Do you feel that your bladder is empty after you urinate/pass water? — ○ Yes ○ No

12. Do you ever push down or strain to urinate/pass water? — ○ Yes ○ No

13. Please list any medications that you are currently taking, either prescribed or purchased over the counter.

14. Who completed this form? — ○ Myself ○ Nurse ○ Someone else

The nurse will talk with you about plans for follow-up.

RU3-B

24277

Figure 2 Basic evaluation form

only the 132 cases for whom baseline (pretreatment) and 4-month (post-treatment) data were available. Differences were examined between women who finished treatment and those who dropped out. The alpha level of 0.05 was set to judge the significant differences.

Table 1 Factors associated with urinary incontinence

Variable	*Continent* (n = 632)	*Incontinent* (n = 842)	F^* or χ^{2**}	*p Value*
Race				
African American	50.4%	49.6%	19.0**	< 0.0001
Hispanic	49.3%	50.7%		
White	36.8%	63.2%		
Age (mean years)	35 ± 15	44 ± 16	117.2*	< 0.0001
Ever having given birth	64.9%	82.0%	53.3*	< 0.0001
Vaginal birth (mean)	1.1 ± 1.4	1.8 ± 1.5	90.6*	< 0.0001
Hysterectomy	0.1%	19.5%	32.8*	< 0.0001

RESULTS

Factors associated with incontinence

The initial sample (n = 1474) was divided into those who reported incontinence and those who did not. Fifty-seven per cent reported some unwanted leakage. The two groups were compared on selected demographic characteristics (Table 1). Age, race, vaginal birth, and history of hysterectomy were significantly different between the continent and incontinent groups. White women were significantly more likely to report incontinence. Incontinent women were more likely to have given birth or to have a history of hysterectomy.

Pretreatment continence status

The pretreatment level of incontinence severity is presented in Table 2. Nearly 25% of those who were incontinent reported unwanted urine loss occurring daily or more frequently. Nearly 40% were losing volumes of urine that they characterized as 'wet' or greater and 41% reported being bothered at the higher levels of the 'bother' scale. When asked about their use of protective pads, 37% of those reporting incontinence indicated that they required this protection, with nearly 42% having to change at least twice a day.

The results presented in the following paragraphs detail the outcome of the hypothesis-testing process and constitute the evaluation of the protocol itself. They demonstrate its effectiveness when carried out by typical providers in ordinary clinical settings as opposed to the more systematic and controlled environment in which conventional research is conducted.

Table 2 Pretreatment continence status (%) among women who reported urinary incontinence (n = 842)

	Women (%)
Frequency of leaking	
< 1/week	43.1
1/week	10.5
> 1/week	21.7
1/day	9.5
> 1/day	15.2
Average amount lost	
Damp	61.5
Wet	33.3
Cupful	3.2
Flood	2.0
Amount bothered by leakage	
1 (not at all)	20.8
2	23.1
3	15.1
4	12.9
5 (very much)	28.1

Practice outcomes

Hypothesis 1 tested for an increase in the percentage of incontinent women identified by routine screening in a clinical setting as compared to those who reported seeking help as documented by previous research. Population-based surveys have found that the percentage of incontinent individuals who report their condition to a health-care provider ranges from 38 to 41%[8,9]. By comparison, 57% (842/1475) of women were identified as incontinent with the routine screening used in the current project. This represents a marked increase when measured against that reported in the literature. In addition to identifying the condition, 63% (529/842) of women who answered affirmatively on one or more of the screening questions completed a basic evaluation and nearly 78% (653/842) of them provided partial information on the basic evaluation. This evidence supports Hypothesis 1, demonstrating that, among ambulatory clinic patients, routine screening and requested completion of basic evaluation information results in the identification of a higher prevalence of incontinence as compared to the proportion of women who typically initiate discussion of incontinence with a health-care provider.

Patient outcomes

The outcome measures of frequency of incontinence episodes, volume of leakage per episode, cost of self-management and quality of life showed improvement from the baseline pretreatment data to the 4-month post-treatment point (Table 3).

Hypothesis 2, that there would be a decreased frequency of episodes of incontinence, was supported. Women experienced significantly fewer episodes in a typical week and in the number of days of leaking in the past week. Hypothesis 3, that there would be a decreased volume of leakage per incontinent episode, was supported. Women selected lower categories to reflect the volume of leakage per incontinence episode over the time of treatment. Hypothesis 4, that there would be a decreased cost of self-management; Hypothesis 5, that there would be a decreased amount of bother associated with incontinence; and Hypothesis 6, that there would be decreased activities avoided due to incontinence, were also supported. All indices specified by the respective hypotheses significantly declined between the pretreatment and post-treatment periods.

DISCUSSION

These results demonstrate the effectiveness of the evidence-based protocol in clinical settings. The participating sites represented a wide range of practice settings, and the overall sample was reasonably diverse. This suggests that the results could be generalized to the larger population in the USA and warrants the implementation of the protocol in general ambulatory women's health-care settings.

Practice outcomes

It should be noted that the reported proportion of women who screened positive for urinary incontinence and subsequently underwent a complete basic evaluation (63%) is artificially low. At least 124 additional basic evaluations were completed, but were inadequately identified. That is, the basic evaluation had been completed, but it was not possible to link it to a specific set of screening questions. Because a woman was to complete the basic evaluation only if her responses to screening questions indicated an incontinence problem, a less conservative estimate of basic evaluation completion would be 78% (653/842). Either proportion is substantially greater than that reflected in previous surveys. This finding demonstrates that routine screening, coupled with a system that facilitates follow-up for basic evaluation, is effective in identifying symptomatic individuals.

Table 3 Changes in continence status pre- and post-treatment among women who reported urinary incontinence

Measure	*Pretreatment* (n = 132)	*Post-treatment* (n = 132)	*F*	*p Value*
Leakage in a typical week	3.0	2.2	7.2	0.002
Number of days of leakage in the past week	2.9	1.9	10.2	0.0001
Average volume of urine lost*	1.6	1.4	4.6	0.03
Micturition frequency during the day	6.1	6.5	1.4	NS
Frequency during the night	1.7	0.9	5.9	0.012
Cost of self-management	$1.18	$0.81	5.75	0.031
Bother score	3.1	2.8	12.31	0.0001
Percentage avoiding activities	14.0%	3.5%	7.96	0.001

*Actual volume was not measured. Respondents indicated one of four categories ranging from a few drops to soaking outer clothes

Patient outcomes

The number of women who provided feedback at the 4-month follow-up ($n = 132$) was markedly lower than the original number who screened positive ($n = 842$). Comparisons of selected baseline characteristics of the original and enduring longitudinal sample are presented in Table 4. Women who persisted in treatment had urinary incontinence of longer duration and greater severity at baseline.

The frequency, volume, and life impact of urinary incontinence decreased following treatment. Given that 57% of the baseline sample of women screened reported some problem with unwanted leakage, replication of this protocol in a wide range of ambulatory sites is likely to benefit diverse types of women across the lifespan.

It is noteworthy that those who were retained to the post-treatment point initially had more severe levels of incontinence, as reflected in longer duration and greater frequency of involuntary loss prior to treatment (Table 4). Others have reported that only 25% of incontinent women start treatment when it is offered[11]. Perhaps the severity of the condition motivates women to accept and persist with behavioral therapy.

Although it was not originally hypothesized, an additional benefit to women's overall well-being was noted. There was a decrease in the frequency of nocturia experienced by women post-treatment. While nocturia is not incontinence, it disrupts sleep and can affect overall well-being. As can be seen in Table 3, the frequency of nocturia declined from a pretreatment level of 1.7 to a post-treatment frequency of 0.9 ($F = 5.9$, $p < 0.012$). This phenomenon has not been reported previously and deserves further investigation.

The statistics and the hypothesis testing reported thus far tell only part of the story. Anecdotal evidence contributed by site co-ordinators provides powerful insights into the impact of the protocol on the lives of individual women. One nurse told of a patient who offered to pay her own way to the AWHONN Convention so that she could explain to other women's health nurses how important the program was. 'You changed my life!' she told the nurse who had implemented the protocol, 'I want other nurses to know about this'. Another woman, whose voiding frequency decreased from about 15 to eight times in the course of a 24-h period, asked of the nurse who helped her, 'Why haven't I heard about this before now?'

Implications for practice

The results of this study demonstrate clear benefits to the health of women when this protocol is incorporated into standard ambulatory patient care. The four recommended screening questions will identify higher numbers of women at risk than will a less systematic approach. Given the significantly greater risk of incontinence in women who have had a hysterectomy, providers should be particularly vigilant when assessing this group.

The basic evaluation questions allow determination of the candidates who will benefit more from referral, such as for treatment of neurological disease, and those who should receive information

Table 4 Comparison of baseline characteristics between the original sample and the enduring longitudinal sample

	Time 1 data only ($n = 842$)	*Retained to time 3* ($n = 132$)	*Statistical difference*
Age (years)	39.9	51.1	$p < 0.001$
Racial distribution of three major groups (%)			
African American	18	7	
Hispanic	10	5	$p < 0.001$
White	72	88	
Duration of incontinence (months)	24.6	39.3	$p < 0.0001$
Frequency of incontinence (times per week)	2.1	3.0	$p < 0.002$
Voiding frequency while awake (times per day)	5.9	6.2	NS
Nocturia frequency (times per night)	1.8	1.3	NS

about the value of bladder and pelvic floor muscle training. Information about available patient education materials and their incorporation into typical practice settings is discussed in detail[7], and updates are available at the AHCPR website http://www.hcfa.gov/medicaid/siq/siqipg.htm.

In summary, this evidence-based protocol, as it was systematically implemented in a variety of ambulatory women's health-care settings, facilitated systematic screening and the obtaining of baseline evaluation data. The simple program of pelvic floor muscle and bladder training yielded significant improvements in women's continence status. The results of this project support widespread incorporation of the protocol into clinical practice in ambulatory care sites.

References

1. Thom D. Variation in estimates of urinary incontinence prevalence in the community: effects of differences in definition, population characteristics, and study type. *J Am Geriatr Soc* 1998;46:473–80
2. Meyer S, Schreyer A, DeGrandi P, Hohlfeld P. The effects of birth on urinary continence mechanisms and other pelvic-floor characteristics. *Obstet Gynecol* 1998;92:613–18
3. Brown JS, Seely DG, Fong J, Black DM, Ensrud KE, Grady D. Urinary incontinence in older women: who is at risk? *Obstet Gynecol* 1996;87:715–21
4. Lagace EA, Hansen W, Hickner JM. Prevalence and severity of urinary incontinence in ambulatory adults: an UPRNet study. *J Fam Pract* 1993;36: 610–14
5. Diokno AC, Brock BM, Brown HB, Herzog AR. Prevalence of urinary incontinence and other urologic symptoms in the non-institutionalized elderly. *J Urol* 1986;136:1022–5
6. Sampselle CM, Wyman JF, Thomas KK, *et al.* Continence for women: evaluation of AWHONN's third research utilization project. *J Obstet Gynecol Neonat Nurs* 1999;29(1)
7. Sampselle CM, Burns P, Dougherty M, Thomas KK, Newman DK, Wyman J. Continence for women: evidence-based practice. *J Obstet Gynecol Neonat Nurs* 1997;26:375–85
8. Burgio KL, Ives DG, Locher JL, Arena VC. Treatment seeking for urinary incontinence in adults. *J Am Geriatr Soc* 1994;42:208–12
9. Goldstein M, Hawthorne ME, Engeberg S, McDowell BJ, Burgio KL. Urinary incontinence: why people do not seek help. *J Gerontol Nurs* 1992;18:15–20
10. Norusis M. *SPSS Advanced Statistics 6.1.* Chicago: SPSS Inc., 1994
11. Samuelsson E, Victor A, Tibblin G. A population study of urinary incontinence and nocturia among women aged 20–59 years. Prevalence, well-being and wish for treatment. *Acta Obstet Gynecol Scand* 1997; 76:74–80

Psychological aspects of the transition to menopause

84

A. Collins

INTRODUCTION

The menopause is associated with biological and psychological changes that affect women's health and well-being, as well as their working capacity. While the menopause as a physiological event has been extensively documented and relatively well described, the psychological and psychosocial factors affecting women at midlife have received much less attention and, therefore, are not as well understood. It should be pointed out that the midlife transition does not only imply a heightened vulnerability to symptoms, but it can also be defined as the 'third developmental phase', a period when women experience an increased sense of personal identity and a confidence in personal efficacy, as well as an increased acceptance of aging.

There continues to be considerable controversy among researchers as to whether mood changes and psychological symptoms are linked to the hormonal changes occurring at the menopause or whether psychosocial factors play a more important role for the development of various symptoms. Earlier research has assumed that there is an association between symptoms such as fatigue, depressed mood, memory problems and decreased sexual interest, and declining estrogen levels. Many clinicians hold the belief that the menopause may be linked to depression and that hormone replacement is effective in improving this condition. This is not surprising, since there are clinical studies that have indicated that estrogen treatment may improve mood and enhance the sense of well-being in some menopausal women[2]. However, many of these studies are based on select groups of women attending menopausal clinics and are lacking in important methodological aspects[3].

Much of the earlier research on the menopause has involved small clinical samples. We know that women who attend menopause clinics are not representative of women in general[4]. Furthermore, many of the earlier studies have focused on the negative aspects of aging, thus contributing to an overly negative view of this life stage. Women themselves have been influenced by these negative stereotypes and images of the menopause. Attitude to the menopause has been shown to be important in affecting symptoms[5-7].

It is not clear that the menopause is associated with an increased incidence of depression[8]. Instead, it seems that the highest incidence of depressed mood occurs in the 30–45-year age range[9]. Studies have shown that episodes of earlier depression may predict depressed mood at the menopause[10]. Women who have suffered from depression previously are more likely to experience depression at the menopause. Depression can also be triggered by distress related to family relationships[11].

Barnett and Baruch[12] have pointed out that women's traditional roles as mothers and wives have been overemphasized in menopause research. A very central aspect of women's lives in today's society that has been overlooked is work role and the quality of work experience. In Sweden, as in many other Western societies, women's participation in the work force has increased tremendously. There has been a heated debate whether this will cause women to suffer from stress-related diseases to the same extent as men. Women's multiple roles may contribute to disease[13]. Previous research on the background of cardiovascular disease has shown that stress and the psychosocial work environment have profound effects on health outcomes in terms of cardiovascular health[14]. Several recent studies show that dissatisfaction with the job and stress at work are related to various physical symptoms[15,16]. There is a need to examine the relationship between the effect of work role and menopausal symptoms.

In our longitudinal study on the menopause, we have brought into focus the relationship between psychosocial and biological factors affecting women's health at the menopause. As far as psychosocial variables are concerned, we thought it important to emphasize the role played by psychosocial factors such as social relationships and job satisfaction, as well as women's experience of the work environment, as central variables in analyzing the factors that are important for women's health and well-being at the menopause. The aim was to examine the interaction of psychosocial and biological factors associated with symptoms and mood change in a population-based sample of Swedish women during the transition to menopause.

METHODS

The Stockholm Menopause Study was carried out using a population-based sample of women. Recruitment of subjects was carried out in two phases. As a first phase of the study, 2011 women were recruited through the Swedish Population Register. They were women aged 48 years who resided in the catchment area of the Karolinska Hospital in Stockholm. They all received a health questionnaire together with a letter and a stamped envelope. A total of 1399 returned the completed questionnaire. A representative sample of 150 women was drawn from this pool of subjects, reflecting the education and parity of the original population of women who had replied. The women were invited to come to the laboratory and were assessed annually over 5 years. The annual follow-up included a general health screening, which involved a gynecological examination, psychological interviews and self-rating scales. The interviews were individual face-to-face, semi-structured, in-depth interviews lasting about 1.5 h. The same interviewer saw the same women each year. Questions that were covered included sociodemographic background and health history, perceived health, experience of symptoms, use of hormonal treatment, social relationships, relationship with parents and with partner, lifestyle, attitude to the menopause, work role, job satisfaction, stress at work and life stress. The answers were transcribed verbatim and coded by each interviewer. Menopausal status was determined based on several questions about menstrual pattern and changes within the past year. The women were classified as pre-, peri- or postmenopausal or HRT users using the same criteria as Avis and McKinlay[17]. The women filled out the Swedish version of the Mensicore Menopause Symptoms Scale and the SL90 depression scale, as well as the CES-D Depression Scale, each year. Relationships with parents were measured using the Quality of Role Scales developed by Rosalind Barnett and translated into Swedish. These ratings were completed at only the fourth and fifth annual visits[18].

RESULTS

As for sociodemographic background, the majority of the women were married or remarried (78%), while 5% were never married, 12% were divorced and 5% were widowed. Thirty per cent had primary education, 40% had secondary education, while 30% had a college or university education. The great majority of women were employed (97%), 77% full-time and 23% part-time. As for menopausal status, 51% were premenopausal, 41% perimenopausal and 8% were postmenopausal at study entry. Six per cent were taking hormonal replacement. None had undergone hysterectomy. At the fifth annual visit, 8% were premenopausal, 31% were perimenopausal and 61% were postmenopausal, and 53% were taking hormone replacement therapy. Seven per cent of the women had undergone hysterectomy with bilateral oophorectomy.

The symptom ratings for baseline symptoms were factor-analyzed using the Varimax criterion. Factor analyses yielded ten independent factors that explained 58% of the variance. These factor dimensions were used in subsequent analyses of the symptom ratings. They included negative mood, vasomotor symptoms, decreased sexual desire, increased sexual desire, vaginal dryness, memory problems, increased vitality, sleep-related problems, joint pain and urogenital symptoms.

Multiple regression analyses of factors associated with symptom ratings[7] completed on the fourth visit showed that only vasomotor symptoms and joint pain had a significant relationship with menopausal status. The other symptom dimensions were explained by a negative attitude to the menopause and to aging, somatic complaints, a lack of regular exercise and a negative relationship with the woman's partner.

Comparison of depression scores over the 5 years using analysis of variance showed that there were no significant differences between menopausal groups or between annual follow-ups[18]. The only group showing elevated depression scores was the small group of women who had undergone a hysterectomy with bilateral oophorectomy. They showed a transient and significant increase in depression during the third annual follow-up. However, the fourth annual follow-up showed no such difference. There were no differences in depression scores between pre- and postmenopausal states. Qualitative analyses of responses to questions in the interviews over the 5 years showed that 14% of the women had a definitively negative attitude to the menopause. These women had significantly higher depression scores than the other women at the fourth and fifth annual visits. They also had higher total SL90 scores, indicating greater general psychopathology than the other women. They had higher anxiety and neuroticism scores than the other women.

A model of multiple regression analyses was created in order to analyze which variables would be significantly associated with depression scores at the fifth annual follow-up. The following variables were included as possibly explaining the variance in depression: menopausal status, education, occupation, somatic complaints, lifestyle (e.g. smoking and regular exercise), job satisfaction and life stress, as well as relationship with partner and with parents. Furthermore, baseline measurements of work satisfaction and earlier depressed mood were included.

The results showed that, for the total group, depressed mood was significantly associated with current health complaints, a negative attitude to the menopause, smoking and postmenopausal status. Variables measured at baseline during the first annual follow-up predicting depressed mood 5 years later were dissatisfaction with work, earlier experience of depressed mood and experience of life stress. It is interesting that the relationship with the woman's partner and with her parents was shown to be of importance. The separate analysis of those women whose mothers were alive and who had completed the quality of parent relationship scale ($n = 59$) showed that a negative attitude to the menopause, a negative relationship with the mother, and current life stress were significantly related to depression scores. Very similar results were derived for those women who completed the scales whose fathers were alive ($n = 34$). Depression was associated with health complaints, a negative attitude to the menopause, a negative relationship with the father and postmenopausal status.

Analysis of responses to questions in the interviews showed that many of the women reported stress and worry about responsibility toward ailing parents and anxiety that the parents would fall ill and require more attention. However, many of the women also expressed joy about their relationship with their parents and rated it to be an important source of happiness.

DISCUSSION

The most important finding was that the majority of women were enjoying good health and did not experience significant mood changes during the transition to menopause. Analysis of background factors showed that psychosocial factors are more important than menopausal status in explaining symptoms and mood changes at the menopause. Thus, the psychosocial environment seems to be more important than hormonal factors in explaining mood changes and symptoms at the menopause.

It is also clear that the great majority of women have a positive attitude to the menopause and only a small group have a negative attitude. Women with a negative attitude to the menopause had significantly higher depression scores. Data from the interviews with the women confirmed these results. The women with a negative attitude expressed considerable negative emotions and reported being unhappy with their lives. In a longitudinal study, Bromberger and Matthews[19] found that pessimism and trait anxiety were associated with more severe problems at the menopause. On the other hand, Caltabiano and Holzheimer[20] found that the presence of dispositional factors, such as optimism and sense of coherence, served as protective buffers for menopausal women.

Our results showed that somatic health, life stress and social relationships, as well as prior depression and dissatisfaction with work, were important. Similar results have been found by Woods and Mitchell[21], who reported from the Seattle Women's Health Study that health status and life stress had a significant effect on depression scores in menopausal women. Dennerstein[10], in a longitudinal population-based study, found that negative mood was mainly explained by health problems, prior premenstrual problems, prior depression and a negative attitude to the menopause.

It is interesting that social and family relationships, particularly the relationship with the mother, proved to be of great importance for the mental health of these women. There has been a debate about women's multiple roles and whether multiple roles are negative for women's health[22]. Earlier research has emphasized the burden of caring for elderly parents, thus adding stress to the already heavy workloads of employed women. Conflicting demands from multiple roles is likely to increase women's total workload and their level of stress. This is particularly true for the proportion of women with ailing parents who have little help from the community or other sources. However, Baruch[23] and Walker and colleagues[24] found that there was very little conflict between caregiving and work role or other social roles among middle-aged women. It is important to emphasize the more positive aspects of the mother–daughter relationship. Results from our interviews showed that many women develop more mature relationships with their mothers at this time in their lives. On the other hand, a proportion of the women had always had emotionally distant or cold relationships with their mothers and they did not seem able to improve their relationships. Others had feelings of guilt and worry about their mothers. The regression analyses showed that a negative and distant relationship with the mother was associated with a higher depression score. It seems that the relationship with elderly parents is important for the well-being of middle-aged daughters.

Our results also showed that experience of the work role was important. Dissatisfaction with work at the entry of the study predicted depression 5 years later. Other research has shown that work role and the psychosocial work environment is of great importance to women's health[25]. A considerable proportion of women are employed in jobs that can be characterized by low control, i.e. the individual has little control over the pace of work or work content, as well as high demands, such as constant deadlines. New data from our ongoing study on work life indicate that perimenopausal women with high-strain jobs have more somatic and psychosomatic symptoms[18] than other women.

In conclusion, our results have shown that the menopause can be seen as a developmental phase in women's lives associated with increased maturity and self-awareness. A certain proportion of women are vulnerable to various symptoms, as well as mood changes, during the menopause. Psychosocial factors, health status, social relationships and perception of work role are more important than menopausal status in explaining these symptoms and changes during the menopause.

References

1. Stewart AJ, Ostrove JM. Women's personality in middle age. *Am Psychol* 1998;11:1185–94
2. Studd J. Depression and the menopause: estrogens improve symptoms in some middle aged women. *Br Med J* 1997;31:977–8
3. Holte A. Menopause, mood and hormone replacement therapy: methodological issues. *Maturitas* 1998;29:5–18

4. Morse CA, Smith A, Dennerstein L, *et al.* The treatment-seeking woman at menopause. *Maturitas* 1994;18:161–73
5. Woods NF, Mitchell ES. Patterns of depressed mood in midlife women: observations from the Seattle Women's Health Study. *Res Nurs Health* 1996;19:111–23
6. Collins A. Menopause from a psychological perspective. In Sjoberg NO, ed. *Menopause and its Treatment.* Carnforth, UK: Parthenon Publishing, 1997
7. Barth Olofsson A, Collins A. Psychosocial factors, attitude to menopause and symptoms in Swedish women at perimenopause. *Climacteric* 2000; in press
8. Collins A. Depression and the menopausal transition. In Studd J, ed. *The Management of the Menopause.* Annual Review. Carnforth, UK: Parthenon Publishing, 1998
9. Hay AG, Bancroft J, Johnston EC. Affective symptoms in women attending a menopause clinic. *Br J Psychiatry* 1994;164:513–16
10. Dennerstein L. Well-being, symptoms and the menopausal transition. *Maturitas* 1996;23:147–57
11. Kaufert P, Gilbert P, Tate R. The Manitoba Project: a re-examination of the link between menopause and depression. *Maturitas* 1992;14:143–55
12. Barnett R, Baruch GB. Women in the middle years: a critique of research and theory. *Psychol Women Q* 1978;3:187–97
13. Waldron I, Jacobs JA. Effects of multiple roles on women's health. Evidence from a longitudinal study. *Women Health* 1989;15:3–19
14. Frankenhaeuser M, Lundberg U, Fredrikson M, *et al.* Stress on and off the job as related to sex and occupational status in white-collar workers. *J Org Behav* 1989;10:321–46
15. Karasek RA, Theorell T. *Healthy Work: Stress, Productivity and the Reconstruction of Working Life.* New York: Basic Books, 1990
16. Perski A. *The Stressed Heart.* Stockholm: Bromberg, 1999
17. Avis NE, McKinlay SM. A longitudinal analysis of women's attutudes towards the menopause: results from the Massachusett's women's health study. *Maturitas* 1991;13:65–79
18. Collins A, Barth Olofsson A. Factors affecting mood changes during transition to menopause. 2000; to be submitted
19. Bromberger JT, Matthews KA. A longitudinal study of the effects of pessimism, trait anxiety and life stress on depressive symptoms in middle-aged women. *Psychol Aging* 1996;11:207–13
20. Caltabiano ML, Holzheimer M. Dispositional factors, coping and adaptation during menopause. *Climacteric* 1999;2:21–8
21. Woods NF, Mitchell E. Pathways to depressed mood for midlife women. *Res Nurs Health* 1997; 20:119–29
22. Barnett R, Davidson H, Marshall N. Physical symptoms and the interplay of work and family roles. *Health Psychol* 1991;10:94–101
23. Baruch GB. The psychological well-being of women in the middle years. In Baruch GB, Brooks-Gunn J, eds. *Women in Midlife.* New York: Plenum Press, 1984
24. Walker AJ, Pratt CC, Wood B. Perceived frequency of role conflict and relationship quality for caregiving daughters. *Psychol Women Q* 1993;17:207–21
25. Hall E. *Women's Work: an Inquiry into the Health Effects of Invisible and Visible Labor.* Stockholm: Akademitryck, 1990

Refounding the knowledge of the psychology of the menopause: longevity without aging

85

L. Zichella

My main aim is to review the scientific knowledge and cultural trends that seem to indicate the need to reconsider the traditional psychological meaning of the menopause. We are facing a period of great social transformations regarding the problem of aging, of which the menopause seems to represent a critical 'precursor'. The number of old people in developed countries has greatly increased during recent years and is still growing. There are multiple reasons for this population change and the consequences represent crucial issues at the economical, political, ethical and individual levels. The main target of medical and preventive intervention should be to maintain individual autonomy and activity during aging, to improve capacity and to reduce or eliminate incapacity and disability.

The menopause has been related to aging: this relationship includes scientific, social, cultural, anthropological and psychological perspectives, and is gradually modified by the evolution of the aging issue. In spite of the substantial scientific and medical research that has been undertaken, many questions still remain about the meaning of the menopause, in both scientific and non-medical disciplines. There is still a major gap between subjective and objective aspects of the problem.

In my opinion, an holistic approach should consider the transition from pure biomedicine to a more complex biocultural dimension[1]. The menopause is not only, as Lock[2] stated, 'a fact' to be compressed into one term that is independent from time space and culture, but also 'a concept', whose significance greatly changes according to the people involved. Nowadays, the predominant significance attributed to the menopause is the 'conclusion' of one important stage of life that is linked to 'getting older'.

In our time, the menopause has been defined and described in many specialized fields of medicine; all of them have contributed to the analysis of some particular aspects of the menopause and have produced an interpretation of its significance. In particular, scientific research about the menopause has been addressed towards the influence that loss of estrogens has on the risk of certain diseases in old women.

Incidentally, most of the widely accepted definitions of the menopause underline that the end of menstruation results from changes in complex relationships between certain hormonal signals and several organs of the body. This is obviously true, but cannot explain the dichotomy between objectivity and subjectivity: the scientific definition of the menopause does not consider the individual subjective experience of this phenomenon, which may be greatly influenced by cultural considerations and certainly have a role in the woman's attitude towards preventive medicine.

It must be considered that disciplines such as anthropology, sociology and politics provide other aspects that are just as important as the scientific approach (Figure 1). The psychological aspects have been traditionally indicated as a part of the menopausal syndrome and include a number of symptoms such as depression, anxiety, fatigue, loss of concentration and loss of self esteem; biologically psychological disturbances at the menopause were generally thought to be due to the decreased levels of ovarian hormones and to the subsequent neurovegetative modifications.

In contrast, hormone replacement therapy (HRT) may positively affect psychological disturbances linked to estrogen deprivation, resulting in both the so-called 'domino effect' (since it eliminates neurovegetative symptoms and, as a consequence, ameliorates psychological symptoms) and

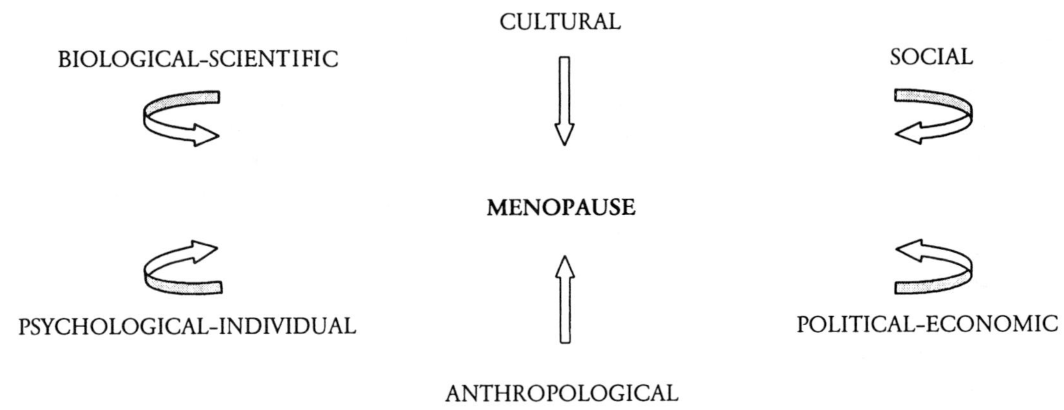

Figure 1 Multiple meanings of the menopause

a direct regulation by estrogens on the brain. However, others have considered psychological symptoms to be independent of a definitive hormonal milieu and linked to a specific individual, familiar and social framework.

Thus, the climacteric has been viewed as a psychological transitional period that includes the end of the parental role, separation from children who reach adulthood, reorganization of close relationships, illness and death of parents and fear of the future. The 'empty nest' syndrome was described as a transitional crisis of the menopause; later on, the menopausal syndrome was related to stressful life events and the positive or negative role of some factors, such as a stable familiar state, and social and working conditions.

The menopause has been designed as a phase in the aging process of women marking the negative transition from the reproductive stage to the non-reproductive stage of life that is coincident with the loss of beauty and sexual appeal. This approach is rightly criticized by the feminist movement. The criticisms are addressed at the masculinist values that consider women to be passive objects of cultural, scientific and economic manipulations, and the menopause to be an unnatural event in striking contrast to the male life-long ability to reproduce.

Last, but not least, according to psychoanalytical theory, the menopause represents a particular moment in which past unconscious conflicts might be revealed. Cultural stereotypes of different societies greatly influence the presence and quality of menopausal psychological disturbances; in fact, the majority of women complaining of climacteric symptoms are found in Western societies, where it seems that youthfulness and beauty are powerful positive values in opposition to aging.

Anthropological transcultural studies have demonstrated that, while primitive cultures share similar symbolism about the loss of reproductive function, major differences are driven by the different cultural developments. According to some philosophical approaches, the link between psyche and cultural environment is very strong: the psyche of a patient is inseparable from the social forces and symbolic systems that constitute his culture, so that selfhood, like illness, is a biocultural construction[1].

This analysis has been extensively developed by postmodernism. From this philosophical perspective, the psychological is always cultural, just as the personal is always political. Even such intrinsically biological stages of human development as puberty, menarche, menopause and old age are affected by the meanings of specific cultures[1], and this is the reason why the cultural influence has become so important in the understanding of the menopause.

In the 1990s, the menopause achieved fundamental political interest, being considered as 'the women's health topic'. The subject of concern has been the progressive aging of so many women and the financial and social effects of such a condition.

The scientific view of the menopause is greatly oriented towards the concept of the 'end of one phase of life', while the cultural interpretations are different; consequently, the concept of the menopause is continually changing as the result of an ongoing dialog between 'biology' and 'culture'. When we try to consider all the aspects, we have to relate the different results deriving from epidemiology, psychology, psychiatry, sociology and anthropology. All these disciplines help to define a universal profile of women that does not necessarily fit with individual experience.

Multiple contrasting interpretations still constitute the complicated picture of the menopause, which still seems to contain several dichotomies that have to be corrected: natural event versus unnatural transition, scientific data versus cultural analysis, objectivity of universal signs and symptoms versus subjectivity of personal experiences, and, finally, different meanings of life cycles between women and men.

The biocultural approach could be used in an attempt to unify all the different meanings. In fact, a biocultural perspective proves invaluable, especially in the opportunities it opens for interdisciplinary collaborations for bringing biomedical knowledge into contact with the insights of anthropologists, sociologists, philosophers, historians and others who make cultural knowledge their field of study[1].

After this long introduction, I will try to suggest some specific motivations that support the refounding of the psychology of the menopause. We should first remind ourselves that the definition of psyche may be integrated with that of behavior and that the psychological conscious and unconscious processes driving individual answers involve many functions such as cognition, memory, perception, intimate experiences and affectivity[3]. In considering this, we can conclude that the psychological dynamics are not only confined to an intra-psychic framework, but have a bipolar relationship with all that is 'external' from the individual psyche.

Second, we have to consider the change in the significance of aging. From the 1960s, scientific research started paying greater attention to aging people. Due to the advances in molecular biology and genetics, aging seems to be viewed as a genetically programmed process. However, an important consequence resulting from the improvement in the pattern of mortality is the abandonment of fatalism and pessimism about growing old and dying, and the discovery of the enjoyment of life and being useful at a greater age[4].

Thus, the dominant model of middle age as the beginning of an unpreventable process of decline should be replaced with a new ideology of aging. Such a transition involves the conceptualization of what Featherstone and Hepworth[4] call the midlife progress novel, where the aging individual is no longer trapped in the experience of the past, but faces the possibility of actively engaging with the processes of biological aging in a struggle to sustain self-identity and discover new sources of personal power and strength.

I agree that aging is not a unitary process determined biologically: biology can be continually modified by culture and is always open to reinterpretation and reconstruction. The greatest effort must be put into reconstructing the social and personal definitions of aging. Although biological life is almost fixed, social and psychological instruments must be directed at creating a new positive energy of life, with a great impact on aging.

As a third point, we have to consider the impact of the enormous development in technology. The relationship between technology and aging has been interpreted in two different ways: on the one hand, technology is capable of transforming the aging process and solving almost all the problems; on the other, the natural process of biological aging should not be resisted.

In the end, this no longer represents a valid dichotomy between nature and culture. Now we must speak of technoculture and, when we consider the relationship between human beings and nature, it makes no sense to see technology as an external factor. Technology cannot be considered as a collection of different instruments that produce artificial forms of nature.

A similar analysis can be extended to other aspects, such as psychology. In fact, until now, we have been thinking of technology as instruments that serve every individual.

Technological development has grown to such an extent that it has become the environment around us and governs our psychological processes. As a consequence, pre-technological psychology must be changed: it is necessary to abandon the individual psychology that considers the human being as a subject and technology as an instrument, and pass to a more active psychology, named 'psychology of action', that takes from technology the instruments useful for its control and the creation of new alternative models[5].

The ever-growing spread of information technology has reduced the impact of cultural diversities; the globalization of this technology could provide, by an anthropological approach, new solutions to the problem of psychology of the menopause.

On the other hand, the increasing medical knowledge concerning women's health has dramatically changed the significance of the menopause for both the individual and society; the problem of prevention in the menopause has broadened from the prevention and treatment of postmenopausal syndrome to that of prevention of many diseases of the third age.

Many years ago, Corman[6], when studying a model of the mechanisms of adaptation in human beings, identified four different phases that occur during the individual's lifetime: passive expansion, active expansion, active retraction and passive retraction. We can easily identify postmenopausal prevention in the period between active expansion and active retraction. All efforts must be directed towards elucidating the so-called 'active retraction' phase during aging.

The reasons for reconsidering the psychology of the menopause have important foundations in the extraordinary changes of the 20th century. The individual (woman or man) must be helped with the powerful educational and informative instruments in resetting his own life program.

Preventive medicine must always consider the subject as a whole and, therefore, must pay attention to all the social and political issues of an aging society. One of the great challenges of our time is to offer to elderly retiring people real opportunities for maintaining an active role, thereby minimizing the negative impact of progressive exclusion from working society.

Reproductive and social 'retirements' no longer have to produce the unhappy coincidence that makes the menopause the starting point of an existential 'Sunset Boulevard'. Women can live for a long time after the menopause and they can, and must, do it well. In conclusion, new definitions of the menopause must be proposed in order to reach the main target of longevity without aging (Figure 2).

Scientific progress aimed at reducing the risk of diseases and their permanent consequences has improved human health in aging; future research and technology will eliminate most of the problems of senescence, i.e. through 'regenerative medicine'. Moreover, advanced technology in assisted reproduction has led to ideal perspectives of women's reproductive longevity after the menopause, giving a scientific background for further discussion of the meaning of the menopause as the end of an important phase of life.

HRT, as a result of new technology applied to humans and appropriate lifestyle, has been shown

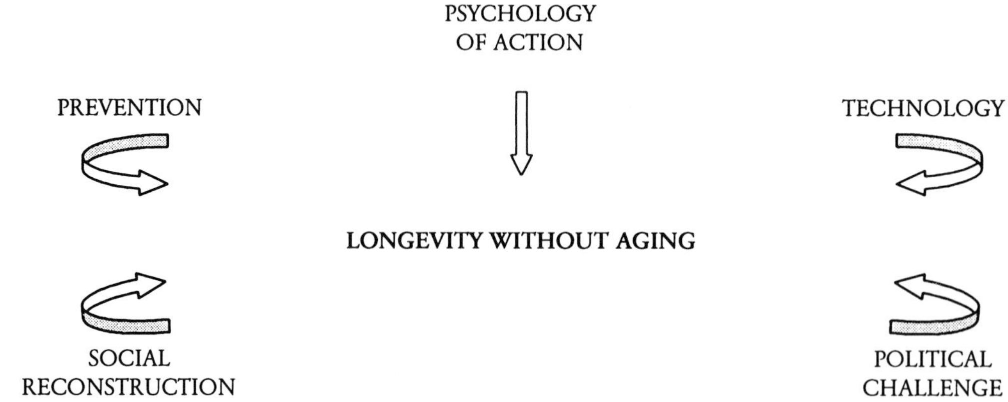

Figure 2 New meanings of the menopause

to be a first-line answer to maintain health and improve well-being in aging women. Medical efforts must be aimed at treating the menopause with the best therapies available in order to preserve both the endocrine and sexual identities that are a unique heritage of every individual at any age.

As a result of our discussion, it is now mandatory that traditional negative psychology of the menopause should be substituted by a new active approach that helps women to achieve a different identity. Of course, social and political changes are necessary to guarantee the reconstruction of a valid social role. Great attention to the psychological and cultural approach modifications in preventive medicine during the menopause are mandatory to achieve long-term compliance with medical treatments and lifestyle behaviors[7-9].

References

1. Morris DB. *Illness and Culture in the Postmodern Age.* Berkeley and Los Angeles, California: University of California Press, 1998
2. Lock M. *Encounters with Aging.* Berkeley and Los Angeles, California: University of California Press, 1993
3. Galimberti U. *Dizionario di Psicologia.* Torino: UTET, 1992:706–70
4. Featherstone M, Hepworth M. Ageing, the life-course and the sociology of embodiment. In Scambler G, Higgs P, eds. *Modernity, Medicine and Health.* London and New York: Routledge, 1998: 147–75
5. Galimberti U. *Psiche e techne. L'uomo nell'età della tecnica.* Milan: Feltrinelli Ed., 1999
6. Corman R. *Le Diagnostique du Temperament par la Morphologie.* Paris: Legrand, 1947
7. Zichella L. The importance of lifestyle after menopause. *Int J Fertil Menopausal Stud* 1995;1:9–15
8. Zichella L, Perrone G. Lifestyle and compliance with HRT. *Eur Menopausal J* 1996;3:250–4
9. Zichella L. LT-HRT challenge: lifestyle, compliance and quality of life. *Menopause Rev* 1998;3:1–2

The psychosocial vulnerability model of the menopause

86

J. G. Greene

INTRODUCTION

There exists in the menopause literature two apparently irreconcilable views regarding the etiology of psychological distress, and in particular depression, at the time of the menopause transition. One view, shared by many gynecologists, attributes such distress directly to hormonal changes. The other view, shared by psychosocial researchers, is that, if there is such a phenomenon as menopausal depression, then it can largely be attributed to stress arising from interpersonal, family, health and social problems. In this paper, the author attempts to reconcile these two viewpoints using a theoretical model derived from life event research.

MENOPAUSE AND DEPRESSION

The belief that there is a direct causal association between the occurrence of the menopause transition and psychological distress, in particular depressed mood, is one that is widely held. There is, in fact, little or no consistent and sound empirical evidence for that belief. The following quotations come from three recent comprehensive and exhaustive reviews of the research literature relating to the association between the menopause and psychological distress in general population samples of climacteric women:

> 'Prospective studies indicate little or no menopausal excess in psychological symptoms, except for depressed mood in one study'[1].
>
> 'There is insufficient evidence at present to maintain that menopause causes depression'[2].
>
> 'The recent well designed studies from around the world show no significant support for the view that psychological problems can be attributed to the effect of the natural menopause transition'[3].

Thus, the consensus among psychosocial researchers, based on the research findings to date, is that there is little foundation for the belief that the menopause itself plays a direct role in the etiology of psychological distress at that time of life.

PSYCHOSOCIAL FACTORS AND DEPRESSION

There is, however, abundant research evidence for an association, at the time of the menopause, between a variety of psychosocial factors and psychological distress. This evidence comes from both cross-sectional studies of general population samples of climacteric women[4], and in more recent times, longitudinal studies[5-11]. The relevant findings from longitudinal studies are summarized in Table 1. As can be seen, a diverse number of psychosocial events from different domains are implicated.

It is a well-established finding that psychosocial factors such as those listed in Table 1 play a role in the etiology of psychological distress among both men and women at all times of life. The research literature on life stress and depression also shows that, for psychosocial factors to induce or exacerbate depression, other factors, designated as vulnerability factors, must be present[12]. A vulnerability factor, by definition, is one that has no effect on its own but acts to induce or exacerbate a condition in the presence of known causal factors, which do have a direct effect on their own. For example, it has been shown that negative life events induce depression among young married women, but that the risk increases if certain vulnerability

Table 1 Summary of the psychosocial findings of longitudinal studies

Reference	*Country*	*Factors associated with depression*
Holte (1992)[5]	Norway	poor social network, negative life events
Hunter (1992)[6]	UK	family problems, bereavement, ill health, negative attitudes
Kaufert *et al.* (1992)[7]	Canada	domestic problems, poor health
Avis *et al.* (1994)[8]	USA	illness, death of family members, negative attitudes, perceived health status
Dennerstein *et al.* (1994)[9]	Australia	interpersonal problems, attitude to aging, current health status, lifestyle
Collins and Landgren (1995)[10]	Sweden	living alone, lifestyle
Woods and Mitchell (1996)[11]	USA	stressful life events, negative attitudes, health status

factors are present. These include having three or more young children in the household, the loss of a mother in childhood, the absence of social support and the lack of a job outside the home[12].

The finding from psychosocial research on the menopause that there is little or no evidence of an association between the menopause transition and depression, but that there is an association between depression and negative psychosocial factors, suggests that, if the menopause is implicated in some way in the etiology of depression, then its most likely mode of action is as a vulnerability or risk factor.

THE MENOPAUSE AS A VULNERABILITY FACTOR

An example of how a vulnerability effect might occur with regard to the menopause and the adverse event of a family bereavement is shown in Table 2. In this example, women not experiencing a bereavement show no evidence of depression, whether they are menopausal or not menopausal. Those experiencing a bereavement, however, show a marked level of depression, but only if they are currently going through the menopause transition. Those not menopausal may be moderately depressed due to the direct effect of the bereavement. Since the menopause coincides with a number of adverse life events characteristic of that age range, such as the decease of the previous generation, then the menopause transition can be an important element in indirectly precipitating or exacerbating depression. The concept of menopausal vulnerability implies that, at the time of the menopause, women become less well able to cope with any personal or social problems they may be experiencing and react to these problems by becoming depressed. The question arises as to why the menopause transition has this effect. Why do women cease to be able to cope with their problems at the time of the menopause? What, in short, are the possible mechanisms by which women are rendered vulnerable?

Table 2 An example of a menopausal vulnerability interaction with bereavement

Menopausal Status	*Bereaved*	*Not bereaved*
Menopausal	extremely depressed	not depressed
Not menopausal	moderately or not depressed	not depressed

Possible mechanisms of vulnerability generally fall into two broad categories, psychological and biological, or, more specifically in the case of the menopause, hormonal.

PSYCHOLOGICAL MECHANISM OF MENOPAUSAL VULNERABILITY

By this it is meant that menopausal vulnerability could be mediated by certain psychological characteristics of women. For example, it has been shown in many studies that women's expectations of, attitude to and perception of the menopause are associated with mood change and psychological distress at that time[6,8,9,11].

Negative expectations are likely to make a woman more sensitive to and more aware of the various physical changes that occur as she moves through the menopause transition, such as vasomotor symptoms, vaginal atrophy and dyspareunia. She may also be fearsome of the possible longer-term effects of the menopause such as osteoporosis and cardiovascular disease. She may have similar fears about the psychological and social consequences of the menopause, perceiving it to be yet another marker in the process of aging. The social and cultural milieu in which she has lived will be influential in this respect.

Thus, in this scenario, such concerns and fears will act to reduce a woman's morale, increase her vulnerability and render her less capable of coping with any interpersonal or psychosocial problems she may be experiencing.

HORMONAL MECHANISMS OF VULNERABILITY

Many researchers have argued that depression among menopausal women is a direct consequence of estrogen deficiency. That is, estrogen has psychotropic properties and consequently hormone replacement therapy is a potential treatment for depression[13]. This effect, it is proposed, operates via specific receptors for sex hormones, such as estrogen, progestogen and androgen, within certain subcortical structures of the brain, in particular the limbic system, which controls mood and other related functions (see Table 3). It is further argued that the main action of gonodal steroids on the central nervous system is mediated by neuroactive transmitters, with sex hormones exerting a modulating effect on the synthesis, release and metabolism of some neuropeptides and neurotransmitters, leading to mood change[14].

However valid this neuroendocrine model may be, to argue that sex hormones have a direct effect on mood is to overlook the fact that psychosocial studies of general population samples of menopausal women have consistently found that psychological distress is restricted to the subgroup of menopausal women exposed to adverse psychosocial factors, leaving the majority of women relatively unaffected.

Table 3 Psychological functions and principal areas modulated by sex steroids. Adapted from reference 14

System	*Area modulated by sex steroids*
Limbic system	mood and affect memory function drive and motivation
Hypothalamus	thermoregulation satiety hunger blood pressure

In other words, the effect of hormone deficiency on the neuroactive transmitters of the limbic system cannot in itself lead to mood changes. For mood change to occur, an essential condition is that adverse psychosocial factors are present. What neuroendocrine changes may well do is to 'destabilize' the limbic system biochemically, thus rendering menopausal women potentially vulnerable to mood change. However, actual mood change will occur only if adverse psychosocial factors are present. Thus, the effect of estrogen deficiency on the integrity of the limbic system may be one of the mechanisms responsible for menopausal women's vulnerability to adverse psychosocial factors. Therefore, the improvement in mood following HRT may be due to the action of sex steroids on the neuroendocrine system reducing vulnerability, thus enabling women to better cope with problems in their life situation.

Figure 1 depicts a schematic representation of the model showing how the psychological and hormonal mechanisms act to produce vulnerability, which in turn mediates the effect of adverse psychosocial factors, leading to mood change.

MOOD OR DRIVE?

The hypothesis that the effect of menopausal vulnerability is to reduce a woman's ability to cope with problems in her life situation raises the question as to what is the primary psychological effect of vulnerability. Is it one of mood change or reduced drive and motivation? Two features would tend to support the view that it is one of reduced drive, with mood change perhaps as a secondary feature.

The first is that receptors for sex steroids are found throughout subcortical structures of the brain, structures which are known to mediate drive and motivation (see Table 3). The second is that, within the psychological symptom picture

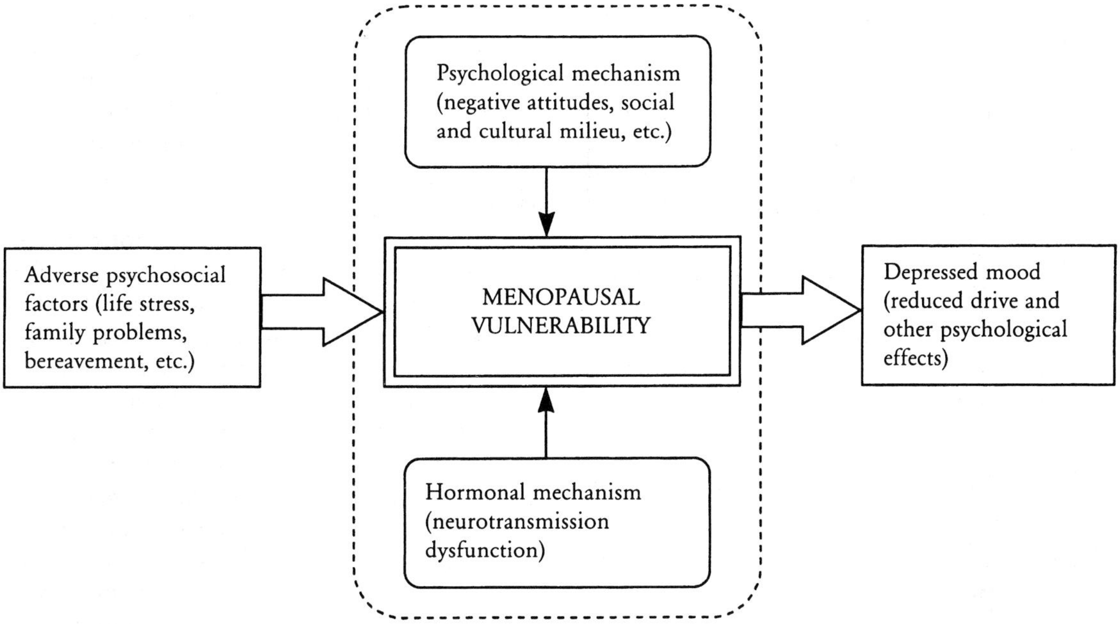

Figure 1 Psychosocial vulnerability model of the menopause

presented by menopausal women, the primary complaint is invariably one of fatigue and tiredness. Most clinicians and women would concur with this. However, it is also a complaint that emerges in all factor analytic studies of menopausal symptoms, and generally has the highest factor loading of all symptoms[15]. It can therefore lay claim to be the most salient of the psychological complaints reported by women at the time of the menopause. Also of relevance to the hypothesis that the behavioral effect of estrogen deficiency is primarily one of drive reduction is the recent finding that among a group of patients diagnosed as having chronic fatigue syndrome, a significant proportion had hormone profiles suggestive of a chronic estrogen deficiency state[13].

CONCLUSION

The consistent lack of evidence from psychosocial research for a direct association between the menopause transition and depression among general population samples of climacteric women would appear to be inconsistent with the implications of the findings that receptors for estrogen have been found in those subcortical structures of the brain which mediate mood. An attempt has been made to resolve these inconsistencies by proposing a model whereby the dysfunctional effects of estrogen deficiency on neurotransmission within these structures do not have a direct role in the etiology of mood change, but act indirectly by rendering menopausal women vulnerable and at risk to depression in response to psychosocial stress.

References

1. Pearce J, Hawton K, Blake F. Psychological and sexual symptoms associated with the menopause and the effects of hormone replacement therapy. *Br J Psychiatry* 1995;67:163–73
2. Nicol-Smith L. Causality, menopause, and depression: a critical review of the literature. *Br Med J* 1996;313:1229–32
3. Morse CA. Menopause transition. In Wren BG, ed. *Progress in the Management of the Menopause.* Carnforth, UK: Parthenon Publishing, 1997:50–7
4. Greene JG. The cross-sectional legacy: an introduction to longitudinal studies of the climacteric. *Maturitas* 1992;14:95–101
5. Holte A. Influences of natural menopause on health complaints: a prospective study of healthy Norwegian women. *Maturitas* 1992;14:127–41
6. Hunter M. The South East England longitudinal study of the climacteric and postmenopause. *Maturitas* 1992;14:117–26
7. Kaufert P, Gilbert P, Tate R. The Manitoba Project: A re-examination of the link between menopause and depression. *Maturitas* 1992;14:143–55
8. Avis N, Brambella D, McKinlay S, *et al.* A longitudinal analysis of the association between menopause and depression: results from the Massachusetts Women's Health Study. *Ann Epidemiol* 1994;4: 214–20
9. Dennerstein L, Smith AMA, Morse C. Psychological well-being, mid-life and the menopause. *Maturitas* 1994;20:1–11
10. Collins A, Landgren BM. Reproductive health, use of oestrogen and experience of symptoms in perimenopausal women: a population-based study. *Maturitas* 1995;20:101–11
11. Woods NF, Mitchell ES. Patterns of depressed mood in mid-life women: observations from the Seattle Mid-life Women's Health Study. *Res Nurs Health* 1996;19:111–23
12. Brown GW, Harris T. *The Social Origins of Depression: A Study of Psychiatric Disorder in Women.* London: Tavistock, 1978
13. Studd JJW, Panay N. Estrogens in the treatment of climacteric depression, premenstrual depression, postnatal depression and chronic fatigue syndrome. In Wren BG, ed. *Progress in the Management of the Menopause.* Carnforth, UK: Parthenon Publishing, 1997:385–92
14. Genazzani AR, Stomati M, Spinetti A, *et al.* Neuroendocrinology of the climacteric period and hormone replacement therapy. In Wren BG, ed. *Progress in the Management of the Menopause.* Carnforth, UK: Parthenon Publishing, 1997:380–4
15. Greene JG. Constructing a standard climacteric scale. *Maturitas* 1998;29:25–31

Psychological perspectives of menopause: themes and images emerging in sandplay therapy

87

S. T. Reece

INTRODUCTION

In general, women tend to avoid becoming consciously aware of the menopause as a specific psychosomatic event occurring sometime during middle age[1]. Both the onset of aging and the mid-life crises that often accompany it are explicit life-cycle experiences and tend to be lived as such, whereas the psychological dimensions of mid-life are more subtle and vague and are therefore more likely to be projected onto relationships within family, marriage and at work. Women typically seek external means of managing aging and menopausal symptoms by shifting toward healthier lifestyles that maximize their quality of life[2,3], but avoid consciously exploring the profound psychological shifts taking place within them. In studies, postmenopausal women have reported experiencing extraordinary dreams[1,4], indicating that significant parallel changes are occurring in the psyche. In this article, I will examine the psychological manifestations of menopause as they are portrayed in Jungian sandplay therapy, which is a non-verbal projective modality that combines art and play therapy[5].

RAMIFICATIONS OF AN UNEXAMINED MENOPAUSE

I worked with five Caucasian perimenopausal women who were undergoing therapy in sandplay training (three were premenopausal, one menopausal, and one postmenopausal). We met for a total of ten sessions, spaced at intervals of 2–3 months, over a period of about 1 year. I documented the therapeutic processes and photographed the trays and then sorted and categorized the images and themes that appeared in the pictures. The Jungian method of amplification was used with the patients to explore their experiences of their sandplay creations.

The sixth woman was a Japanese patient, now residing in the USA, who was referred by her physician for a severely incapacitating depression and the physical symptom of tinnitus. She underwent weekly counselling and sandplay therapy sessions concomitantly for about 6 months.

Issues and concerns of daily life described by these women in our training/therapeutic sessions related to three main areas: external world, family/marital relationships and relationship to self. Concerns about external world issues involved overextending themselves and becoming consumed by the demands of outer life; the indiscriminate use of their energies and talents; and over-identification with ego issues of power and control.

Problematic familial/marital relationships included concerns about being overinvolved with family members' needs, yet feeling disconnected from them on an emotional level; diminished intimacy with their partner, resulting in anxiety, tension and dissatisfaction; and increasing gaps and/or distancing in communication, in some cases culminating in separation. Regarding their relationship to self, the women all expressed, in one way or another, feeling lost, alienated, lonely and dissatisfied. The loss of feeling their 'center' or 'core' or 'true self' was lamented by all.

In general, at the beginning of treatment, these women felt that their partners did not understand what they were going through and were not able to meet their needs. The larger truth was that they themselves did not understand what they were experiencing and had not been able to articulate their needs, even to themselves. By losing touch with the complex psychobiological movements taking place within themselves, they concomitantly lost the ability to communicate honestly and effectively with others. By translating their inchoate turmoil into sand-tray pictures, however, they were able to see the archetypal forces operating within themselves, which, in turn, empowered them to face the areas in their lives that needed redefining and rebalancing.

SANDPLAY THERAPY PROCEDURES

Sandplay therapy provides a safe space for patients to express anything that rises to the surface, including distressing problems of any sort and the emotions triggered by them. More importantly, the process is itself a means of coping with both the distressful feeling and the situation engendering it[6].

Sandplay materials include a box or tray that measures 57 × 72 × 7 cm, and dry and/or wet sand. In addition, multitudinous miniature figurines are displayed on nearby shelves. The patient is given the following direction: 'Please make a picture in the box using these miniatures anyway you want. There is no right or wrong way to play'. The therapist records any story told after the person has finished creating the tray and then takes photos of the completed tray.

EXPLORING SAND-TRAY CREATIONS

Table 1 summarizes the images produced in the patients' sand trays in terms of three categories of archetypal motifs: themes of transition, internal reorganizational processes and imagistic representations of symptoms.

The archetypal themes and images produced by the menopausal women reveal the climacteric biopsychosocial changes taking place during the transition periods of middle age and older age. In *Rites of Passage*, van Gennep[7] identifies three archetypal stages that comprise a rite of passage marking an important transitional period. First comes the stage of isolation in which the person withdraws from society, often seeking closer contact with nature. Next comes the ordeal of severance, an event involving physical or symbolic confrontation with loss and death, whereby the individual is forced to rely solely upon his/her resources in undergoing, in essence, the 'trial by fire'. Finally, having endured the ordeal, the individual emerges reborn, renewed, and returns to society as a changed individual[7].

Psychologically, menopausal women face a total change in identity and in individuality with the cessation of blood flow and the loss of fertility[8]. Yet women in menopause have no rites of passage to guide and sustain them while they undergo the ordeal of these huge physical and psychological alterations. In most civilized cultures, they face this crucial stage of life alone, without the solace of prescribed rites, and often bombarded by horrific media tales of suffering and doom. This is one adult identity crisis that has been generally ignored in the literature[9]. Women who do not face and explore the psychological meaning of this major physical shift may remain stuck in their old identity, longing for what was but will never be again. This lack of psychological development causes pervasive imbalances in all domains of personal life[10]. In severe cases, denial of menopausal realities may render a woman too disturbed and 'out of synch' with herself to function at home or at work with any degree of adequacy, let alone fulfilment.

The sandplay process functions as a rite of passage whereby women can experience, consciously and unconsciously, the three stages of van Gennep's rite of passage and find their own center in the midst of the life-altering change.

In formulating the archetypal thematic categories regarding internal reorganization within the psyche, I referred to Perry's earlier work in this area[11]. Here, again, the sandplay modality is ideally suited as a venue for expressing the often ineffable stirrings that mark the subtle shifts of the psyche's movement. Sandplay therapy provides a three-dimensional experience of the problem (symptom), its resolution and the means by which the resolution is attained. This comprehensive function of sandplay is well illustrated by the trays of these menopausal women. By creating tableaux in the sand that depicted inexpressible psychic states, these women got in touch with their inner

Table 1 Archetypal motifs expressed in sandplay therapy with menopausal women

	Perimenopausal women		*Premenopausal women*			*Postmenopausal women*
Image categories	*Hana*	*V**	*W**	*X**	*Y**	*Z**
Transition themes						
Death, destruction, chaos: images of shipwreck, car collision, death mask	✓	✓			✓	✓
Birth: images of mother and baby, birth of new central figure (ego → self → Self)	✓	✓	✓			✓
Journey to new place: images of vehicle on path, bridge, Indian village	✓	✓	✓		✓	✓
Rituals: images of wedding, shaman's healing dance, meditation hut	✓	✓		✓		✓
Internal reorganizational themes						
Integration and differentiation: images of mounds, island, mandala, spirals	✓	✓	✓	✓	✓	✓
Symmetry and balance-hands (right/left): images of two concentric circles, two divided worlds	✓	✓	✓	✓	✓	✓
Separation and reunion of opposites: images of man/woman in separate worlds, wedding	✓	✓	✓		✓	✓
Wholeness: images of ceremonial circle, vehicle moving in circle, starfish	✓	✓	✓	✓		
Symptoms and recovery						
Tinnitus, emotionality: images of dwarves	✓					
Hot flushes, night sweats: images of fire, volcano, wells	✓	✓	✓		✓	✓
Alienation, depression: images of desert, underground, tunnel	✓					
Expansion and wholeness: images of multiplicity and complexity	✓	✓	✓	✓	✓	✓

*The letters V, W, X, Y and Z represent clients in these categories

center as they struggled to cope with the subtle – and not-so-subtle – shifts in their lives, image by image, sand tray by sand tray.

A BRIEF CASE EXAMPLE

'Hana', a Japanese married woman with no children, was the owner of a successful business. Six months prior to seeking therapy, she lost her business partner and overworked herself to exhaustion, attempting to compensate for the loss. In her highly stressed state, she was forced to acknowledge self-limits previously unknown to her, which she attributed to aging and which frightened her excessively. She became severely depressed, refused all sexual contact with her husband, lost sleep and appetite, and began suffering from tinnitus. Finally, she became completely incapacitated, was not able to work or even do daily chores, and was forced to ask her elderly mother for help in maintaining the household.

Hana's initial sand tray depicted the themes and images underlying her present condition and also what sort of inner work she needed to do by way of altering her current undesirable state. In Figure 1, her lethargy is expressed through a desolate, static symmetry, in which her psychic energy flow is virtually paralyzed, unmoving. In Figure 2, a bridge appears with two children on it, suggesting movement and a rebalancing process[12], especially

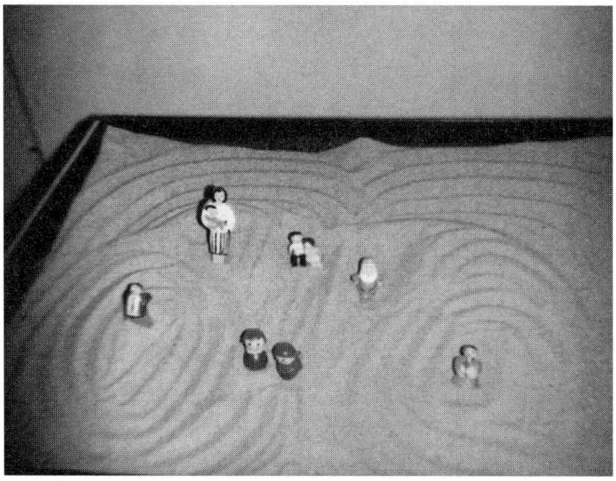

Figure 1 The client's lethargy is expressed through a desolate, static symmetry in which her psychic energy flow is virtually paralyzed

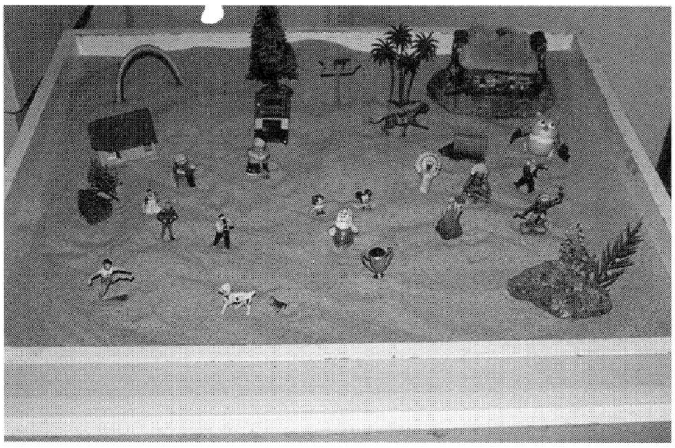

Figure 2 The client's tray begins to show expansion, movement and a rebalancing process, though her world is still divided. A dwarf appears near the center in both Figures 1 and 2

between the masculine and feminine poles. Loving attention to her inner happenings (dwarf's noises) needed to supplant her preoccupation with managing the external world. Her grief over the absence of mature intimacy (she was in a dependent position) needed to be seen freshly (depicted in the mother-child image suggesting the death-rebirth theme). Over time, she created images and themes expressive of the three thematic categories in Table 1. Experiencing the healing and psychological development that was concretized in the sand trays, she returned to work on a trial basis. She was deeply delighted to 'rediscover' her own talent and her enjoyment of her customers' genuine appreciation of her services. She now experiences her work activities as involving energizing mutual exchanges. By reconnecting with this valuable internal reality, she was able to rejoin her husband and her world with new hope and purposefulness.

It is also interesting to note that Hana and a Caucasian woman (designated 'V' in the table) expressed images and themes in the same categories, suggesting the possibility that the psychological processes of menopause are not subject to the impact of cultural differences.

FINAL THOUGHTS

The sandplay modality was instrumental in evoking the unconscious themes and images active within a small group of perimenopausal women, allowing them to become conscious of, and active participants in, the psychological processes paralleling the physical ones. In the absence of a culturally sponsored rite of passage, these women individually produced images that portrayed the ordeal of changing from one state to another, with all the confusing reorganization of internal processes and symptom production that occurs alongside such an ordeal. Their sand trays capture the soulful experiences of the passage of modern women through the menopause[13].

ACKNOWLEDGEMENTS

I would like to thank Patrick Lee, PhD, and Barbara Nelson, PhD, for allowing me to use their unpublished dissertations on working with menopausal women in sandplay therapy. I am also grateful to the women in the Sandplay Study Group in Lafayette, LA, USA.

Finally, I would like to extend my thanks to my patient who allowed me to use her therapy material for this study.

References

1. Mankowitz A. *A Change of Life: A Psychological Study of Dreams and the Menopause*. Toronto: Inner City Books, 1984:11-28
2. Compton MS. *Women at the Change: The Intelligent Woman's Guide to Menopause*. St. Paul, MN: Llewellyn Publications, 1998
3. Sugiyama M. *Konenki no Hoken-gaku*. Tokyo: Daiichishuppan, 1995:94-101
4. Signel K. *Wisdom of the Heart: Working with Women's Dreams*. New York: Bantam Books, 1990:246-59
5. Kalff D. *Sandplay: A Psychotherapeutic Approach to the Psyche*. Boston: Sigo Press, 1980:23-39
6. Bradway K. Sandplay is meant for healing. *J Sandplay Ther* 1994;2:9-12
7. van Gennep A. *The Rites of Passage*. Translated by Vizem M and Caffee G. Chicago: University of Chicago Press, 1960
8. Harding EM. *The Way of All Women*. New York: Harper & Row, 1975:241-63
9. Compton MS. *Women at the Change: The Intelligent Woman's Guide to Menopause*. St. Paul, MN: Llewellyn Publications, 1998:20
10. Henderson JL. *Thresholds of Initiation*. Middletown, CT: Wesleyan University Press, 1967:4-19
11. Perry JW. *The Far Side of Madness*. Dallas, TX: Spring Publications, 1992:25-36, 98-105
12. Perera SB. *Descent to the Goddess: A Way of Initiation for Women*. Toronto: Inner City Books, 1981:85-8
13. Harding ME. *Woman's Mysteries, Ancient and Modern*. New York: Putnam's Sons, 1971:10-19

Index